PATHOLOGY OF INFERTILITY
Clinical Correlations in the Male and Female

PATHOLOGY OF INFERTILITY
Clinical Correlations in the Male and Female

EDITED BY

BERNARD GONDOS, M.D.
Director of Pathology
Sansum Medical Clinic
Santa Barbara, California

DANIEL H. RIDDICK, M.D., PH.D.
Professor and Chairman
Department of Obstetrics and Gynecology
University of Vermont
Burlington, Vermont

1987
Thieme Medical Publishers, Inc., New York
Georg Thieme Verlag, Stuttgart · New York

Thieme Medical Publishers, Inc.
381 Park Avenue South
New York, New York 10016

Cover design by Wendy Ann Fredericks

PATHOLOGY OF INFERTILITY
Bernard Gondos
Daniel H. Riddick

Library of Congress Cataloging-in-Publication Data
Pathology of infertility.
   Includes index.
   1. Infertility.   I. Gondos, Bernard.   II. Riddick,
Daniel H.   [DNLM: 1. Infertility—etiology.   2. Infertil-
ity—physiopathology.   WP 570 P297]
RC889.P33   1987   616.6'92   87-6514

Important note: Medicine is an ever-changing science. Research and clinical experience are continually
broadening our knowledge, in particular our knowledge of proper treatment and drug therapy. Insofar as
this book mentions any dosage or application, readers may rest assured that the authors, editors, and
publishers have made every effort to ensure that such references are strictly in accordance with the state of
knowledge at the time of production of the book. Nevertheless, every user is requested to carefully examine
the manufacturers' leaflets accompanying each drug to check on his own responsibility whether the dosage
schedules recommended therein or the contraindications stated by the manufacturers differ from the
statements made in the present book. Such examination is particularly important with drugs that are either
rarely used or have been newly released on the market.

Some of the product names, patents, and registered designs referred to in this book are in fact registered
trademarks or proprietary names even though specific reference to this fact is not always made in the text.
Therefore, the appearance of a name without designation as proprietary is not to be construed as a
representation by the publisher that it is in the public domain.

Typeset by Bi-Comp, Inc., York, PA, USA.
Printed and bound by Kingsport Press, Kingsport, TN, USA.
Printed in the United States of America.

5 4 3 2 1

TMP ISBN 0-86577-248-7
GTV ISBN 3-13-677001-3

Preface

The expanding field of reproductive science encompasses striking new advances in clinical infertility management and rapidly increasing knowledge on the pathogenesis of fertility problems. In contrast to only a few short years ago, understanding of the basis for disorders of fertility now requires an extended multidisciplinary approach drawing on the experience of authorities in a variety of areas.

The purpose of this book is to provide a comprehensive review of the most current information on the pathogenesis of the major causes of infertility, as presented by recognized authorities in their specific fields. Major emphasis is on a combined basic and clinical science approach. Newer research techniques, diagnostic methods, and conceptual advances in disease classification have received full consideration. The editors have decided to present the information in a traditional organ system approach in dealing with the female and male reproductive systems. We have attempted at the same time to stress common underlying mechanisms of pathophysiology as they apply to different disease processes.

The book is intended for the use of pathologists, gynecologists, urologists, endocrinologists and others involved in the diagnosis and management of fertility disorders. For such individuals, keeping up with the tremendous number of journal articles and professional meetings in the area of reproduction has become a virtually insurmountable task. Our intention is that this textbook will address that problem and make it more manageable. In providing a reference source on the basis of fertility disorders, the various chapters stress methods of diagnosis and evaluation rather than treatment, although the latter is given some consideration as it relates to basic understanding. More complete information on treatment of infertility can be found elsewhere.

It is also hoped that the book will be of use to veterinary reproductive scientists and basic investigators in the reproductive sciences. The countless examples of experimental disease models, the expanding application of new research techniques to clinical diagnosis and the value of comparing similar diseases in different species reflect the general need for understanding of problems in human reproduction. With this in mind, we have attempted to select contributors whose interests and expertise span the basic and clinical sciences.

The authors have been encouraged to treat their subjects as comprehensively as possible, considering major disease processes and related, perhaps less well known, entities. Inevitably, there will be some overlap and even some difference of opinion from one chapter to another. We hope that the reader will appreciate our reasons for permitting and, in fact, encouraging this. There are certainly benefits in seeing how different individuals develop similar ideas, particularly when the views are based on extensive experience from different clinical perspectives. That in some instances the views may arouse controversy is indeed a healthy sign in a field expanding as rapidly as the reproductive sciences.

We are indebted to the authors for their considerable time and effort. It is particularly gratifying and not unexpected that those working in the area of infertility have a special interest in providing their views on mechanisms of pathogenesis. The high quality of the contributions is an indication that a book on this important subject is particularly timely. The expert manner in which the different chapters are presented will provide a valuable and much needed review of current knowledge on problems of infertility.

Bernard Gondos
Daniel H. Riddick

Foreword

This thoroughly modern book fulfills the opening statement in the preface; it is multi-authored and multi-disciplinary including obstetrics and gynecology, pathology, endocrinology, urology, genetics and basic science. All of the authors contribute well their respective talents and knowledge. Considering its multi-authorship, the style and form of the chapters are surprisingly uniform. It stresses new concepts of the increasingly important and expanding problems of the infertile couple. It emphasizes new techniques and guides to treatment, but not the details thereof; they are to be found elsewhere. It cites animal models, pathophysiology, endocrinology, and other basic aspects of the whole field of reproduction. One learns to understand this exceedingly complex field of biology by realizing how the various species handle these problems. For, after all, animals and humans share many, if not most, of the basic mechanisms involved in reproduction.

This book lays to rest for all time the opprobrium attached since biblical times to the "barren woman" by bringing to light the complex problems in the female and male that combine to frustrate the fertility rightfully expected by the average normal couple.

This splendid comprehensive book is indeed "ein handbuch" in the true Germanic sense of the word. It brings to hand all the modern knowledge of a complex subject. Your writer in his medical youth thought that a handbook (handbuch) was a volume which could be easily held in the hand, and even read in bed at night; but no, it is a compendium of all pertinent knowledge on the subject and not a how-to-do-it sort of volume.

The tabular data and illustrations are well planned, pertinently placed and add significantly to the value of the volume. The bibliographic references are extensive and modern. Older references, when germane, are also included.

Your writer has been in the field of Obstetrics-Gynecology and its clinical aspects, its pathology, embryology, primate research and teaching nearly all of his professional life—57 years. He has, for many of those years, been consulted on the problems of Ob-Gyn pathology including interpretation of endometrial biopsies. The chapter on the latter subject is a splendid example of how this book addresses the problems of infertility.

It has been a pleasure, privilege and an honor to have been asked to write the foreword for this book. Needless to say, I warmly recommend it to the many professionals in the field.

Arthur T. Hertig, M.D.
Winchester, Massachusetts

Contributors

Nancy J. Alexander, Ph.D.
Institute for Reproductive Medicine
Eastern Virginia Medical School
Norfolk, Virginia

Shalender Bhasin, M.D.
Division of Endocrinology
Harbor/UCLA Medical Center
Torrance, California

Richard A. Bronson, M.D.
Department of Obstetrics and Gynecology
Cornell University Medical College
New York, New York

R. Jeffrey Chang, M.D.
Department of Obstetrics and Gynecology
University of California at Davis
Sacramento, California

Carolyn B. Coulam, M.D.
Department of Obstetrics and Gynecology
University of Pittsburgh
Pittsburgh, Pennsylvania

Douglas C. Daly, M.D.
Department of Obstetrics and Gynecology
University of Massachusetts
Worcester, Massachusetts

Dominique de Ziegler, M.D.
Department of Obstetrics and Gynecology
UCLA School of Medicine
Los Angeles, California

Shirley G. Driscoll, M.D.
Department of Pathology
Harvard Medical School
Boston, Massachusetts

Gregory F. Erickson, Ph.D.
Department of Reproductive Medicine
University of California at San Diego School of
Medicine
La Jolla, California

Bernard Gondos, M.D.
Department of Pathology
Sansum Medical Clinic
Santa Barbara, California

A. F. Haney, M.D.
Department of Obstetrics and Gynecology
Duke University Medical Center
Durham, North Carolina

Avner Hershlag, M.D.
Department of Obstetrics and Gynecology
George Washington University Medical Center
Washington, D.C.

E. Horvath, Ph.D.
Department of Pathology
University of Toronto
Toronto, Ontario, Canada

Keith A. Horvath, M.D.
Department of Pathology
University of Chicago
Chicago, Illinois

Mohamed Ishakia, D.V.M., Ph.D.
Institute of Primate Research
University of Nairobi
Nairobi, Kenya

Howard W. Jones, Jr., M.D.
Institute for Reproductive Medicine
Eastern Virginia Medical School
Norfolk, Virginia

Neil L. Kao, B.S.
Department of Pathology
University of Chicago
Chicago, Illinois

K. Kovacs, M.D., Ph.D.
Department of Pathology
University of Toronto
Toronto, Ontario, Canada

Donald B. Maier, M.D.
Department of Obstetrics and Gynecology
University of Connecticut Health Center
Farmington, Connecticut

Kamran S. Moghissi, M.D.
Department of Obstetrics and Gynecology
Wayne State University School of Medicine
Detroit, Michigan

Peter T. Nieh, M.D.
Department of Urology
Lahey Clinic
Burlington, Massachusetts

Robert W. Rebar, M.D.
Department of Obstetrics and Gynecology
Northwestern University Medical School
Chicago, Illinois

B. Jane Rogers, Ph.D.
Department of Obstetrics and Gynecology
Vanderbilt University
Nashville, Tennessee

Lonnie D. Russell, Ph.D.
Department of Physiology
Southern Illinois University School of Medicine
Springfield, Illinois

Robert J. Stillman, M.D.
Department of Obstetrics and Gynecology
George Washington University Medical Center
Washington, D.C.

Ronald S. Swerdloff, M.D.
Division of Endocrinology
Harbor-UCLA Medical Center
Los Angeles, California

Thomas H. Tarter, Ph.D.
The Population Council
Rockefeller University
New York, New York

Ting-Wa Wong, M.D., Ph.D.
Department of Pathology
University of Chicago
Chicago, Illinois

J. Donald Woodruff, M.D.
Department of Gynecology and Obstetrics
Johns Hopkins University School of Medicine
Baltimore, Maryland

Luciano Zamboni, M.D.
Department of Pathology
Harbor-UCLA Medical Center
Los Angeles, California

Contents

1. Inflammatory and Traumatic Conditions of the Cervix

Kamran S. Moghissi

The uterine cervix plays a unique and important role in the process of reproduction. The cervix and its mucous secretion are involved in aiding sperm migration to the upper reproductive tract, protecting sperm from the hostile environment of the vagina and from phagocytic action, supplementing the energy requirements of sperm, filtering out abnormal sperm, functioning as a sperm reservoir, and aiding sperm capacitation.

The cervix is also a major site of pathological changes, including the common neoplasms of the pelvic organs. Many pathological conditions of the cervix affect the anatomical or functional integrity of the cervix and may be associated with impaired fertility. In this chapter, the traumatic, inflammatory, and neoplastic disorders of the cervix which may interfere with normal reproductive process will be reviewed.

ANATOMY AND PHYSIOLOGY

The cervix represents the terminal portion of the uterus and separates the vagina from the uterine cavity (Figure 1–1). It is a thick-walled, cylindrical structure that tapers at its inferior extremity. The canal of the cervix is 2.5 to 3 cm in length, fusiform in shape, and flattened posteriorly; its middle third is slightly dilated. The average transverse diameter at its widest point is 7 mm. The external os is the opening in the portio vaginalis that connects the cervical canal with the vagina.

Histologically the cervix differs from the corpus uteri. The pars vaginalis of the cervix is lined by stratified squamous epithelium similar to that lining the vagina, and it normally shows no keratinization. The epithelial cells of the endocervix comprise different types of nonciliated secretory and ciliated cells. The latter are tall columnar, rest on a thin basement membrane, and form a single layer; their nuclei are oval and located basally. Secretory cells are covered by microvilli and contain large numbers of cytoplasmic granules and clear droplets of mucus. Some ciliated cells have been observed via both transmission and scanning electron microscopy. Columnar epithelium from the ectocervix has very few ciliated cells, whereas endocervical epithelium has many ciliated cells.[1] The active beating of cilia may facilitate the orientation and flow of mucus from the surface of secretory cells to the upper vagina.

There are no true glands in the cervix. Early studies by Fluhmann[2] suggest that, instead of glands, the basic epithelial structure of the cervical mucosa is an intricate system of crypts or grooves which, grouped together, give an illusory impression of glands. These crypts may run in an oblique, transverse, or longitudinal direction; they never cross one another, although they may bifurcate or extend downward. The arrangement of the crypts in the endocervical canal resembles that of the trunk and branches of a tree. There is considerable variation in the size of the crypt openings. The smallest openings are 40 to 50 μm and the largest range from 300 to 600 μm.

The junction of columnar epithelium and squamous epithelium is known as the squamocolumnar junction. Unless active metaplasia is present, the junction is very sharp.

Extensive studies of cervical crypts at different levels of the endocervical canal and under different hormonal conditions have been reported.[3] The mean total number of crypts per cervix has been estimated to be 28,000 for estrogen-pretreated cervices and 23,000 for gestagen-pretreated cervices.[3] This finding is in contrast to the figure reported by Odeblad,[4] who suggested there are approximately 100 mucus-secreting, glandlike units (crypts) in the cervical canal.

Cyclic changes in the shape and diameter of the cervix have been described. In the immediate premenstrual period and during menstruation, the isthmus of the cervix (the narrow part of the canal between endocervix and the endometrial cavity) is short, wide, and atonic. Isthmic tone gradually increases during the follicular phase, which particularly affects the lower segment of the isthmus. In the luteal phase, progressive lengthening and narrowing of the isthmus give a hypertonic, tubular appearance that persists until the immediate premenstrual phase.

The cervix, like the rest of the uterus, is clearly derived from the müllerian ducts; however, its epithelial lining is continuous with that of the vagina. There is some controversy about when the two epithelia, that is, squamous and columnar, normally join, whether prenatally or postnatally. There is some doubt about the origins of both the

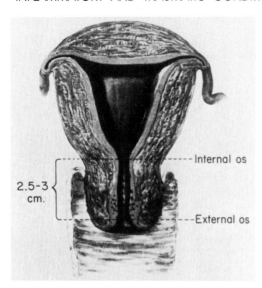

Figure 1–1. Human uterus.

vaginal epithelium at the upper end and of the portio vaginalis of the cervix.

The blood supply of the cervix is derived primarily from the uterine artery, and azygous arteries of the vagina and ascending branches of the vaginal arteries also contribute to it. The venous drainage parallels arterial vessels and communicates with the vascular network of the bladder neck. Veins from the cervix join the uterine and ovarian venous plexuses and empty finally into the hypogastric veins. The major source of blood supply to mucus-producing endocervical epithelium is from the first branches of the uterine arteries as they descend along the body of the cervix.[4]

The nerve supply of the cervix is derived from three plexuses of the pelvic autonomic system: the superior, middle, and inferior hypogastric plexuses.

Numerous nerve fibers, following the vascular network in the submucosa and independent of the vascular system, are found in the endocervix.[5] Collateral branches of these terminal nerves are in contact with endocervical crypts. Other nerve fibers traverse the submucosa of the cervical crypts and form a dense network around the epithelial invagination. These fibers are in intimate contact with the crypts and actually appear to enter into columnar cells.

Nerve fibers positive for cholinesterase-specific staining are most numerous in relation to cervical crypts, arterial vessels, and strands of smooth muscle.[6] An extensive adrenergic network, at the internal os where smooth muscle is abundant, and throughout the cervix in relation to blood vessel walls, has been demonstrated. The precise function of this neural network is unclear. Clinical observations, however, indicate that these nerves may be involved in pain perception resulting from the stretching of the endocervix, particularly the internal os. Adrenergic and cholinergic nerve fibers may also play a role, directly or indirectly, in the secretory function of the epithelial cells through their action on blood vessels.

CERVICAL SECRETION

Cervical mucus is a complex secretion produced constantly by the secretory cells of the endocervix. A small amount of endometrial, tubal, and possibly follicular fluid may also contribute to the cervical mucus pool. Debris from uterine and cervical epithelial cells and leukocytes is also present.

Endocervical epithelial cells produce a mucous secretion at the rate of 20 to 60 mg/day in normal women of reproductive age. During midcycle the amount increases 10- to 20-fold and may reach up to 700 mg/day.[7] Cyclic variation in the physical properties and chemical content, as well as the amount, of the cervical constituents has been reported.

PHYSICAL AND BIOCHEMICAL PROPERTIES OF CERVICAL MUCUS

Cervical mucus is a heterogeneous secretion with a number of rheologic properties, including viscosity, flow elasticity, spinnbarkeit, thixotropy, and tack or stickiness.[8]

Human cervical mucus usually is about 92% to 94% water. At ovulation, when the mucus is most abundant, the water content rises to 98%.[8] Human cervical secretion contains 1% inorganic salts, of which the principal constituent is NaCl (0.7%). Traces of potassium, magnesium, calcium, copper, zinc, iron phosphates, sulfates, and bicarbonate are also present.[10] The mucus is isotonic with saline throughout the cycle. The salt content of dry mucus, however, shows an increase coinciding with the time of ovulation. Since the concentration of salt remains constant while the gross amount changes cyclically, the water content of the mucus must change in the same proportion as the salt to maintain a constant concentration. In other words, there is a relative increase in the secretion of water and salt and a decrease in the amount of organic material in the dry weight of the midcycle mucus; this, incidentally, favors the occurrence of the fern phenomenon. The osmotic pressure of cervical mucus remains the same throughout the cycle.

Low Molecular-Weight Organic Compounds

Cervical mucus contains the free simple sugars (glucose, maltose, mannose) and other reducing substances.[10] The free sugars decrease during the ovulatory period.

Lipids are also present in cervical mucus. Serial determination of lipids has revealed a decrease in the amount of total lipids, cholesterol, and lipid phosphorous at midcycle, whereas the ratio of cholesterol to lipids remains the same.

Human cervical mucus contains large amounts of prostaglandins, ranging between 1 to 5 ng/mg of wet weight.

These include PGE_1, PGE_2, PGD_2, $PGF_1\alpha$, and $PGF_2\alpha$. The origin and biologic significance of cervical mucus prostaglandins are not known.[13]

Free amino acids have been detected in cervical secretion. A decrease in the concentration of the various amino acids is noted during the midcycle phase. This may reflect the aqueous dilution of the mucus at this period.[9]

High Molecular-Weight Components

Ultracentrifugation of the mucus results in two fractions: the supernatant, which contains the soluble macromolecules (polysaccharides, enzymes, and serum-type proteins), and the sediment (gel), which consists mainly of high-molecular-weight glycoproteins (mucins).

Glycogen is the principal polysaccharide of cervical secretion. An enzyme capable of reducing glycogen to utilizable glucose, amylase, has been found in the mucus.

Large numbers of enzymes have been detected in human cervical secretion. The levels of many of these enzymes, including alkaline phosphatase, esterase, amino peptidase, lactic dehydrogenase, and guaiacol peroxidase, have a marked preovulatory decrease and postovulatory rise, and seem to show a response to progesterone in the luteal phase. It has been suggested that assay of some of the enzymes that exhibit preovulatory decline and postovulatory rise may be used to predict or detect ovulation.[10]

Proteins

Pooled human cervical mucus contains about 1% to 3%[9] protein in two basic forms, soluble proteins and mucin. The soluble proteins comprise 55% of the total proteins and resemble serum proteins; albumin and γ-globulin (IgG) are the major components. By immunodiffusion and immunoelectrophoretic studies of human cervical mucus, 15 additional proteins, including lactoferrin, secretory IgA, and α_1-antitrypsin, have been identified. Cyclic variation in the amount of several proteins in cervical mucus has been described. In general there appears to be a preovulatory decrease and a postovulatory increase in the amount of albumin, α_1-antitrypsin, and immunoglobulins.[9,11]

Most serum proteins in the cervical mucus probably originate in blood serum.[8,10]

Such soluble proteins as secretory IgA and lactoferrin are obviously synthesized by cervical epithelium since they are absent in the blood.

Mucins comprise 45% of proteins in the cervical mucus. Mucin is a hydrogel that is rich in carbohydrates and belongs to a special class of glycoprotein. It is responsible for the distinctive viscoelastic and sperm-transport properties of cervical mucus. Purified human cervical mucin is a high molecular weight glycoprotein that is approximately 80% carbohydrate and 20% protein. The pH of cervical mucus is between 6.3 and 8.5. Serial determinations have revealed an increase in alkalinity at midcycle. The optimal pH for sperm penetration is also in the range of 7 to 8.5.

CYCLIC CHANGES OF CERVICAL MUCUS AND THEIR RELATION TO OVULATION

The secretion of cervical mucus is regulated by ovarian hormones. Estrogen stimulates the production of copious amounts of watery mucus, while progesterone inhibits the secretory activity of cervical epithelial cells. The physical properties and certain chemical constituents of cervical mucus show cyclic variations; their determination may be used to evaluate indirectly the amount of circulating sex hormones which can then be used to detect the occurrence of ovulation. Cyclic alterations in the constituents of cervical mucus may also influence sperm penetrability, nutrition, and survival. Figure 1–2 shows serial determinations of important properties of human cervical mucus, tested during a normal menstrual cycle in 10 women, in relation to pituitary and ovarian hormone secretion and *in vitro* sperm penetration. These data clearly demonstrate that optimal changes of cervical mucus properties, such as increase in quantity, spinnbarkeit, ferning, pH, and decrease in viscosity and cell content, occur immediately prior to ovulation and reverse after ovulation. Preovulatory mucus is most receptive to sperm penetration.[12] The proportion of saline in cervical secretion directly determines the consistency of the mucus and the rate of sperm penetration.

SPERM MIGRATION THROUGH CERVICAL MUCUS

For many years, reproductive biologists and clinicians have attempted to clarify the factors responsible for the passage of spermatozoa through the human cervix and to the upper reproductive tract. Studies in animal species in which the cervix and its secretions are similar to those in the human provide much useful information. Caution should be exercised, however, when extrapolating from animal data to humans.

Information on the mechanism of sperm migration and survival in the human female reproductive tract is derived from clinical observations and indirect data. Many areas remain obscure.

Approximately 200 to 500 million sperm are deposited on the cervix and posterior vaginal fornix during a normal coitus. Human semen coagulates immediately after ejaculation and traps most sperm cells until seminal proteolytic enzymes bring about liquefaction. The first portion of the ejaculate contains three-fourths of the sperm, which, under favorable conditions, quite promptly penetrate the cervical secretion.[13,14] Because spermatozoa are

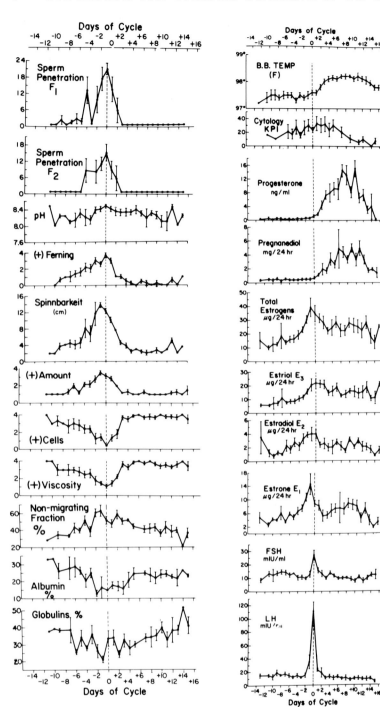

Figure 1–2. Composite profile of serum gonadotropin and progesterone levels; urinary estrogens and pregnanediol levels; basal body (B.B.) temperature; karyopyknotic index (KPI) of vaginal cells; and cervical mucus properties throughout the menstrual cycle in 10 normal women. Day 0 is day of LH peak (dotted line). Vertical bars represent 1 SEM. F_1 and F_2 indicate the number of sperm in the first and second microscopic fields (200X) from the interface, 15 minutes after the start of *in vitro* sperm-cervical mucus penetration test.

quickly destroyed by vaginal acidity, their entrapment in the coagulum until liquefaction takes place may be considered a protective device to prevent their demise.

In vitro studies have shown that nonliquefying semen samples are lysed when treated with an acid buffer. Thus it is possible that vaginal acidity enhances liquefaction of the seminal coagulum. Indeed, complete liquefaction of the seminal clot *in vivo* appears to occur somewhat faster than ejaculation.

Vaginal content is usually acid, with a pH of about 3 to 5. However, cervical secretions coating the upper part of the vagina and its fornices considerably increase the alkalinity of the vaginal milieu. They provide a favorable medium for sperm survival and appear to promote their motility and longevity.

Seminal plasma, an alkaline fluid, has a buffering effect on the vaginal acidity and changes the vaginal pH, thus smoothing the transition of sperm from the semen into the cervical mucus.[15]

Sperm migration through the cervix involves three distinct but interrelated factors: first, the ability of sperm to penetrate the mucus by their intrinsic motility; second, the fibrillar structure of cervical mucin, which enables it to participate actively in the process of sperm transport;

and third, the morphological configuration of cervical crypts, which contributes to the storage and preservation of sperm in the cervical canal and their sustained and prolonged release to the upper tract. Various studies have shown that there is an excellent correlation between the ability of sperm to penetrate in cervical mucus and sperm density, percentage of the normal forms (oval sperm), and sperm motility. Sperm motility and normal morphology appear to be the most important factors.[9]

Based on studies in cattle and subhuman primates, it has been conjectured for many years that cervical crypts may play an important role in sperm penetration and storage in the cervix.[16,17] Such a process could cause aggregation of a large number of sperm in the crypts of the cervical canal, where they are stored and released at a constant rate into the uterus.

Certain similarities between the epithelial structures of the human cervix and cervical mucus and those of subhuman primates suggest that an identical or closely related process may also be operative in women.

Some clinical reports lend further support to the concept of the cervix as a site of sperm storage.[3] For example, in some studies spermatozoa have been recovered from the cervix of women as long as 48 hours after artificial insemination.[18]

Sperm penetrability of human cervical mucus can begin on approximately the ninth day of a normal cycle and it increases gradually to a peak at ovulation. It is usually inhibited within 1 to 2 days after ovulation but may persist to a lesser degree for a longer period.[9]

Two phases of sperm migration through the cervix have been recognized: First, a rapid phase, during which the leading spermatozoa penetrate the central portion of the cervical canal and advance in a line parallel to mucin fibrils originating in the vicinity of the internal os; Second, a delayed phase, during which sperm enter the cervical mucus around the periphery of the central core, are oriented by mucin fibrils originating from the crypts, and

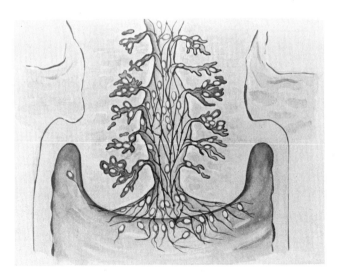

Figure 1–3. Schematic representation of current concept of sperm transport through the cervix. Note long mucus filaments, sperm penetration along the molecular line of strains, and aggregation of spermatozoa in the crypts and clefts of the cervical canal.

colonize the crypts.[19] The latter process is responsible for the storage of sperm in the cervical crypts and their gradual release over an extended period into the uterus and oviducts (Figure 1–3).

INFLAMMATORY DISEASES OF THE CERVIX

Bacterial Infections

Inflammatory cervical lesions are of specific interest to clinicians interested in infertility since they have the potential of interfering with sperm transport through the cervix and impairing fertility. The cervix is also a primary site of contamination by many infectious organisms which might be transmitted to the upper reproductive tract.

A wide variety of bacterial organisms may affect the cervix. Acute cervicitis may result from direct infection by nonspecific microorganisms or by secondary invaders. The former group includes streptococci, staphylococci, and enterococci. During the puerperium, the cervix is most susceptible to infection by these bacteria. The most common secondary invaders include gram-negative diplococci, *Neisseria gonorrhoeae, Trichomonas vaginalis* and *Candida albicans.*

Insertion of foreign bodies such as pessaries and tampons into the vagina may also lead to acute cervico-vaginal inflammation.

Clinically, acute cervicitis is characterized by purulent, malodorous vaginal discharge, which is yellowish green (*Trichomonas* infection) or whitish, colorless, with cottage cheese appearance (*Candida*). The cervix is usually edematous, reddened, and inflamed. Histologically, there is extensive stromal edema with polymorphonuclear leukolytic infiltration and often focal type of mucous membrane. When the endocervix is involved, cervical crypts show evidence of acute inflammatory and exudative reaction. Cervical mucus may appear turbid or grossly purulent and thick, even in the preovulatory period, and will contain increased amounts of protein and pus cells. Preovulatory spinnbarkeit and ferning (crystallization) may be considerably decreased or absent. In gonorrheal infection, the organism penetrates the endocervical epithelium and produces an acute inflammatory reaction in the subjacent stroma which, by the third or fourth day, is associated with a marked vascular and exudative reaction. This inflammatory reaction consists initially of polymorphonuclear leukocytes with small but increasing number of lymphocytes and plasma cells surrounding the cervical crypts. Eventually, the surface epithelium shows a patchy degeneration and desquamation, with marked tissue edema and serous exudate. The exudate, along with inflammatory and epithelial cell debris, forms the characteristic discharge which contains the typical gram-negative intracellular diplococci.

Cervical crypts are commonly infected during the acute inflammatory phase. The acute inflammation may either subside spontaneously or persist as a chronic process interfering with the drainage of the secretory products of crypts. Inflammatory involvement of crypts may serve as a focus of persistent or latent infection which further facilitates the local or distant spread of the infection to the upper reproductive tract.[20,21]

Acute cervicitis may interfere with fertility in several ways: First, during the acute phase which is invariably associated with acute vaginitis, coital activities may be extremely painful. Second, the inflammatory exudate may totally alter the normal appearance and function of the cervical secretion. Studies *in vitro* and *in vivo* have shown that sperm penetration in purulent cervical mucus containing a large number of leukocytes is impaired. Finally, with persistence of infection, the involvement of the upper reproductive tract leading to endometritis and salpingitis is a distinct possibility.

Chronic Nonspecific Cervicitis

Chronic cervicitis is a common gynecological disorder which occurs almost exclusively in women of reproductive age, it being infrequent after the menopause and virtually nonexistent in prepubertal girls. The condition is usually associated with a low-grade infection in a cervix distorted by minor lacerations, exposure of the cervical canal to the lower pH of the vaginal secretions, and altered bacterial flora. Inflammation of cervical crypts produces structural changes such as edema and fibrosis which impair drainage of mucus and perpetuate optimal conditions for continuing infection. The condition is clinically characterized by a whitish, greenish, commonly yellowish discharge. Grossly, the cervix may appear hypertrophic and has nabothian cysts. It frequently shows a markedly irregular erosion composed of an ectocervical area of columnar and metaplastic squamous epithelium. On colposcopic examination, cervical mucosa is hyperemic because of an increased number of terminal vessels.

Microscopically, there is a variable degree of submucosal chronic inflammatory infiltration consisting of lymphocytes and plasma cells.

The bacteria most commonly cultured from the cervices of women with chronic cervicitis include *Staphylococcus aureus, Aerobacter aerogenes, Enterococcus faecalis, Streptococcus viridans, E coli,* and *Proteus vulgaris.*[22] Normal cervical mucus was found to be sterile in one-third of women who were examined. Cervical mucus from the remaining two-thirds showed scanty flora. Lactobacilli, diphtheroids, coagulase-negative staphylococci, non-hemolytic streptococci, *E coli,* and yeast, all common contaminants of the vaginal flora, were the most important organisms.[22]

Some older studies have suggested that cervical mucus may have bacteriostatic and bactericidal properties against certain strains of bacteria such as staphylococci and *Streptococcus hemolyticus* (*S pyogenes*), but it enhances the growth of certain strains of *Neisseria gonorrhoeae in vitro.*[23] More recent reports have not substantiated these findings but have detected muramidase (lysozyme) activity in cervical secretion.[24] Muramidase is an enzyme capable of hydrolyzing the structurally impor-

tant beta 1 to 4 linkage between N-acetylmuramic acid and N-acetylglucosamine in the cell walls of certain bacteria. Serial determinations of muramidase show a marked decrease coinciding with the time of ovulation and a postovulatory increase.

Toth and colleagues[25] reported that various bacteria were unable to migrate in a capillary tube filled with ovulatory cervical mucus. Nonetheless, aerobic and anaerobic bacteria obtained from semen specimens or added to semen could easily penetrate the cervical barrier when active spermatozoa were present. No bacterial migration could be demonstrated when luteal phase or pregnancy cervical mucus was used. Similarly, mucus collected from women taking oral contraceptives showed only minimal penetration by spermatozoa and bacteria. The conclusion drawn from these *in vitro* observations was that microorganisms migrate through the cervical mucus with moving spermatozoa. The importance of these observations relating to the protective effect of cervical mucus against bacterial invasion of the upper reproductive tract is thus clear.

Martin and associates[26] demonstrated that cervical mucus from uninfected, healthy women converted gonococci susceptible to killing by fresh human serum to a resistant state after 3 hours' incubation at 37° C. This serum resistance could play an important role *in vivo* in the survival of gonococci in the initial stages of urogenital infection. Bactericidal activity of the human cervical mucus is present during all phases of the menstrual cycle but is least pronounced at ovulation.[27]

Chronic cervicitis has been incriminated as a factor contributing to infertility in women. Certain bacteria such as *E coli,* β-hemolytic streptococci (*S viridans*), *S hemolyticus, Aerobacter,* and others have been found to have spermicidal properties *in vitro.* The spermicidal action of these bacteria does not appear to be an absolute deterrent to sperm transport and fertility, since conception can and does occur frequently in women who have chronic cervicitis. However, in a study of 350 infertile patients, Sobrero[22] found that treatment of chronic cervicitis significantly increased the subsequent chance of the women to conceive.

Granulomatous Infections of the Cervix

Sexually transmitted granulomatous diseases commonly encountered in the vulva may also involve the cervix. These include syphilis, either as the primary chancre, secondary mucous patches, or tertiary gumma, lymphogranuloma venereum, granuloma inguinale, and chancroid. In addition, tuberculosis of the cervix may occasionally be seen. Syphilis, a chronic, sexually transmitted disease caused by *Treponema pallidum,* gains access to the cervix through the mucous membranes. It spreads rapidly to regional lymph nodes, causing a lymphadenitis. In the female, the primary chancre occurs on the cervix in about 40% of the cases.

Clinically, the primary chancre is characterized by a single punched-out ulceration which is painless and nontender. It tends to ooze serum and, since there is associated endarteritis obliterans, it does not bleed. The histologic appearance of the lesion is that of typical syphilitic, diffuse, chronic inflammation with marked vascular and reparative tissue changes.

Tuberculosis of the cervix is almost always secondary to tuberculous salpingitis and endometritis. The incidence of cervical lesions among populations infected with genital tuberculosis varies from 2% to 60%, with an incidence of 5% in the United States.[28]

Clinically, the cervix is patulous, red, and friable, and may show severe ulceration resembling that of cervical carcinoma. Histologically, tuberculous infection of the cervix is recognized by the presence of multiple granulomata or tubercles. These are characterized by a central caseous necrosis surrounded by epithelioid histocytes and multinucleated giant cells of Langhans in which the nuclei are distinctly distributed at the periphery of the cytoplasm. The periphery of the tubercles is heavily infiltrated by lymphocytes and plasma cells. Granulomatous lesions of cervical tuberculosis are to be distinguished from foreign body giant cell granulomata due to suture or cotton, lymphogranuloma venereum, schistosomiasis, and sarcoidosis.

With the exception of tuberculosis, there is no evidence that granulomatous lesions of the cervix either interfere with sperm transport or impair fertility. The effect of tuberculous cervicitis on fertility is an indirect one. Concomitant tuberculous involvement of endometrium and fallopian tubes commonly leads to infertility.

Parasitic Infections of the Cervix

Parasitic infections of the cervix are uncommon in the United States and developed countries, and they have been reported mostly from Africa, South America, and some Asian countries.

Schistosomiasis of the cervix generally caused by *S. haematobium* is particularly prevalent in Africa (Egypt). Clinically, the cervix may appear ulcerated or indurated. Polypoid masses masquerading clinically and histologically as verrucous carcinoma may be present. Microscopically, the cervical lesions are produced by the inflammatory response to the ova and are characterized by noncaseating granulomata (pseudotubercles), with ova sometimes calcified, surrounded by multinucleated giant cells.

Schistosoma infestation has been reported to induce sperm antibody production and cause infertility.[29]

Approximately 100 cases of amebiasis of the cervix uteri have been described.[30] The condition is characterized by a purulent vaginal discharge, induration and ulceration of the vulva, vagina, and cervix. There is usually severe pain, tenderness, and associated diarrhea. Impairment of fertility, though not documented, is entirely feasible.

Other parasitic infections of the cervix are rare and include pinworm (*Oxyuris vermicularis*) and echinococcosis. These may be associated with severe anatomic distortions of the cervix and cause functional disorders leading to infertility.

Chlamydial Infections

The chlamydia are obligate intracellular parasites containing both RNA and DNA and possessing a cell wall. They include the causal organism of psittacosis, trachoma, and inclusion conjunctivitis. In the reproductive tract they cause lymphogranuloma venereum and a considerable proportion of nonspecific infections. *C trachomatis* is a major cause of sexually transmitted diseases (STD) worldwide. Those most susceptible to chlamydial infections appear to be young, sexually active women. Twelve to 27% of women attending veneral disease clinics yield a positive culture for *C trachomatis*. In those who were contacts of men with nongonococcal urethritis, rates reached approximately 87%.[31,32]

The association of chlamydial infection, salpingitis, and infertility has been repeatedly documented. In one report, 64% of infertile women with tubal abnormalities as a cause had serologic evidence of prior chlamydial infection. Other studies have reported similar findings. It is now believed that half to two-thirds of tubal infertility is consequent to chlamydial salpingitis.

Less clear is the link between infertility and chlamydial cervicitis. Battin and associates[33] examined the effect of *C trachomatis* infection on cervical mucus and sperm-cervical mucus interaction in 63 consecutive infertile patients undergoing a midcycle postcoital test in the San Francisco area. They found no evidence of acute infection in this small group of patients, nor could they demonstrate any correlation between previous exposure to *C trachomatis* as demonstrated by positive IgG chlamydial antibody titer and abnormal PCT or tubal disease. Unfortunately, the findings of this report are at variance with other studies in regard to the association of tubal disease and *C trachomatis* infection.

Thus, the association between acute chlamydial infection, cervical mucus abnormality, and sperm-cervical mucus interaction remains unclear. However, it appears that previous exposure to the disease may not affect the function of the cervix. Of related interest is the recent demonstration that oral contraceptives promote chlamydial cervicitis and do not protect against ascending infection to the oviducts, contrary to their protective effect in bacterial infection.[34]

Mycoplasma Infections

The genus *Mycoplasma* comprises a group of self-replicating prokaryotes that lack cell walls. They form the taxonomic class Mollicutes. Their minimal reproductive units are the size of large viruses and contain both ribosomal RNA and double-stranded DNA. Over 60 species of mycoplasma organisms have been described. *Ureaplasma urealyticum,* once called T-mycoplasma, has been separated from the genus *Mycoplasma* because of its distinctive capacity to hydrolyze urea. Among mycoplasmas, only *M hominis* and *U urealyticum* have been isolated from genital infections with any degree of frequency and will be considered here.[35]

The frequency of recovery of mycoplasmas varies depending on age, sexual activity, and populations screened. In young girls the frequency is about 10%. With puberty the frequency of colonization rises. A strong correlation exists between the onset of sexual activity, frequency of sexual activity, number of partners, and the incidence of positive cultures. In the healthy, sexually-active adult woman, *M hominis* and *U urealyticum* can frequently be found in the cervical opening, vagina, and distal urethra. The frequency of *U urealyticum* in cervical mucus of fertile women and those with unexplained infertility varies considerably (Table 1–1). Generally, however, the highest frequency has been observed among patients with unexplained infertility.[35,36]

Several studies have indicated decreased sperm motility in ejaculates containing *U urealyticum* organisms.[36] The demonstration that genital mycoplasma organisms can attach to sperm has led to the suggestion that these organisms may interfere with sperm transport as well as sperm metabolism and sperm–egg interaction. In support of the latter process, it has been shown that exposure of sperm samples to mycoplasma resulted in a diminished zona free hamster penetration rate.[37] This occurred without a change in sperm motility. Further studies have suggested that genital mycoplasma organisms in the vagina may produce a factor that impairs sperm function.[35]

The impact of mycoplasma infection on fertility may also be assessed by the results of fertility restoration among treated and untreated patients. Unfortunately controversies also exist in this area. Most studies indicate an improved pregnancy outcome, but only a few controlled studies have been conducted. Among these, some show an improved pregnancy rate, whereas others do not.[35,36]

Collectively, the epidemiologic studies fail to provide persuasive evidence that either *M hominis* or *U urealyticum* is causally related to infertility. However, the conflicting reports and clinical trials lead one to conclude that couples with unexplained infertility have a greater yield of positive cultures for *U urealyticum* than normal controls or couples whose infertility is based on identifiable factors. Furthermore, in selected groups of patients with positive cultures, treatment for *U urealyticum* may be associated with an increased chance of conception. Remaining, however, is a relatively large percentage of couples in whom ureaplasma infection apparently has no deleterious effect on reproductive function and, if infertile, the colonization is not responsible for their inability to achieve conception.

Viral Infections

Common viral infections affecting the cervix are condylomata acuminata resulting from human papilloma virus (HPV) and herpes infections. Two distinct types of biological response are produced by these virus infections. The first reaction involves cellular degeneration and necrosis; the second consists of cellular stimulation and proliferation leading to hyperplasia and sometimes to overt neoplasia.[20]

Herpes genitalis may result in spontaneous abortion and fetal morbidity and mortality. HPV has been linked to cervical carcinoma. Neither virus, however, has been directly incriminated in inhibition of conception. Nevertheless, because of interference with normal coital activities, an indirect effect may be suspected.

ECTROPION (CERVICAL EROSION)

The term *ectropion* or erosion is applied to areas of columnar epithelium extending from the cervical canal over the external os onto the portio. This occurs twice as commonly on the anterior as on the posterior lip, but both lips may be involved simultaneously. The everted endocervical mucosa appears as a red, velvety zone which bleeds easily on touch. The term *cervical erosion* is actually incorrect since there is no loss of surface epithelium. The pathogenesis of endocervical eversion is unclear. It develops during fetal life and can occur at the time of puberty and during the reproductive years, but is absent in postmenopausal women.

The dynamics of events by which the columnar epithelium extends onto the portio are uncertain. The squamous transformation of ectopic endocervical tissue is probably stimulated by the acid vaginal pH and provides a protective surface for underlying endocervical tissue. The movement of endocervical epithelium and its squamous transformation are presumably under the influence of the local (vaginal) environment as well as hormonal status. Accordingly, the physiologic squamocolumnar junction of the transformation zone is topographically inconstant and follows the movement of the transformation zone.[21] It is commonly influenced by the hormonal environment and occurs frequently in pregnancy and among oral contraceptive users.

Because cervical ectropion occurs in a large number of women, it is regarded as a normal physiologic process and is not believed to have an important effect on fertility. However, the exposed endocervix is more susceptible to infection and when endocervicitis and alterations of normal midcycle cervical mucus occur, interference with sperm penetration and fertility may result.

Table 1–1. Recovery of *Ureaplasma urealyticum* in Cervical Mucus of Fertile and Infertile Women

Type	Frequency (%)
Fertile control	23–68
Infertile women	35–52
Women with unexplained infertility	52–91

TRAUMATIC AND CONGENITAL CONDITIONS OF THE CERVIX

Cervical Lacerations and Trauma

Obstetrical and nonobstetrical lacerations of the cervix, when adequately repaired, heal promptly and leave little or no residual scarring and should not interfere with fertility. Unrecognized or neglected cervical tears will result in splitting of the cervix, exposure of the endocervix to the vaginal environment, infection, and possibly incompetence. In addition to their unsightly appearance and the presence of leukorrhea, these neglected tears may, in fact, impair fertility. Traumatic ulcerations of the cervix may result from the use of a cervical cap, tampons, or other foreign bodies.[38] Fertility impairment will occur only if these ulcers are not recognized and become infected.

Cervical fistula is an abnormal opening in the cervix and lower uterine segment usually caused by a rupture or laceration during midtrimester abortion.[39] It may also result from perforation by an intrauterine device. These injuries do not alter fertility potential, but they may cause complications during labor.

Amputation of the cervix, an operation commonly performed in conjunction with the Manchester operation in the past, may cause excision of the entire mucus-producing epithelium and result in "dry cervix," a condition associated with considerable impairment of fertility. Similarly, it is common clinical experience that deep conization and cauterization of the endocervix may destroy or significantly reduce mucus-producing cells and interfere with sperm transport. Laser surgery of the cervix, if extended deeply within the endocervical canal, may have similar effects. Controlled studies, however, are not available to document these clinical observations.

Cryotherapy of the cervix is believed to be less traumatic and, in fact, might be beneficial. Cryotherapy probes are relatively shallow and generally destroy only the superficial epithelium of the exocervix.[40]

Cervical Incompetence

Cervical incompetence does not cause infertility but may be the cause of repeated abortion and reproductive failure. Classically, the condition occurs in the second trimester of pregnancy and is characterized by painless dilatation and/or effacement of the cervix, rupture of the amniotic sac prior to any significant contractions, or the relatively painless passage of the gestational sac.

The precise cause of cervical incompetence is in most instances difficult to establish. Dilatation of the cervix for diagnostic curettage or abortion, cervical surgery, previous traumatic obstetric deliveries with the use of forceps, and maternal exposure to diethylstilbestrol are commonly elicited in the patient's past history and are incriminated. Congenital cervical incompetence occurs in approximately 2% of women.

Histologic studies have shown that the human cervix is composed predominantly of fibrous connective tissue. Isolated and attenuated strands of smooth muscle are found in the cervix and are embedded in a heavy collagenous matrix. These strands vary in amount in different cervices and are irregularly scattered, except in the most peripheral areas of the portio vaginalis where they tend to be concentrated.[41] In women with cervical incompetence there is an abnormal ratio of muscular to connective tissue in the region of the anatomic internal os of the cervix and the isthmic region of the uterus.[38] In clinical practice, the diagnosis of cervical incompetence is arrived at from historical data and is based on the degree of anatomic cervical distortion by hysterosalpingography and/or ultrasonography.[42] A high rate of fetal salvage has been claimed when cervical incompetence has been corrected by cerclage operation during pregnancy.[43] However, controlled clinical trials are needed to document further the effectiveness of these procedures.[44]

Congenital Anomalies of the Cervix

Congenital malformation of the cervix results from failure of development or union of the müllerian ducts. In its most severe form, the corpus and the cervix may be absent. Congenital atresia of the cervix may also occur in the presence of the corpus.

Structural abnormalities of the cervix have also been associated with prenatal DES exposure. These anomalies are described elsewhere in this volume. (See Chapter 4.)

Cervical Stenosis

Cervical stenosis may be congenital or follow surgical treatments of the cervix such as conization and cauterization. Clinically, these cervices are characterized by a "pinhole" cervical os with considerable diminution or absence of cervical mucus.

Although pregnancies are known to occur in women with cervical stenosis, infertility may result because of the absence of cervical mucus, which is essential for sperm penetration and normal vaginal lubrication.

NEOPLASTIC CHANGES AND THEIR EFFECT ON FERTILITY

Benign Neoplasms

Benign lesions of the cervix include polyps, microglandular endocervical hyperplasia, leiomyoma, fibroadenoma, adenomyoma, hemangioma, and condylomatous lesions.

Polyps

Endocervical polyps are not true neoplasms and should be considered pseudotumors. They constitute the most common new growth of the endocervix. They usually cause profuse leukorrhea, metrorrhagia, and postcoital bleeding. Clinically, cervical polyps are characterized as rounded or elongated structures with a red, smooth, or lobulated surface which can measure a few millimeters or several centimeters.

Histologically, cervical polyps contain a variety of structural patterns. The most common type is the endocervical mucosal or mucous type, composed of mucus-secreting epithelial infoldings and crypts with or without cystic or adenomatous glandular changes. Occasionally they are mainly fibrous and are referred to as cervical fibrous polyps. Cervical polyps are considered as focal protrusions of endocervical folds, including epithelium and substantia propria. They may affect fertility in several ways. Polyps can interfere with sperm penetration and migration by obstructing the cervical canal, by producing local infection, and possibly by producing abnormal mucus secretion.

Other Benign Tumors

Cervical leiomyoma represents about 8% of all uterine myomas. They usually occur singly, may produce unilateral enlargement of the cervix, or may be pedunculated and obstruct the cervical canal.

These tumors unquestionably interfere with normal cervical function and, if pregnancy occurs, may cause complications during pregnancy, labor, or postpartum. Histologically, they are similar to uterine leiomyomas.

Other neoplasms of the cervix are uncommon and will affect fertility only if they are located in or arise from the endocervix, or when their size is large enough to cause anatomical distortion of the cervix.

Malignant Tumors of the Cervix

These include squamous cell carcinoma, adenocarcinoma and rarely, sarcoma of the cervix. Carcinoma of the cervix is one of the most common malignancies affecting the female. In its preinvasive forms, dysplasia and carcinoma *in situ*, these lesions do not interfere with cervical function. Invasive carcinoma of the cervix is occasionally encountered in early pregnancy, indicating an absence of the effect of the neoplastic process in reproductive function. Advanced carcinoma of the cervix, however, may cause considerable structural deformity and disruption of cervical function, and it is usually incompatible with normal fertility.

ENDOMETRIOSIS

Ectopic endometrial implants appear as one or more small, bluish or red nodules on the portio or, occasionally, in the endocervical canal. These lesions may occur in conjunction with pelvic endometriosis or as isolated foci of the disease. Histologically, the glands and stroma are similar to those of endometrium but usually have a proliferative pattern. Endometriosis of the cervix probably exerts little or no influence on fertility.

References

1. Jordan JA: Scanning electron microscopy of the physiological epithelium. *In* JA Jordan, A Singer (eds): The Cervix. Philadelphia, WB Saunders Co., 1976.
2. Fluhmann CF: The cervix uteri and its disease. Philadelphia, WB Saunders Co, 1961.
3. Insler V, Glezerman M, Bernstein D, *et al.*: Cervical crypts and their role in storing spermatozoa. *In* Insler V, Bettendorf G (eds): Advances in Diagnosis and Treatment of Infertility. New York, Elsevier-North Holland, 1981.
4. Zinser HK: La vascularisation du col utérin. *In* Les Fonctions du Col Utérin. Paris, Masson et Cie, 1964.
5. Giro C: Contribution a l'étude du système nerveux, terminaux des glandes cervicales des rongeurs et de la femme. *In* Les Fonctions du Col Utérin. Paris, Masson et Cie, 1964.
6. Rodin M, Moghissi KS: Intrinsic innervation of the human cervix: a preliminary study. *In* Blandau RJ, Moghissi KS (eds): The Biology of the Cervix. Chicago: University of Chicago Press, 1973.
7. Moghissi KS, Syner FN: Cyclic changes in the amount of sialic acid of cervical mucus. Int J Fertil 21:246, 1976.
8. Moghissi KS: Composition and function of cervical secretion. *In* Gripp R (ed): Handbook of Physiology: Endocrinology II. Washington, DC: American Physiology Society, 1973, Part 2, Chapter 31.
9. Moghissi KS: The function of the cervix in human reproduction. Current Probl Obstet Gynecol VII:4–58, 1984.
10. Moghissi KS: Prediction and detection of ovulation. Fertil Steril 34:89, 1980.
11. Schumacher GFB: Biochemistry of cervical mucus. Fertil Steril 21:697, 1970.
12. Moghissi KS, Syner FN, Evans TN: A composite picture of the menstrual cycle. Am J Obstet Gynecol 114:405, 1972.
13. Macleod J, Hotchkiss RS: Distribution of spermatozoa and certain chemical constituents in the human ejaculate. J Urol 48:225, 1942.
14. Sobrero AJ, Macleod J: The immediate postocital test. Fertil Steril 13:184, 1962.
15. Fox CA, Meldrum SJ, Watson BW: Continuous measurement by radiotelemetry of vaginal pH during human coitus. J Reprod Fertil 33:69, 1973.
16. Mattner PE: The distribution of spermatozoa and leucocytes in the female genital tract in goats and cattle. J Reprod Fertil 17:253, 1968.
17. Jaszczak S, Moghissi KS, Hafez ESE: Effect of prostaglandin $F_2\alpha$ on sperm transport in the reproductive tract of female macaques (*M fascicularis*). Arch Androl 4:17, 1980.
18. Hanson FW, Overstreet JW, Katz DF: A study of the relationship of motile sperm numbers in cervical mucus 48 hours after artificial insemination with subsequent fertility. Am J Obstet Gynecol 143:85, 1982.
19. Moghissi KS: Sperm migration through the human cervix. *In* Insler V, Bettendorf G (eds): The Uterine Cervix in Reproduction. Stuttgart, Georg Thieme Publishers, 1977.

20. Slavin G: The pathology of cervical inflammatory disease. *In* Jordan JA, Singer A (eds): The Cervix. Philadelphia, WB Saunders Co, 1976, p 251.

21. Ferenczy A: Benign lesions of the cervix. *In* Blaustein A (ed): Pathology of the Female Genital Tract, Second Edition. New York, Springer-Verlag, 1982, p 136.

22. Sobrero AJ: Bacteriological findings in the midcycle endocervical mucus in infertile women. Ann NY Acad Sci 97:591, 1962.

23. Pommerenke WT: Cyclic changes in physical and chemical properties of cervical mucus. Am J Obstet Gynecol 52:1023, 1946.

24. Rozansky R, Persky S, Bercovici B: Antibacterial action of human cervical mucus. Proc Soc Exp Biol Med 110:876, 1962.

25. Toth A, O'Leary WM, Ledger W: Evidence for microbial transfer by spermatozoa. Obstet Gynecol 59:556, 1982.

26. Martin PMV, et al: Induction in gonococci of phenotypic resistance to killing by human serum by human genital secretions. Br J Vener Dis 58:363, 1982.

27. Enhorning G, Huldt L, Melen B: Ability of cervical mucus to act as a barrier against bacteria. Am J Obstet Gynecol 106:532, 1970.

28. Schaefer C: Tuberculosis of female genital tract. Clinic Obstet Gynecol 13:965, 1970.

29. El Mahgoub S: Antispermatozoal antibodies in infertile women with cervicovaginal schistosomiasis. Am J Obstet Gynecol 112:781, 1972.

30. Cohen C: Three cases of amoebiasis of the cervix uteri. J Obstet Gynecol Brit Cwlth 80:476, 1973.

31. Grump DW: A growing danger—chlamydial infertility. Contemporary Ob/Gyn 24:39, 1984.

32. Grump DW, Gibson M, Ashikaga T: Evidence of prior pelvic inflammatory disease and its relation to *Chlamydia trachomatis* antibody and intrauterine contraceptive device use in infertile women. Am J Obstet Gynecol 146:153, 1983.

33. Battin DA, Barnes RB, Hoffman DI, *et al: Chlamydia trachomatis* is not an important cause of abnormal postcoital tests in ovulating patients. Fertil Steril 42:233, 1984.

34. Washington AE, Gove S, Schachter J, *et al.*: Oral contraceptives, *Chlamydia trachomatis* infection, and pelvic inflammatory disease. JAMA 253:2246, 1985.

35. Styler M, Shapiro SS: Mollicutes (mycoplasma) in infertility. Fertil Steril 44:1, 1985.

36. Friberg J: Mycoplasmas and ureaplasmas in infertility and abortion. Fertil Steril 33:351, 1980.

37. Busolo F, Zanchetta R: The effect of *Mycoplasma hominis* and *Ureaplasma urealyticum* on hamster egg *in vitro* penetration by human spermatozoa. Fertil Steril 43:110, 1985.

38. Weissberg S, Dodson MG: Recurrent vaginal and cervical ulcers associated with tampon use. JAMA 250:1430, 1983.

39. Fleury F: Recognizing and treating the cervical fistula. Contemporary Ob/Gyn 10:25, 1977.

40. Creasman WT: Does cryosurgery affect fertility? Contemporary Ob/Gyn 4:81, 1974.

41. Danforth DN: The distribution and functional activity of the cervical musculature. Am J Obstet Gynecol 68:1261, 1954.

42. Barford DAG, Rosen MG: Cervical incompetence: Diagnosis and outcome. Obstet Gynecol 64:159, 1984.

43. Peters WA, Thiagarajah S, Harbert G: Cervical cerclage: twenty years' experience. South Med J 72:933, 1979.

44. Rush RW, Isaacs S, McPherson K, *et al.*: A randomized controlled trial of cervical cerclage in women at high risk of spontaneous preterm delivery. Br J Obstet Gynecol 91:724, 1984.

2. Immunologic Abnormalities of the Female Reproductive Tract

Richard A. Bronson

The locus of action of many of those immune events within the female reproductive tract that lead to infertility is at the level of the gametes, derived from the male as well as the female. These highly specialized cells of evanescently short lifespan are especially liable to damage as a result of immune perturbation. This chapter will focus upon mechanisms by which immunities to sperm and ova can play a role in altering three aspects of early reproduction: fertilization, ovulation, and nidation.

FERTILIZATION—ANTISPERM ANTIBODIES

Sperm-reactive antibodies have been detected in the serum of men and women of all ages, including children before the onset of puberty, and appear to be directed against intracellular antigens, some of which are common to both spermatozoa and bacteria.[1,2] In contrast to this high background level of "naturally occurring" antibodies, which appear to play no role in reproduction, a small minority of infertile women have been found to possess immunoglobulins directed against sperm surface antigens, either intrinsic to the plasma membrane[3,4] or derived from seminal plasma.[5] There is increasing clinical and experimental evidence that such antibodies play a pathologic role in reproduction, impairing sperm transport within the female reproductive tract and those early events of gamete interaction that lead to fertilization.[6,7] Antisperm antibodies originating in the male may also lead to impaired sperm penetration into and survival within the female reproductive tract. Sperm entry from semen into cervical mucus is impaired when antisperm autoantibodies are present on the sperm surface.[8] Should these sperm enter the mucus, they would also be liable to complement-dependent damage.[9] Price and Boettcher, using hemolysis of red blood cells sensitized with anti-RBC antibody, have shown complement activity to be present within cervical mucus at 10% the level seen in serum.[10] Yang and associates have also recently demonstrated the presence of a complete complement cascade within the oviductal secretions of the rhesus monkey.[11] In addition to complement-mediated cell lysis, spermatozoa may also be opsonized by the presence of antibodies on

their surface, and an increased ability of macrophages to destroy these antibody-bound sperm has also been demonstrated.[12] The lifespan of the sperm population within the female reproductive tract following coitus might then be shortened in such a manner.

REGULATION OF IMMUNOGLOBULIN SECRETION WITHIN THE REPRODUCTIVE TRACT

Antisperm antibodies may be present within the female reproductive tract as a result of both transudation and local secretion. Wira and Sullivan have examined the influence of the sex hormones on levels of IgA and IgG, as well as secretory component, in cervicovaginal and uterine secretions of ovariectomized rats.[13,14] Administration of estradiol resulted in a significant decline, in a dose-dependent manner, in the cervicovaginal content of IgA, IgG and secretory component. Treatment of rats with progesterone also lowered levels of IgA and secretory component.

In contrast, estradiol stimulated the appearance of IgA-positive cells and increased tissue and intraepithelial content of IgA in the rat uterus. Estradiol also induced an increase in production of secretory component, which appears to control the movement of polymeric IgA into luminal secretions. Immunoglobulins produced by tissue lymphocytes within the endometrium are joined to secretory piece produced by the endometrial epithelium, prior to their transport into the uterine lumen. These responses were blocked by progesterone when administered with estradiol. The effect of estrogen upon the uterine secretion of immunoglobulins is opposite to that noted at the level of the cervix and vagina, indicating that each compartment of the female reproductive tract responds differently to hormonal stimulus.

Studies performed by Schumacher *et al.* in the rhesus monkey also indicated that antibodies directed against specific antigens, as well as total immunoglobulin levels, vary within both oviductal secretions and cervical mucus throughout the reproductive cycle, reaching a nadir near ovulation at the time of high endogenous estradiol levels.[15] These experiments, unfortunately, were performed under gonadotropin stimulus, and superphysiologic levels of estradiol were often encountered. The actual magnitude of changes in the concentration of immunoglobulins within oviductal secretions during spontaneous ovulation is thus not clear.

We have compared the presence of antisperm antibodies detected within serum with those present in vaginal secretions and utero-tubal lavages as well as peritoneal fluid collected at laparoscopy.[16] Washes of vaginal secretions were collected by flushing the vagina with 2 cc of Ringer's lactate after three days of sexual abstinence. Sperm-reactive antibodies were studied, by immunobead binding, following *in vitro* antibody transfer to known antibody-negative donor sperm, in vaginal secretions and serum of 170 women. Forty-one women (24.3%) were found to have antisperm antibodies in both vaginal secretions and serum. Seventy-nine women had positive circulating humoral antibodies directed against sperm but negative vaginal washes. Conversely, antisperm antibodies were found within the vaginal wash, yet were absent from serum in only a small minority (2.9%) of women (Table 2–1). The latter figure compares closely with that reported by Clarke, who detected, by immunobead binding, antisperm antibodies within cervical mucus when none were detected in serum in 4.9% of cases.[17] Chen and Jones have documented the presence of complement-dependent sperm-immobilizing activity within 10% of cervical mucus samples from infertile couples in the absence of humoral antisperm antibodies.[18] The incidence of sperm agglutinins within cervical mucus extracts is said to be considerably higher, at 30%, but whether this represents a true antibody-mediated aggregation of sperm is unclear.[19]

The presence of such sperm-reactive antibodies within vaginal or cervical secretions, in conjunction with their absence in serum, and the predominance of IgA's[20] suggest local production within the reproductive tract (Table 2–2). Local production of antisperm antibodies is also suggested by the finding of unique classes of immunoglobulins directed against regions of the sperm surface (head versus tail) in these fluids that were not present in serum. In contrast, sperm-reactive antibodies detected in peritoneal fluid reflect those seen in serum, consistent with their nature as transudates. As there may be exchange of fluid between the free peritoneal cavity and distal ampulla of the oviduct, sperm may be exposed at the site of fertilization to complement-fixing antibodies derived from the peritoneum.

A comparison of the isotypes and regional binding specificities of antisperm antibodies present within vaginal, cervical, utero-tubal and peritoneal fluids indicates, as suggested by the data derived from animal studies, that the mix of these antibodies in each reproductive tract compartment can vary considerably and may not be a reflection of those seen in serum. The isolated local secretion of such sperm-reactive antibodies within the reproductive tract, in conjunction with their complete absence in serum, appears uncommon. In addition, the concentration of these antibodies appears to vary throughout the reproductive cycle. These considerations illustrate the difficulty in determining for the individual woman whether the presence of antisperm antibodies plays any role in impaired reproduction.

COMPLEMENT-MEDIATED SPERM DAMAGE WITHIN THE FEMALE REPRODUCTIVE TRACT

Sperm immobilization within cervical mucus of normal pH (7.0–7.4) containing antisperm antibodies is a slow process requiring four to six hours to become apparent. The mixture of immunoglobulin classes of those antibodies present within the reproductive tract will determine their aggregate effect upon spermatozoa. Sperm-reactive antibodies of the IgA class, the major isotype present within mucosal secretions, do not fix complement and cannot mediate complement-dependent sperm immobilization.[21] Localized binding to the sperm surface of antibodies known to fix complement, however, may also not be associated with loss of sperm motility. The difficulty of judging the reproductive consequences of the presence of antisperm antibodies is graphically illustrated by a comparison made of the ability of two sera obtained from different women, each containing high levels of head-directed antisperm antibodies to damage sperm. Following transfer *in vitro* to a highly motile population of sperm selected by swim up from ejaculates of known fertile men, sperm immobilization was rapid in one case in the presence of guinea pig serum as a source of complement but totally lacking in the second case. Studies of the immotile sperm by transmission electronmicroscopy revealed disruption of the plasma membrane over the

Table 2–2. Immunoglobulin Classes of Sperm-Reactive Antibodies Detected in Vaginal Flush

Isotype	No. Cases (% Total)
IgA	34 (73.9%)
IgG	25 (54.5%)
IgM	7 (15.2%)

Table 2–1. Detection of Antisperm Antibodies[a] in 170 Women at Risk for Immunity to Spermatozoa

Serum	Vaginal Flush	
	Positive	Negative
Positive	41 (24.1%)	79 (46.4%)
Negative	5 (2.9%)	45 (26.4%)

[a] Sperm-reactive antibodies were detected by immunobead binding following *in vitro* antibody transfer to known antibody-negative donor sperm.

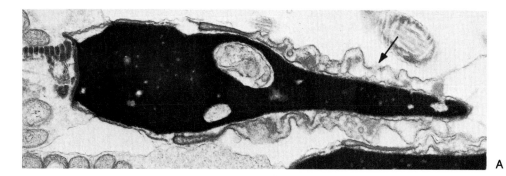

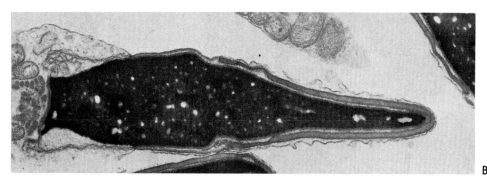

Figure 2–1. A highly motile population of sperm selected by swim up from the ejaculate of a fertile donor was exposed to human serum containing antibodies of the IgM and IgG class reactive with the sperm head and tail and either guinea pig serum (1:32 dilution) as a source of complement (A) or heat-inactivated (56°C × 30 minutes) guinea pig serum (B). Disruption of the acrosome with loss of acrosomal contents (arrow) in association with sperm immobilization was seen in the presence of active complement. (Bronson RA, Cooper GW, Phillips D: Unpublished observations.)

sperm head, with loss of acrosomal contents, but retention of normal sperm ultrastructure following exposure to the second serum and complement (Figure 2–1). Antisperm antibodies of the IgM class predominated in the first instance while IgG's were present, perhaps of a non-complement-fixing subclass, in the serum that did not mediate sperm membrane damage.[22] Both of these sera would have been declared strongly positive by any of several tests available for the detection of antisperm antibodies (ELISA, TAT, MAR, and immunobead binding) and yet their biological effects differed greatly.

That sperm immobilization within cervical mucus is complement-dependent has been previously demonstrated by adding a source of complement, such as guinea pig serum, to heat-inactivated human cervical mucus extracts.[18] As guinea pig serum contains hetero-antibodies that react with the human sperm tail, sperm immobilization may occur within cervical mucus previously shown to support sperm survival.[23] Hence, if guinea pig serum is to be used as a source of complement, it must be absorbed with human spermatozoa. Complement activity of serum also varies between individual animals as well as between species (Figure 2–2).

These considerations led us to demonstrate, by an alternate means, that sperm immobilization within cervical mucus was complement-dependent and, indeed, mediated by the classical pathway of complement activation. Cervical mucus was extracted following addition of an equal volume of phosphate-buffered saline by sonication and high speed centrifugation. A motile population of sperm selected by swim up from the ejaculate of a fertile donor was exposed to the mucus extract in the presence of increasing amounts of antiserum raised in rabbits against human C4. Neutralization of sperm immo-

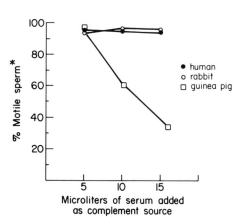

*60 minutes incubation at 37°C

Figure 2–2. Motile spermatozoa selected by swim up from the ejaculate of a fertile donor were exposed to heat-inactivated human serum containing complement-fixing sperm-reactive antibodies and either human, rabbit, or guinea pig serum as a source of complement. Guinea pig serum had been preabsorbed with human spermatozoa to remove cross-reacting antibodies.

bilization occurred with the addition of increasing amounts of anticomplement antibody (Table 2–3), demonstrating the process to be complement-dependent. As C4 plays no role in the alternate pathway of complement activation, sperm immobilization must have been mediated through activation of the classical complement cascade.[24]

These observations, as well as the prior study of Price and Boettcher,[10] do not exclude the possibility of antibody-independent, alternate pathway-mediated sperm immobilization. The alternate pathway sets in motion, in the absence of antibody, a sequence of events leading to formation of the same membrane attack unit (MAC) as the classical antibody-dependent complement pathway.[24] The interaction of MAC with membranes results in a local reorganization of the lipid bilayer, leading to lysis of erythrocytes, bacteria, and nucleated cells. A crucial step in the activation of the alternate pathway is the binding of C_3 to cells and its subsequent degradation to C_3a and C_3b split products by C_3 convertase. When factor B binds to C_3b at the cell surface, it becomes susceptible to cleavage by factor D, resulting in the formation of alternate pathway C_3 convertase. As C_3b, a cleavage product of the C_3 converting enzyme, becomes a subunit of that enzyme, a positive feedback loop is established. Deposition of a few molecules of C_3b on the cell surface may result in the formation of many molecules of C_3 convertase.

Control of this chain reaction occurs through the binding of an inhibitor, beta 1H, to the cell surface. The presence of beta 1H inhibits C_3 convertase formation by preventing binding of C_3b to Bb. It also allows access of a C_3 convertase inhibitor to bind to the cell surface. The ratio of binding of beta 1H to C_3b will determine then whether a particular cell surface will activate the alternate pathway or not. Using radiolabeled beta 1H and bound C_3b, their relative binding to the cell surface can be determined. This ratio, termed the restriction index, was defined as 1.0 for sheep erythrocytes, a cell known not to activate

the pathway.[25] Activators of the alternate pathway, such as rabbit erythrocytes, have a low restriction index (0.1), indicating that beta 1H-C_3b interaction on those surfaces is only one-tenth that seen for sheep erythrocytes.

Cell surfaces may be modified by several means including incorporation of chemically defined lipopolysaccharides or by removal of sialic acid residues. It is possible to convert nonactivators of the alternate pathway, such as sheep erythrocytes, to activators by removing cell-bound sialic acid with concomitant reduction of the restriction index from 1.0 to 0.3.[26]

The restriction index of spermatozoa is not known, nor is it known whether this might vary between ejaculates of different men. As neuraminidases may be secreted by bacteria, it is possible that the composition of the local vaginal flora in the presence of cervicitis or vaginitis could influence whether the alternate pathway is activated on the sperm surface or not, leading to membrane damage and immobilization in the absence of antisperm antibodies.

We have attempted to determine whether or not the alternate pathway exists within human cervical mucus by exposing human or rabbit erythrocytes to mucus extracts. The latter are known to activate the alternate pathway, while the former do not. Since there was little difference in the degree of hemolysis noted between erythrocytes of both species, evidence could not be obtained that the alternate pathway of antibody-dependent complement-mediated damage exists.

ETIOLOGY OF IMMUNITY TO SPERM IN WOMEN

The repeated intravaginal insemination of women at coitus with millions of spermatozoa is usually not associated with the development of immunity to sperm leading to impaired fertility. That spermatozoa possess antigens to which the immune system may react has been demonstrated in many species by the development of antisperm antibodies following experimental immunization. The female reproductive tract is also capable of mounting an immune response. This has been documented experimentally in rhesus monkeys by intravaginal inoculation with glycopolysaccharide or *S. typhosa* or T4 coliphage.[28] Intravaginal insemination of rabbits with xenogenic sperm has also been associated with development of sperm-reactive antibodies.[29] Secretory IgA directed against *Candida* has been found in women following yeast vaginitis,[30] and intravaginal inoculation with polio virus leads to the production of locally produced antiviral antibodies within the vaginal secretions,[31] indicating that the human female reproductive tract is not an immune privileged site.

Germ cells obtained from testicular suspensions in mice, when injected intravenously into syngeneic recipients, lead to reduced natural killer cell activity, reduced mixed lymphocyte reactivity, and decreased potential to generate cytotoxic T-lymphocyte responses to modified

Table 2–3. Neutralization of Sperm Immobilization by Cytotoxic Cervical Mucus with Anticomplement Antiserum[a]

Experimental Category	% Motile Sperm[b]
1. Unheated cervical mucus extract[c]	5%
2. Heated cervical mucus extract	94.5%
3. Unheated cervical mucus extract + 5 μg anti-C4	5%
4. Unheated cervical mucus extract + 100 μg anti-C4	10%
5. Unheated cervical mucus extract + 150 μg anti-C4	33%
6. Heated cervical mucus extract + 100 μg anti-C4	87%

[a] Guinea pig serum (1:32) has previously absorbed with human spermatozoa.
[b] Following 90 minutes incubation at 37°C.
[c] Human cervical mucus collected in the late follicular phase was extracted by sonification and configuration.

cell surface allogen antigens. Mice injected with allogeneic spermatozoa are also immune-suppressed.[32] Seminal fluid has been shown to contain several immunosuppressive substances.[33] A high molecular weight immunosuppressive factor has been partially purified from human semen by Lord *et al.*[34] Anderson and Tarter have noted a relative lack of antigenicity of epididymal sperm in mice after their incubation in seminal fluid when compared with saline. They proposed that seminal fluid-derived immunosuppressive factors might adsorb to the sperm surface and alter their reactivity with lymphocytes or macrophages.[35] Alternatively, antigenic sites on the sperm surface could have been occluded by coating proteins at ejaculation. In support of the latter hypothesis, O'Rand has found evidence for the disappearance of a specific antigen, detected with a fluoroscein conjugated monoclonal antibody probe, when epididymal sperm are mixed with seminal fluid, and the reappearance of this antigen following sperm residence within the uterus.[36]

Could nature then provide the means, through concomitant exposure at coitus, to seminal fluid immunosuppressants of preventing the development of immunity to spermatozoa? We hypothesized that a lack of immunosuppressive activity of seminal fluid might lead to the development of allo-antibodies which reacted with the sperm surface leading to subsequent infertility. To test this hypothesis, immunosuppressive activity of semen obtained from men in couples diagnosed to be free of sperm-reactive antibodies was compared with that from husbands whose wives were found to have high or low levels of immunity to sperm.[37]

Tests for antisperm antibodies were performed when less than five motile sperm per high power field were seen in well-estrogenized cervical mucus, in the face of normal semen quality, or when altered sperm motion within cervical mucus was noted (shaking, vibration, or restricted tail beat) at post-coital testing. Spermatozoa from the ejaculate of the husband were tested for surface bound immunoglobulins by immunobead binding. Sera from husband and wife were also tested by immunobead binding following *in vitro* antibody transfer to either the husband's spermatozoa (if antibody negative) or known antibody negative sperm of a fertile donor. Spermatozoa were separated from seminal fluid, one to six hours following ejaculation, by centrifugation, and residual sperm-free seminal fluid were stored at −70° for further study.

The ability of seminal fluid to suppress phytohemagglutinin-stimulated activation (PHA) of normal lymphocytes was compared in four clinical groups: 1) men and women free of detectable sperm-reactive antibodies, 2) couples in whom wives had high levels of antisperm antibodies, including their presence within vaginal secretions, 3) couples in whom wives had low levels of sperm-reactive antibodies confined to serum, and 4) couples in whom husbands were autoimmune to spermatozoa.

A wide range in the ability of seminal fluid to suppress mitogen-stimulated lymphoblast formation was noted among men whose wives were free of antisperm antibod-

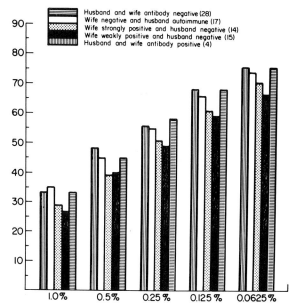

Mean Response* to Phytohemagglutinin of Normal Lymphocytes in the Presence of Seminal Plasma

Husband and wife antibody negative (28)
Wife negative and husband autoimmune (17)
Wife strongly positive and husband negative (14)
Wife weakly positive and husband negative (15)
Husband and wife antibody positive (4)

FINAL CONCENTRATION SEMINAL FLUID IN LYMPHOCYTE CULTURE

*As % control response [³H thymidine uptake by 2 x 10⁵ lymphocytes in presence of dilute seminal fluid/uptake in absence of seminal fluid] x 100

Figure 2–3. The ability of seminal fluid to suppress mitogen-stimulated lymphoblast formation was compared in couples with and without immunities to spermatozoa. No differences between groups were apparent.

ies (Figure 2–3). No difference was seen in levels of immunosuppression caused by semen samples of husbands whose wives were highly sensitized to sperm versus nonimmune wives. In those cases in which concurrent semen analyses of ejaculates submitted for mitogenesis studies were available, there was no correlation between either sperm concentration or total ejaculate sperm and immunosuppressive activity. The percent of control response of normal lymphocytes to PHA in the absence of seminal plasma was no different over the five seminal plasma concentrations studied for wives free of sperm-reactive antibodies compared with wives in whom such antibodies were detected in either serum alone or serum and vaginal secretions.

These findings failed to demonstrate a relationship between immunosuppressive activity of seminal fluid and the presence of sperm-reactive antibodies in women. These data, as well as the wide variation observed in the ability of seminal fluid of different individuals to suppress PHA-stimulated blast formation, did not support the hypothesis that a deficiency of semen immunosuppressors plays a role in the etiology of the abnormal immunologic response of certain women against sperm antigens. A more direct assay of B cell function, however, such as *in vitro* antibody stimulation by the polyclonal activator pokeweed mitogen, or preferably by sperm antigens themselves, might demonstrate such a relationship.

CAN ABNORMAL SPERM TRANSPORT IN FEMALE REPRODUCTIVE TRACTS PREDISPOSE TO SPERM IMMUNIZATION?

Spermatozoa have been found on the fimbrial surfaces of the fallopian tube as well as within peritoneal fluid of women after coitus.[38] The isthmus of the oviduct is known to regulate the number of sperm within the ampulla.[39] While millions of spermatozoa are present within seminal plasma, only tens to hundreds are present within the distal fallopian tube.[40] As has been shown in mice, intraperitoneal administration of intact spermatozoa in the absence of adjuvants can lead to the production of sperm antibodies.[41] Abnormal transport of large numbers of spermatozoa to the peritoneum, either due to altered tubal function or following intrauterine insemination, could then in theory lead to immunity to spermatozoa. To investigate this possibility, we tested the sera of 20 women undergoing repeated intrauterine insemination for the presence of humoral antisperm antibodies. These women had undergone at least 3 cycles, and as many as 16 cycles, of intrauterine insemination with a highly motile population of husband's spermatozoa, selected by swim up and washed free of seminal fluid. In the majority of couples, intrauterine insemination was performed in the face of poor penetration and survival of sperm within abnormal cervical mucus. In those, 18 women, essentially free of antisperm antibodies, remained so following a series of inseminations, and there was no change in antibody levels in the remaining patients who initially demonstrated immunity to sperm.

The route of inoculation of antigen also appears to be important in determining the isotypes of those antibodies present within the reproductive tract. This has been demonstrated in experiments in which women were inoculated either intravaginally or orally with polio virus.[31] The distribution of isotypes of antipolio virus within vaginal secretions following intravaginal inoculation was different from that seen following intraoral inoculation and consisted primarily of IgA's, indicating their local production. We have obtained similar results studying the distribution of isotypes of sperm-reactive antibodies in infertile women when compared with that seen in sera of heterosexual and homosexual men.

Sixty unselected sera from admitted homosexual males were compared with sera of 180 infertile couples selected for study on the basis of abnormal sperm swimming behavior within cervical mucus at postcoital testing.[42] Antisperm antibodies were detected in a greater proportion of sera of known homosexual men (78.3%) than from men in infertile couples (44.4%). Head-directed antibodies were present in 65.9% of positive sera of homosexuals versus 32.7% of heterosexual men. These antibodies were primarily of the IgM class in the sera of homosexuals (63.6%), but not in heterosexual men (35%). Sera from infertile females contained comparable levels of high titer head-directed antibodies (83.2%) to those in homosexuals (85.7%). This compared with 38.5% of sera from heterosexual men of infertile couples. As all the homosexual men studied were predominantly exposed to oral sex, the gastrointestinal route of exposure to semen may lead to an antigen processing that closely mimics the female, leading to a difference in distribution of antisperm isotypes when compared to men with autoantibodies to sperm.

The antigens to which sperm-reactive antibodies are directed have not yet been well characterized. A tissue-specific antigen secreted by the seminal vesicles has been identified in the rat which binds to spermatozoa at the time of ejaculation.[43] Sperm-reactive antibodies may then be directed against coating proteins present within the seminal fluid which bind to sperm at ejaculation, or to intrinsic antigens of the sperm plasma membrane. Evidence for the former possibility has been provided by Isojima and associates.[44] They have produced monoclonal antibodies to human seminal plasma antigens from azoospermic men which were subsequently purified by immuno-affinity chromatography. An IgM monoclonal antibody that possesses the ability to block fertilization *in vitro* and leads to sperm immobilization in the presence of complement has been identified. Monoclonal antibodies have also been developed against specific integral protein antigens of both rabbit[45] and human spermatozoa.[46] At least one of these antigens, in the rabbit, appears to be located near the sperm-zona receptor, since antibodies raised against it have been found to block binding of sperm to the zona pellucida and subsequent fertilization. Similar results have been obtained in the pig.[47] Certain human sera of infertile men also possess antisperm antibodies directed against the sperm head that similarly block binding of human sperm to the human zona pellucida.[48]

FERTILIZATION FAILURE— ANTIOVUM ANTIBODIES

The oocyte is surrounded by an acellular elastic sphere, the zona pellucida, which first appears during intrafollicular growth of the oocyte, remains through preimplantation embryonic growth, and is shed by the blastocyst within the uterus at the time of implantation. The zona also plays a role, as has been shown in mice, in protecting the precompaction embryo from disaggregation as it is transported through the oviduct.[49,50] Species-specific receptors are present on the outer surface of the zona, to which sperm bind prior to zona penetration.

Evidence has accumulated that the acrosome reaction occurs following attachment of sperm to the zona pellucida of the mouse. Florman and Storey have shown that the acrosome reaction is accelerated when sperm are exposed to acid-solubilized zona components.[51] Binding of sperm to the zona and induction of the acrosome reaction are mediated by one of three specific sulfated glycoproteins of the zona pellucida.[52,53] In the hamster[54] and guinea pig,[55] however, the acrosome reaction appears to occur as sperm pass through the outermost of the egg vestments, the cumulus oophorus, rather than on the zona surface.

Wolgemuth and associates have raised antibodies against the zona proteins purified by high resolution two-dimensional polyacrylamide gel electrophoresis, and they used these as a probe to study intrafollicular formation of the zona.[56] Zona pellucida proteins, as judged by immunoperoxidase localization of these antibodies, were first observed early in follicular maturation at the periphery of the cytoplasm of oocytes when surrounded by a thin granulosa cell layer. No staining was initially observed in granulosa cells during early follicular development. Zona proteins were localized within the cytoplasm of the inner layer of granulosa cells, however, later in follicular development when the zona matrix would be distinguished into inner and outer regions.

Several species have been immunized, including subhuman primates, with either whole ovaries, solubilized whole zona pellucida, or purified zona proteins.[57,58] Polyclonal antisera to solubilized zona pellucida have produced temporary sterility, as has a monoclonal antibody directed against ZP3, the murine sperm zona receptor.[59] These monoclonal antibodies were detected on the zona of intrafollicular oocytes following passive immunization of mice, and these eggs, subsequently ovulated, were impenetrable to sperm in vitro. Monoclonal antizona antibodies were no longer detected on the surface of ovarian oocytes 80 days following administration of antibody; this observation correlated with the restoration of fertility.

Interestingly, several species immunized with solubilized zonae or purified zona proteins have been found to develop ovulatory dysfunction. Immunization of subhuman primates with either heat-solubilized porcine zona pellucida or purified zona antigen has been associated with abnormalities of ovulation and follicular maturation.[60,61] Rabbits immunized with solubilized porcine zona pellucidae that developed antibodies against zona proteins failed to form functional corpora lutea in response to HCG administration. All immunized animals showed elevated serum levels of FSH and LH, and numbers of developing follicles in these animals were markedly reduced within seven weeks of immunization.[62]

ANTIZONA PELLUCIDA ANTIBODY: REPRODUCTIVE SIGNIFICANCE IN HUMANS

Given evidence that impaired fertility could be induced experimentally by either active or passive immunization against the zona pellucida proteins, several investigators have attempted to determine whether such antibodies occur spontaneously in women. Several problems in methodology, however, have resulted in a failure of consensus. Human zona pellucidas are difficult to obtain. The target antigen used to detect antizona antibodies must be provided by some other means. The zona pellucida of the pig, cow, and human share antigenicity,[63] and porcine zonas have been used to test for the presence of antizona antibodies in human sera. Whether those antigens present between species are epitopes of zona pellucida receptors for spermatozoa is unclear and their relevance to fertility unknown.[64] Common antigens may also be shared with other tissues, including red blood cells, and false positive reactions due to cross-reactive antibodies may then be present. Finally, the zona possesses a pore-like microstructure which is liable to promote nonspecific adsorption of proteins, including fluoroscein conjugated antiglobulins.

In a preliminary study, Shivers and Dunbar tested the sera of 23 infertile women for antisperm antibodies.[65] Six of the sera produced strong, and nine produced minor, immunofluorescent reactions when exposed to porcine zona pellucida. Subsequent studies unfortunately have produced contradictory results. Sacco and Moghissi have studied sera from 125 fertile and infertile women for autoantibodies to zona pellucida, using an indirect immunofluorescent technique similar to that described by Shivers and Dunbar.[66] A high incidence of positive reactions was found in sera of all groups examined, suggesting that this observation may not represent an autoimmunity by specific zona component, but rather a nonspecific reaction of no reproductive consequence. In contrast Nishimoto et al., who tested 735 human sera against porcine zonas using similar techniques,[67] found 13 of 135 samples from patients with unexplained infertility but none of 141 samples of fertile men and women to contain antizona antibodies. Kamada and associates have also tested human sera for antizona activity, using passive hemagglutination. Bovine erythrocytes coated with purified porcine zona substance were used as indicator cells.[68] Eight of 88 serum samples from infertile sera gave a positive reaction, whereas only 1 of 99 control sera were positive. Following absorption with porcine erythrocytes, however, antizona activity was retained in only 4 of these serum samples (4.5%). In an unpublished study of clinically defined sera provided by the WHO Reference Bank, the same group has found an incidence of antizona autoantibodies of only 3%.[69]

Karuchi et al. have developed a radioimmunoassay to detect antibodies to the zona pellucida, using I^{125} labeled purified porcine zona as antigen.[70] Antibodies were detected using this method in 3 of 11 sera from women with unexplained infertility, 4 of 12 fertile women, and 3 of 10 fertile men. As antibody titers in the infertile women were no higher than that in fertile couples, it would appear that antizona autoantibodies detected in human sera by this method would not play a role in impaired reproduction.

Following solubilization of the porcine zona pellucida and the purification of several components by high resolution two-dimensional polyacrylamide gel electrophoresis, it had been hoped that one of these proteins might be the putative zona receptor to which spermatozoa bind. This could then be utilized in an enzyme-linked immunosorbent assay for the detection of antizona antibody. Proof awaits, however, that the purified material binds to the zona receptor of the sperm plasma membrane in a saturable manner, indicating specific binding, and that sperm exposed to this purified protein demonstrate an impaired attachment to intact zonas.[71]

ANTIOVARY ANTIBODIES AS A CAUSE OF OVARIAN FAILURE

The etiology of primary ovarian failure in younger women can be divided into two broad groups: 1) those cases associated with an abnormality of the X chromosome, where the gonad is dysgenetic, and 2) those associated with a normal karyotype. Abnormally-shaped ovaries of small volume are also found in the majority of the latter instances,[72] but a subgroup of these women have been identified in whom ovarian volume is normal, as judged at laparoscopy or by sonography. Ovarian failure could be on an autoimmune basis in these instances, with blockade of gonadotropin action at the granulosa cell level, rather than due to an absence of follicles. These women often exhibit resistance to gonadotropins when tested with human menopausal gonadotropins as a provocative stimulus of follicular maturation, suggesting that failure of follicular maturation is not on the basis of bioinactivity of endogenous gonadotropins. Could autoantibodies directed against ovarian gonadotropin receptors play a role in the failure of follicular development?

Autoimmune antireceptor antibodies have been detected in serum in other endocrinopathies that may result in either blockade of target cell function (myasthenia gravis)[73] or hyperstimulation (Graves' disease).[74] Primary ovarian failure has been documented in association with myasthenia[75] as well as other autoimmune diseases, sug-

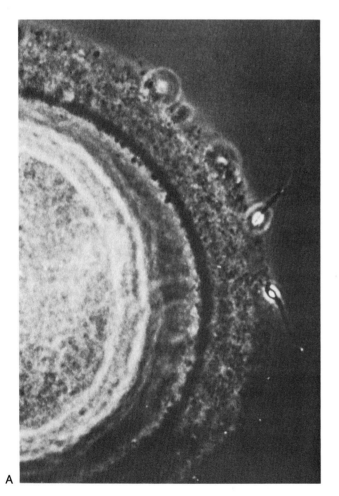
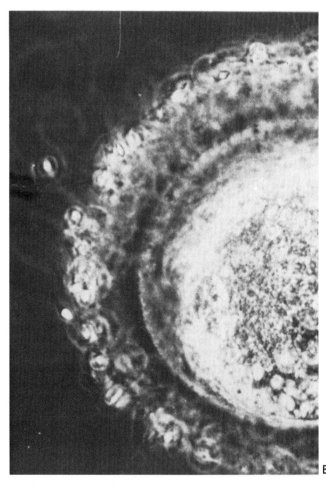

A   B

Figure 2–4. The ability of serum obtained from a woman with primary ovarian failure and myasthenia gravis to inhibit binding of human spermatozoa to the human zona pellucida was studied. Unfertilized, salt-stored human oocytes were first exposed to patient's serum (1 : 1 dilution) or each of six sera from women with regular menses, and then inseminated with human spermatozoa capacitated by overnight incubation in Biggers-Whittingham-Whitten medium containing 10 mg/ml HSA. The number of sperm attached to the zona pellucida was markedly reduced in each of three replicate experiments by patient serum (A) when compared with controls (B). (Yanagimachi R, Bronson RA, Emanuel N: Unpublished observations)

gesting a generalized breakdown in the immune mechanisms of tolerance to self-antigens of these individuals.

In an attempt to determine the prevalence of circulating antibodies directed against ovaries of women with primary ovarian failure, Coulam and Ryan have studied 110 sera of women under the age of 35 years with amenorrhea[76] in the presence of elevated serum gonadotropins. Antiovary antibodies were detected by incubating patient serum with I^{125} labeled proteins extracted from ovaries of normal premenopausal women. Following precepitation of the radiolabeled protein with an antihuman antiglobulin, the percentage of specific bound counts was determined. Twenty-seven percent of the sera were found to be positive for circulating antiovarian antibodies. Sera from 24 women with polycystic ovaries, which were studied as a control, were found to be free of antiovary autoantibodies. Whether these autoantibodies are the cause or the result of ovarian failure remains unclear. Evidence for the latter has been provided by Mathur and associates, who also found high titers of antiovary antibodies in women with gonadal dysgenesis and Turner's syndrome.[77]

Autoantibodies against the zona pellucida were found in a 28-year-old woman with primary ovarian failure manifesting abnormal follicular maturation in association with secondary amenorrhea.[78] After an uneventful term pregnancy and two first-trimester spontaneous abortions, menses ceased. A diagnosis of myasthenia gravis was made one year later, following gradual onset of diplopia, ptosis, dysarthria, and proximal muscle weakness. Symptoms were controlled with Mestinon.

There was no withdrawal bleeding following administration of Provera, and serum gonadotropins were found to be elevated at FSH/LH 56/41 and 41/200 miu/ml. Serum T4 and T3 resin uptake were normal, antithyroid antibodies were negative, and a normal adrenal response to cortrosyn was observed. Antinuclear and antiparietal antibodies were negative. Peripheral blood karyotype was 46, XX. Laparoscopy revealed ovaries of normal dimension, but with no evidence of follicular maturation. A factor was present in her serum which prevented binding of human spermatozoa to the human zona pellucida. Zona-intact salt-stored human eggs[78] were preincubated for 20 to 30 minutes in patient serum diluted 1:1 or control serum in each of six women who were menstruating regularly. Eggs were washed free of serum and then inseminated in vitro with preincubated, capacitated human spermatozoa. In each of three separate experiments, sperm binding to the zona pellucida was impaired following preincubation of eggs with patient serum, so that only few sperm were adherent when compared with eggs that had been exposed to control serum (Figure 2–4). This observation is of particular note in light of the abnormal follicular maturation previously described after immunization of laboratory animals with zona proteins.

Spontaneous menses occurred three to four months following thymectomy, and gonadotropins returned to normal, at the time, at FSH/LH 18/15 miu/ml. Thereafter, amenorrhea recurred and gonadotropins fluctuated between elevated and normal levels over the next several months. These clinical observations and the previously noted experimental studies suggest that antibodies directed against zona pellucida glycoproteins might impair ovarian function by reacting with granulosa cells, which synthesize and secrete zona proteins during follicular maturation. Antizona autoantibodies might block the binding of gonadotropins to their receptors, at the granulosa cell surface with the result that aromatization of androgens to estradiol and LH receptor development was impaired.

ANTIOVUM ANTIBODIES: THE OOCYTE PROPER

We have investigated whether some women in couples with unexplained infertility might possess autoantibodies directed against the egg proper, rather than the zona pellucida. Given the ethical concerns in using human eggs as reagents, we have studied the heterologous interaction of human sera with either unfertilized zona-free hamster eggs or fertilized zona-free and zona-intact mouse eggs during their preimplantation development.

Fifty-six sera of women and 13 sera of men from infertile couples were screened for complement-dependent hamster egg cytotoxicity. Following removal of the egg vestments with hyaluronidase and trypsin, three to five zona-free hamster eggs were distributed individually in microtiter plate wells containing 15 microliters of heat-inactivated human test serum (1:10 dilution) in the presence or absence of active complement. Serum from male guinea pigs, at 1:20 or 1:30 dilution, was used as a source of complement, and either heat-inactivated guinea pig serum (56°C × 60 minutes) or serum neutralized with goat anti-guinea pig C3 antiserum was used as a control. Complement activity of guinea pig serum was assessed by testing for immobilization of human spermatozoa in the presence of human serum containing antisperm antibodies of IgM or IgG class directed against the principal piece of the sperm tail. Following incubation of eggs in serum, 2 to 3 drops of 0.2% trypan blue in phosphate-buffered saline were added to each well. Eggs were incubated an additional sixty minutes and transferred through three washes of PBS/HSA and observed for dye uptake.

In the presence of cytotoxic serum and active complement, zona-free hamster eggs became increasingly granular in appearance, the oolemmal edge lost its sharp border, and progressive swelling occurred. Lucent areas appeared within the periphery, and distribution of cytoplasmic granules became nonuniform. These eggs took up trypan blue (Figure 2–5).

Twenty-three of 56 sera from women (41.1%) and 1 of 13 (7.7%) from men with unexplained infertility were found to be cytotoxic. Eighteen sera from women submitted for pregnancy testing in which chorionic gonadotropin was detected were studied as controls for antioocyte, complement-dependent cytotoxicity, and none of the exposed eggs demonstrated trypan blue uptake.

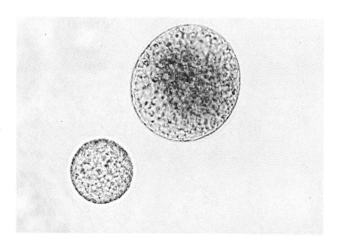

Figure 2–5. Two zona-free hamster eggs are compared, one of which has swollen and taken up trypan blue. Both eggs were exposed to the same heat-inactivated human serum from a woman with unexplained infertility. The larger egg was exposed to guinea pig serum (1:32 dilution) as a source of active complement, while the smaller egg was exposed to heat-inactivated guinea pig serum.

That egg cytotoxicity was complement-dependent was demonstrated both by heat inactivation of complement as well as neutralization with anti-C3 antibody. The zona pellucida appeared to protect embryos against the cytotoxic antibodies present, an observation previously noted by Heyner *et al.*, who exposed zona-intact and zona-free preimplantation mouse embryos to experimentally induced antiembryo antibodies.[79] No relationship was noted between the presence of antisperm antibodies in these sera and egg cytotoxicity. When two sera were studied by immunoperoxidase staining, reaction product was noted on the oolemmal surface, suggesting that the cytotoxic factor was, indeed, an immunoglobulin. These antibodies, should they be true autoantibodies directed against the human egg, could act at two loci: either during follicular development prior to formation of the zona pellucida; or, should conservation of egg surface antigens be present through preimplantation development, at the time of hatching of the embryo from the zona during nidation.

Evidence for the latter was provided by a study of six of the 23 sera found to be cytotoxic to fertilized hamster eggs. In each case, when zona-free mouse blastocysts were exposed to sera in the presence of complement, collapse of the blastocoele was noted, with cytoplasmic blebbing, and lysis of trophectoderm occurring within ninety minutes. No evidence of cytotoxicity was noted when zona-intact mouse blastocysts were exposed to these sera and complement. To eliminate the possibility that one of the components of complement might not traverse the zona pellucida, zona-intact blastocysts were preincubated with test serum in the absence of guinea pig serum. The zona pellucida was then dissolved with pronase, the eggs washed and placed in guinea pig serum. No evidence of cytotoxicity was noted, suggesting

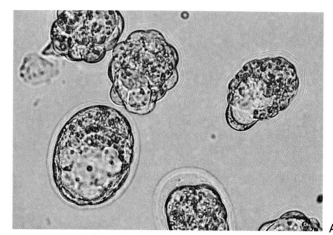

A

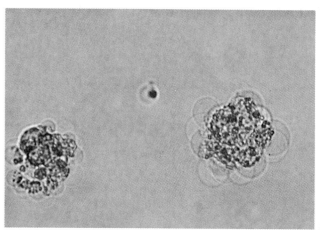

B

Figure 2–6. A. Zona-intact and zona-free blastocysts from oviducts of the mouse at the two-cell stage and cultured *in vitro* for 72 to 96 hours. B. Zona-free mouse blastocysts, following *in vitro* hatching, were exposed to heat-inactivated human serum from a woman with unexplained infertility, and guinea pig serum as a source of complement. Collapse of the blastocoele and cytoplasmic blebbing of trophectoderm were apparent in the presence of complement but not in its absence. See the Color Plate after page 84.

that the cytotoxic factor itself was impermeable to the zona pellucida (Figure 2–6).

POSTIMPLANTATION EVENTS: EFFECT OF SPERM-REACTIVE ANTIBODIES

Menge and associates have performed a series of experiments in rabbits which indicated that embryo survival as well as fertilization is impaired in females immunized with washed spermatozoa or sperm extracts. Menge, Rosenberg, and Burkons immunized female rabbits both systemically with rabbit semen and Freund's adjuvants and by transvaginal injection of washed sperm with polyadenylic acid and polyuridylic acids as adjuvants.[80] These animals also received intrauterine suspensions of washed sperm with similar adjuvants. The percentage of rabbit morulae developing to blastocysts *in vitro* in medium containing uterine fluid of immunized animals was substantially reduced when compared with controls, at 46.1% versus 19.4%. Serum containing antisperm antibodies, however, failed to impair blastocyst development. Secretory IgA's isolated from uterine fluid of immunized rabbits markedly inhibited blastocyst development, while IgG's were without effect, and by the third day of culture, the majority of embryos exposed to SIgA were collapsed and degenerated. Indirect immunofluorescence with goat antirabbit SIgA antiserum demonstrated the presence of immunoglobulins bound to these blastocysts. When SIgA was absorbed with washed rabbit spermatozoa, the majority of blastocysts cultured went on to hatch *in vitro,* with normal expansion, and failed to demonstrate antibody bound to their cell surface by indirect immunofluorescence. Goat antirabbit SIgA antiserum could also be shown to neutralize the inhibitory effect of these sperm-induced antibodies on blastocyst growth. Transplantation antigens did not appear to play a role in embryo toxicity, as absorption of uterine fluid with paternal lymphocytes failed to remove the antiembryo activity.

In a later experiment Menge, Peegel, and Riolo solubilized surface antigens of the rabbit's sperm plasma membrane with lithium diiodosalicylate and reported that immunization with this extract led to impaired fertility due to inhibition of fertilization.[81] Immunization with a nonionic detergent, NP 40, extract of the remaining sperm pellet, following LIS extraction, also impaired fertility, but at a postfertilization level.

Immunized rabbits were artifically inseminated with dilute semen. Two to four cell embryos were also transferred from superovulated donors to oviducts of immunized recipients. In rabbits immunized with LIS extracts, the percentage of ovulated ova implanting based on corpora lutea counts was 3% versus 78% for the control group. Failure of fertilization was also observed in estrous rabbits artifically inseminated with sperm exposed *in vitro* to serum from rabbits immunized with the LIS sperm extract. In rabbits immunized with the NP 40 extract to the sperm pellet, the percentage of ovulated eggs implanting was also depressed at 15%. One day following insemination, the majority of animals were found to contain cleaving fertilized ova after their oviducts were flushed. In these rabbits, but not those immunized with the LIS extract, there was also a significant reduction in the percent of preimplantation embryos transferred to their oviducts from unimmunized animals which subsequently implanted. Antibodies of the IgA class, which reacted with blastocysts, were found by indirect immunofluorescence within the uterine fluid of rabbits immunized against the NP 40 extract of sperm.

Menge and associates postulated that lithium diiodosalicylate extracted sperm surface antigen moieties were capable of inducing an immune response which blocked fertilization, while nonionic detergent extracted antigens which cross-reacted with the cell surface of preimplantation embryos. In that they were not solubilized by LIS, but rather by the nonionic detergent NP 40 containing 1

millimolar dithiothreotol, the immunogens responsible for inducing postfertilization infertility appear to have originated from a subsurface site on spermatozoa.

Sera of rabbits immunized with epididymal mouse sperm were shown, by indirect immunofluorescence, to contain antibodies which reacted with the cell surface of unfertilized and fertilized mouse ova, two- and four- cell embryos and blastocysts.[82] Serum absorbed with spleen, kidney, liver, and brain of adult mice continued to react with ova and preimplantation embryos as well as sperm. Further absorption of serum with mouse ovary, however, removed the reactivity against unfertilized and fertilized ova as well as two-cell embryos, but immunofluorescent staining of later preimplantation embryos was unaffected. These results suggested that at least two distinct sperm antigen moieties exist, one cross-reacting with the ovary, and the other with an antigen arising after fertilization, at the four- to eight-cell stage.

Seki and Mettler have shown that iso-antibodies raised in mice against spermatozoa also cross-react with preimplantation mouse embryos,[83] confirming the prior results of Menge and Fleming using xenoantibodies raised in rabbits against sperm.

The cross-reacting antigen(s) present on the plasma membrane of preimplantation embryos could have arisen at the time of fertilization from the incorporation of sperm plasma membrane,[84] or through expression of the paternal genome. The latter is not activated, however, until after the second cleavage division following fertilization and could not account for the previous observations made on one- and two-cell eggs.[85] Another likely candidate against which these antisera might be directed are the oncofetal antigens, present on cell lines derived from teratocarcinomas and other primitive tumors.[86] They have been detected on normal fetal tissues but not adult tissue, except for mature spermatozoa of several species, including man, rabbit, and mouse. Preimplantation embryos of several species also express these antigens in a stage-specific manner, and they appear to be conserved throughout nature.[87]

Beer and associates have raised the question of whether antisperm antibodies might play a role in the etiology of recurrent spontaneous abortions in humans.[88] They analyzed sera of 167 recurrent aborters by four different assays: radiolabeled antiglobulin, tray agglutination, sperm immobilization, and dot immunobinding. Forty-eight (28%) sera were positive for sperm-reactive antibodies in at least one assay. Although this figure is substantially higher than the incidence of antisperm antibodies in the sera of unselected infertile couples (8%), no difference in the mean number of abortions was seen in those women antisperm-antibody-positive versus those antibody-negative. A combination of abnormal maternal response to paternal lymphocytes in mixed lymphocyte culture in the face of maternal sperm-reactive antibodies, however, carried a poor prognosis for subsequent fertility. The number of living children and pregnancies was significantly greater in this group following immunization with paternal lymphocytes. These results suggested that the antisperm antibodies detected in their study cross-reacted with antigens on the developing blastocyst or feto-placental unit and might play a role in pregnancy loss. Beer and associates postulated that women with recurrent abortion who manifest immunologic abnormalities, including the presence of sperm-reactive antibodies, when immunized with paternal leukocytes, mount an immune response which might be protective of the feto-placental unit by blocking antigenic sites previously seen by antisperm antibody.

We have failed, however, to find an increased risk of spontaneous abortion in women with antisperm antibodies detected by immunobead binding who have conceived spontaneously following a delay in conception. Given the experimental findings of Menge and coworkers previously noted, the antibodies detected in our studies might be directed against sperm surface antigens rather than those subsurface antigens that cross-react with embryos or trophoblast.

POSTIMPLANTATION EVENTS: AUTOIMMUNITY TO ENDOMETRIUM

Mathur and coworkers have demonstrated the presence of autoantibodies to endometrium in women with endometriosis.[89] By a passive hemagglutination technique which used human O Rh positive erythrocytes coated with endometrial antigens, 11 of 13 patients with endometriosis were found to have serum antiendometrial antibodies. In 10 of these women, endometrial biopsies tested by immunofluorescence were found to be strongly positive for IgA and IgG antibodies. In contrast, endometria from normal, healthy controls were negative for IgG's and only weakly positive for IgA's. When normal endometrium was layered with sera at 1:10 dilution from patients with endometriosis, versus 10 normal controls, all controls were negative for IgG and IgM antibodies. Four were slightly positive for IgA's. The sera of all 13 patients with endometriosis were positive for antibodies to endometrium.

In more recent work Chihal, Mathur, and associates reported that circulating antiendometrial antibodies were detected in 75% of women with active endometriosis diagnosed at laparoscopy but not present in normal men and women.[90] High titers of circulating endometrial antibodies were observed in women with residual endometriosis unsuccessfully treated with Danazol, while they were negative in women with complete resolution of endometriosis following hormonal therapy. Although women with mild endometriosis diagnosed at laparoscopy were not found to have autoantibodies to endometrium,[91] antibody titers did not correlate with the stage of endometriosis.

Patients with moderate to severe endometriosis have also been found to exhibit a decrease in T-lymphocyte-mediated cytotoxicity toward homologous endometrial cells,[92] but whether an underlying immune defect is the cause or the result of endometriosis is unclear. During the early stages of nidation, changes in the cell surface of both trophectoderm and the endometrial epithelium are necessary for successful implantation.[93] Antiendometrial autoantibodies might so alter the close apposition of these cells that trophectoderm attachment and penetration of the endometrial epithelium is unsuccessful.

POSTIMPLANTATION EVENTS: PROTECTIVE ROLE OF TROPHOBLAST

Three to five days after fertilization the mammalian preimplantation embryo develops into a blastocyst. The inner cell mass, from which the fetus is derived, becomes surrounded by a sphere of trophectoderm. These highly invasive cells have been shown to play a role in hatching of the blastocyst from its zona pellucida, attachment to the endometrial epithelium, and invasion of the conceptus into the endometrial stroma.[93] A body of experimental evidence has accumulated recently, indicating that trophoblast also plays a role in those mechanisms that protect the implanting embryo from immunologic attack by the mother.

The transfer of blastocysts of one species into the uterus of a closely related species is associated initially with successful implantation, but subsequent embryo resorption occurs.[94,95] That resorption is mediated through a maternal immune response has been suggested by studies of pregnancies occurring when blastocysts of *Mus caroli*, an Asian species of mouse, were transferred to the uterus of the species *Mus musculus*. By the ninth day of pregnancy, *Mus caroli* embryos were resorbed, and maternal lymphoid cells isolated from resorption sites have been shown to possess cytotoxic activity against mitogen-stimulated *Mus caroli* lymphoblast cells.[96]

Mus musculus trophectoderm is protective of *Mus caroli* inner cell mass, suggesting that invasion of maternal cytotoxic T cells is dependent upon the genotype of the trophoblast. This was documented by injecting *Mus caroli* inner cell masses within *Mus musculus* blastocysts, which survived within the *Mus musculus* uterus, leading to viable chimeric embryos. The converse combination of *Mus musculus* inner cell mass within *Mus caroli* trophoblast was resorbed when transferred to the pregnant *Mus musculus* uterus.[97]

In response to, or concomitant with, invasion of trophoblast, the endometrium of the uterus undergoes a series of changes known as decidualization.[98] Cytoplasm of the endometrial stromal cells becomes prominent, cell to cell contact is made, with tight junction formation, and a variety of other cells including macrophages and small lymphocytes make their appearance within the stroma.[99] These lymphoid cells, as well as lymphocytes in the draining lymph nodes of the uterus, have been shown to contain a population of suppressor cells capable of inhibiting cytolytic T cell generation and of releasing a suppressor factor in culture.[100] Suppressor cells are absent at implantation sites of *Mus caroli* embryos within the *Mus musculus* uterus on day 9 of pregnancy, while present at the implantation sites of *Mus musculus* embryos in the contralateral horn. Indeed, lymphoid infiltration of these xenoembryos is noted prior to the onset of the resorption in association with decidual suppressor cell deficiency.

Clarke and associates have found evidence that decidualization in itself is not sufficient to recruit local suppressor cells.[101] Both intrauterine and subcutaneous grafts of a paternally derived tumor were rejected in pseudopregnant animals previously challenged systemically with paternal allografts to generate cytolytic lymphocytes. Examination of the decidua of these animals failed to demonstrate the presence of suppressor cells.

Chimeras of *Mus musculus* and *Mus caroli* can also be produced by aggregation of preimplantation embryos. The composite trophectoderm contains elements of both species in varying proportions. Some of these chimeric embryos implant and survive to term within the *Mus musculus* uterus. It is possible that the presence of *Mus musculus* trophoblast within the chimeric blastocyst exerts a protective effect on the embryo by recruiting suppressor cells to the decidua. Evidence in support of this thesis has recently been presented by Slapsys and associates.[102] They examined the role of *Mus musculus* trophoblast in the intrauterine recruitment of suppressor cells. When decidualization is induced in estrogen-progesterone treated mice by intrauterine installation of oil or by teratocarcinoma cells, suppressor cells were not found within the decidual tissue. A cell line cultured from C3H placenta, which shows characteristics of trophoblast, however, was successful in recruiting a suppressor cell population. These results suggest that interaction of the trophoblast and decidua is required for accumulation of non-T suppressor cells. Clarke and associates have postulated that the trophoblast, rather than acting as a barrier, or by directly suppressing cells of the maternal immune system, recruits a population of maternally derived suppressor cells to the implantation site, blocking maternal rejection mechanisms at that level.

POSTIMPLANTATION EVENTS: ANTITROPHOBLAST ANTIBODIES

Chavez and McIntyre have attempted to determine, using preimplantation mouse embryos, whether naturally occurring antitrophoblast antibodies might play a role in impaired reproduction.[103] They found that heat-inactivated sera from women who habitually abort—but not from controls—promoted disruption of trophoblast cells. When these toxic sera were absorbed with human trophoblast membranes, they did not subsequently inhibit trophoblast outgrowth, suggesting that the toxic factor is an antibody directed against trophoblast antigens.

Naturally occurring antibodies to oncofetal antigens, however, have been demonstrated in the sera of multiparous women[104] as well as in autoimmune illnesses.[105] In addition, we have demonstrated the presence of trophoblast-directed, complement-dependent cytotoxicity in one-quarter of umbilical cord sera obtained following uncomplicated pregnancy and delivery. The complement-dependent nature of this cytotoxicity suggests that it is mediated by an immunoglobulin. These results must

then call into question the reproductive significance of such antitrophoblast toxicity.

References

1. Tung KSK, Cooke WD Jr, McCarty TA, *et al.*: Human sperm antigens and antisperm antibodies. II. Age-related incidence of antisperm antibodies. Clin Exp Immunol 25:73–79, 1976.
2. Rodman TC, Lawrence J, Pruslin FH, *et al.*: Naturally occurring antibodies reactive with sperm proteins: apparent deficiency in AIDS sera. Science 228:1211–1215, 1985.
3. Jones WR: Immunologic infertility—fact or fiction? Fertil Steril 33:577–586, 1980.
4. Bronson R, Cooper G, Rosenfeld D: Sperm antibodies: their role in infertility. Fertil Steril 42:171–183, 1984.
5. Koyama K, Takada Y, Ikuma K, *et al.*: Isolation of a human seminal plasma-specific antigen responsible to sperm immobilization in sterile women by immunoaffinity chromatography on bound monoclonal antibody to human seminal plasma. Second International Congress of Reproductive Immunology, Kyoto, August 17–20, 1983.
6. Alexander NJ: Antibodies to human spermatozoa impede sperm penetration of cervical mucus or hamster eggs. Fertil Steril 41:433–439, 1984.
7. Bronson RA, Cooper GW, Rosenfeld DL: Sperm-specific iso- and auto-antibodies inhibit binding of human sperm to the human zona pellucida. Fertil Steril 38:724–729, 1982.
8. Bronson RA, Cooper GW, Rosenfeld DL: Autoimmunity to spermatozoa: effect on sperm penetration of cervical mucus as reflected by postcoital testing. Fertil Steril 41:609–614, 1984.
9. Bronson RA, Cooper GW, Rosenfeld DL: Complement-mediated effects of sperm head-directed human antibodies on the ability of human spermatozoa to penetrate zona-free hamster eggs. Fertil Steril 40:91–95, 1983.
10. Price RJ, Boettcher B: The presence of complement in human cervical mucus and its possible relevance to infertility in women with complement-dependent sperm immobilizing antibodies. Fertil Steril 32:61–66, 1979.
11. Yang SL, Schumacher GFB, Greer J, *et al.*: Sperm antibodies and complement in oviductal fluid of rhesus monkeys. Thirty-first Annual Meeting, Society for Gynecologic Investigation, San Francisco, March 21–24, 1984.
12. London SF, Haney AF, Weinberg JB: Diverse humoral and cell-mediated effects of antisperm antibodies on reproduction. Fertil Steril 41:907–912, 1984.
13. Wira CR, Sullivan DA: Estradiol and progesterone regulation of immunoglobulin A and G and secretory component in cervico-vaginal secretions of the rat. Biol Reprod 32:90–95, 1985.
14. Sullivan DA, Wira CR: Hormonal regulation of immunoglobulins in the rat uterus: uterine response to multiple estradiol treatments. Endocrinol 114:650–658, 1984.
15. Schumacher GFB: Humoral immune factors in the female reproductive tract and their changes during the cycle. *In* DS Dhindsa, GFB Schumacher (eds): Immunological Aspects of Infertility and Fertility Regulation. New York, Elsevier/North Holland, 1980, pp 93–142.
16. Bronson RA, Cooper GW, Rosenfeld DL, *et al.*: Correlation between the presence of antisperm antibodies in serum

and within vaginocervical secretions. Fertil Steril 39:411, 1983.

17. Clarke GN: Detection of antispermatozoal antibodies of IgG, IgA and IgM immunoglobulin classes in cervical mucus. Am J Reprod Immunol 6:195–197, 1984.

18. Chen C, Jones WR: Application of a sperm micro-immobilization test to cervical mucus in the investigation of immunologic infertility. Fertil Steril 35:542–545, 1981.

19. Shulman S: Sperm antibodies in women: local immunity. Am J Reprod Immunol 3:197, 1983.

20. Ingerslev HJ, Moller NPH, Jager S, et al.: Immunoglobulin class of sperm antibodies in cervical mucus from infertile women. Am J Reprod Immunol 2:296–300, 1982.

21. Bronson RA, Cooper GW, Rosenfeld DL: Correlation between regional specificity of antisperm antibodies to the spermatozoan surface and complement-mediated sperm immobilization. Am J Reprod Immunol 2:222–224, 1982.

22. Kratz HJ, Brosos T, Isliker H: Mouse monoclonal antibodies at the red cell surface. II. Effect of hapten density on complement fixation and activation. Mol Immunol 22:229–235, 1985.

23. Witkin SS, Brown CA, Good RA, et al.: Sperm immobilization by sera from unimmunized guinea pigs: requirements for immunoglobulin and complement. J Reprod Immunol 2:65–72, 1980.

24. Muller-Eberhard HJ, Schreiber RD: Molecular biology and chemistry of the alternative pathway of complement. Adv Immunol 29:1–53, 1980.

25. Pangburn MK, Morrison DC, Schreiber RD, et al.: Activation of the alternative complement pathway: recognition of surface structures on activators bound by C_3b. J Immunol 124:977–982, 1980.

26. Kazatchkine MD, Fearon DT, Austen KF: Human alternative complement pathway: membrane-associated sialic acid regulates the competition between B and BlH for cell-bound C_3b. J Immunol 122:75–81, 1979.

27. Schreiber RD, Muller-Eberhard HJ: Assembly of the cytolytic alternative pathway of complement from 11 isolated plasma proteins. J Exp Med 148:1722–1727, 1978.

28. Schumacher GFB, Yang SL, Broer KH: Specific antibodies in oviduct secretions of the rhesus monkey. In FK Beller, GFB Schumacher (eds): The Biology of the Fluids of the Female Genital Tract. New York, Elsevier/North Holland, 1979, pp 389–398.

29. Edwards RG: Antigenicity of rabbit semen, bull semen, and egg yolk after intravaginal or intramuscular injections into female rabbits. J Reprod Fertil 1:385–401, 1960.

30. Waldman RH, Cruz JM, Rowe PS: Immunoglobulin levels and antibody to Candida albicans in human cervicovaginal secretions. Clin Exp Immunol 10:427, 1972.

31. Ogra PH, Ogra SS: Local antibody response to polio vaccine in the human female genital tract. J Immunol 110:1307–1311, 1973.

32. Hurtenbach U, Shearer GM: Germ cell-induced immune suppression in mice: effect of inoculation of syngeneic spermatozoa on cell-mediated immune responses. J Exp Med 155:1719–1729, 1982.

33. James K, Hargreave TB: Immunosuppression by seminal plasma and its possible clinical significance. Immunol Today 5:357–367, 1984.

34. Lord EK, Sensabaugh GF, Stites DP: Immunosuppressive activity of human seminal plasma. I. Inhibition of in vivo lymphocyte activation. J Immunol 118:1704–1711, 1977.

35. Anderson DJ, Tarter TH: Immunosuppressive effects of mouse seminal plasma components in vivo and in vitro. J Immunol 128:535–539, 1982.

36. O'Rand MG: Modification of the sperm membrane during capacitation. Annals NY Acad Sciences 383:392–402, 1982.

37. Bronson RA, Cooper GW, Stites DP, et al.: Unpublished data.

38. Templeton AA, Mortimer D: The development of a clinical test of sperm migration to the site of fertilization. Fertil Steril 37:410–415, 1982.

39. Thibault C: Physiology and physiopathology of the fallopian tube. Int J Fertil 17:1–13, 1972.

40. Ahlgren M: Sperm transport to, and survival in, the human fallopian tube. Gynecol Invest 6:206–214, 1975.

41. McLaren A: Immunological control of fertility in female mice. Nature 201:582–585, 1964.

42. Bronson R, Cooper G, Rosenfeld D, et al.: Comparison of antisperm antibodies in homosexual and infertile men with auto-immunity to spermatozoa. Thirtieth Annual Meeting, Society for Gynecological Investigation, Washington, DC, March 17–20, 1983.

43. Dravland E, Joshi MS: Sperm-coating antigens secreted by the epididymis and seminal vesicles of the rat. Biol Reprod 25: 649, 1981.

44. Isojima S, Koyama K, Shigata M, et al.: Purification of human seminal plasma antigens relevant to sperm immobilization, agglutination, and blocking fertilization. Am J Reprod Immunol 7:139, 1985.

45. O'Rand MD: Inhibition of fertility and sperm-zona binding by antiserum to the rabbit sperm membrane auto-antigen RSA-1. Biol Reprod 25:621–628, 1981.

46. Wolf DP, Sokoloski JE, Dandekar P, et al.: Characterization of human sperm surface antigens with monoclonal antibodies. Biol Reprod 29:713–723, 1983.

47. Peterson RN, Russell L, Bundman D, et al.: Sperm-egg interaction: evidence for boar sperm plasma membrane receptors for porcine zona pellucida. Science 207:73–74, 1980.

48. Bronson RA, Cooper GW, Rosenfeld DL: Sperm-specific iso-antibodies and auto-antibodies inhibit the binding of human sperm to the human zona pellucida. Fertil Steril 38:724–729, 1982.

49. Bronson RA, McLaren A: Transfer to the mouse oviduct of eggs or blastocysts with and without the zona pellucida. J Reprod Fertil 22:129, 1970.

50. Modlinski J: The role of the zona pellucida in the development of mouse eggs in vivo. J Embryol Exp Morphol 23:539–547, 1970.

51. Florman HM, Storey BT: Mouse gamete interactions: zona pellucida is the site of the acrosome reaction leading to fusion in vitro. Dev Biol 91:121–130, 1982.

52. Bleil JD, Wasserman PM: Structure and function of the zona pellucida: identification and characterization of the proteins of the mouse oocyte's zona pellucida. Dev Biol 76:185–202, 1980.

53. Bleil JD, Wasserman PM: Sperm-egg interactions in the mouse: sequence of events and induction of the acrosome reaction by a zona pellucida glycoprotein. Dev Biol 95:317–324, 1983.

54. Yanagimachi R, Phillips DM: The status of acrosomal caps of hamster spermatozoa immediately before fertilization in vivo. Gamete Res 9:1–19, 1984.

55. Huang TTF, Fleming AD, Yanagimachi R: Only acrosome-reacted spermatozoa can bind to and penetrate zona pellucida: a study using the guinea pig. J Exp Zool 217:287–290, 1981.

56. Wolgemuth DJ, Celenza J, Bundman DS, et al.: Formation of the rabbit zona pellucida and its relationship to ovarian follicular development. Dev Biol 106:1–14, 1984.

57. Gwatkin RBL, Williams DT, Carol OJ: Immunization of mice with heat-solubilized hamster zonae: production of anti-zona antibody and inhibition of fertility. Fertil Steril 28:871–877, 1977.

58. Mahi-Brown CA, Yanagimachi R, Hoffman JC, et al.: Fertility control in the bitch by active immunization with porcine zona pellucida: use of different adjuvants and patterns of estradiol and progesterone levels in estrous cycles. Biol Reprod 32:761–772, 1985.

59. East IJ, Mattison DR, Dean J: Monoclonal antibodies to the major protein of the murine zona pellucida: effects on fertilization and early development. Dev Biol 104:49–56, 1984.

60. Gulyas BJ, Gwatkin RBL, Yuan LC: Active immunization of cynomolgus monkeys (Macaca fascicularis) with porcine zona pellucidae. Gamete Res 4:299–307, 1983.

61. Sacco AG, Subramonian MG, Yurewicz EC, et al.: Heteroimmunization of squirrel monkeys (Scimiri sciureus) with a purified zona antigen (PPZA): immune response and biologic activity of antiserum. Fertil Steril 39:350–358, 1983.

62. Skinner SM, Mills T, Kirchick HJ, et al.: Immunization with zona pellucida proteins results in abnormal ovarian follicular differentiation and inhibition of gonadotropin-induced steroid secretion. Endocrinology 115:2418–2432, 1984.

63. Sacco AG, Yurewicz EC, Subramonian MG, et al.: Zona pellucida composition: species cross-reactivity and contraceptive potential of antiserum to a purified pig zona antigen (PPZA). Biol Reprod 25:997–1008, 1982.

64. Drell DW, Dunbar BS: Monoclonal antibodies to rabbit and pig zonae pellucidae distinguish species specific and shared antigenic determinants. Biol Reprod 30:435–444, 1984.

65. Shivers CA, Dunbar BS: Autoantibodies to zona pellucida: a possible cause for infertility in women. Science 197:1082–1084, 1977.

66. Sacco Ag, Moghissi KS: Anti-zona pellucida activity in human sera. Fertil Steril 31:503–506, 1979.

67. Nishimoto T, Mori T, Yamada I, et al.: Autoantibodies to zona pellucida in infertile and aged women. Fertil Steril 34:552–556, 1980.

68. Kamada M, Hasebe H, Irahara M, et al.: Detection of anti-zona pellucida activities in human sera by the passive hemagglutination reaction. Fertil Steril 41:901–906, 1984.

69. Kameda M, Mori T: Unpublished data.

70. Karuchi H, Wakimoto H, Sakumoto T, et al.: Specific antibodies to porcine zona pellucida detected by quantitative radioimmunoassay in both fertile and infertile women. Fertil Steril 41:265–269, 1984.

71. Sacco AG, Subramonian MC, Yurewicz QE: Association of sperm receptor activity with a purified pig zona antigen. J Reprod Immunol 6:89–104, 1984.

72. McDonough PG, Byrd JR, Tho PT, et al.: Phenotypic and cytogenetic findings in 82 patients with ovarian failure-changing trends. Fertil Steril 28:638–641, 1977.

73. Gomez CM, Richman DP: Monoclonal antiacetylcholine receptor antibodies with differing capacities to induce experimental autoimmune myasthenia gravis. J Immunol 135:234–241, 1985.

74. Kidd A, Okita N, Row VV, et al.: Immunologic aspects of Graves' and Hashimoto's diseases. Metabolism 29:80–99, 1980.

75. Escobar ME, Cigornaga SB, Chiauzzi VA, et al.: Development of the gonadotropic-resistant ovary syndrome in myasthenia gravis: suggestion of similar auto-immune mechanisms. Acta Endocrinol 99:431–436, 1982.

76. Coulam CB, Ryan RJ: Prevalence of circulating antibodies directed toward ovaries among women with premature ovarian failure. To be published.

77. Mathur S, Jerath RS, Mathur RS, et al.: Serum immunoglobulin levels, autoimmunity, and cell-mediated immunity in primary ovarian failure. J Reprod Immunol 2:83–92, 1980.

78. Yanagimachi R, Bronson RA, Emanuele N: Unpublished observations.

79. Heyner S, Brinster R, Palm J: Effect of iso-antibody on preimplantation mouse embryos. Nature 222:783, 1969.

80. Menge AC, Rosenberg A, Burkons DM: Effects of uterine fluids and immunoglobulins from semen-immunized rabbits on rabbit embryos cultured in vitro. Proc Soc Exp Biol Med 145:371–378, 1974.

81. Menge AC, Peegel H, Riolo ML: Sperm fractions responsible for immunologic induction of pre- and post-fertilization infertility in rabbits. Biol Reprod 20:931–937, 1979.

82. Menge AC, Fleming CH: Detection of sperm antigens on mouse ova and early embryos. Dev Biol 63:111–117, 1978.

83. Seki M, Mettler L: Influence of spermatozoal antibodies on the reproduction of mice. Am J Reprod Immunol 2:225–232, 1982.

84. O'Rand MG: The presence of sperm-specific surface isoantigens on the egg following fertilization. J Exp Zool 282:267–273, 1977.

85. Van Blerkom J, Bell H: Regulation of development in the fully grown mouse oocyte: chromosome-mediated temporal and spatial differentiation of the cytoplasm and plasma membrane. J Embryol Exp Morphol 93:213–230, 1986.

86. Jacob F: Mouse teratocarcinoma and embryonic antigens. Immunol Rev 33:3–32, 1977.

87. Johnson LV, Calarco PG: Mammalian preimplantation development: the cell surface. Anat Rec 196:201–219, 1980.

88. Beer AE, Quebbeman JF, Semprini AE: Immunopathological factors contributing to recurrent spontaneous abortion in humans. To be published.

89. Mathur S, Peress MR, Williamson HO, et al.: Auto-immunity to endometrium and ovary in endometriosis. Clin Exp Immunol 50:259–266, 1982.

90. Chihal HJ, Mathur S, Holtz G, et al.: Endometrial antibodies in the detection and evaluation of therapy of endometriosis. Pacific Coast Fertility Society Meeting, 1985.

91. Halme J, Mathur S: Lack of local autoimmunity in mild endometriosis. Int J Fertil. To be published.

92. Steele RW, Domanski WP, Marner DJ: Immunologic aspects of human endometriosis. Am J Reprod Immunol 6:33–36, 1984.

93. Schlafke S, Enders AC: Cellular basis of interaction between trophoblast and uterus at implantation. Biol Reprod 41:65–75, 1975.

94. Tarkowski AK: Interspecific transfers of eggs between rat and mouse. J Embryol Exp Morphol 10:470–495, 1962.

95. Dent J, McGovern PG, Hancock JL: Immunological implications of ultrastructural studies of goat and sheep hybrid placentae. Nature 231:116–117, 1971.

96. Croy AB, Rossant J, Clark DA: Histological and immunological studies of post implantation death of *Mus caroli* embryos in the *Mus musculus* uterus. J Reprod Immunol 4:277–293, 1982.

97. Rossant J, Mauro VM, Croy BA: Importance of trophoblast genotype for survival of interspecific murina chimeras. J Embryol Exp Morphol 69:141–149, 1982.

98. Bell SC: Decidualization and associated cell types: implications for the role of the placental bed in the materno-fetal immunological relationship. J Reprod Immunol 5:185–194, 1983.

99. Bulmer JN, Johnson PM: Immunohistological characterization of the decidualization leucocyte infiltrate related to endometrial gland epithelium in early human pregnancy. Immunol 55:35–44, 1985.

100. Slapsys RM, Clark DA: Active suppression of host-versus-graft reaction in pregnant mice. I. Kinetics, specificity, and *in vivo* activity of non-T suppressor cells. Am J Reprod Immunol 3:65–71, 1983.

101. Nagarkatti PK, Clarke DA: *In vitro* activity and *in vivo* correlates of alloantigen-specific murine suppressor T-cells induced by allogeneic pregnancy. J Immunol 131:638–643, 1983.

102. Slapsys RM, Beeson JH, Clark DA: The role of the trophoblast in the localization of decidua-associated suppressor cells. Fifth Annual Meeting, Society for the Immunology of Reproduction. Durham, North Carolina, 1984.

103. Chavez DJ, McIntyre JA: Sera from women with history of repeated pregnancy losses cause abnormalities in mouse preimplantation blastocysts. J Reprod Immunol 6:273–282, 1984.

104. Hamilton MS: Maternal immune responses to onco-fetal antigens. J Reprod Immunol 5:249–264, 1983.

105. Salinas FA, Quismorio FB, Friou GJ: Serum antibodies to fetal antigens in systemic lupus erythematosis and rheumatoid arthritis. Clin Immunol Immunopathol 11:388–405, 1978.

3. Congenital Anomalies of the Uterus

Howard W. Jones, Jr.

This chapter will deal primarily with those anomalies of the müllerian ducts which have special relevance to infertility. In some instances a particular anomaly will be mentioned briefly although its relevance to infertility may be somewhat indirect—congenital anomaly of the uterus or the Rokitansky-Kuster-Hauser syndrome is an example. Other anomalies are of importance only in a preventive sense; that is, therapy can prevent infertility, especially if it is timely. Such an example would be an obstructive transverse vaginal septum.

No mention will be made of anomalies of the müllerian ducts caused by intrauterine exposure to diethylstilbestrol (DES) since these are covered in a separate chapter.

CLASSIFICATION

A simple classification of anomalies of the müllerian ducts comprises three groups.

   I. Agenesis (partial)
  II. Problems of vertical fusion
     A. Obstructive
     B. Nonobstructive
 III. Problems of lateral fusion
     A. Obstructive
     B. Nonobstructive

AGENESIS OF THE MÜLLERIAN DUCTS

Agenesis of the müllerian ducts is sometimes categorized under the heading of congenital absence of the vagina; however, with absence of the vagina, the uterus most often is not present. Perhaps a more accurate term for the condition would be partial aplasia or dysplasia of the müllerian ducts. The disorder is sometimes referred to as the Rokitansky-Kuster-Hauser syndrome.

Agenesis is always partial, as no case has been described with absolutely no derivative of the ducts. The uterus is characteristically absent, but the ovaries and fallopian tubes are quite normal. Such patients seek the physician around the time of puberty or after because of failure of the onset of menstruation. The external genitalia are quite normal except that the vaginal opening is absent or, as mentioned above, only a very shallow vagina is present.

Internally, the müllerian ducts seem to fail to fuse. At the proximal end of each fallopian tube there is a muscular thickening. The muscular thickening on each side joins in the midline by palpable and visible strands, suggesting a diminutive and undeveloped double uterus. On very rare occasions there may be enough endometrial tissue in one of these rudimentary anlagen to accumulate menstrual blood. When this occurs, cyclic lower abdominal pain will be encountered and the rudimentary horn which has functional endometrium must be surgically removed.

Absence of the uterus and vagina is associated with anomalies of the urinary tract in a significant number of cases. This includes congenital absence of the kidney, malrotation and malposition of the kidney, including pelvic kidneys. An intravenous pyelogram is indicated for all patients who have müllerian anomalies.

Anomalies of the bony system are not uncommon and are mostly of the spine (fusion), but they may involve maldevelopment of any bone.

The diagnosis of congenital absence of the uterus and vagina is usually self-evident. The only confusion in the differential diagnosis is with the androgen insensitivity syndrome. (See Chapter 14.) Scant or absent pubic and axillary hair will usually distinguish androgen insensitivity, but when in doubt a karyotype will make the distinction. Visualization of the internal organs by laparoscopy is not a necessary part of the diagnostic work-up.

In the Rokitansky-Kuster-Hauser syndrome there is no known therapy which can provide for normal reproduction. However, a functioning vagina can be provided. On theoretical grounds, if a patient were anxious to reproduce with her own gametes, it should be possible to aspirate eggs, fertilize them *in vitro,* and transfer them to the uterus of a surrogate. This, however, is for the future, if ethical and other concerns can be resolved.

The creation of a vagina can sometimes be done by mechanical dilatation by the patient, but most often some surgical procedure is necessary. A split thickness graft placed in the space developed between the bladder and rectum works exceedingly well. Patients can expect to have normal vaginal function although reproduction is not possible.

TRANSVERSE VAGINAL SEPTUM—OBSTRUCTIVE

An obstructive transverse vaginal septum may sometimes be encountered in infants. Occasionally a large volume of mucus will collect above the obstruction causing hydromucocolpos. If such an obstruction is not promptly relieved, there is serious potential for impairment of the urinary tract and, with the development of hydronephrosis, some deaths have been reported.

Hydromucocolpos seems to be due to a rare autosomal recessive gene. The site of the obstruction may be anywhere along the vaginal canal but it most frequently occurs at the junction of the middle and upper third of the vagina. The diagnosis in infancy is not easy as there is no bulging from the vaginal opening. Often these patients are thought to have some intra-abdominal problem because they have a large mass in the lower abdomen. The most effective therapy is a surgical approach from below to remove the obstructive membrane.[1]

Most often there are no symptoms of an obstructed transverse vaginal septum until after the onset of menstruation. The symptoms therefore are associated with obstruction to the outflow of menstrual blood. Curiously

enough, the thickening of the obstructing membrane seen in adults is often greater than that in infants. It is not clear why in some infants a large amount of mucus collects above the obstructing membrane while in others it does not. Whether this discrepancy is associated with the character of the obstructive membrane is uncertain, but in adults the transverse vaginal septum often is quite thick and its removal is more difficult. Indeed, as mentioned above under agenesis of the müllerian ducts, if a considerable segment of the vagina is undeveloped, the patients are often described in the literature as having congenital absence of the vagina with a functioning uterus present. However, the condition is quite different from the Rokitansky-Kuster-Hauser syndrome in that patients with the transverse vaginal septum do not have anomalies of the urinary tract or of the skeletal system.

There are several variations in the amount of deficiency of the uterus. The uterus may be present but have no functioning endometrium and no vagina (Figure 3–1). A very troublesome situation occurs when the defect in development includes the cervix. In this situation there may be a functioning but obstructed uterine corpus and a defect in cervical and vaginal development (Figure 3–2). Preservation of reproductive potential in this situation has seldom been achieved. There seems to be but a single documented case of successful reproduction.[2] Attempts to keep open a fistulous opening between the endometrial cavity through the maldeveloped cervix and the vagina have usually been doomed to failure. After repeated dilatations over a number of years, it is usually

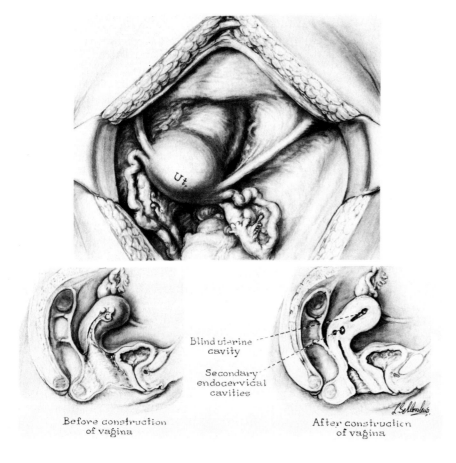

Blind uterine cavity

Secondary endocervical cavities

Before construction of vagina

After construction of vagina

Figure 3–1. An unusual example of a congenital deformity: a uterus with nonfunctioning endometrium and congenital absence of the vagina.

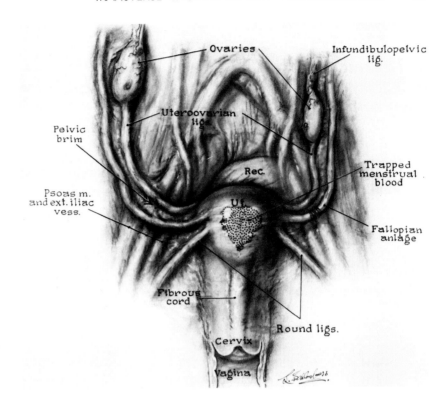

Figure 3–2. A drawing showing congenital absence of the cervix but with a small, well-formed upper uterus with functioning endometrium. In this case the vagina was relatively normal, although generally, in cases with congenital absence of the cervix, the vagina will be absent too.

necessary to solve the problem by removal of the corpus of the uterus. Because of this experience, one can only reluctantly recommend that if the cervix is absent the problem be immediately solved by performing a removal of the malformed uterus. It should be noted that at the time of definitive surgery, the matter of future reproduction has often been settled because of maldevelopment of the fallopian tubes or because of widespread endometriosis.

As a result of the accumulation of menstrual blood, symptoms are marked by cyclic pain requiring therapy in adolescence. The preferred method of treatment is to approach the problem from below. In some instances, there is such a large defect between the small upper vagina and any lower vagina that it is not possible to anastomose the two directly. For this situation special lucite stents are very helpful in providing a framework along which the epithelia from the upper vagina and the lower vagina can grow and communicate. These special stents have a bulbous end placed in the upper vagina near the cervix so that they self-retain. They are allowed to stay in place for a matter of six months or more and usually can be removed in a second operation without a great deal of difficulty (Figure 3–3).

TRANSVERSE VAGINAL SEPTUM—NONOBSTRUCTIVE

Oftentimes a transverse vaginal septum will not be complete and hence accumulation of menstrual blood or mucus does not become a factor. However, such a partial

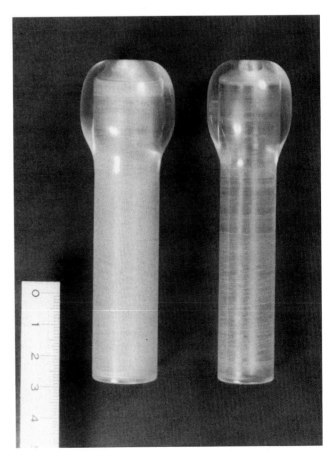

Figure 3–3. Custom-made lucite forms useful in the treament of congenital absence of the vagina with the uterus present.

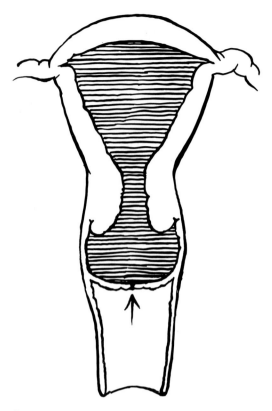

Figure 3–4. Diagram of a transverse vaginal septum with a pinhole opening that caused no problem until infection occurred subsequent to a pregnancy.

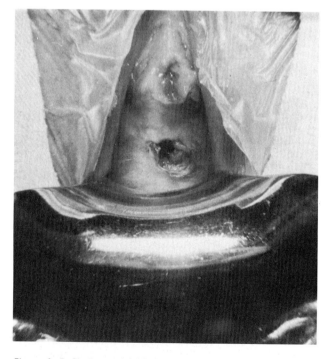

Figure 3–5. Photograph of the situation diagrammed in Figure 3–4. The pinhole opening photographed here had to be enlarged to allow the drainage of the purulent material which had obstructed the pinhole opening.

transverse vaginal septum may cause dyspareunia or develop complications that compromise reproduction.

Occasionally, the opening in the transverse vaginal septum is so small that its identification is extremely difficult. Sometimes the transverse vaginal septum gives no dyspareunia and indeed is not identified until after a pregnancy has occurred. Lochia has been known to obstruct the pinpoint opening through the transverse vaginal septum, causing infection and the necessity for emergency surgical drainage (Figures 3–4, 3–5).

PROBLEMS OF LATERAL FUSION—OBSTRUCTIVE

The uterine anlagen may fail to fuse at several different points along their length. In extreme cases, no fusion at all occurs, resulting in a double vagina and uterus. If the failed fusion involves obstruction on one side, menstrual blood will accumulate causing cyclic menstrual pain soon after puberty.

The resulting symptoms are very much related to the site of obstruction. When there is development of a uterus didelphis, that is, a double vagina and uterus, but with an obstruction low in the vagina on one side, a very large amount of blood may accumulate and the condition may go unrecognized for a number of years. Apparently the distensible vagina can accommodate the increment of blood of each menstruation by absorbing enough fluid between the menstrual periods so that succeeding menstrual periods add to the accumulated blood without the production of excruciating pain. When this unfortunate situation exists, retrograde involvement of the tubes may also occur and the development of a rather large tuboovarian accumulation of menstrual blood is often associated with endometriosis and impairment of future reproductive potential (Figure 3–6). If the septum is removed before the tubes and ovaries are compromised by endometriosis, reproduction may be consistent with the reproduction in a uterine duplication.

If obstruction occurs in the region of the cervix, the reservoir-like action of the vagina is lost and symptoms are very acute from the retention of blood within the endometrial cavity. Such patients seek help immediately and will seldom have more than three or four periods before severe pain demands attention. If the cervix is well-formed on the unobstructed side, consideration may be given to anastomosing the obstructed side to the nonobstructed side (Figure 3–7).

At times the obstruction involves what amounts to an isolated horn of the uterus with minimal connection to the unobstructed side. When this occurs, removal of the rudimentary horn is required and should be done as early as possible so that retrograde menstruation will not cause endometriosis and compromise of subsequent reproduction (Figures 3–8, 3–9). A few examples of pregnancy have been observed in an obstructed rudimentary horn. Essentially all of these have been in very young individuals who were exposed to pregnancy before the monthly accumulation of trapped menstrual blood had

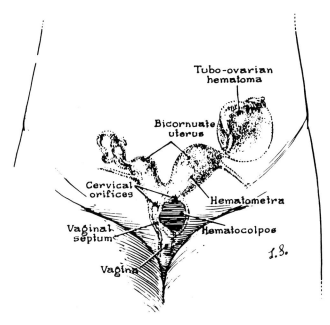

Figure 3–6. Diagram of a blind left vagina which caused an accumulation of blood requiring a salpingo-oophorectomy. There was extensive endometriosis.

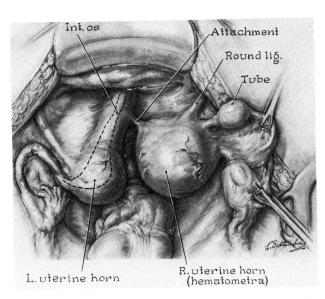

Figure 3–8. Drawing of a rudimentary uterine noncommunicating horn. Note that the abnormality of the tube which was obstructed prevented retrograde menstruation and prevented the development of endometriosis.

an opportunity to cause endometriosis and destroy reproductive function. Of necessity the sperm ascended the normal side. All such patients had symptoms of an ectopic pregnancy (Figure 3–10).

A special situation exists when, in addition to the unilateral obstruction in the vagina, there is also a lateral communication between the two horns of the uterus. This lateral communication is usually through the cervix (Figure 3–11). In this situation the obstructive symptoms are not pressing and the patient often complains of a

disappearing mass at the vaginal outlet as the blind vagina fills with menstrual blood and has it slowly emptied through the lateral communication in the uterus. Treatment of this particular situation involves only removal of the vaginal septum. No treatment is needed for the lateral communication, and reproduction is consistent with that of a duplicated uterus.

Every imaginable variation may occur, including some that are not easy to interpret from embryological considerations (Figures 3–12, 3–13). When there is unilateral obstruction of the müllerian ducts, absence of the ipsilateral kidney is the rule. Therefore, an intravenous pyelogram is not only a routine matter but a very useful diag-

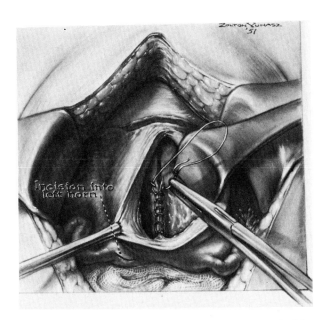

Figure 3–7. Drawing of an anastomosis between a patent horn and an obstructed horn.

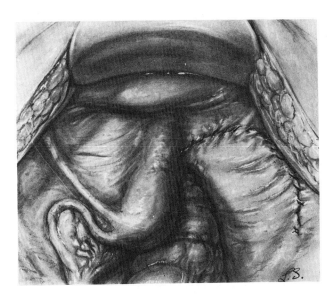

Figure 3–9. Drawing of the situation shown in Figure 3–8 subsequent to the removal of the rudimentary horn.

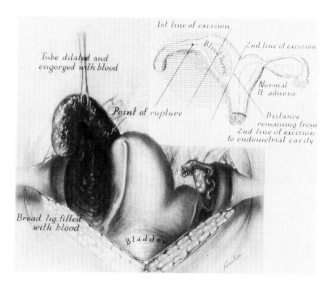

Figure 3–10. Diagram showing a pregnancy which occurred in a blind horn.

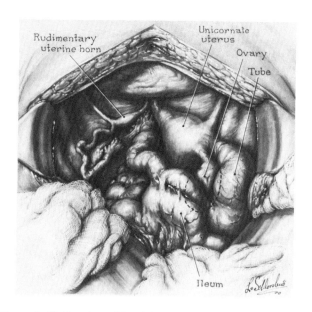

Figure 3–12. Drawing of the internal situation of a very unusual double uterus with a rudimentary uterine horn on one side and a unicornuate uterus on the other, but with obstruction of the unicornuate uterus low in the vagina as shown in Figure 3–13.

nostic tool that may clarify the diagnosis in obscure circumstances.

The epithelium of an obstructed vagina is almost always composed of cuboidal cells which testify to the müllerian origin of the epithelium. When the vaginal septum is removed in obstructed cases, the newly opened vagina lined with glandular epithelium slowly undergoes metaplasia so that after two or three years the vagina attains its normal adult squamous composition.

PROBLEMS OF LATERAL FUSION—NONOBSTRUCTIVE

Didelphic and Unicornuate Uterus

In nonobstructive failure of lateral fusion involving both the uterus and vagina, there are no symptoms related to

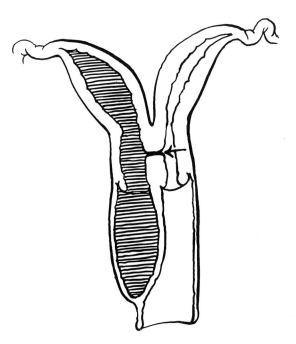

Figure 3–11. Diagram of a lateral communicating uterus associated with a blind vagina.

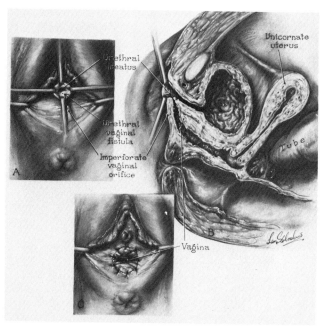

Figure 3–13. Diagram from the case shown in Figure 3–12, illustrating the pinpoint opening with obstruction at the vaginal outlet in a very unusual anomaly.

menstruation. This is the classic uterus didelphis (Figure 3–14). However, due to narrowness of one or another of the vaginae, dyspareunia may be another problem. If so, removal of the septum may be required. At times there is asymmetry of the two vaginal cavities, so that vaginal function is normal and satisfactory on one side but quite impossible on the other.

Although precise contemporary data are lacking, overall reproduction seems to be modestly compromised in patients with didelphic uteri. It is remarkable that there is no major series of cases describing reproduction in the uterus didelphis. Information is almost anecdotal and consists of case reports or small series. A number of examples of simultaneous pregnancies in each side of the uterus have been reported. The older literature contains examples of deliveries from below with sequential labor and remarkable intervals between the birth of each child. Intervals up to 24 hours are not unusual, and intervals of several days and indeed several weeks have been reported. There is no indication for surgical intervention on the didelphic uterus.

Information about reproduction in the unicornuate uterus is also sparse. As judged by the report of small series, reproduction is somewhat compromised by infertility, pregnancy wastage, and premature labor. Treatment for problems of pregnancy wastage in the unicornuate uterus is difficult. Removal of the anlage attached to the unicornuate uterus has some beneficial effect.[3]

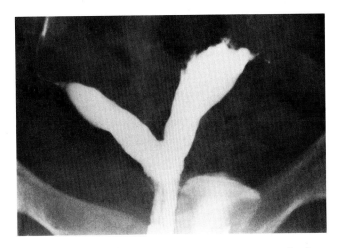

Figure 3–15. Hysterogram showing a double uterus. From the hysterogram it is impossible to tell whether this is a bicornuate or a septate uterus.

Bicornuate and Septate Uterus

A symmetrical non-obstructed double uterus may cause a problem in reproduction. Generally there seems to be no problem in becoming pregnant, but miscarriage, often repeated, or premature labor occurs many times. Primary infertility in a patient with a symmetrical double uterus is sometimes observed, but the causal relationship between the infertility and the anomaly is an unresolved problem. Nevertheless, there are anecdotal examples of

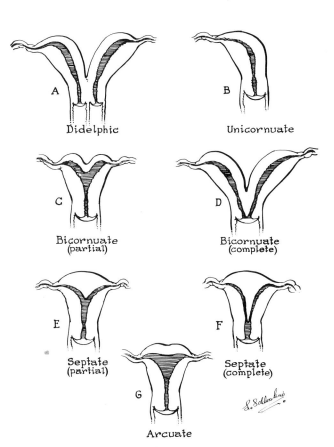

Figure 3–14. Diagram of the various forms of double uteri.

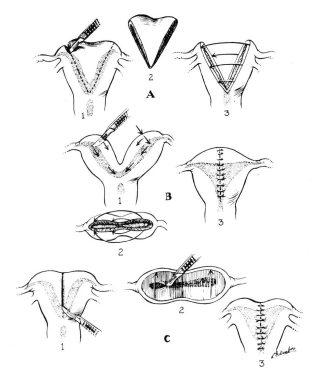

Figure 3–16. A. Wedge resection operation for a septate uterus. B. The typical Strassman procedure suitable for a bicornuate uterus. C. The Tompkins modification of a double uterus operation.

the resolution of infertility with the correction of the double uterus.

In symmetrical double uterus without obstruction a precise classification is of utmost importance as it has very important clinical implications. It is necessary to distinguish between the bicornuate uterus and the septate uterus. The bicornuate causes only minimal problems for reproduction whereas the septate uterus is almost always associated with reproductive failure (Figure 3–14). This distinction cannot be made by a hysterosalpingogram because the shadows of the cavities are exactly the same (Figure 3–15). It is the exterior configuration of the uterus which is of importance. In the bicornuate uterus two distinct horns can be felt. In the septate uterus the external configuration of the uterus is essentially normal, although the uterus may oftentimes seem somewhat broad. It is therefore necessary to perform a very good bimanual examination to determine this point. Ultrasonography may be helpful but it too is not always reliable.

The diagnosis of a reproductive problem attributable to a double uterus is made essentially by exclusion. As mentioned before, there is considerable uncertainty about the relationship of primary infertility to a double uterus. Most often the problem is that of repeated miscarriage. Hence it becomes necessary to exclude all other causes for miscarriage, including male factors and female factors such as cervical incompetence, chronic illness, luteal phase defects, genetic problems, and endocrine disorders of the adrenal and thyroid. It needs to be mentioned that placental endocrine defects sometimes cannot be identified except by following a patient during pregnancy.

The history of the miscarriage is particularly helpful.

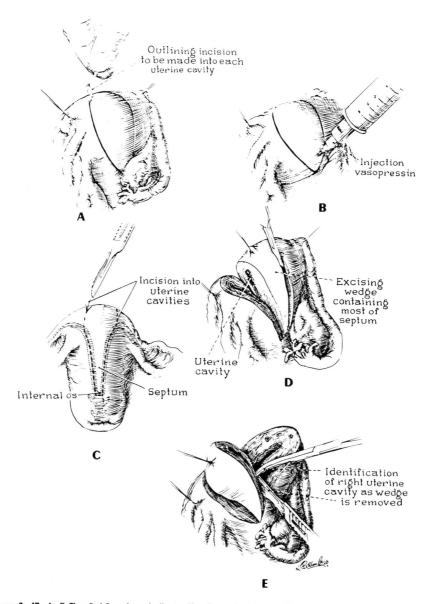

Figure 3–17. A–E. The first five steps in the unification of a uterus with the wedge resection technique.

The characteristic story is that of an early mid-trimester loss associated with what amounts to a mini-labor. However, exceptions to this rule can occur[4].

Pregnancy loss secondary to a septate uterus usually occurs in the first trimester of pregnancy. Clinically, spontaneous abortion secondary to a septate uterus and that resulting from other causes are not distinguishable. Thus, as with the bicornuate uterus, exclusion of all other causes of miscarriage must be assured.

It is of particular note that the evaluation of endometrial histologic maturity may be confused by the presence of a septum. If the endometrial biopsy is obtained from the septum itself, the endometrium will be similar to that of the lower uterine segment, i.e., it will be significantly immature by comparison with the endometrium from the anterior fundal region away from the septum. This important difference must be recognized to avoid treating an unrecognized septate uterus with progesterone suppositories or Clomid in an attempt to improve the endometrium. The hysterosalpingogram and pelvic examination will avoid this confusion.

TREATMENT

Where a correctable endocrine or metabolic cause of reproductive loss can be identified, such disorder should be corrected and a pregnancy attempted before any surgical procedure is considered. In the event that no endocrine, metabolic, or other disorder can be identified, or if correction does not result in a viable pregnancy, surgical correction can be considered.

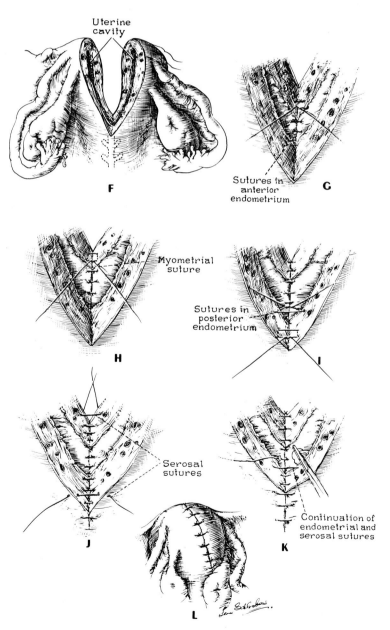

Figure 3–17. F–L. The final seven steps in the unification procedure using the wedge technique.

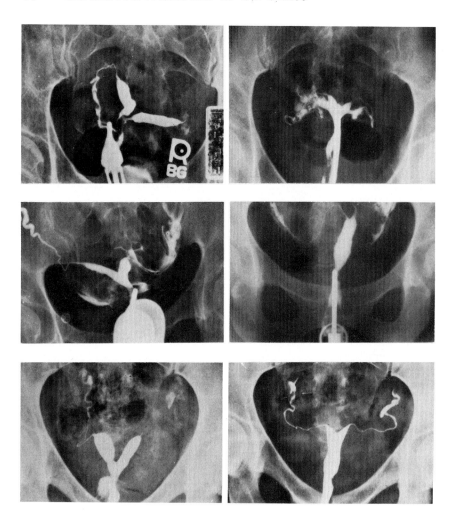

Figure 3–18. Before- and after-hysterograms of patients with double uterus treated by the wedge operation. In all instances the patients had had multiple miscarriages preoperatively and subsequent to operation had at least one term delivery.

TECHNIQUE OF SURGICAL CORRECTION

The classical Strassman procedure for unifying a uterus was devised at the turn of the century, before hysterosalpingography was available. This procedure is unsuitable for correcting the defect due to a septate uterus, which is the type of uterus associated with reproductive disorders. Therefore, the Strassman procedure has little application in contemporary practice.

The abdominal approach to correction of a septate uterus can be accomplished by initiating the procedure with a sagittal midline incision opening the two horns and reanastomosis (Figure 3–16). A similar and equally satisfactory method of construction is to excise the septum by wedge and to anastomose the remaining halves in the midline (Figure 3–17). This alternative method does, however, remove some myometrial tissue along with the septum.

A highly satisfactory and alternative approach to abdominal excision of a uterine septum has recently been described using the operative hysteroscope, thus avoiding an abdominal procedure and its longer hospitalization, greater expense, and greater morbidity.[7,8,10] The septum is simply incised under direct vision through the hysteroscope, utilizing either the long flexible hysteroscopic scissors, or using cautery in conjunction with a resectoscope.

The viable pregnancy rate utilizing either the abdominal approach or the hysteroscopic approach is approximately 80%.[4,5,6,7,8,9] Vaginal delivery is expected following hysteroscopic resection of the septum, whereas cesarean section delivery is recommended after the abdominal approach. There have been, however, few uterine ruptures which might have been associated with the abdominal procedure (Figure 3–18).

References

1. Mandell J, Stevens PS, Lucey DT: Diagnosis and management of hydrometrocolpos in infancy. J Urol 120:262, 1978.

2. Zarou GS, Esposito JM, Zarou DM: Pregnancy following the surgical correction of congenital atresia of the cervix. Int J Gynecol 11:143, 1973.

3. Andrews MC, Jones HW, Jr: Impaired reproduction performance of the unicornuate uterus: intrauterine growth retardation, infertility and recurrent abortion in five cases. Am J Obstet Gynecol 144:173, 1982.

4. Muasher SJ, Acosta AA, Garcia JE, *et al.:* Wedge metroplasty for the septate uterus: an update. Fertil Steril 42:515, 1984.

5. Rock JA, Jones HW, Jr: The clinical management of the double uterus. Fertil Steril 28:798, 1977.

6. Rock JA, Schlaff WD: The obstetric consequences of uterovaginal anomalies. Fertil Steril 43:681, 1985.

7. Daly DC, Walters CA, Soto-Albors CE, *et al.:* Hysteroscopic metroplasty: surgical technique and obstetric outcome. Fertil Steril 39:623, 1983.

8. DeCherney AH, Russell JB, Graebe RA, *et al.:* Resectoscopic management of müllerian fusion defects. Fertil Steril 45:726, 1986.

9. Musich JR, Behrman SJ: Obstetric outcome before and after metroplasty in women with uterine anomalies. Obstet Gynecol 52:63, 1978.

10. Chervenak FA, Neuwirth RS: Hysteroscopic resections of the uterine septum. Am J Obstet Gynecol 141:251, 1981.

4. Pathology of Infertility and Adverse Pregnancy Outcome After In Utero Exposure to Diethylstilbestrol

Robert J. Stillman and Avner Hershlag

In the late 1940s the synthetic estrogen diethylstilbestrol (DES) began the legacy now associated with its use following reports of a benefit in treating a wide variety of pregnancy disorders. These disorders included threatened or habitual abortions, toxemia, premature deliveries, postmaturity, and stillbirth.[1,2] It is estimated that in the early 1950s approximately 10% of offspring were exposed to DES *in utero,* while in the later 1950s and 1960s its use declined to 1% to 2%. Between the late 1940s and 1971, approximately 2 to 3 million women were prescribed DES during their pregnancies, thereby exposing a total of approximately 1–1.5 million male and 1–1.5 female progeny to the drug *in utero.*[3]

Examination of papers published between 1948 and 1955 which claimed to demonstrate efficacy of DES revealed studies widely flawed by their lack of appropriate, or any, control groups.[1,2] In contrast, controlled studies from the same period almost uniformly demonstrate the lack of clinical utility of DES as definitive or prophylactic therapy for pregnancy disorders.[4–6] More recent reevaluation of the statistical analysis of one of these controlled studies actually demonstrated that DES ingestion in pregnancy was associated with a significantly greater frequency of abortions, premature deliveries, and stillbirths.[6,7] The adverse affects on offspring exposed *in utero* to DES might have been predicted from animal studies during the years prior to and during its use in humans, but these adverse effects have only come to light with the passage of time from exposure. What should have been recognized, even during its early years of use, was the drug's lack of efficacy for the indications for which it was prescribed.[5] It was not until 1971, however, following reports of 8 women who developed clear cell adenocarcinoma of the vagina after *in utero* exposure to DES that its use in pregnancy was banned by the Federal Drug Administration.[3] As the male and female offspring exposed *in utero* to DES now pass though and beyond the reproductive age, a wider scope of adverse affects are being manifested. (Table 4–1).[3] In addition, late sequelae in the mothers who ingested the drug may also become apparent.[9]

PATHOGENESIS OF DES EFFECTS ON THE DEVELOPING FEMALE REPRODUCTIVE TRACT

According to most researchers the vagina has a double ancestry from both the fused lower end of the müllerian ducts and from the urogenital sinus. The former grows downward and meets the posterior wall of the urogenital sinus at the müllerian tubercle. The primitive vagina is initially lined by müllerian columnar epithelium before squamous epithelium grows upwards from the urogenital sinus to replace it.[10,11] At about the tenth gestational week, squamous cells derived from the urogenital sinus invade the common tube from below and grow up the muscular scaffold to completely replace the müllerian epithelium to the level of the external cervical os.

Evidence that the stroma of the female genital tract has specific inductive effects on the development of the overlying epithelium raises the possibility DES may affect the stroma primarily, leading to secondary induction of abnormal epithelial changes.[12]

A direct effect of DES on the stroma during any period from at least the ninth gestational week through the fifth month also may explain the various vaginal, cervical, and uterine structural abnormalities. The various mesenchymal layers of the cervix and uterine corpus fail to segregate, becoming clinically manifest in the young adult as stromal hyperplasia (ridges), hypoplasia (hypoplastic fornices), or abnormally contoured uterine cavities. In an experimental model, genital tracts from aborting fetuses may be grafted into athymic nude mice and then exposed to DES or other hormones (such as progesterone) and compared to those not exposed. In reproductive tracts exposed to DES, profound changes appeared in the

Table 4–1. Summary of Adverse Effects of *In Utero* Exposure to DES[a]

Effects of *in utero* exposure to DES on female progeny

I. Anatomic abnormalities

  A. Lower müllerian tract

    1. Adenosis and clear cell adenocarcinoma

    2. Cervicovaginal structural abnormalities

      a. Collars, hoods, septa, and cockscombs

      b. Cervical mucus effects

      c. Cervical stenosis (after "therapy")

      d. Cervical incompetence

  B. Upper müllerian tract

    1. Uterine structural abnormalities

    2. Fallopian tube structural abnormalities

II. Reproductive abnormalities

  A. Menstrual dysfunction

  B. Reproductive dysfunction

    1. Infertility

    2. Adverse pregnancy outcome

      a. Spontaneous abortion

      b. Ectopic pregnancy

      c. Premature delivery

      d. Perinatal death

      e. Term delivery

      f. Summary: Overall adverse pregnancy outcome

Effects of *in utero* exposure to DES on male progeny

I. Anatomic abnormalities

II. Reproductive dysfunction

  A. Altered semen analysis

  B. Altered fertility potential

[a] From Stillman RJ[3]: Am J Obstet Gynecol 142:905, 1982.

stroma rather than in the epithelium. In humans, the uterine stroma differentiates into two distinct compartments about the third month of development—one of which will become the endometrial stroma, the other the myometrium. DES impedes development and differentiation. In the lower genital tract, DES affects the stroma and, in effect, makes it inhospitable to the normal upward growth of squamous epithelium from the urogenital sinus. The original columnar epithelium lining the müllerian ducts is not replaced and persists to become the analog of what is known later as adenosis (Figure 4–1).

PATHOLOGIC CHANGES IN THE LOWER GENITAL TRACT

The term vaginal epithelial changes (VEC) is often used to encompass adenosis, ectropion, and associated squamous metaplasis in reference to DES-exposed females (Figure 4–2). In the DES Adenosis (DESAD) Project, VEC was reported in 34% of 1275 exposed individuals, most closely associated with earlier weeks in pregnancy when therapy was initiated, total dose administered, and the

length of intrauterine exposure to DES. Cervical ectropion is the presence of glandular (columnar) epithelium or its mucinous products in the ectocervix. While ectropion is found in 40%–65% of nonexposed females, it is seen in over 95% of exposed patients, and is also more extensive in these patients.[8,11]

Vaginal adenosis is the presence of glandular (columnar) epithelium or its mucinous products in the vagina. Clinically detectable adenosis is uncommon except in association with *in utero* DES exposure, where it is recognized in from 35% to 90% of patients. It is found most commonly in the anterior vaginal fornix (81%) and usually limited to the upper vagina (86%). In about 10% of patients with adenosis, columnar epithelium is found on the surface only, sometimes with a papillary configuration. More commonly there exists a combination of surface and lamina propria involvement. In 85% of biopsy specimens, columnar cells found in areas of adenosis may be mucinous and histologically similar to cells of endocervical glands. The columnar cells in adenosis may however be mucin-free and similar to the glandular configuration of the endometrium or the fallopian tubes.[11] Colposcopic follow-up and histologic verification demonstrate that adenosis is a dynamic lesion that undergoes progressive squamous metaplasia over time. Ultimately, adenosis may disappear completely in some patients, to be replaced by a normally glycogenated mucosa.[12a]

During a follow-up period of 3 years, the extent of VEC can decrease in 29.2% of patients, increase in 6.6%, and not change in 54%.[12a] A sharp decline in the frequency of VEC is noted in the latter half of the third decade of life, with a concomitant increase in squamous metaplasia. The "healing" or transformation of columnar epithelium comprising adenosis begins as a "reserve cell" proliferation and advances through immature squamous metaplasia. The end result is a normal-appearing, fully glycogenated squamous epithelium. The glands are converted into squamous pegs. A small pool or tiny droplet of mucin may comprise the final vestige.

The area between the old and new squamo-columnar junctions is defined as the transformation zone. This area of intense mitotic metaplastic activity may be prone to dysplastic transformation, resulting in cervical or vaginal squamous dysplasias or carcinomas. This may occur especially after exposure to those oncogens associated with sexual contacts. This process is well described in patients not exposed *in utero* to DES. However, increased risk of squamous dysplasias in DES-exposed offspring is being reported. A larger transformation zone simply may have a greater chance for dysplastic alteration. As the DES-exposed cohort enters into an age range where squamous dysplasias are more commonly seen, careful surveillance to detect any further increase is of obvious importance and need.[13]

An important question addresses the premalignant nature of adenosis and its progression into clear cell adenocarcinoma. In two documented cases, clear cell adenocarcinoma was found in the same area where adenosis has been previously diagnosed. Indirect evidence is obtained by serial blocks done on surgical specimens from patients with clear cell adenocarcinomas. Foci of

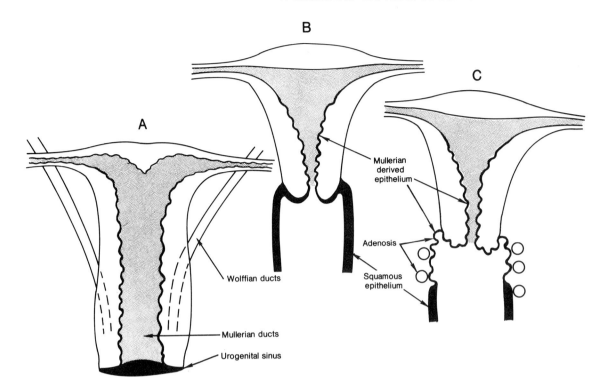

Figure 4–1. Schematic representations of the embryologic development of the vagina in the unexposed and DES-exposed woman. A. Cephalad progression of urogenital sinus-derived squamous epithelium (solid black) over müllerian duct-derived columnar mucosa (stippled) early in gestation. The wolffian ducts are regressing without testosterone stimulation. B. Vaginal canal lined by squamous epithelium up to the endocervical canal as found in late gestation in normal female fetuses. C. DES exposure before the nineteenth week of gestation, often causing retention of the müllerian mucosa over parts of the cervix and vagina (adenosis) by interference with the normal migration of squamous epithelium. This may also lead to structural changes in the vagina, cervix, and/or uterus. (From Stillman RJ, Am J Obstet Gynecol 142:905, 1982, with permission.)

atypical tubuloendometrial epithelium were found in 80% of the cases, almost always adjacent to the tumor. The coexistence of atypical vaginal adenosis and atypical cervical ectropion, with clear cell adenocarcinoma at the proximity to its margin, may support a hypothesis that these lesions are precursors of clear cell carcinoma.[11]

However, in patients followed longitudinally, adenosis commonly regresses spontaneously, rather than proceeding to an atypical and then malignant state. The fortunately low frequency of adenocarcinoma (1/1000–1/10,000 exposed females) compared to the high frequency of adenosis in DES-exposed females mitigates strongly against adenosis itself as a premalignant lesion.[11] The analogy of progression of squamous dysplasia to squamous carcinoma is not appropriate. In the latter, intervention to eradicate the dysplasia before progression is warranted. Aggressive management of adenosis has been employed, including partial vaginectomy, radiation, biopsy, and cautery. However, our current understanding of the lack of malignant transformation of adenosis makes these therapies overzealous. Combined with the record of spontaneous regression of adenosis and risks of intervention (like cervical stenosis), appropriate cytologic evaluation and observation of these generally benign lesions seems far more prudent.[3]

Clear Cell Adenocarcinoma

Intrauterine exposure to DES may be followed by the appearance of adenocarcinoma of the vagina or cervix, almost always of the clear cell type. The major age-associated increase in clear cell carcinoma is at age 12, with peak at age 19, and decrease thereafter. Occasional cases are found well into the third decade of life. The nature of the second stimulus which is associated with a sharp increase in frequency of this otherwise rare cancer one-and-a-half decades after intrauterine exposure to DES is speculative, but the hormonal events in the peripubertal period have been implicated because of the temporal association to the tumor's detection. While an age-associated decrease in occurrence has been noted after age 19, a second increase later in the life span of the exposed females is possible and of obvious concern. To date this has not been observed and the frequency of the tumor remains low compared to the many individuals exposed.[11]

DES may act as a tumor promoter or cocarcinogen through a mechanism other than stimulating cell proliferation of the altered target cells. Some *in vitro* studies show that DES at a certain dose range can actually inhibit cell proliferation. An alternative mechanism involves the

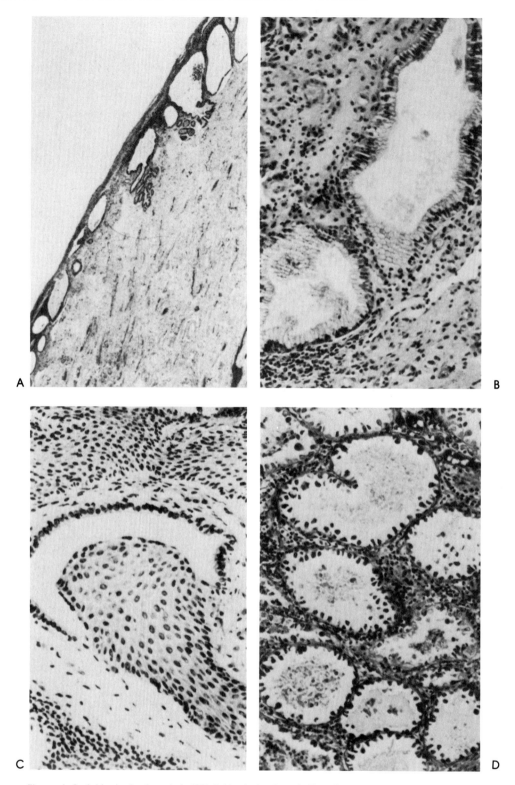

Figure 4–2. A. Vaginal adenosis (×100). B. Vaginal adenosis. The glands are lined by endocervical-type epithelium (×200). C. Active squamous metaplasia involving surface epithelium and underlying gland as a squamous peg (×250). D. Clear cell adenocarcinoma. The cysts are lined by hobnail cells (×180). (From Scully R and Welch W, Pathology of the Female Genital Tract after Prenatal Exposure to DES. *In* Chapter 3 of Developmental Effects of DES in Pregnancy, AL Herbst and HA Bern [eds.] New York: Thieme-Stratton Inc., 1981, with permission.)

metabolism of stilbestrol estrogens to quinone intermediates which may then interact with cellular targets such as DNA. Some support for this mechanism is provided by studies which show that DES can induce chromosome abnormalities such as aneuploidy and increase the level of sister chromatid exchange. While the mechanism is unclear, the direct association of DES exposure *in utero* to the appearance of this otherwise rare tumor is not.

According to the FIGO criteria, 57% of the clear cell adenocarcinomas described following DES exposure were vaginal. If the tumors were classified based on their predominant location, the ratio of vaginal: cervical clear cell carcinomas was 7:3. The cervical carcinomas are predominantly on the ectocervix, while the vaginal carcinomas are usually located on the anterior wall and the upper third portion.[11]

In the past, there was much support for the mesonephric origin of clear cell adenocarcinoma, leading to the term "mesonephroma" as a synonym. Support for the mesonephric origin was based on the following observations: the clear cell component resembles the solid form of clear cell carcinoma; the neoplasms occur along the course of the wolffian ducts; and the origin of 3 out of 13 cases of clear cell carcinoma of the cervix was found to be from mesonephric remnants.

In recent years the tendency has been to relate the tumor to a müllerian origin, based on the following facts: A high association of pelvic endometriosis with clear cell carcinoma of the ovary (25%). Clear cell adenocarcinomas of the endometrium arise within the endometrium or endometrial polyps and may be admixed with endometrial adenocarcinoma. The origin of 4 out of 13 clear cell adenocarcinomas was from the epithelial lining of endometriosis cysts. Small cell adenocarcinomas originate in the superficial layers of the cervix and vagina, where epithelium of the müllerian type is found in over 90% of the cases in the form of cervical ectropion and vaginal adenosis. Most clear cell adenocarcinomas of the vagina involve primarily the anterior wall, where adenosis is also primarily situated. Histologically the clear cell is the most predominant. This is a large polyhedral cell with a clear cytoplasmic appearance. The "hobnail" cells (Figure 4–2) are also found lining the tubules, cysts, and papillae. They are characterized by a bulbous nucleus that protrudes into the lumen beyond the apparent cytoplasmic limits of the cell. Electron microscopic studies revealed the presence of cytoplasmic glycogen and short blunted surface villi. Cytologic examination is positive or suspicious for carcinoma in about 80% of the cases.[11]

Clear cell carcinomas spread locally, lymphatically, and hematogenously. These carcinomas spread outside the abdominal cavity more often than squamous carcinomas arising at the same site. Pelvic nodal involvement occurs in 17% of vaginal Stage I clear cell carcinoma. Pelvic nodes are involved in 50% of Stage II vaginal and Stage IIb cervical clear cell carcinoma. Over one-third of recurrences have been in the supraclavicular nodes or in the lungs, while only 10% of squamous cell carcinomas recur in these sites. Persistent or recurrent disease has been described in over 25% of the cases, most of them within three years of primary therapy, and most patients have

died. Treatment with both surgery and radiation has been effective, though guidelines for the optimal approach have not yet been established. Prognosis is most favorable when the microscopic pattern is tubulocystic, with a five-year survival rate of 88%, while with other patterns, such as solid or papillary, it is 73%. Mitotic activity and grading of the tumor also help in gauging the prognosis.

Cervicovaginal Structural Abnormalities

Besides mucosal changes of adenosis and adenocarcinoma, the fibromuscular and stromal development of the lower müllerian tract are influenced by *in utero* DES exposure. As mentioned earlier, mucosal changes may be influenced by DES effects on stromal development underlying these tissues. In some recent reports structural abnormalities were identified in 25% of subjects identified by review of records, 43% of patients who referred themselves, and 49% of patients referred by physicians. These latter groups are, of course, more likely to contain a relatively biased population, which may account for the greater frequency of abnormalities found.

Structural defects of the cervix and vaginal fornix (Figure 4–3) include,[14] among others, Cockscomb: a raised ridge, usually on the anterior cervix; Collar: a flat rim involving part to all of the circumference of the cervix; Pseudopolyp: polypoid appearance of the cervix due to circumferential constricting groove, thickening of the anterior or posterior endocervical canal (includes endocervical stromal hyperplasia); Hypoplastic cervix: cervix less than 1.5 cm in diameter.

Structural defects of the vagina include complete or partial absence of the pars vaginalis, abnormality of the fornix, fusion of cervix to vagina, partial or complete forniceal obliteration, transverse or longitudinal septum, and vaginal bands, constriction rings, or narrowing. The presence of cervicovaginal structural anomalies is generally associated with higher total administered dose of DES and the gestational week in which DES exposure began. The highest incidence of anomalies may be seen when the drug was administered in gestational weeks 13 to 22. As with adenosis, longitudinal follow-up with patients demonstrates spontaneous regression of some cervicovaginal structural abnormalities.[15]

Cervical Stenosis (After Surgery)

Adenosis and ectropion, with their extensive areas of columnar epithelium on the cervix and vaginal portio, often result in mucoid discharge in DES-exposed women. The areas of exposed columnar epithelium can also be associated with vaginal infections and resultant inflammation. In combination with cervicovaginal structural abnormalities, the hypermucorrhea and inflammation may give a disturbing appearance on vaginal examination. Inflammation or inflammatory atypia may be seen on exfoliative cytology. Patient complaints of discharge or odor and

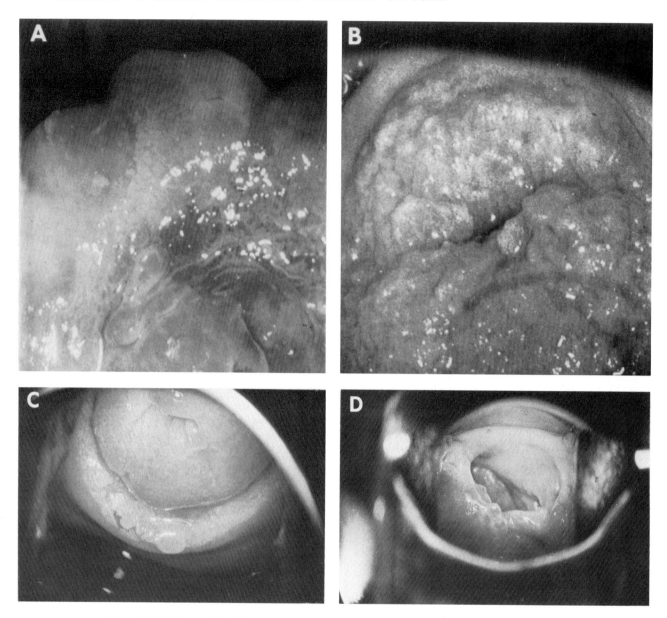

Figure 4–3. Colposcopic photomicrographs of cervicovaginal changes seen in female progeny in response to in utero exposure to DES. A. Cockscomb cervix. B. Adenosis on cervix and portio vaginalis. C. Annular cervical hood or collar. D. Transverse vaginal septum. (From Burke L and Mathews B: Colposcopy in Clinical Practice, Philadelphia: F.A. Davis Co., 1977, with permission.)

concerns about precancerous nature of adenosis led clinicians commonly to resort to cryotherapy for treatment. It is now recognized, however, that even minor gynecologic surgery on the cervix and vagina, including cryotherapy, is not without risk. The healing process in the DES-exposed offspring is abnormal, since up to 80% of these patients will subsequently develop cervical stenosis, compared to approximately 1% of non-DES-exposed patients undergoing the same procedure for cervical dysplasia[16–18] (Table 4–2). Cervical stenosis may lead to subsequent cervical-mucus factor infertility and/or may be associated in some patients with endometriosis due to increased retrograde menstruation.[17]

As discussed previously, because much of the columnar epithelium of adenosis and ectropion will heal spon-taneously by squamous metaplasia and is not a precancerous lesion, cryotherapy as treatment for these abnormalities must be weighed against significant risk of cervical stenosis. Considering the risk-benefit ratio involved with cryotherapy and other "minor" gynecologic procedures in the DES-exposed population, these should be employed only for clear-cut and conservative indications, such as biopsy-proven moderate dysplasia or worse. Use of point cautery or laser therapy to a small colposcopically defined lesion, rather than generalized pericervical therapy, should be emphasized to minimize the area of destruction. Careful evaluation of colposcopic, cytologic, and histologic changes by clinicians and pathologists experienced in DES-associated alterations will also minimize aggressive therapies by differentiating

Table 4–2. Summary of Effects of Minor Cervical Surgery[a] in DES-exposed Females

Author	(No.) DES	Surgery (No.)	Surgery (%)[b]	Stenosis (No.)	Stenosis (%)[c]	Endometriosis (No.)	Endometriosis (%)[d]
Schmidt[16]	276	51	18	38	75	—	—
Stillman[17]	20	6	30	5	83	3	60
Haney[18]	33	11	33	9	82	8	89
Total	329	68	21	52	76	11[e]	79[f]

[a] Includes cryotherapy, cautery, and conization.
[b] Of those with DES.
[c] Of those with surgery.
[d] Of those with stenosis.
[e] All with infertility.
[f] 11 of 14 patients with stenosis (from Stillman and Haney only).

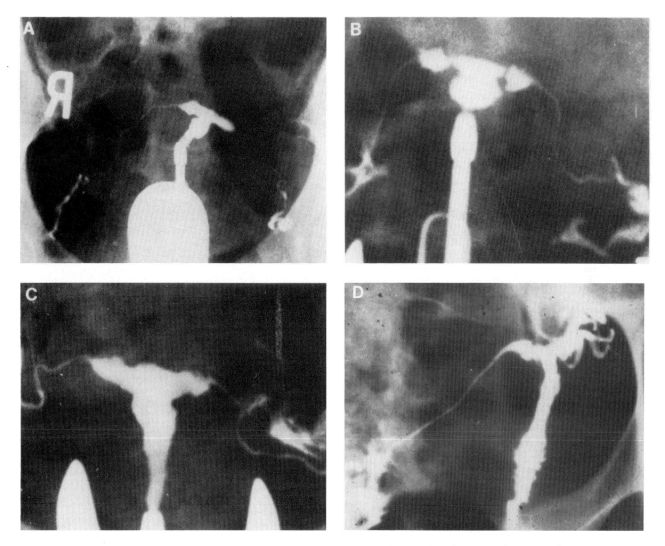

Figure 4–4. Examples of upper mullerian tract abnormalities found in female progeny in response to in utero exposure to DES as demonstrated by hysterosalpingography. A. T-shaped uterus. B. Constriction rings. C. Irregularity of uterine cavity. D. Small and irregular uterine cavity. (From Kaufman RH, Adam E, Binder GL, et al.: Upper genital tract changes and pregnancy outcome in offspring exposed in utero to diethylstilbestrol, Am J Obstet Gynecol 137:299, 1980, published by C.V. Mosby Company, with permission.)

what in DES-exposed patients are benign from other lesions.

PATHOLOGIC CHANGES IN THE UPPER GENITAL TRACT

Uterine abnormalities have been associated with DES exposure in up to 41.6% of record review patients and in 61.5% of walk-in, referral, and other patients. The most common anomalies are uterine cornual constriction rings, a T-shaped uterus, irregular uterine margins, and hypoplastic uterus (Figure 4–4). Other anomalies reported include a wide lower segment, arcuate uteri, unicornuate uteri, and filling defects, synechiae, and others.[19] Significant alterations in the cervical canal, upper and lower segment ratios, and overall uterine size compared to nonexposed patients exist on hysterosalpingographic (HSG) evaluation.[20]

The frequency of uterine abnormalities is increased in the presence of vaginal epithelial changes and cervical structural changes. Both may serve as general markers for the presence of uterine anomalies. DES-exposed women with structural alterations of the lower genital tract are four-and-a-half times more likely to have "abnormal" hysterosalpingogram than non-DES-exposed women. When uteri from DES-exposed women were examined after a hysterectomy, isolated areas of myometrial thickening were observed to produce indentations into the endometrial cavity, resulting in the roentgenogram observed.

The fallopian tubes usually appear normal, both histologically and on HSG. Shortened distorted tubes with pinpoint ostia were found in one small series of surgical specimens.[21] Functional abnormalities of the fallopian tubes as demonstrated by frequent ectopic gestation may be more common than obvious structural changes.[3]

REPRODUCTIVE ABNORMALITIES

Concern that DES could cause functional reproductive abnormalities and infertility increased as evidence of anatomic abnormalities in the reproductive system of females exposed to DES *in utero* accumulated. Mice treated with different doses of DES injected subcutaneously on days 4 through 16 of gestation demonstrate a dose-related decrease in reproductive capacity, ranging from minimal subfertility in the lower DES dose to a total sterility at the highest dose. Reduced fertility was reflected by both a decrease in the number of litters and smaller litter sizes.[22] The component of sterility seen with higher doses was oviductal-ovarian, since the number of ova recovered from the oviductal ampullae after induced ovulation was less than 30% of that of controls. In addition, structural abnormalities of the oviduct, uterus, cervix, and vagina were observed which contributed to infertility.

Drawing conclusions for humans from data obtained in rodents must be done with caution, but analogous anatomical abnormalities and analogous reproductive dysfunction after DES exposure support the utility of many such studies.[11] A primate animal model has great value, but the expense prohibits the number of animals necessary for appropriate statistical analysis.[23]

Evaluation of reproductive dysfunction in the female should be separated into two general categories—namely, the effects of *in utero* exposure to DES on (a) fecundability, and (b) pregnancy outcome in those women who do conceive. The capability or the diminished capability to conceive of the female exposed to DES *in utero* is still a controversial issue. Fertility might be affected in DES-exposed offspring in one or more of a variety of ways.

FECUNDABILITY

Ovulatory Factor

Menstrual irregularities and oligomenorrhea have been described in DES-exposed females.[24–27] Oligomenorrhea or oligi-ovulation imply the possibility of ovulatory factor infertility. The significant increase in oligomenorrhea in DES-exposed subjects compared to control subjects may diminish with time, as the cycles of the DES-exposed patients tend to become more regular over the 10 to 15 years following menarche. Thus, as DES-exposed women enter their mid-twenties, an age when they are first attempting conception, cycle and ovulatory regularity may be established. As a group, the age at first pregnancy might not be delayed by an ovulatory factor which had been present earlier.[27] Berger noted that among 50 infertile DES patients, significantly fewer were diagnosed as having ovulatory disorders compared to 50 concurrently-evaluated, matched infertile controls.[28]

Uterine Factor

Uterine malformation as described on HSG may imply a failure of implantation. Berger found that significantly more infertile DES-exposed patients had uterine abnormalities (96%) than infertile controls (6%).[28] Haney found 64% of infertile DES-exposed patients had HSG abnormalities,[20] not dissimilar to rates found in DES patients who were not specifically seen for infertility but having HSGs performed.[19] A direct effect of uterine abnormalities in DES-exposed females to primary infertility is difficult to detect. However, with some severe uterine malformations, even implantation would be difficult to envision.

Peritoneal Factor

Tubal factor infertility may be hypothesized by anatomic abnormalities of the tubes. Despite patency, the higher frequency of ectopic gestation serves as evidence of their dysfunction.[3] Certainly secondary infertility after surgery from ectopic gestation might occur and must be considered contributing to tubal factor infertility.

Table 4–3. *In Utero* DES Exposure Associated with Endometriosis in Infertile Females

	Endometriosis	Infertile		DES-Exposed with Endometriosis	DES-Exposed		NonDES-Exposed with Endometriosis	NonDES-Exposed	
	(No.)	(No.)	(%)	(No.)	(No.)	(%)	(No.)	(No.)	(%)
Stillman[17]	156	397	39	10	20	50	146	377	39
Haney[18]	13	33	39	13	33	39	—	—	—
Berger[28]	52	100	52	32	50	64	20	50	40
Cramer[29a]	268	1,550[b]	17	14	75	19	254	1,475	17

[a] Of 268 primary infertile women with endometriosis, 14 (5.2%) also had DES exposure, significantly greater (p = .0001) than their control group of 3,794 delivery controls, of whom 62 (1.6%) had DES exposure *in utero*.

[b] Not all infertile women had laparoscopy to evaluate for endometriosis.

Endometriosis is found in a high proportion of all infertile women, but especially so in the DES exposed[17,18,28,29] (Table 4–3). Retrograde menstruation with subsequent implantation and growth is a common theory explaining pelvic endometriosis. Factors which increase the retrograde menstruation and/or predispose to implantation might increase the frequency of endometriosis. In comparing infertile DES-exposed women to nonexposed, more endometriosis is found in the exposed cohort.[17] Many patients with DES exposure have a decrease in the width of the cervical canal. This may become evident or exacerbated by the effects of cryotherapy in a large majority of those patients undergoing these procedures.[18] Cervical narrowing and/or post-therapy stenosis may lead to increasing retrograde menstruation and predispose to endometriosis.[17] Speculatively, abnormal configuration of the cornual region of the uterus may predispose to increased retrograde egress of menstruum. The effect of *in utero* exposure to DES on peritoneal mesothelial differentiation, another theory on the etiology of endometriosis, is unknown.

Endometriosis was found in 13 of 33 DES-exposed infertile women (39%) by Haney and Hammond.[18] Eight of these 13 had cervical stenosis following minor cervical surgery, including cryotherapy. These 8 are among the total of 11 patients who had cervical surgery and 9 who developed stenosis. In a controlled study, 10 of 20 (50%) DES-exposed infertile females who had undergone laparoscopy or laparotomy had endometriosis. This was higher, but not significantly greater, then the 39% found in a group of 377 nonDES-exposed infertile women identically evaluated.[18] In a larger group of 50 DES-exposed infertile women, 64% were found to have endometriosis, significantly greater than 40% of matched infertile controls[28] (Figure 4–5).

A multicenter collaborative study compared 268 patients with primary infertility and endometriosis to 3,794 matched delivery controls. A highly significant association between DES exposure and endometriosis was found.[29] It appears, therefore, that a growing body of evidence supports an increase in the frequency of endometriosis among DES-exposed infertile patients com-

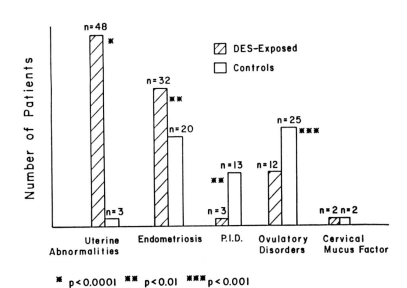

Figure 4–5. Fertility factors in 50 DES-exposed women and 50 controls. (From Berger MJ and Alper MM: Intractable Primary Infertility in DES-exposed Women, J Reprod Med, 31:231, 1986, with permission).

pared to infertile or delivery control patients. Many of these patients also have cervical stenosis (Table 4–2). Information on the frequency of endometriosis in noninfertile DES-exposed patients is not readily available, in part due to lack of indication for their surgical evaluation.

Thus an individual woman exposed *in utero* to DES may have ample reason for difficulty in conceiving—from possibilities of ovulatory dysfunction to cervical, uterine, tubal, and peritoneal (endometriosis or postoperative adhesions) factors. However, while one or more of these factors certainly may play an etiologic role in the infertility of a particular individual, whether or not infertility itself exists more frequently in the DES-exposed population overall compared to nonexposed is unsettled.

Fertility, as assessed by the incidence of pregnancy, mean gravidity, or frequency of infertility problems, did not differ between the DES-exposed population and a control group according to Cousins and associates.[26] In addition, there were no differences in the ability to conceive between DES patients with, and those without, gross cervicovaginal changes: 41% of the total DES study group, 46% of the DES subgroup with gross cervicovaginal changes, and 46% of the control patients had been pregnant at least once.

Most studies have evaluated only fertility (Table 4–4) in DES-exposed females as opposed to its converse, infertility (Table 4–5). Large studies carefully defining fecundability and infertility which compare DES-exposed patients to control patients need to be published. Infertility must be defined as inability to conceive after at least one year of regular intercourse without contraception, not the patient's perception of difficulty conceiving. The proportion of patients seeking pregnancy for this one-year minimum but unable to conceive must be known, as well

Table 4–5. Infertility in DES Daughters

Author	DES Patients	Infertility[a]	
		DES (%)	Control (%)
Berger[30]	69	33.3	—
Herbst[35]	338	15.7	6.4
Schmidt[31]	106	29.2	—

[a] Inability to achieve pregnancy after one or more years of attempts.

as the proportion in an appropriate control population. The results of a multicollaborative study from infertility centers may address this issue and would be a welcome addition to the data currently available.

Berger and Goldstein observed 89 sexually active women, all of whom demonstrated DES-associated cervicovaginal abnormalities.[30] Over a nine-year period 46 patients in this selected group conceived. No controls were evaluated. In another uncontrolled study, Schmidt and associates reported that 106 DES-exposed female progeny conceived 129 pregnancies, but 31 patients (29%) remained infertile for one to eight years. No etiologies for the infertility were discussed.[31]

Barnes and colleagues stated that fertility, as measured in terms of pregnancies achieved, did not differ between the women exposed to DES and the control subjects. There were no differences in the percentages of those women who became pregnant, the distribution of ages at first pregnancy, or the number of pregnancies between the two groups. Comparison of DES versus control groups, with consideration of such variables as a history of pelvic inflammatory disease, race, previous use of contraception, use of an intrauterine contraceptive device, years of sexual activity, and marital status, failed to reveal any differences in the percentage of women conceiving. Barnes and colleagues addressed an earlier paper which presented conflicting results.[32] Their results pertaining to fertility differ from those of Bibbo.[24,33] Whereas Bibbo found almost a two-fold difference in the percentage of women who had become pregnant (33% among controls versus 18% among women exposed to DES), Barnes *et al.* could find no difference (50% controls versus 47% to DES). They restricted their consideration to sexually active women, where Bibbo was concerned with an overall pregnancy rate in a younger group of patients with different follow-up methods.

Herbst and colleagues presented more data from the University of Chicago[34] which followed the offspring of patients enrolled in the 1953 double-blind, placebo-controlled study of DES efficacy published by Dieckmann.[5] The proportion of women who had been pregnant at least once was significantly higher in the placebo-exposed group (58%) than in the DES-exposed subjects (39%, P value less than .0005). When those who had been sexually active or those who had been using contraceptives were excluded, there remained a statistically significant different conception experience between the two groups (86% vs. 67%, P < .001). The difference

Table 4–4. Fertility in DES Daughters

Author	DES Patients	Fertility[a]	
		DES (%)	Control (%)
Barnes[32]	618	47	50
Bibbo[33]	229	18[b]	33
Cousins[26]	71	41	46
Herbst[34]			
All study pts.	226	39[b]	58
Women at risk for pregnancy	132	67[b]	86
Herbst[35]			
Women at risk for pregnancy	338	75[b]	92
Schmidt[16]	276	71	—

[a] Proportion of women pregnant at least once during the period under study. The length of this period varies among the studies. Fertility statistics in these studies do not measure infertility (inability to achieve pregnancy after one or more years of attempts), because they do not report the percentage of women seeking pregnancy but unable to conceive within a year's time.

[b] Statistical significance reported by author.

Note: Tables 4–4 through 4–9 modified from and used with permission of Joan Emery of DES Action.

remains significant when the groups were further limited to only married women who had not used regular contraception. Their results[34,35] support those of Bibbo.

Differences in study-design, population, control groups, and means of statistical assessment may account for discrepancies between the studies of Barnes and Herbst. Despite the lack of certainty regarding fertility in the overall DES population, an individual woman who has been exposed to DES who is also infertile may have any of the factors enumerated earlier as the etiology for that infertility. Each of these factors must therefore be carefully evaluated and treated. Unfortunately, Berger and Alper[28] refer to the "intractability" of infertility in DES-exposed patients. Only 4% of 50 DES exposed females with primary infertility were found to have conceived in one to four years of follow-up after complete evaluation and treatment by infertility specialists. This compares to conception in 44% of 50 matched controls similarly evaluated and concurrently treated. Reports of successful use of *in vitro* fertilization techniques to overcome infertility in the DES-exposed female have been published, with pregnancy at the rate of 19% per embryo transfer.[36] Further study is needed to evaluate how best to treat individual patients with the variety of infertility problems that may be associated with *in utero* DES exposure.

ADVERSE PREGNANCY OUTCOME

In 1978 Goldstein suggested that "it is plausible to postulate that DES exposure *in utero* can impair the normal development of the entire müllerian tract sufficiently to predispose the patient to miscarriages, incompetent cervix, and even ectopic pregnancy because of abnormalities of the tubes, uterus, and cervix."[37] A number of studies published since that time have proven some of these speculations to have been accurate in those DES-exposed females who do conceive.[3,38]

An increased rate of early spontaneous abortions is reported in DES daughters, in both controlled and uncontrolled studies[8,19,26,30,31,32,35,39,40] (Table 4–6). The ectopic tubal pregnancy rate is also found to be significantly greater in DES-exposed daughters compared to controls[3,8,32,35] (Table 4–7). According to a collective review of the number of studies for a total of 960 pregnancies, the rate of ectopic pregnancy was 3.4% in the DES-exposed population and 0% among the control. When first-pregnancy experience only was considered, those rates were 6% and 0%, respectively. Some studies put the ectopic pregnancy rate between 6% to 8%. The high frequency of ectopic tubal gestation is generally unaccompanied by abnormalities on HSG. A functional tubal abnormality is therefore suggested. However, tubal and paratubal anatomic abnormalities have been noted on laparoscopy and laparotomy that seem consistent with a transmüllerian effect of DES exposure. These may be associated with the tubal dysfunction.

Preterm delivery is also found more frequently in studies of DES daughters[3] (Table 4–8). The rate ranges from 10%–30% in comparison to 0% to 5% in control groups, with preterm delivery defined either as delivery before week 37 of gestation or an infant weight of 2,500 gm. An increase in perinatal death rate may be occurring in DES-exposed patients, probably associated with prematurity of preterm delivery. Several studies have attempted to link the reported increase in adverse pregnancy outcome to specific anatomic abnormalities associated with DES. While this generally cannot be done, the outcomes of pregnancies in DES-exposed women with an abnormal HSG were significantly worse than those of the DES-exposed with normal HSG, suggesting the abnormal cavity dimensions may play a role in early or late pregnancy loss.[38] Of 99 women exposed to DES who had normal HSGs, 75% had normal pregnancy outcomes, compared

Table 4–6. Miscarriage in DES Daughters

Author	DES Dtrs. with 1 Pregnancy	Evaluable Pregnancies[a]	Spontaneous Abortions	
			DES (%)	C (%)
Barnes[32]	289	220	25.9[b]	16.1
Berger[30]	46	62	48.3	—[c]
Cousins[26]	29	27	18.5	8.8
Herbst[35d]	150	114	21[b]	11
Kaufman[19]	210	260	32[b]	8
Mangan[40]	98	164	18.3[b]	8.4
Sandberg[39]	167	164	22	—
Schmidt[16]	75	93	25.8	—

[a] For this and all other tables in this series, "evaluable pregnancies" refers to all pregnancies with outcomes other than therapeutic abortion. Percentages in the last two columns are based on the number of evaluable pregnancies.

[b] Statistical significance reported by author.

[c] In this and all subsequent tables, a - is used to indicate absence of a control group.

[d] First pregnancies only.

Table 4–7. Ectopic Pregnancies in DES Daughters

Author	Total Pregnancies	Evaluable Pregnancies[a]	Ectopics	
			DES (%)	Control (%)
Barnes[32]		220	3.6	1.3
Berger[30]	80		3.8	—
Cousins[26]	43		4.7	0
Herbst[34]	149		2.7	0
Herbst[35]		212	5.7[b]	.3
Kaufman[19]	344		2.6	0
Mangan[40]	179		4.9[b]	.03
Sandberg[39]	225		3.6	—
Schmidt[16]	129		5.4	—

[a] Total number of pregnancies minus the number of therapeutic abortions.

[b] Statistical significance reported by the author.

Table 4–8. Preterm Deliveries in DES Daughters

Author	DES Dtrs. with 1 Pregnancy	Evaluable Pregnancies	Preterm Deliveries DES (%)	Preterm Deliveries Control (%)
Barnes[32]	289	220	7.7	4.5
Berger[30]	46	62	13	—
Cousins[26]	29	27	30[a]	0
Herbst[34]	89	116	24[a]	4.4
Herbst[35b]	150	114	20[a]	6
Kaufman[19]	210	260	10.7[a]	3.4
Mangan[40]	98	164	7.3[a]	2.2
Sandberg[39]	167	164	16	—
Schmidt[16]	75	93	12.9	—

[a] Statistical significance reported by author.

[b] Gives preterm statistics for first pregnancies only.

Table 4–9. Total Pregnancy Outcome in DES Daughters

Author	DES Dtrs. with 1 Pregnancy	Evaluable Pregnancies	Viable Pregnancy Outcome DES (%)	Viable Pregnancy Outcome Control (%)
Berger[30]	46	62	42	—
Cousins[26]	29	27	58	88
Herbst[34]	89	116	65	90
Herbst[35]	122	212	67	84
Kaufman[19]	210	260	75	92
Mangan[40]	98	164	75	90
Sandberg[39]	167	164	69	—
Schmidt[16]	75	93	62	—

Note: Authors did not report on statistical significance for these pregnancy outcome statistics.

to only 51% among 70 DES-exposed women who had abnormal HSGs.

Early but uncontrolled reports linked premature deliveries to cervical incompetence and led to suggestions for prophylactic cervical cerclage in DES-exposed patients. While some cervical incompetence may be associated with cervicovaginal changes of DES, most premature delivery follows premature labor in these patients. Premature labor may be associated with decreased dimensions of the uterine cavity to accommodate the growing fetus. Cervical cerclage for cervical incompetence should, therefore, not be employed without a classic history of silent dilatation of the cervix without labor. It should certainly not be used as a prophylaxis against incompetency in a woman without prior pregnancy loss. This is particularly important because of the potential risks associated with minor gynecologic surgery in the DES-exposed female.[3]

Overall, consistently low term-pregnancy rates of 47%, 41%, 57%, and 40% were reported in various DES-exposed populations among first pregnancies. The 47% rate is contrasted with an 85% term-delivery rate among first pregnancies in placebo-exposed patients. Thus, the term-pregnancy rates among DES-exposed women range between 40% and 50% and may even be lower in DES-exposed patients with HSG abnormalities. These rates are much lower than the 80% to 90% term deliveries in control women.[3] Eventually 81 to 82% of the DES-exposed women do deliver a term, live-born infant compared to 93 to 95% of a control population.[8,32,34] It has been reported, however, that while 81% of pregnancies in these DES-exposed women were delivered of a live-born infant, only 60% were delivered at term. The rates for overall viable pregnancy outcome (preterm and term) are summarized in Table 4–9.

Thus, significantly more women who were exposed to DES than non-exposed women will have an adverse pregnancy outcome. Although their reproductive history may, therefore, be more complicated than that of women not exposed to DES (i.e., preceded by more abortions, ec-

topic pregnancies, or premature deliveries), fortunately about 82% of those DES-exposed women who do conceive will eventually carry a pregnancy which results in a live-born infant. Overall the subgroup of DES-exposed women with HSG and cervicovaginal changes appear at greater risk of adverse pregnancy outcome than other DES-exposed women.

EFFECTS OF *IN UTERO* EXPOSURE TO DES ON MALE PROGENY

Approximately one-half of the offspring exposed *in utero* to DES were male. Because of the well-known reproductive tract teratogenicity of other exogenous steroids in the male subjects, investigation of the male reproductive tract and reproductive performance is important. Experimental evidence in male animals exposed *in utero* or neonatally to DES supports these concerns.

Pubertal development, secondary sexual characteristics, and hormonal levels are similar in DES-exposed men and controls. However some anatomic abnormalities have been reported to occur more frequently in a DES-exposed group. Epididymal cysts, hypoplastic testes, capsular enduration, Leydig cell hyperplasia, microphalius and prostatic utricle hypertrophy (in the fetus) have all been reported.[41–43] In contrast, a recent report from the DESAD project disputes whether these benign urogenital abnormalities are occurring with increased frequency.[44] Subject selection and eligibility differ among these studies and may account for the discrepancy in findings. Most studies do support an increased occurrence of a variety of anatomic abnormalities in DES-exposed males.

Concerns have been raised about the frequency of testicular cancer in DES-exposed males. Anecdotal reports have detailed seminoma and embryonal cell carcinoma in these men. However, in comparing these reports to the usual incidence of these testicular cancers, there is currently no information to suggest an increased risk for testicular cancers in the DES-exposed population. A recent controlled study from the DESAD project found no increase in testicular tumors in DES-exposed males compared to controls.[44] Careful follow-up must continue, but any suggestion of increased association must be accompanied by appropriate controls from the nonexposed population.

Dispute exists regarding reproductive dysfunction in males. Altered semen analyses have been reported in DES-exposed males. The sperm density in 88 adult men exposed to DES evaluated by Gill and associates was found to be 83 million/ml compared to 123 million/ml in 85 placebo-exposed men (p < 0.02). In addition, the total sperm count, the motility grade, the total number of motile sperm, the percentage of normal morphology, and overall quality score were all statistically lower in DES-exposed men. Hormonal analyses have revealed no major differences in luteinizing hormone, or testosterone levels between these groups.[45] More recent evaluation by these same authors in an expanded study population revealed less dramatic differences between DES-exposed and control males.

Stenchever et al also reported that the mean sperm count among DES-exposed men was significantly lower than among random control men (66.4 million/ml versus 101.7 million/ml; p < 0.05). No differences in morphology or motility were found.[46] In contrast, no differences in semen parameters were noted by Andonian and Kessler, who compared 24 DES-exposed men to 24 age-matched control men.[43] This is supported by the DESAD project recent report which found no abnormalities on semen analysis comparing DES-exposed to control males. This includes evaluation of count, motility, motility grade, morphology, and overall Eliasson score. The fertility potential of the DES-exposed versus control males was unaltered, based on reports of pregnancies fathered by either group.[44]

Little other information on fertility rates of DES-exposed men has been published. Older reports detail that a significantly higher number of DES-exposed men compared to control men have Eliasson semen scores rated as severely pathologic (23% versus 5%). This semen score, which combines many aspects of semen qualities, correlates with fertility potential. In addition, only DES-exposed men were found to have azoospermia, and 20.5% compared to only 3.5% of placebo-exposed men had sperm counts less than 20 million/ml.[45] These abnormalities are contested by recent data.[44]

Using the zona-free hamster egg sperm penetration assay, the sperm from 14 of 17 DES-exposed men (82%) failed to penetrate hamster oocytes adequately (with ≤ 15% of the eggs penetrated). This is contrasted to only 17% of 12 randomly selected nonDES-exposed control men, and none of 11 fertile control men in whom penetration was below 15%. While there is some potential selection bias in the small groups, these initial results suggested a decrease in fertilizing capacity among men exposed in utero to DES. However, as seen with other study groups, as this study population was expanded, the statistical significance of decreased sperm penetration in DES-exposed males was lost.[47]

Thus, even firm data on anatomical genital tract abnormalities in males have recently met with some challenge, as have data on the alterations in semen analysis and fertility potential. Further studies of DES-exposed men to evaluate genital tract and semen abnormalities and fertility potential are certainly warranted. True infertility studies for men exposed to DES, which include evaluation of the female partner, also need to be performed. This can also include a long-term follow-up of the incidence of prostatic and testicular disorders and malignancies in these men. Complete history and physical examination of both partners of an infertile couple (always important in assessing the various factors that decrease fertility potential) should include seeking evidence of in utero DES-exposure of the male.

COMMENT

The legacy of in utero exposure of men and women to DES continues to unfold. The tragedy of clear cell adenocarcinoma in a young female population has been somewhat mitigated by the low incidence of the disorder compared to the total number of DES-exposed progeny. Also, the marked decrease in its occurrence after 19 years of age is encouraging in that the period of risk for the large majority of the exposed population may be over. The strong evidence that benign DES-associated vaginal and cervical changes do not progress to clear cell carcinoma, and even regress spontaneously through squamous metaplasia, is also encouraging. In addition, since the drug was banned for use in pregnancy in 1971, in utero exposure has ceased and no further cases of DES exposure should occur. The legacy should, therefore, be self-limited. However, what the future holds for those progeny who were exposed to DES as they continue to age is unknown. Some current areas of concern include the impact of oral contraceptive use in these patients, the psychological effects of DES exposure,[48] frequency of cervical squamous dysplasias,[13] and the use of DES for postcoital contraception. In addition, theoretical concerns exist about malignant effects on hormone-responsive tissues, especially the breast, the prostate, and the endometrium and stroma of the uterus. The mothers who ingested the drug during pregnancy are being followed to detect late adverse sequelae, especially recent concerns of increases in frequency of breast carcinoma.[9]

As the exposed progeny now proceed through the reproductive age range, the spectrum of reproductive abnormalities has emerged (Tables 4–10 and 4–11). Still controversial are infertility rates. More solidly established in female offspring are increased frequencies of spontaneous abortions, ectopic pregnancies, premature deliveries, perinatal deaths, and overall adverse pregnancy outcome. While more than 80% of DES-exposed women will eventually succeed in delivering a term live-born infant, this is significantly less than the rate in comparable control subjects and is undoubtedly lower in the subgroup who demonstrated DES-associated cervicovaginal and/or HSG changes. Anatomic abnormalities and abnormalities in semen analyses of the men exposed in utero

Table 4–10. Summary of the Currently Recognized Effects of *In Utero* Exposure to DES on Female Progeny[a]

Anatomic		Reproductive	
Lower Müllerian	Upper Müllerian	Menstrual	Fertility Potential
Clear cell carcinoma	Uterine structural changes	Cycle irregularities	Infertility
Adenosis	T-shape	Dysmenorrhea	Adverse pregnancy outcome
Cervicovaginal structural changes	Small cavity	Shorter menstrual flow	First-trimester spontaneous abortion
Transverse ridges	Constriction rings		Second-trimester spontaneous abortion
Cockscomb	HSG filling defects		Ectopic gestation
Cervical hoods and collars	Tubal structural changes		Premature delivery
Cervical mucus effects			Perinatal death
Cervical incompetence			
Cervical stenosis (after "therapy")			
Squamous dysplasia			

[a] The statistical significance of these effects may not be unanimously accepted. From Stillman RJ[3]: Am J Obstet Gynecol 142:905, 1982.

to DES have also been described by most authors, but have recently been disputed, as has the impact on the frequency of infertility in these progeny. Now that the evaluation of the reproductive histories of these women and men has progressed to this point, treatments will be sought. As mentioned, caution must be exercised in the use of unindicated or prophylactic therapies, especially those that would involve operative procedures on the cervix or uterus, such as cryotherapy, cerclage, or metroplasty.[3] The side effects and adverse outcomes of these procedures may outweigh the potential benefits unless clear indications exist.

If DES had been successful in decreasing pregnancy wastage and the complications of late pregnancy for which it had been prescribed, a philosophical risk/benefit argument might now be waged: should a couple risk taking the medication in pregnancy, possibly to deliver an offspring prone to the late adverse effects summarized above, versus possibly not having that particular offspring at all?[3] We know from strong evidence provided even by 1954, that it is a moot point, for the drug was not efficacious.[4–7] Although given by physicians with the hope only of benefiting their patients, we see that DES presented risk without benefit. Now we can only hope that sound epidemiologic follow-up may lead to effective and rational therapies of the abnormalities in those offspring who were so unfortunately exposed.

References

1. Smith OW: Diethylstilbestrol in the prevention and treatment of complications of pregnancy. Am J Obstet Gynecol 56:821, 1948.
2. Smith OW, Smith G: The influence of diethylstilbestrol on the progress and outcome of pregnancy based on a comparison of treated with untreated primigravidas. Am J Obstet Gynecol 58:994, 1949.
3. Stillman RJ: *In utero* exposure to diethylstilbestrol: Adverse effects on reproductive tract and reproductive performance in male and female offspring. Am J Obstet Gynecol 142:905, 1982.
4. Ferguson JH: Effect of stilbestrol on pregnancy compared to the effect of a placebo. Am J Obstet Gynecol. 65:592, 1953.
5. Dieckmann WJ, Davis ME, Rynkiewicz LM, et al.: Does the administration of diethylstilbestrol during pregnancy have therapeutic value? Am J Obstet Gynecol 66:1062, 1953.
6. Spodick DH: Randomized controlled clinical trials. JAMA 247:2258, 1982.
7. Brackbold Y, Berendes HW: Dangers of diethylstilbestrol: Review of a 1953 paper. Lancet 2:520, 1978.
8. Herbst AL, Poskanzer DC, Robboy SJ, et al.: Prenatal exposure to stilbestrol: A prospective comparison of exposed offspring with unexposed controls. N Engl J Med 292:334, 1975.
9. Greenburg ER, Barnes AB, Resseguiel LJ: Breast cancer in

Table 4–11. Summary of the Currently Recognized Effects of *In Utero* Exposure to DES on Male Progeny[a]

Anatomic		Reproductive	
Testicular	Other	Semen Analyses	Fertility Potential
Cryptorchidism	Microphallus	Decreased concentration	Diminished Eliasson score
Hypoplasia	Epididymal cysts	Decreased count	
Capsular induration	Prostatic utricle hypertrophy (fetus)	Decreased motility grade and % motile	
Leydig cell hyperplasia (fetus)		Decreased normal morphology	

[a] The statistical significance of some of these effects may not be unanimously accepted. From Stillman RJ[3], Am J Obstet Gynecol 142:905, 1982.

mothers given diethylstilbestrol in pregnancy. N Engl J Med 311:1393, 1984.

10. Ulfelder H, Robboy SJ: The embryologic development of the human vagina. Am J Obstet Gynecol 126:769, 1976.

11. Herbst AL, Bern HA, (eds): Developmental effects of diethylstilbestrol in pregnancy. New York, Thieme-Stratton Inc, 1981.

12. Cunha GR, Fujii H: Stromal parenchymal interactions in normal and abnormal development of the genital tract. Chap 14. In AL Herbst, HA Bern, (eds) Developmental effects of diethylstilbestrol (DES) in pregnancy. New York, Thieme-Stratton Inc, 1981.

12a. Burke L, Antonioli D, Friedman FA: Evolution of diethylstilbestrol-associated genital tract lesions. Obstet Gynecol 57:79, 1981.

13. Robboy SJ, Noller KL, O'Brien P, et al.: Increased incidence of cervical and vaginal dysplasias in 3,980 diethylstilbestrol-exposed young women. JAMA 252:2979, 1984.

14. Sandberg EC: Benign cervical and vaginal changes associated with exposure to stilbestrol in utero. Am J Obstet Gynecol 125:777, 1976.

15. Antonioli DA, Burke L, Friedman EA: Natural history of diethylstilbestrol-associated genital tract lesions: Cervical ectopy and cervicovaginal hood. Am J Obstet Gynecol 137:847, 1980.

16. Schmidt G, Fowler WC: Cervical stenosis following minor gynecologic procedures on DES-exposed women. Obstet Gynecol 56:333, 1980.

17. Stillman RJ, Miller LC: Diethylstilbestrol exposure in utero and endometriosis in infertile females. Fertil Steril 41:389, 1984.

18. Haney AF, Hammond MG: Infertility in women exposed to diethylstilbestrol in utero. J Reprod Med 28:851, 1983.

19. Kaufman RH, Adam E, Binder GL, et al.: Upper genital tract changes and pregnancy outcome in offspring exposed in utero to diethylstilbestrol. Am J Obstet Gynecol 137:299, 1980.

20. Haney AF, Hammond CB, Soules MR, et al.: Diethylstilbestrol-induced upper genital tract abnormalities. Fertil Steril 31:142, 1979.

21. DeCherney AH, Cholst I, Naftolin F: Structure and function of the fallopian tubes following exposure to diethylstilbestrol (DES) during gestation. Fertil Steril 36:741, 1981.

22. McLachlan JA, Newbold RR, Bullock B: Reproductive tract lesions in male mice exposed prenatally to diethylstilbestrol. Science 190:991, 1975.

23. Hendrickx AG, Benirschke K, Thompson RS, et al.: The effects of prenatal diethylstilbestrol (DES) exposure on the genitalia of pubertal Macaca mulatta, I: Female offspring. J Reprod Med 22:233, 1979.

24. Bibbo M, Haenszel WM, Wied GL, et al.: A twenty-five-year follow-up study of women exposed to diethylstilbestrol during pregnancy. N Engl J Med 298:763, 1978.

25. Barnes AB: Menstrual history of young women exposed in utero to diethylstilbestrol. Fertil Steril 32:148, 1979.

26. Cousins L, Karp W, Lacey C, et al.: Reproductive outcome of women exposed to diethylstilbestrol in utero. Obstet Gynecol 56:70, 1980.

27. Barnes AB: Menstrual history and fecundity of women exposed and unexposed in utero to diethylstilbestrol. J Reprod Med 29:651, 1984.

28. Berger MJ, Alper MM: Intractable primary infertility in DES-exposed women. J Reprod Med 31:231, 1986.

29. Cramer D, Wilson E, Stillman RJ, et al.: Association of endometriosis with maternal diethylstilbestrol (DES) exposure. Fertil Steril: Abstr. Supp:65:185, 1986.

30. Berger MJ, Goldstein DP: Impaired reproductive performance in DES-exposed women. Obstet Gynecol 55:25, 1980.

31. Schmidt G, Fowler WC, et al.: Reproductive history of women exposed to diethylstilbestrol in utero. Fertil Steril 33:21, 1980.

32. Barnes AB, Colton T, Gundersen J, et al.: Fertility and outcome of pregnancy in women exposed in utero to diethylstilbestrol. N Engl J Med 302:609, 1980.

33. Bibbo M, Gill WB, Azizi F, et al.: Follow-up study of male and female offspring of DES-exposed mothers. Obstet Gynecol 49:1, 1977.

34. Herbst AL, Hubby MM, Blough RR, et al.: A comparison of pregnancy experience in DES-exposed and DES-unexposed daughters. J Reprod Med 24:62, 1980.

35. Herbst AL, Hubby MM, Azizi F, et al.: Reproductive and gynecologic surgical experience in diethylstilbestrol-exposed daughters. Am J Obstet Gynecol 141:1019, 1981.

36. Muasher SJ, Garcia JE, Jones HW: Experience with diethylstilbestrol-exposed infertile women in a program of in vitro fertilization. Fertil Steril 42:20, 1984.

37. Goldstein DP: Incompetent cervix in offspring exposed to diethylstilbestrol in utero. Obstet Gynecol (Suppl.) 52:738, 1978.

38. Stillman RJ: Pregnancy prospects of DES daughters. Contemp Obstet Gynecol October 1984, p. 47.

39. Sandberg EC, Riffle NL, Higdon JV, et al.: Pregnancy outcome in women exposed to diethylstilbestrol in utero. Am J Obstet Gynecol 140:194, 1981.

40. Mangan CE, Borow L, et al.: Pregnancy outcome in 98 women exposed to diethylstilbestrol, their mothers, and unexposed siblings. Obstet Gynecol 59:315, 1982.

41. Gill WB, Schumacher GFB, Bibbo M.: Structural and functional abnormalities in the sex organs of male offspring of mothers treated with diethylstilbestrol (DES). J Reprod Med 16:147, 1976.

42. Gill WB, Schumacher GFB, Bibbo M.: Association of diethylstilbestrol exposure in utero with cryptorchidism, testicular hypoplasia, and semen abnormalities. J Urol 122:36, 1979.

43. Andonian RW, Kessler R: Transplacental exposure to diethylstilbestrol in men. Urology 13:276, 1976.

44. Leary FJ, Resseguie LJ, Kurland LT: Males exposed in utero to diethylstilbestrol. JAMA 252:2984, 1984.

45. Gill WB, Schumacher GFB, Bibbo M: Genital and semen abnormalities in adult males two and one-half decades after in utero exposure to diethylstilbestrol. Chap. 7. In AL Herbst (ed) Intrauterine Exposure to Diethylstilbestrol in the Human. Chicago, American College of Obstetricians and Gynecologists, 1978.

46. Stenchever MA, Williamson RA, Leonard L, et al.: Possible relationship between in utero diethylstilbestrol exposure and male infertility. Am J Obstet. Gynecol 140:186, 1981.

47. Shy KK, Stenchever MA, Karp LE, et al.: Genital tract examinations and zona-free hamster egg penetration test for men exposed in utero to diethylstilbestrol. Fertil Steril 42:772, 1984.

48. Burke L, Apfel RJ, Fischer S, et al.: Observations on the psychological impact of diethylstilbestrol exposure and suggestions on management. J Reprod Med 24:99, 1980.

5. Endometrium in Infertility

Shirley G. Driscoll

Adequately prepared endometrium is a *sine qua non* of nidation, implantation, and support of the conceptus until parturition. The blastocyst confronts the endometrium about six days following fertilization and, in successful cases, becomes embedded in the endometrial stroma, subsequently decidualized. The cycling endometrium reflects hormonal output of the ovary, dictated principally by the maturing follicle and the corpus luteum, which evolves following ovulation. Close correspondence between the ovarian cycle and the endometrial cycle was predicted more than three-quarters of a century ago, corroborated by the seminal observations of Hertig and colleagues,[1] and reinforced with repetition and refinement of those studies and related investigations.[2-9] It is not unreasonable to consider possible endometrial causes of infertility. In some instances, the endometrium will reflect disorders or dysfunctions located in the hypothalamus, adenohypophysis, or ovary. In others, endometrial lesions occur in concert with generalized pelvic disease. In still others, intrinsic endometrial disease is a factor in reproductive failure. Systemic diseases, also impairing fertility, are rarely reflected in endometrial structure.

ENDOMETRIAL BIOPSY

As a practical consideration it is important that the endometrium is readily available for sampling in the intact patient, at little risk, with minimal discomfort and small expense. In general the methods of evaluating a sample are reliable and reproducible, and require care and simple tools but no sophisticated methodology. On the other hand, new knowledge has naturally led to the implementation of increasingly sophisticated measures in the evaluation of the endometrium of normal early pregnancy and, of course, in infertility.

The risks of endometrial biopsy seem to be few. Livengood and coworkers,[10] however, described streptococcal endocarditis in a patient with rheumatic valvular heart disease as a complication of endometrial sampling. Subsequent studies demonstrated transient bacteremia in 4 of 24 nonpregnant, premenopausal women subjected to endometrial brushing and biopsy. On the basis of these observations he recommended consideration of prophy-

lactic antibiotic therapy for women who risk endocarditis if they are subjected to such procedures.

The purpose of the endometrial biopsy is to assure that endometrial structure is normal and to assess its response to the cyclic secretions of the ovary. Endometrial dating, the detailed histologic evaluation of the response to ovarian hormones, should not be attempted if the specimen is abnormal or if it does not include stratum functionale, the superficial region of the endometrium.

Detectable endometrial abnormalities influencing the capacity of the woman to conceive encompass endocrine dysfunctions (endogenous or exogenous), inflammatory diseases, intrinsic structural defects, disorders of growth, and rare miscellaneous disturbances. Occasionally, repetitive inapparent first trimester abortions masquerade as infertility. The accessibility of the uterine lining for sampling can be exploited toward understanding infertility in all such circumstances.

Among infertile women, histologic evaluation of the endometrium serves mainly to *exclude* the presence of occult endometrial disease potentially inimical to implantation. Inferences concerning a woman's hormonal status from a single small sample of endometrium may be questioned. Such samples have greatest value when repeated, analyzed objectively, and then evaluated in context with other data relative to the subject's endocrine status.

To interpret endometrial samples one must be familiar with the histological features of the normal uterine mucosa at various sites. The specimen may include, or even be limited to, the lower uterine segment, where the complex, finely tuned postovulatory responses do not occur. One must also avoid attempting interpretation of endometrium lacking stratum functionale, or obtained from an abnormal site. It is also unwise to attempt dating a diffusely abnormal endometrium. Such tissues may not conform to the profiles of regularly cycling endometria, rendering the resultant report meaningless. When evaluating infertility, it is usually satisfactory to sample the endometrium rather than to perform an exhaustive curettage. Sampling may not yield a true aliquot because some endometrial abnormalities occur only focally. A lesion found in a small tissue fragment is usually interpretable, but such a sample does not exclude focal disease elsewhere in the uterine lining.

DATING THE ENDOMETRIUM

Familiarity with the normal histological features of the endometrium leads to some valid generalizations.[1,2,5,7–9] During the proliferative phase of the endometrium and the follicular phase of the ovary, usually lasting about two weeks, the endometrium—glands, luminal epithelium, stroma, and blood vessels—grows. Gradual thickening of the mucosa occurs as these components proliferate, the glands becoming more tortuous. Gland lumina contain a thin mucoid secretion prior to ovulation. At ovulation the glandular epithelium contains minute subnuclear vacuoles and mitotic activity is brisk. Until then it is appropriate to designate endometrium as early, mid-, and late proliferative if the specimen is adequate for interpretation. Two alternative conventions are used when reporting normal secretory endometria: that which refers to the first day of menses as Day 1 and is based on a 28-day cycle, and that which reports the post-ovulatory day. For example: early stromal predecidua indicates "Secretory endometrium, Day 23" or "Postovulatory, Day 9." Either is satisfactory when used consistently. Beginning on the second day following ovulation, under the stimulus of progesterone, secretory activity becomes evident and increasingly prominent. For the first of two weeks, changes in the glandular epithelium predominate: Cytoplasmic vacuolation becomes greater, vacuoles appear above the nuclei and are then discharged into gland lumina, the secretory product gradually become inspissated, and dilated glands collapse. The second week of the secretory phase is dominated by changes in the stroma. Mitotic activity having ceased in all cellular components by day 19, mitoses resume in the stroma on Day 23 as the stromal cells manifest nuclear and cytoplasmic enlargement. These changes are first noticeable around the spiral arterioles, then involve the stroma under the luminal epithelium (stratum compactum), becoming nearly confluent before regression supervenes. The latter is manifested in the stroma, where intrinsic cells become dissociated, endometrial granulocytes appear, and an influx of inflammatory cells heralds the onset of menstruation, usually beginning on the twenty-eighth day.

Scattered lymphocytes are normally found in the endometrial stroma but are especially numerous as small clusters close to or within the stratum basalis, particularly in the proliferative phase. Such clusters lack germinal centers. Geppert[11] has demonstrated intra-epithelial lymphocytes in normal, cycling endometria. These cells are more numerous in the secretory than in the proliferative phase. Their significance is unknown.

Conventional "routine" evaluation of endometrial samples has been extremely useful. Systematic study of the principal components—glandular epithelium, interglandular supportive stroma and blood vessels—has provided a wealth of clinically valuable information. Consideration of other normal constituents—the luminal epithelium, lymphocytes, macrophages, and neutrophils—has been relatively scant, even using the classical tools of histologic sectioning and ordinary stains. Ultrastructural studies of these components have also been infrequent and unsystematic. Immunohistochemical and -cytochemical evaluation of the stroma and of its various cellular constituents has been minimal. Thus we have a large fund of knowledge about the histological features of glandular epithelium and distinctive endometrial stromal cells during normal cycles and in abnormal states, but we lack information about the more subtle attributes of the tissue. We would expect these to be of physiological importance and to be disturbed in functional derangements of the uterine lining.

Some additional comments are in order concerning the study of the endometrium in relation to infertility. Endometrial dating should follow a consistent system familiar to the pathologist. Fixation (preferably in Bouin's solution), processing into paraffin, and staining (usually with hematoxylin/eosin) should be standardized to assure objective comparisons. The specimen should be evaluated without prior knowledge of the dates of the last menstrual period, the expected next menstrual period, and the shift in basal body temperature. The pathologist should avoid rendering a diagnostic interpretation unless the specimen is obtained from the stratum functionale and is adequate for the purpose intended. When the normal, adequate sample of functionale has been examined and some interpretation made, information concerning the last menstrual period and the presumed time of ovulation should be noted.

The use of this method by experienced pathologists leads to agreement between examiners of plus or minus two days during the secretory phase. If the endometrium, in relation to the timing of ovulation, seems less developed than expected by two days or more it is considered *underdeveloped*. On the other hand, if development is two days or more in advance of what is expected, it is considered *overdeveloped*. This system cannot be applied to endometria appearing more advanced than Day 26 (of a 28-day-cycle) since we lack criteria to recognize over-ripe premenstrual endometrium. Because the reproducibility of the current system is plus or minus two days, a diagnosis that straddles a date, as, for example, 20 to 22 days, is not helpful. This implies a range of 18 to 24 days, useless beyond stating that it is secretory, post-ovulatory, and not premenstrual, endometrium.

ENDOMETRIAL SAMPLING

It is conventional for clinicians attending infertile patients to obtain samples of endometrium for histologic evaluation and for comparison with published and previously observed norms. Opinions among observers differ as to the optimal time when a sample should be taken. Those who prefer it taken at or close to the onset of menstruation minimize the risk of inadvertent interruption of an early pregnancy, while observing endometrial maturation at its fullest and prior to spontaneous breakdown and sloughing. Others prefer to sample before retrogressive changes occur and select a date five or six days prior to expected menstruation as the optimal time. Still others target several times during the postovulatory interval.[12]

According to Jones,[13] an appropriate time for biopsy is late in the luteal phase, around Day 25, before degenerative changes have supervened to obscure the morphologic evidence of appropriate endometrial maturation in response to progesterone secretion. Others suggest that the appropriate day is about Day 7 postovulatory, i.e. when the blastocyst and the endometrial mucosal surface would interact to commence implantation. On Day 12 following ovulation the morphological features of the endometrium normally have peaked, the degenerative changes have not begun, and dating should be easier. The risk of interrupting pregnancy by ill-timed biopsy—when the blastocyst has just been implanted—is denied in some publications. It has even been suggested that biopsy during the cycle of conception may be advantageous because of enhanced decidual reaction following trauma.[7] Of course, hormonal treatment influences target organs, and responses to such treatment may modify endometrial structure, influencing interpretation of samples.

On the assumption that the important criteria to establish are those appropriate for implantation, Noyes recommends that endometrial biopsies be taken on the sixth and ninth days following the shift of basal body temperature and in two successive menstrual cycles.[14] He points out that animal studies, as well as a few isolated observations in human beings, suggest that the blastocyst may survive in, and even prefer to confront, underdeveloped endometrium rather than overdeveloped endometrium.[15] Experimental transfer of embryos in rats, mice, rabbits, and sheep support the view that the blastocyst is not well maintained if it is placed in the uterus when the endometrium is overdeveloped.

In many laboratory animals, localized trauma to the prepared endometrium induces deciduoma formation.[16] It has long been known that focal enhancement of predecidual change, even frank decidualization of endometrial

stroma, also occurs in the human female, in response to intrauterine foreign bodies and occasionally at the surface of a polyp. Dallenbach-Hellweg used a simple probe to produce focal, superficial endometrial trauma in healthy women at various times during the endometrial cycle.[17] Focal decidualization was induced in secretory endometrium. Dallenbach-Hellweg suggests that such premature decidualization may occur as the cleaving zygote is inserted into the uterus following *in vitro* fertilization, and thus may explain some failures of subsequent implantation. The implications of these observations seem even broader, since a similar response may follow endometrial biopsy in the secretory phase and thus preclude or diminish the probability of implantation of an unsuspected blastocyst conceived a few days prior to instrumentation. It should be noted that decidual transformation of the human endometrium does not normally begin until several days following implantation.

In summary, while assessment of endometrial structure is critical in the diagnostic approach to female infertility, optimal use of this approach cannot be realized *in vacuo*. The value of endometrial sampling is significantly increased in a context of clinical correlation involving both the gynecologist and the pathologist. (Table 5–1).

LUTEAL PHASE DEFECTS

This subject is dealt with separately in Chapter 11, but some comments regarding effects on the endometrium are briefly presented here.

That ovarian secretions may fail to sustain endometrial development in some cycles and in some women is intuitively appealing. The diagnosis, "inadequate luteal phase" or "luteal phase defect," has been applied to functional defects that might be responsible for infertility or early spontaneous abortion.[13,18–21] Unfortunately, documentation beyond morphology and simple clinical data has often been unsatisfactory. To expect precise repetition of biological events that are exquisitely responsive to the stresses of everyday life may be naive. Also, confident interpretation of an endometrial biopsy requires an adequate specimen, representative of the functional layer, prepared and read expertly. These specifications are not met in every case. Once limitations of the morphological approach, observer errors, and biological variations are taken into account, confirmation of a significant luteal phase defect mandates successive biopsies during consecutive cycles, interpreted by clinician and pathologist in concert.

Biochemical studies of endometrium[22,23] have been of interest in relation to infertility but have not been of practical value. Similarly, fine structural details[24] have not been illuminating, except in the rare individual case. Of interest is the case report of Pedersen[25] who detected the absence of dynein arms in endometrial cilia in a case of infertility. Such rare associations provide documentation of one component of a clinical complex and satisfy the need of the clinician and patient to understand the basis of the patient's problem as well. Perhaps one effect of an infectious process on endometrium impairing fertility

Table 5–1. Factors Limiting Diagnosis of Endometrial Samples

Attributable to referring *clinician*

Clinical data not provided or inaccurate

Sample procured at inappropriate time

Sample not representative of functional endometrium

Sample insufficient for evaluation

Sample handled or fixed improperly

Attributable to *pathologist*

Inadequate examination of specimen

Sample processed improperly

Poor preparation of microscopic slides

Inadequate care in evaluation of slides

Inadequate experience with endometrium

Observer bias

Attributable to *tissue sample*

Inadequate in quantity

From a non-representative site

Condition of interest occurs only focally

Limited repertoire of histopathologic response

Functional defects without morphological counterpart

might also be mediated through damage to cilia, correctable with appropriate antibiotics.

Possible explanations of the endometrium being unprepared for the blastocyst (in a patient who is ovulating or, obviously, there would be no blastocyst) include inadequate gonadotropic preparation of the developing follicle during the follicular phase or failure to maintain it in the luteal phase and deficiencies of hormone receptors in the endometrium generally or in the area selected by the blastocyst. It has been recommended that the diagnosis of luteal phase defect be invoked when the morphological features of the endometrium imply deficient amounts, or duration, of progesterone secretion by the corpus luteum. Such deficiency is suggested when the endometrium is more than two days out of phase with expectations, based on the time of ovulation. In other instances the secretory endometrium is abnormal: glands and stroma have developed asynchronously and are "out of phase," or some foci of synchronous glands and stroma are in one phase while other foci, also synchronous, are in another phase.[8]

A caveat concerning hypotheses relative to endometrial preparation for blastocyst implantation can be derived from ectopic implantation. The normal oviduct is not supplied with a lamina propria from which to form any substantial quantity of decidua, yet in many instances the blastocyst becomes implanted in the tubal mucosa. Also relevant is the fact that human implantation normally begins before decidualization, or even predecidualization. Thus, while a partnership of the blastocyst and a prepared site are necessary for successful implantation, stromal decidual change is not a prerequisite for this to occur.

Considerable speculation and investigation have focused on aberrations of endocrine preparation of the endometrium that may relate to a woman's capacity to conceive and bear a viable child. Of course, if ovulation fails, fertilization is impossible even though the endometrium has been prepared by progesterone from an unruptured follicle. Similarly, a defective but viable oocyte may be fertilized and cleavage may commence—development then continuing briefly—and sufficient trophoblast may form to sustain the corpus luteum for a short time. The classic work of Hertig and Rock demonstrated morphological defects in a surprisingly high proportion of early conceptuses, both pre- and post-implantation.[25]

ENDOCRINE DISORDERS

Primary disorders of the ovary, the adrenal gland, adenohypophysis, or central nervous system may be reflected in endometrial structure. For example, some tumors of the ovary have effects that mimic those of normal female gonadal secretions. Hyperthecosis and the polycystic ovary syndrome (see Chapter 10) are associated with abnormal endometrial cycles and impaired fertility. Disorders of the adrenal gland and of other endocrine organs also interfere with cyclic endometrial maturation and regression. Finally, some therapeutic tactic or drug may influence the endometrium, either directly or indirectly.

Growth disturbances of the endometrium include abnormal proliferations in response to abnormal levels of trophic and other stimulatory hormones. These tend to occur in women who are not ovulating regularly, but there are also women who complain of infertility in whom focal endometrial hyperplasia or even neoplasia is found at biopsy.[27-34] Aksel et al.[30] described two patients with anovulatory infertility whose endometrial biopsies disclosed very atypical proliferation, one adenomatous and suspected of being localized to a polyp, and the other diagnosed as atypical hyperplasia progressing to a well-differentiated adenoacanthoma. Their observations, like those of others, emphasize that infertility and endometrial neoplasia are linked in many cases to ovarian dysfunction. Although the majority of infertile women are not at increased risk of endometrial carcinoma, a by-product of a thorough diagnostic study may be the chance discovery of an early tumor. According to Barber and Sommers,[34] while less than 5% of cases of endometrial carcinoma occur in women younger than 40 years of age, women at special risk have certain characteristics which include the following: a high incidence of infertility, disturbance of menstruation with menorrhagia, intervals of amenorrhea, abnormal menarche, marked irregularity of cycles, and often polycystic ovary syndrome. Associated ovarian hyperthecosis or excessive follicular luteinization may produce androgens, a source of endogenous hyperestrogenism through peripheral conversion to estrogens. While these changes may reflect a general endocrinopathic diathesis, the condition may be discovered only incidentally during investigations of infertility.

One of the most difficult challenges in gynecologic pathology is that of separating severely atypical endometrial hyperplasia from neoplasia. Conservative management of the young patient with a borderline lesion includes a carefully tailored regimen of progestagen therapy and judiciously timed sampling of the uterine lining. Preservation of reproductive potential leads to gratifying success in some cases. Spontaneous correction of ovarian dysfunction may explain the rare authentic coincidence of pregnancy with endometrial adenocarcinoma. Cutler[35] reported three patients with gonadal dysgenesis treated with diethylstilbestrol who developed adenosquamous carcinoma of the endometrium.

BINDING OF STEROIDS, RECEPTOR CONTENT

Quantifying receptor content of tissue samples is fraught with pitfalls. From their participation in postovulatory differentiation and proliferation, endometrial stromal cells seem likely to develop progesterone receptors. The temporal course of development of receptors in the discrete endometrial components, i.e., the glandular epithelium, luminal epithelium, stromal cells and vessels, has not been delineated. If one considers the small sample of tissue usually obtained at biopsy and its variable content of these constituents, physiologic inferences from analyses of whole specimens seem unwise. Morphological

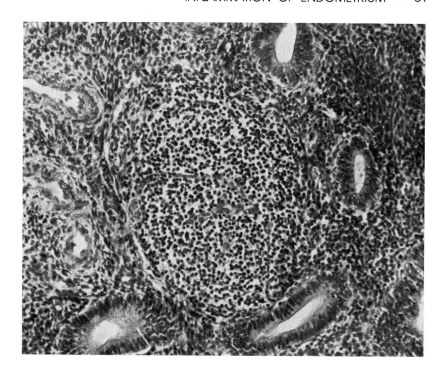

Figure 5–1. Chronic endometritis with dense aggregates of inflammatory cells. The infiltrate of mononuclear cells is located within the stroma adjacent to vascular channels. H & E (×150).

demonstration of the presence, the waxing, and the waning of receptors in the endometrium is a more useful goal in normal and abnormal circumstances.[36–39]

INFLAMMATION OF ENDOMETRIUM

The inflammatory processes affecting fertility are embraced by the term *endometritis* (Figure 5–1). In some communities tuberculous endometritis is commonplace among women suffering from infertility.[40,41] The inflammatory and infectious sequelae of abortion and of the puerperium and reactions to the intrauterine contraceptive device may also initiate inflammatory changes in the endometrium (Figure 5–2). Because the endometrium is sloughed, thus debrided, every four weeks or so when cycles are intact, many infections of the female reproductive organs involve the endometrium only transiently. On the other hand, infection may impair the capacity of the glands to secrete and the stroma to differentiate while

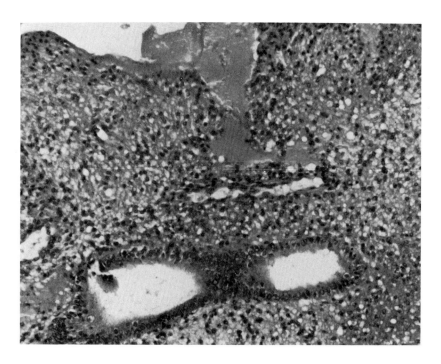

Figure 5–2. Endometrial response to intrauterine device includes breakdown of surface epithelium, stromal edema, and diffuse infiltration of inflammatory cells. H & E (×150).

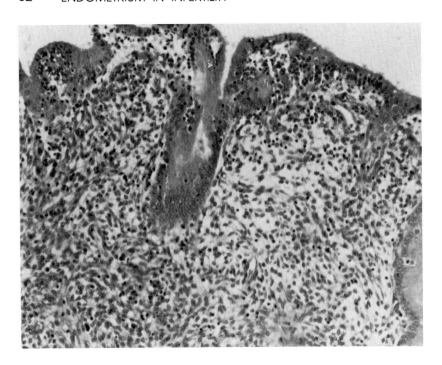

Figure 5–3. Nonspecific chronic endometritis with prominent inflammatory process immediately beneath the surface epithelium. H & E (×150).

recruiting inflammatory cells, including many phagocytes—a reasonable basis for failure of the blastocyst to survive or to implant.[42–46] One mechanism by which the intrauterine contraceptive device exerts contraceptive effects may be that of marshaling inflammatory cells, including phagocytes, to the site where they act against the blastocyst, the spermatozoa, or both.

Myriad species of microorganisms have been implicated in the pathogenesis of endometritis. Actinomyces has been a culprit in pelvic infections associated with intrauterine devices. Bacteria, mycoplasmas, viruses, and protozoa have variously been cited as causes.[47–50] In most cases, the histopathologic picture is nonspecific (Figures 5–3, 5–4) and antibiotic therapy seems to offer reason-

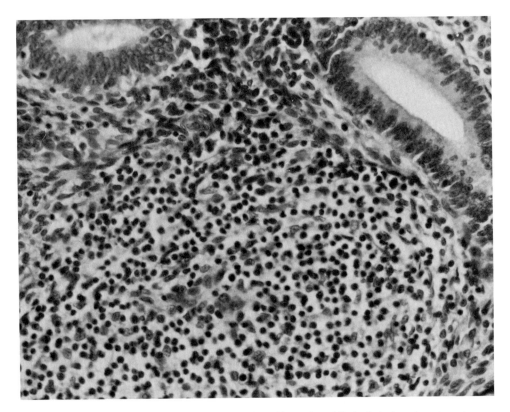

Figure 5–4. Chronic inflammatory cells encountered in endometritis include lymphocytes, plasma cells, and macrophages. H & E (×400).

able prospects for cure. Cultures may be helpful in individual cases when a conventional regimen of treatment has failed. Whether chemical irritation of the endometrium or immune reactions can give rise to endometritis and thus explain infertility is speculative.

While endometritis *per se* may indicate a condition unfriendly to the blastocyst, the concomitant salpingitis in many instances may have greater impact on the capacity of the individual to conceive and carry a pregnancy. Since a variable percentage of patients who have pelvic infections do not cycle regularly, it is difficult to assess the overall impact of endometritis on fertility.

It is commonly believed that the presence of plasma cells in the endometrium constitutes evidence of an abnormal condition. Meticulous survey of normal endometria from asymptomatic women demonstrates rare plasma cells in all specimens, but the presence of numbers sufficient to be easily recognizable is abnormal. During the normal puerperium, however, there is a clinically occult interval of acute, then chronic, endometrial inflammation, characterized first by neutrophils and then by a mixture of lymphocytes, macrophages, and plasma cells. In such circumstances the presence of inflammatory cells does not necessarily imply abnormality. Whether they interfere with implantation is unknown.

Several reports indicate that some women who appear to be infertile actually experience occult early spontaneous abortion.[51,52] Careful monitoring of serum levels of chorionic gonadotropin reveals clinically unsuspected pregnancy, subsequently lost. In some cases endometrial sampling demonstrates a conceptus, indicating a spontaneous miscarriage masquerading as infertility. Whether these processes are related is uncertain. An underlying endometrial abnormality has been suspected which would explain some of them.

SYSTEMIC DISORDERS

Diverse systemic diseases may influence the ovary and its target organs without necessarily contributing significantly to infertility. Those effects may sometimes be suspected from examination of the uterine lining at biopsy or curettage. Bleeding disorders, leukemias, lymphomas, metastatic neoplasms, and sarcoidosis are examples.

IMMUNE PHENOMENA

Recent investigations have addressed issues concerning the relevance of abnormal infiltrates of lymphocytes in the endometrium in the context of various disorders including infertility.[53-56] None of these has reached a level of clinical practicality. The role, if any, of immune phenomena in female infertility is yet to be fully defined. The normal presence of varying populations of lymphocytes, with or without other inflammatory cells, suggests that the immune system of the endometrium is dynamic and important. Immunocytochemical observations may be expected to shed light on this matter.

INTRINSIC UTERINE LESIONS

An intrinsic structural abnormality of the uterus, such as atrophy overlying a submucosal myoma or changes in vascularity, may render the endometrium abnormal.[55-59] Endometrial polyps are sometimes found during the diagnostic evaluation of the infertile patient. Relevance of such lesions to infertility is conjectural. The presence of a polyp may interfere with implantation or influence motility of the uterus. That the uterine mucosa overlying a septum or lining a miniature or malformed uterus can be adequately prepared for implantation and fully evolved placentation seems dubious. One must also take into account reduction of mucosal surface area and diminution in uterine capacity resulting from obliterative endometrial synechiae following trauma or other severe endometrial damage.

References

1. Noyes RW, Hertig AT, Rock J: Dating the endometrial biopsy. Fertil Steril 1:3–25, 1950.
2. Noyes RW, Hertig AT, Rock J: Dating the endometrial biopsy. Am J Obstet Gynecol 122:262–263, 1975.
3. Wagner D, Richart RM, Terner JY: DNA content of human endometrial gland cells during the menstrual cycle. Am J Obstet Gynecol 100:90–97, 1968.
4. Blaustein A: Interpretation of Biopsy of Endometrium. New York, Raven Press, 1980.
5. Hendrickson MR, Kempson RL: Surgical Pathology of the Uterine Corpus. Philadelphia, WB Saunders, 1980.
6. Robertson WB: The Endometrium. London, Butterworths, 1981.
7. Cove H: Surgical Pathology of the Endometrium. Philadelphia, Toronto, Lippincott, 1981.
8. Dallenbach-Hellweg G: Histopathology of the Endometrium (3rd Edition). Berlin, Springer-Verlag, 1981.
9. Dallenbach-Hellweg G, Poulsen H: Atlas of Endometrial Histopathology. Philadelphia, W.B. Saunders, 1985.
10. Livengood CH III, Land MR, Addison WA: Endometrial biopsy, bacteremia, and endocarditis risk. Obstet Gynecol 65:678–681, 1985.
11. Geppert M, Geppert J: Lymphocytes in the epithelial layers of decidua and normal or abnormal endometrium. Arch Gynecol 233:47–51, 1982.
12. Shangold M, Berkeley A, Gray J: Both midluteal serum progesterone levels and late luteal endometrial histology should be assessed in all infertile women. Fertil Steril 40:627–630, 1983.
13. Jones GS: The luteal phase defect. Fertil Steril 27:351–356, 1976.
14. Noyes RW: The underdeveloped secretory endometrium. Am J Obstet Gynecol 77:929–945, 1959.
15. Noyes RW: Normal phases of the endometrium. *In* HJ Norris, AT Hertig, MR Abell, (eds) The Uterus. Ch. 7, pp 110–135. Baltimore, Williams and Wilkins, 1973.
16. Finn CA, Porter DG: The Uterus. Reproductive Biology Handbooks. Vol. 1, pp 74–80. Acton, MA, Publishing Sciences Group, 1975.
17. Dallenbach-Hellweg G, Hohagen F: On the problem of premature decidualization induced by the embryo transfer. Lab Invest 52:17A, 1985.

18. Rosenfeld DL, Garcia CR: A comparison of endometrial histology with simultaneous plasma progesterone determinations in infertile women. Fertil Steril 27:1256–1266, 1976.

19. Shepard MK, Senturia YD: Comparison of serum progesterone and endometrial biopsy for confirmation of ovulation and evaluation of luteal function. Fertil Steril 28:541–548, 1977.

20. Andrews WC: Luteal phase defects. Fertil Steril 32:501–509, 1979.

21. Wentz AC: Endometrial biopsy in the evaluation of infertility Fertil Steril 33:121–124, 1980.

22. Maeyama M, Sudo I, Saito K, et al.: Glycogen estimation by a rapid enzymic method in very small samples of human endometrium: Glycogen content in the endometrium of infertile patients during the menstrual cycle. Fertil Steril 28:159–162, 1977.

23. Soutter WP, Allan H, Cowan S, et al.: A study of endometrial RNA polymerase activity in infertile women. J Reprod Fertil 55:45–52, 1979.

24. Gore BZ, Gordon M.: Fine structure of epithelial cell of secretory endometrium in unexplained primary infertility. Fertil Steril 25:103–107, 1974.

25. Pedersen H: Case Report: Absence of dynein arms in endometrial cilia: cause of infertility? Acta Obstet Gynecol Scand 62:625–627, 1983.

26. Hertig AT, Rock J, Adams EC: A description of 34 human ova within the first 17 days of development. Am J Anat 98:435–499, 1956.

27. Sommers SC, Hertig AT, Bengloff H: Genesis of endometrial carcinoma: II Cases 19–35 years old. Cancer 2: 957–971, 1949.

28. Jackson RL, Dockerty MB: The Stein-Leventhal syndrome: Analysis of 43 cases with special reference to association with endometrial carcinoma. Am J Obstet Gynecol 73:161–173, 1957.

29. Chamlian DL, Taylor HB: Endometrial hyperplasia in young women. Obstet Gynecol 36:659–665, 1970.

30. Aksel S, Wentz AC, Jones GS: Anovulatory infertility associated with adenocarcinoma and adenomatous hyperplasia of the endometrium. Obstet Gynecol 43:386–391, 1974.

31. Fechner RE, Kaufman RH: Endometrial adenocarcinoma in Stein-Leventhal syndrome. Cancer 34:444–452, 1974.

32. Wood GP, Boronow RC: Endometrial adenocarcinoma and polycystic ovary syndrome. Am J Obstet Gynecol 124:140–142, 1976.

33. Dockerty MB, Lovelady SR, Foust GT: Carcinoma of the corpus uteri in young women. Am J Obstet Gynecol 61:966–981, 1951.

34. Barber HRK, Sommers SC: Carcinoma of the Endometrium; Ch 21, pp 175–178. New York, Masson, 1981.

35. Cutler BS, Forbes AP, Ingersoll FM et al.: Endometrial carcinoma after stilbestrol therapy in gonadal dysgenesis. N Engl J Med 287:628–631, 1972.

36. Laatikainen T, Andersson B, Karkkainen J, et al.: Progestin receptor levels in endometria with delayed or incomplete secretory changes. Obstet Gynecol 62:592–595, 1983.

37. Maynard PB, Symonds EM, Johnson J, et al.: Nuclear progesterone uptake by endometrial tissue in cases of subfertility. Lancet, Aug. 6, 310–312, 1983.

38. Press MF, Nousek-Goebl N, King WJ, et al.: Immunohistochemical assessment of estrogen receptor distribution in the human endometrium throughout the menstrual cycle. Lab Invest 51:495–503, 1984.

39. Bergqvist A, Ekman R, Ljungberg O: Binding of estrogen and progesterone to human endometrium in the different phases of the menstrual cycle. Am J Clin Pathol 83:444–449, 1985.

40. Mukerjee K, Wagh KV, Agarwal S: Tubercular endometritis in primary sterility. J Obstet Gynaecol India 17:619–624, 1967.

41. Bazaz-Malik G, Maheshwari B, Lal N: Tuberculous endometritis: a clinicopathological study of 1,000 cases. Br J Obstet Gynaecol 90:84–86, 1983.

42. Dumoulin JG, Hughesdon PE: Chronic endometritis. J Obstet Gynaecol Br Emp 58:222–235, 1951.

43. Rotterdam H: Chronic endometritis: A clinicopathologic study. In SC Sommers, PP Rosen (eds) Pathol Annu Pt. II, 209–231. New York, Appleton-Century-Crofts, 1978.

44. Greenwood SM, Moran JJ: Chronic endometritis: morphologic and clinical observations. Obstet Gynecol 58:176–184, 1981.

45. Paavonen J, Kiviat N, Brunham R. et al.: Prevalence and manifestations of endometritis among women with cervicitis. Am J Obstet Gynecol 152:280–286, 1985.

46. Czernobilsky B.: Endometritis and infertility. Fertil Steril 30:119–130, 1978.

47. Gump DW, Dickstein S, Gibson M.: Endometritis related to Chlamydia trachomatis infection. Ann Intern Med 95:61–63, 1981.

48. Winkler B, Gallo L, Revmann W, et al.: Chlamydial endometritis, a histologic and immunohistochemical analysis. Am J Surg Pathol 8:771–778, 1984.

49. Horne HW, Hertig AT, Kundsin KB, et al.: Subclinical endometrial inflammation and T-Mycoplasma, a possible cause of human reproductive failure. Int J Fertil 18:226–231, 1973.

50. Robb JA, Benirschke K: Intrauterine herpes simplex virus infection in spontaneous abortions: chronic persistent infection detection by glucose oxidase-avidin-biotin immunohistochemistry. Lab Invest 50:50A, 1984.

51. Braunstein GD, Karow WG, Gentry BS: Subclinical spontaneous abortion. Obstet Gynecol 50:41s–44s, 1977.

52. Cline DL Unsuspected subclinical pregnancies in patients with luteal phase defects. Am J Obstet Gynecol 134:438–444, 1979.

53. McDermott MR, Bienenstock J: Evidence for a common immune system I: migration of B immunoblasts into intestinal, respiratory, and genital tissues. J Immun 122:1892–1898, 1979.

54. Daly DC, Tohan N, Doney TJ, et al.: The significance of lymphocytic-leukocytic infiltrates in interpreting late luteal phase endometrial biopsies. Fertil Steril 37:786–791, 1982.

55. Winter AJ: Microbial immunity in the reproductive tract. J Am Vet Med Assoc 181:1069–1073, 1982.

56. Wira CR, Sullivan DA, Sandoe CP: Estrogen-mediated control of the secretory immune system in the uterus of the rat. In JR McGhee, J Mestecky (eds) The Secretory Immune System. Ann NY Acad Sci 409:534–551, 1983.

57. Deligdish L, Loewenthal M: Endometrial changes associated with myomata of the uterus. J Clin Pathol 23:676–680, 1970.

58. Candiani GB, Fedele L, Zamberletti D, et al.: Endometrial patterns in malformed uteri. Acta Eur Fertil 14:311–318, 1983.

59. Burchell RC Creed F: Vascular anatomy of the human uterus and pregnancy wastage. Br J Obstet Gynaecol 85:698–706, 1978.

6. The Fallopian Tube and Infertility

J. Donald Woodruff

The fallopian tube is the site of many of the biological processes which culminate in a normally implanted pregnancy. The principal functions of the tube are gamete transport and provision of a suitable environment for the gametes and for the fertilized ovum during early development. Interference with these functions can result in impaired fertility, or prevention of successful pregnancy outcome if fertilization does occur. In this chapter, consideration is given to the normal physiology of the fallopian tube and to pathophysiologic alterations, particularly as they relate to fertility.

Named by Fallopius in 1561 because of its similarity to the tuba, the fallopian tube represents the cephalic end of the paramesonephric duct. At this terminus, it is compressed between the receding pronephros and the large mesonephric body with its adjacent gonad[1] (Figure 6–1). This compression accounts for the development of fimbria and the frequency with which accessory lumina, demonstrated most dramatically by the hydatid of Morgagni, are found in the ampulla and infundibulum of the tube.

Dilatation of these accessory lumina produces a majority of the paraovarian cysts[2] (Figure 6–2). Such lesions were previously felt to originate from the mesonephric duct and its tubules. In retrospect, the latter thesis is unrealistic. There is a firm musculature around the mesonephric structures, thus limiting the possibility of dilatations, and there is little secretory activity of the epithelium. Thus, the possibility of cyst formation is unlikely.[3] Nevertheless, these structures are routinely present in the paratubal region, more specifically between the tube and ovary (Figure 6–3). The secretory cells of the fallopian tube are extremely active cyclically and with the occlusion of distal and/or proximal ends of the accessory lumen, will dilate and form a hydrosalpinx[4] (Figure 6–4). Such structures, occluded at the terminal end but patent to the main lumen, could represent a nidus for the development of a tubal pregnancy. This situation is, undoubtedly, uncommon since the fertilized egg would have to be diverted in its passage down the tube into one of the diverticula and this sequence of events would represent an action against the main stream, i.e., from fimbriated end to uterus. Nevertheless, examples of pregnancy in accessory lumina have been undeniably demonstrated.

In addition to the mesonephric tubules noted in the paraovarian area, other unique structures are occasionally noted adjacent to the tube. Adrenal rests are not uncommon and are usually found in the paratubal rather than the paraovarian region. What part these structures play in the genesis of the adrenal tumor is still controversial.[5] Peritoneal inclusions adjacent to the tube commonly demonstrate squamous metaplasia and these foci are known as Walthard's islets or rests (Figure 6–5). This shows clearly that such processes, more commonly demonstrated in the Brenner tumor, are representative of squamous metaplasia, on peritoneal surfaces, rather than of urothelial origin.

ANATOMY

Anatomically, the tube is divided into the cornual portion, approximately 1 cm in length, the isthmus 1–2 cm, the ampulla 3–5 cm, and the infundibulum with its fimbriated end approximately 1 cm. Thus, the entire length of the normal fallopian tube varies from 6–15 cm with an average length of 8–10 cm.[6,7]

The cornual portion of the tube actually lies within the uterine wall and the lumen in this area with the adjacent isthmus is approximately 100–500 μm in diameter (Figure 6–6). As a result, it is obvious that the fertilized egg, usually 200–250 μm by the time it enters the uterine cavity, could be mechanically obstructed at this point. In the cornual portion, the lumen of the fallopian tube is lined originally by endometrium as it enters into the uterine cavity. Although the autochthonous musculature of the fallopian tube is circular, at the cornua the extension of the adjacent myometrium is demonstrated by longitudinal bundles of uterine smooth muscle in the subserosal region. Consequently, although the peristalsis is largely a segmental "milking process," there is action by the longitudinal element which assists in the propulsion of intraluminal material. The extension of the muscle into the fimbria undoubtedly assists in ovum pick-up. In this area and extending throughout the isthmus into the fimbria is a longitudinal smooth muscle band beneath the epithelium.

The endometrial lining in the cornual portion and the

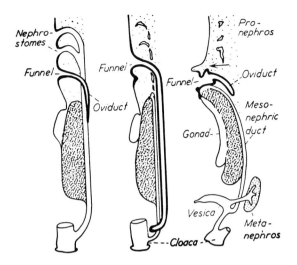

Figure 6–1. Demonstration of the embryology in the region of the developing oviduct. Note the compression between the pronephros and the mesonephric body. (From Witschi.[1])

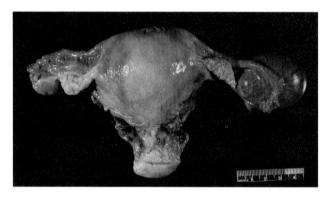

Figure 6–2. Bilateral parovarian cysts, larger on right, two small cysts on left.

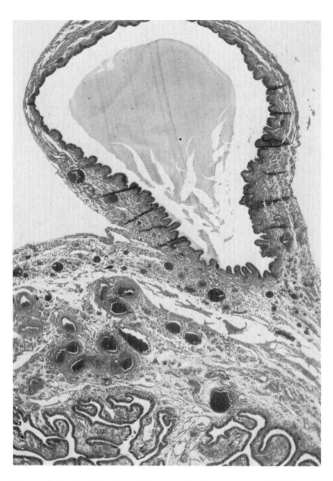

Figure 6–4. Paratubal cyst showing flattened mucosal folds with attenuated muscle surrounding the lumen.

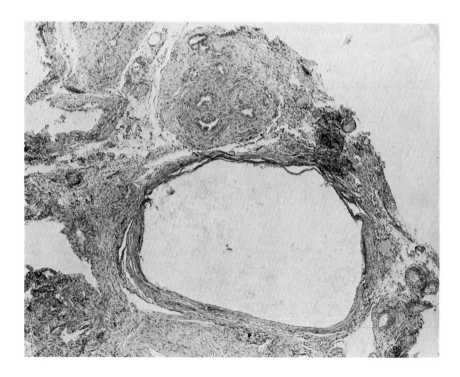

Figure 6–3. Mesonephric tubules (upper center) with dilated mesonephric duct below.

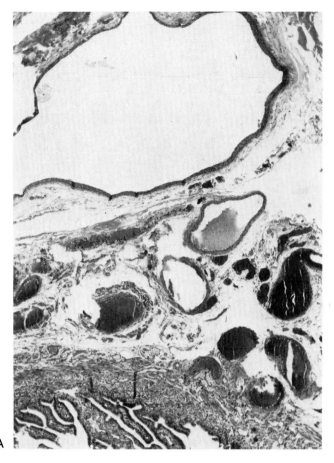

A

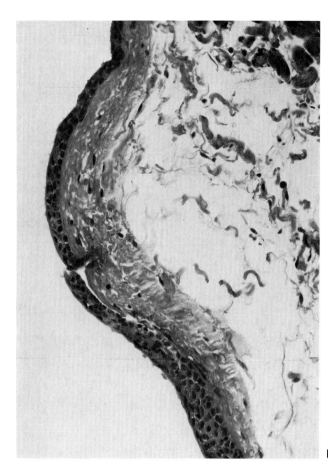

B

Figure 6–5. A. Peritoneal inclusion adjacent to fallopian tube. Note beginning squamous metaplasia. B. High power of metaplasia seen in peritoneal inclusion cyst in Figure 6–5A.

immediately adjacent isthmus explains the frequency with which "tubal polyps" have been reported. These gradually disappear, to be supplanted by the scant periarterial muscle. The luminal folds in this region appear in the so-called "Grecian cross configuration" with its four indentations into the small lumen. Endometrial stroma commonly extends into the isthmus, and "invasion" of the muscle by the endometrium, similar to the pattern seen in adenomyosis, is undoubtedly the process producing "salpingitis isthmica nodosa" (Figure 6–7). The decidual reaction in this endometrium during pregnancy could decrease the luminal diameter and represent an additional contribution to the development of ectopic pregnancy. Many investigators have noted the frequency with which salpingitis isthmica nodosa is found in the patient with tubal pregnancy in the absence of any definitive evidence of a true infectious process.

Progressing into the ampullary portion of the tube, its longest component, the inner longitudinal muscle is lost and the circular muscle becomes predominant. The only longitudinal muscle in this area is vascular musculature. The mucosal folds in the ampulla become more complex and intricate. There is a minimal amount of musculature present in the mucosal folds and it is particularly concentrated where the blood supply, present usually at a solitary thickened focus, enters from the mesosalpinx at the antimesenteric border (Figure 6–8). Classically, the vessels are branches from the ovarian and ascending branches of the uterine arteries.

The musculature is well defined in the infundibulum as it progresses into the fimbria. It is in this area that the accessory lumina are more commonly found and they can be demonstrated by the presence of an epithelial lining consisting of ciliated, secretory, and mesothelial cells, and a minimal amount of circular muscle;' the last feature demonstrating a tubal origin to the structure (Figure 6–4). The fimbria are delicate finger-like projections extending from the infundibulum into the abdominal cavity. Each has its individual muscular component which helps in encompassing the ovary at the time of ovulation, thus assisting in ovum pick-up. The importance of the fimbria cannot be overemphasized. Without their presence, tuboplastic procedures are rarely, if ever, successful.

As would be expected, the tube has both a sympathetic and parasympathetic nerve supply; the former is derived from L1-L4 and the latter from S1-S2. Consequently, a sphincter is produced. This was felt to be important in the progression of the fertilized egg through the tube with a delay of 24–36 hours at the ampullary-isthmic junction due to this nerve supply. Although such a delay is appreciated, as is a similar physiologic obstruction at

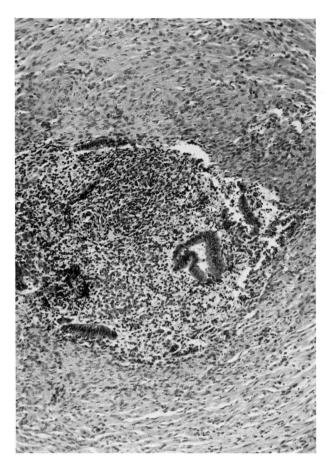

Figure 6–6. Cornual portion of tube as it enters uterus. Stroma and glands are endometrial.

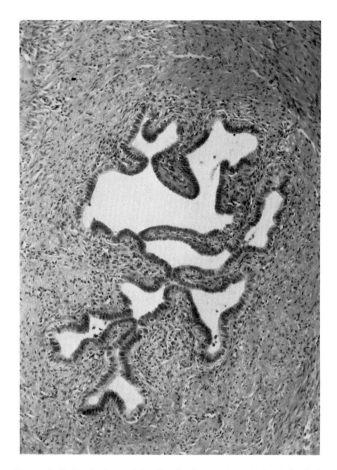

Figure 6–7. Beginning salpingitis isthmica nodosa. Note similarity to superficial adenomyosis. Also note endometrial stroma.

the cornua, recent studies cast doubt on the significance of the neural pathways.

HISTOLOGY

The cellular components of the fallopian tube are divided into four varieties (Figure 6–9).[6,7] The ciliated and secretory cells are found throughout; however, near the fimbriated end, the ciliated component is most prominent and, conversely, the secretory elements stand out in the isthmus. This is functionally appropriate since ciliated action at the fimbria assists in "ovum pick-up" while the secretory cells contribute to nutrition of the fertilized egg as it progresses toward the uterus. The fimbria ovarica are extensions of the normal fimbria and progress over the adjacent peritoneal surface (Figure 6–10). These may assist in directing the ovum into the tubal lumen.

The ciliated cells remain constant in their size throughout the length of the fallopian tube as well as throughout the cycle. In contrast, the secretory cells demonstrate the cyclic alterations by actively secreting during the progestational phase. These definitive cell types are easily identified. The ciliated cell has a centrally placed nucleus with a perinuclear halo and definable surface cilia, usually 9–

11 in number. In contrast, the nucleus of the secretory cell varies in its position depending on the cycle and, during the progestational phase, the nucleus may actually be extruded into the lumen. The intercalary, or peg, cell represents a secretory cell which has extruded its secretion and the cell walls have collapsed around the residual nucleus. One of the most interesting of the cell types is the controversial undifferentiated (indifferent) cell. This cell is recognized readily throughout the upper genital canal. In the cervix it is known as the reserve or subcolumnar cell and in the tube as the indifferent cell. Although poorly recognized in the endometrium, it is nevertheless present and takes part in regeneration of the surface epithelium. In the fallopian tube this basally placed cell has been studied metabolically by the use of tritiated thymidine and acridine orange fluorescence; it is the most active of the epithelial elements. Since mitoses are rarely if ever seen in the normal fallopian tube, this indifferent cell may be of significance in replication of the epithelium. It is quite proliferative in the infected tube and thus may contribute to repair of the damaged surface as in the endometrium.

Other alterations in the epithelium of the fallopian tube demonstrate its relationship to the paramesonephric system. Endometriosis is not uncommon. Sim-

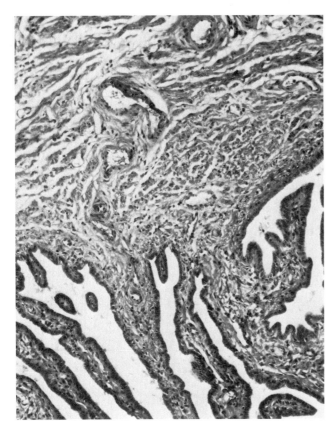

Figure 6–8. Entering core of vessels from mesosalpinx, main focus of vascularity in normal tube. There are a few inner longitudinal muscle bundles. Beyond, the circular muscle.

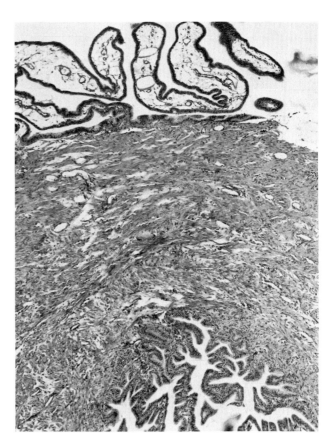

Figure 6–10. Tubal lumen with fimbria ovarica on serosal surface adjacent to fimbria.

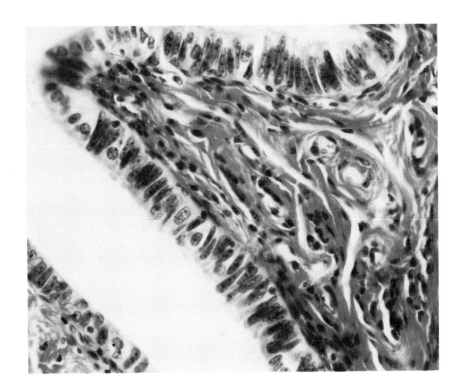

Figure 6–9. Normal tubal epithelium: ciliated cells with perinuclear halos, groups of secretory cells with nuclei at luminal border, peg cell in low middle, and indifferent cells at base (small round nuclei).

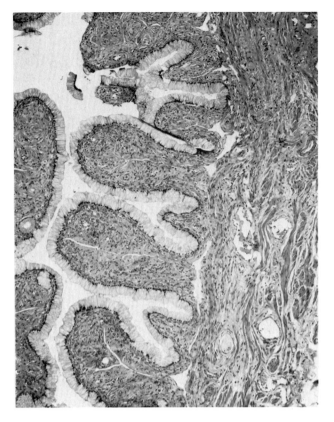

Figure 6–11. Normal tube lined by metaplastic mucin-secreting (endocervical type) epithelium.

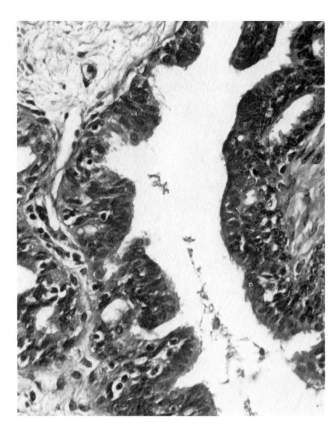

Figure 6–12. Proliferation of the tubal epithelium in a patient with endometrial carcinoma.

ilarly, mucus-secreting epithelium, a type of endocervical metaplasia, is recognized on rare occasions (Figure 6–11). Finally, neoplastic changes similar to those found in the endometrium may be seen in the fallopian tube. On rare occasions, adenocarcinoma of the endometrium

and/or epithelial ovarian neoplasia are found in conjunction with tubal malignancy.[8] They represent multifocal disease and in most instances are *not* demonstrations of metastatic cancer but rather examples of the responsiveness of the paramesonephric epithelia to proliferating

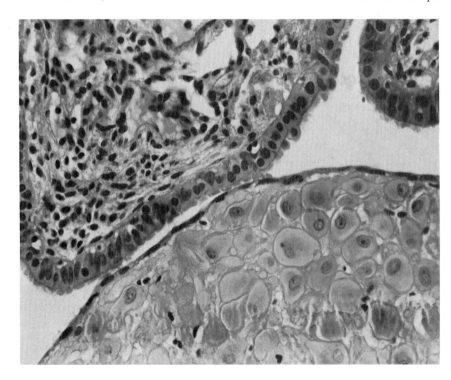

Figure 6–13. Marked decidual reaction in fallopian tube. Note relatively low epithelial cells in the tube during pregnancy.

stimuli. In addition to these neoplastic alterations at multiple sites in the upper genital canal, epithelial proliferations are seen in response to prolonged estrogen stimulation and are similar to those associated with endometrial hyperplasia and well differentiated uterine cancer (Figure 6–12).

HORMONE RESPONSES AND REACTIONS TO MEDICATIONS

The fallopian tube demonstrates well-defined histologic alterations in response to cyclic estrogen and progester-

one, as noted above. Similarly there are classic alterations in response to the hormones of pregnancy. Decidual reactions are frequent, most commonly seen in the cornual portion, but they may be noted in other areas (Figure 6-13). The postpartum residua of these decidual reactions may be demonstrated by a fibrotic hyalinized nodule impinging on the tubal lumen (Figure 6–14). The latter has been misinterpreted as leiomyoma but actually represents fibrosed decidua, a condition similar to that seen in the peritoneal surfaces and identified as leiomyomatosis peritonealis disseminata.

Epithelial changes during pregnancy are typical. Both varieties of epithelial cells are lower and less active. In

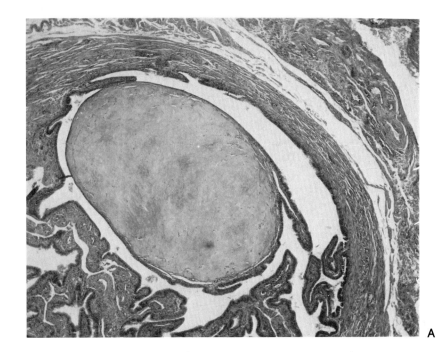

A

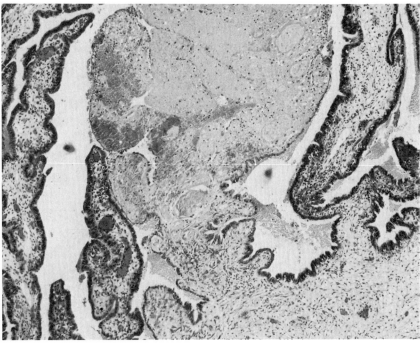

Figure 6–14. A. Fibrotic hyaline nodule in lumen of tube, probably representative of hyalinized decidua. B. Focus of degenerating decidua in tube suggestive of tubal polyp or myoma.

B

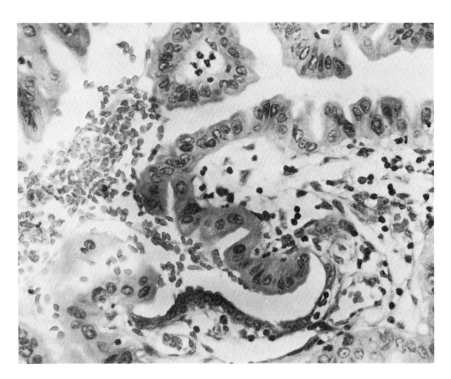

Figure 6–15. Flat epithelium of the tube during pregnancy in low middle area, in contrast to the large clear cells in center. The so-called "metaplastic tumor" seen in association with pregnancy.

contrast, the lesion known as metaplastic tumor of the fallopian tube represents a unique response to hormones of pregnancy simulating the Arias-Stella reaction in the endometrium. The cells are large with abundant clear cytoplasm and often hyperchromatic nuclei appear at the luminal edge (Figure 6–15). Thus, the metaplastic tumor of the fallopian tube is not a neoplasm but a reaction to pregnancy. The largest number of such cases have been found in tubes removed in the process of sterilization, giving circumstantial evidence to validate this thesis. Furthermore, there are no reports of subsequent development of adnexal neoplasia in tubes resulting from such lesions.[8]

Oral contraceptives produce reactions in the fallopian tube similar to those seen during pregnancy. The epithelial cells, both secretory and ciliated, are relatively flat and there is a lack of secretory activity. Undoubtedly, this lack of normal activity plays a pertinent role in the effectiveness of the medication, although anovulation is the major factor.

Demonstrations of reactions to estrogen are noted most prominently in patients with endometrial hyperplasia and carcinoma. The typical features of estrogen stimulation are multilayering of the epithelium and a rare mitosis. With these demonstrations of abnormal proliferation, there is no evidence of secretory activity and both secretory and ciliated cells are of similar height.

FUNCTIONS OF THE FALLOPIAN TUBE[9,10]

Sperm Transport

Normal ejaculates contain about 100 million sperm, nearly all of which die and are absorbed. Only thousands enter the oviduct, and only tens reach the site of fertiliza-

tion. The chief sites of elimination are the cervix, the utero-tubal junction, and the isthmus. The need for millions of sperm in the ejaculate may be related to the mechanism of transport to the ampulla.

Sperm have been recovered from human oviducts within five minutes after being placed on the cervix. The ascent of sperm from the vagina to the oviduct thus occurs more rapidly than the intrinsic motility of the sperm would explain.

Capacitation

Freshly ejaculated sperm or epididymal sperm have poor fertilizing ability. The enhancement of fertilizing ability is called "capacitation." Capacitated sperm can be decapacitated by exposure to seminal or epididymal fluid and then recapacitated in the fallopian tubes.

Ovum Pick-up

The infundibular portion of the tube is brought into apposition with the ovary at ovulation by movement of the tubal musculature. The tubal fimbria hold the inferior pole of the ovary for several minutes, during which time the ovum is conducted into the ampulla by action of the fimbria on the cumulus mass. Pick-up of the ovum can also occur from the cul-de-sac in some cases, as women with an ovary on one side and an oviduct on the other side sometimes become pregnant. Currents caused by cilia and direct cilial mechanisms are involved.

Ovum Capacitation

The ovum has a finite fertilizable life span which varies with the species tested. Some pregnancy wastage has been attributed to fertilization of an aged ovum. Removal of the corona radiata from rabbit tubal ova affects the fertilizing ability of the egg. When exposed to sperm two to four hours after ovulation, 50% of denuded eggs are fertilized as compared with 88% of eggs that retain the corona. If exposure is delayed until the sixth hour, only 12% of the eggs without the corona are fertilized, as compared with 60% of the eggs with corona. Denudation of the corona may limit the length of time during which the ovum can be fertilized.

Fertilization

Besides causing physiologic changes in the ovum prior to fertilization, tubal fluid provides a *sufficient* environment for *in vitro* fertilization of the rabbit egg. However, the tubal environment is not *necessary* for fertilization, providing the spermatozoa have been previously capacitated.

Zygote Transport

Once fertilized, the ovum pauses at the ampullary-isthmic junction. The duration of the pause appears to be rather precisely timed and successful nidation depends upon this timing within fairly narrow limits. The delay in ovum transit is an integral part of the sequence of events leading to successful implantation.

Ovum transport into the rabbit uterus can be accelerated by the prior injection of progesterone and delayed by injection of estrogen. The mechanisms by which the ovarian hormones alter ovum transport rates are currently under investigation.

Transport of Particulate Material

Fragments of endometrium are commonly noted in the lumen of the tube, particularly during the menses. Bits of tumor may be transported from the pelvic cavity into the vagina and subsequently noted in cytologic preparations. The most common finding is the so-called psammoma body. Finally, foreign material will be carried from the vagina into the abdominal cavity via the tube. This material is subsequently noted in various sites throughout the pelvic cavity, most commonly in the ovarian cortex, and erroneously called psammoma bodies. Recent studies identify this material as being largely magnesium, calcium, and aluminum. Thus, foreign material deposited in the vagina will reach the abdominal cavity if the tubes are patent, depending on particle size, in approximately 25 minutes. Talc appears to be the most common material containing these elements.

ENDOMETRIOSIS

As noted previously, physiologic changes in the fallopian tube simulate those described in the endometrium during the normal cycle, as well as those present during pregnancy and associated with neoplasia. Endometriosis is common at the cornual portion where extensions of the endometrium from the corpus may result in the production of endometrial polyps, often erroneously interpreted as tubal polyps, although no pathologic study has documented the histopathologic features of such lesions. Finally, true tubal polyps have rarely been identified.

It must be re-emphasized that salpingitis isthmica nodosa is for the most part not infectious in origin but is representative of endometriosis or adenomyosis. Such adenomatous changes may extend throughout a somewhat thickened wall of the tubal isthmus. The association of salpingitis isthmica nodosa and tubal pregnancy must be noted and may well be related to reduction in the caliber of the lumen by the adenomatous process and the decidual changes during early pregnancy.

Although the cornu is the most common site at which endometrium is found within the fallopian tube, it is by no means the only site of endometriosis. Rarely, large segments of tubal mucosa may consist of typical endometrium (Figure 6–16). Since the tube and its lamina propria are part of the paramesonephric system, such findings are demonstrations of the multipotency of this system. Finally, endometriosis is noted on the peritoneal surfaces of the tube and may exhibit normal tubal function and contribute to the infertility so commonly associated with this protean disease.

One of the most interesting aspects of fallopian tube endometriosis has been recognized in patients who have had prior tubal ligations and are being studied for the feasibility of reanastomosis.[11] Hysterosalpingography performed in such cases has commonly demonstrated a

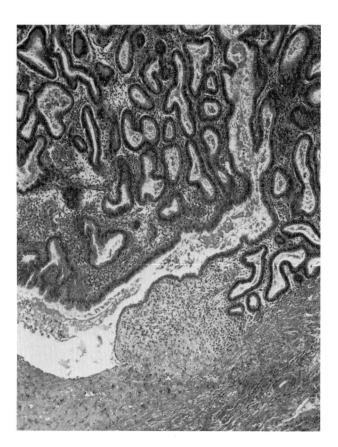

Figure 6–16. Extensive endometriosis of the fallopian tube.

fistulous tract extending from the site of tubal occlusion through the tubal wall and into the peritoneal cavity. This fistulous tract is lined by endometrium—a magnificent demonstration that desquamated endometrium, lodged at a particular point in the tube or on any peritoneal surface, may convert that surface epithelium (mesothelium) into an endometrial type, probably by the process of metaplasia. This basic thesis was presented in 1931 by Everett[12] who suggested a possible tubal origin of endometriosis. The current findings following tubal ligation demonstrate the validity of Everett's point of view.

Desquamated endometrium is commonly seen in the fallopian tube at the time of menstruation. Typically this endometrium passes through the fallopian tube into the abdominal cavity where it may irritate the peritoneal surfaces, with the subsequent development of endometriosis. Obviously, this would be an uncommon finding if the fallopian tube were occluded at the cornual portion by salpingitis or any obstructive process. Usually the endometrium desquamated into the fallopian tube is found during the menstrual period. Nevertheless, on occasion, endometrium at various stages of the cycle may be found in the lumen (Figure 6–17). It is possible that irregular shedding, trauma, or endometrial polyps may account for such findings.

Lastly, it seems quite possible that endometriosis in the fallopian tube, responding to the hormones with production of decidua, may either by mechanical obstruction or the presence of suitable tissue for implantation or both be related to the development of tubal pregnancy.

SPONTANEOUS OR IATROGENIC TRAUMA TO THE FALLOPIAN TUBE

Torsion

Torsion of the fallopian tube[13,14] is more common than usually recognized and should be appreciated as a cause of acute pelvic pain (Figure 6–18A), not infrequently associated with pregnancy. Torsion is most commonly associated with a pre-existing essentially normal tube; although on rare occasions such a process develops with hydrosalpinx. Ordinarily it would seem unlikely for such a problem to develop in the diseased adnexa since the associated adhesive disease would prevent movement to a major degree. The most common cause of torsion is that associated with an ovarian tumor, particularly the dermoid cyst. These lesions are freely movable and may, in the process of normal patient activity, arrive at a position anterior to the broad ligament. In such a situation, with prolapse over the broad ligament, the blood supply is jeopardized. Thus, both the tube and tumor may be infarcted. On rare occasions such infarction may lead to autoamputation of the tube and the occasional finding of a calcified mass in the cul-de-sac associated with absent adnexa is indicative of such a sequence of events (Figure 6–18B). To differentiate between the autoamputated adnexa and the congenital absence of one adnexa, it is important to appreciate the stump of the adnexa at the cornu in the former situation.

Tubal Ligation

The trauma associated with tubal ligation, particularly the application of such instruments as the fallope ring, is usually found when the patient is operated on for reanastomosis of the tube. Scarring is found in the area, and often a dilated tube can be recognized in the proximal portion (Figure 6–19). It has already been noted that a fistula may develop following procedures such as tubal ligation in approximately 25% of the cases within two years; such fistulae are lined by endometrium. This sequence of events dramatically demonstrates the ability of desquamated endometrium, when it is contained in a closed space, to convert the paramesonephric epithelium into an endometrial type.

NEOPLASIA

Benign tumors of the fallopian tube are extremely uncommon, and rarely, if ever, a cause of infertility or eccyesis. Nevertheless, they should be recognized for their uniqueness and unusual histopathology. The metaplastic tumor, previously mentioned, is an Arias-Stella-like reaction to pregnancy and thus not a true neoplasm. Further-

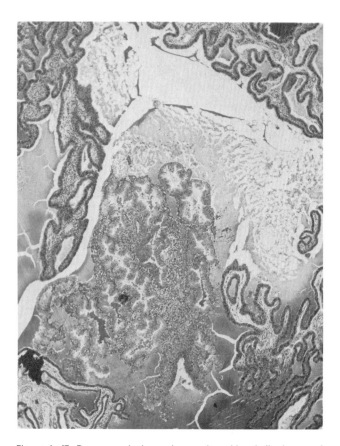

Figure 6–17. Desquamated secretory endometrium in the lumen of a normal tube.

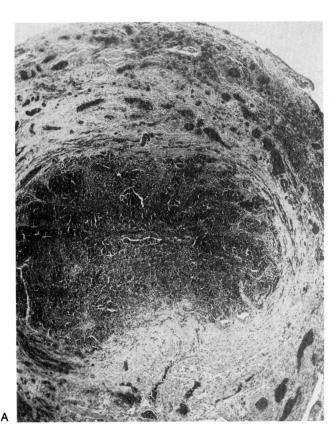 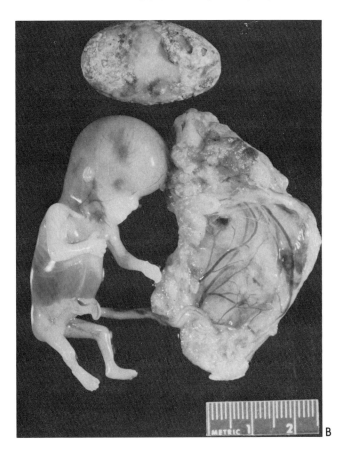

Figure 6–18. A. Acutely infarcted tube. Note vascularity of subserosal vessels and obliteration of lumen. B. Unilateral extrauterine pregnancy. Opposite tube and ovary were absent. Note calcified mass in upper portion of illustration resulting from autoamputation of contralateral adnexa.

more, most of the myomas of the tube are probably fibrotic reactions in pre-existing decidua. The most common true benign tubal neoplasm is the adenomatoid lesion. This tumor has been identified for years and often misdiagnosed as angioma, lymphangioma, or low-grade adenocarcinoma. Currently, on the basis of electron-microscopic studies, it is classified as being of mesothelial origin (Figure 6–20). This lesion is rarely more than 1.5–2 cm in size, is asymptomatic, and is usually an incidental laboratory finding. The most significant feature of the adenomatoid tumor is the recognition that, in spite of its glandular pattern, it is benign.[15] The same lesion may be found in areas adjacent to the tube, specifically on the posterior surface of the uterus and the peritoneal surface of the ovary. The latter could be erroneously misinterpreted as metastases.

Malignant tumors are uncommon, making up only a 3% to 5% of all pelvic malignancies. They occur most often in the 6th decade of life and so do not represent a threat to the infertile patient.

INFLAMMATORY DISEASE

Inflammatory disease of the tube and adjacent ovary represents one of the major challenges to our society, not only medically but economically. Currently, about 250,000 patients with PID (pelvic inflammatory disease) are admitted to hospitals in the United States each year. Treatment costs about 4 billion dollars a year. Consequently, it is of major importance that such lesions be identified early and treated adequately to avoid lengthy, expensive hospitalizations and destructive surgery, and often removal of the pelvic organs (Figure 6–21). The question of whether early admission of the patient with PID and the institution of appropriate therapy in a controlled environment would avoid more disastrous sequelae remains to be determined.

The varieties of salpingitis have been well identified. Acute infection generally ascends from the lower genital canal. Although approximately 25% to 40% are gonococcal in origin, currently Chlamydia has been implicated more commonly, and a mixed bacterial flora, including the coliform bacilli, streptococci, and staphylococci, and the anaerobes, are frequently cultured. It is obviously important to identify the agent or agents in order to institute the most appropriate therapy.

In addition to the ascending infections there are postabortal or postpartum inflammatory reactions. The latter are not uncommon and may result in parametritis and associated perisalpingitis. Under such circumstances the endosalpinx may be relatively unaffected and intrauterine pregnancy is more of a postinfection possibility. Fur-

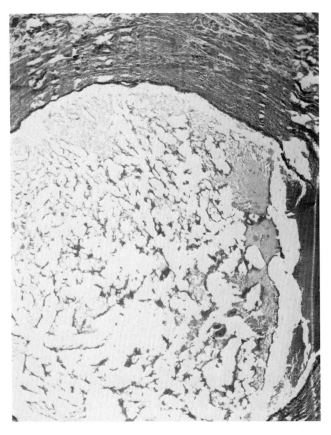

Figure 6–19. Dilatation of tubal lumen in area of resection post-tubal ligation.

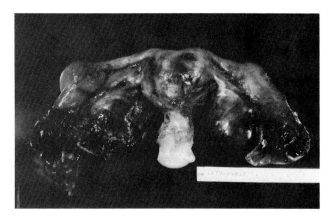

Figure 6–21. Bilateral tuboovarian inflammatory masses (PID).

thermore, particularly in those inflammatory conditions associated with an IUD, it is not uncommon to find one adnexal region relatively uninvolved. Thus, the tube may be salvaged, a rare possibility with the usual endo-salpingitis associated with the common ascending infections.

In the patient with the typical acute endosalpingitis, the tube is edematous and the fimbria are patent. Microscopic study reveals a lumen filled with an exudate of polymorphonuclear cells (Figure 6–22). Nevertheless, in contrast to the pyosalpinx, there is little or no agglutination of the mucosal folds and the myosalpinx is not thickened. Adhesions, if present, are filmy in contrast to the

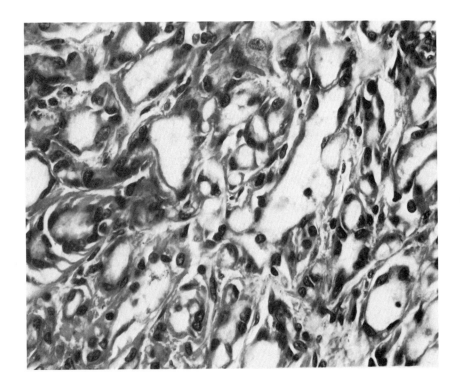

Figure 6–20. Adenomatoid tumor of the fallopian tube. Pattern suggests malignancy but lesion is a benign tumor of mesothelial origin.

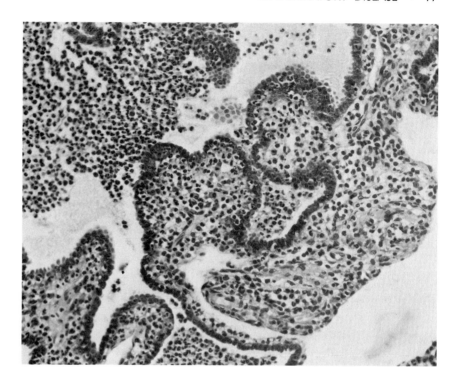

Figure 6–22. Endosalpingitis, acute, with purulent material in lumen and dilated edematous folds but no agglutination.

dense fibrous reaction seen in the recurrently infected organ.

Adequate treatment during the initial phase of the acute disease results in minimal distortion of the tube. There is an approximate 85% possibility for a normal intrauterine pregnancy.[16] Conversely, after three or more episodes, fertility is reduced to 10% to 15%. It should be noted that the current increase in tubal pregnancy may well be related to the early treatment of tubal disease with resultant tubal patency but disturbances in the normal passage of the fertilized egg.

Chronic tubal disease is classically demonstrated by agglutination of the mucosal folds, thickening of the lamina propria and muscularis, and often a perisalpingitis due to the associated peritonitis. The adenomatous pattern in the lumen produced by this chronic inflammatory process may be misinterpreted as neoplastic (Figure 6–23). The proliferation of the epithelium, particularly the indifferent cell, emphasizes this histologic atypicality (Figure 6–24). The submucosal infiltrate is characterized by the plasma cell, although lymphocytes and polymorphonuclear elements are frequently recognized, particularly in the recurrently infected tube.

Follicular salpingitis usually results from a relatively mild insult to the mucosal surfaces. The agglutination of the folds is minimal and the fimbriated end is often patent. As a consequence, fertilization is quite possible. Nevertheless, the intricate pattern results in the formation of blind pockets and a resultant obstruction to the normal passage of the fertilized egg (Figure 6–25). Follicular salpingitis is a common finding in the tube adjacent to an eccyesis.[17]

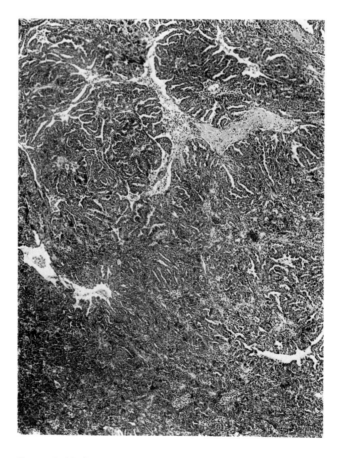

Figure 6–23. Severe chronic salpingitis showing adenomatous change suggestive of malignancy.

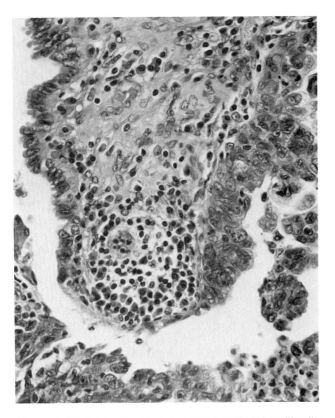

Figure 6–24. Salpingitis showing marked epithelial proliferation suggestive of neoplasia.

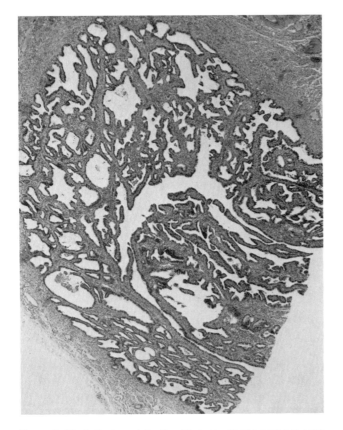

Figure 6–25. Follicular salpingitis with many small pockets in folds and questionably patent lumen.

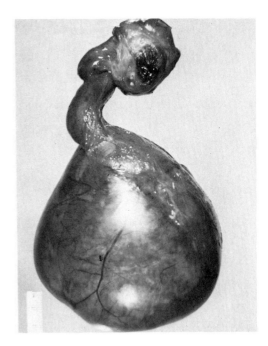

Figure 6–26. Large hydrosalpinx.

Hydrosalpinx, simplex or follicularis, and pyosalpinx are other varieties of chronic disease. These are due to obstruction at both the cornual and fimbriated ends of the tube. Hydrosalpinx simplex is the result of an acute process which occludes both ends of the tube (Figure 6–26). The purulent material thus acutely distends the lumen. With resorption of the pus, there is a residual clear or cloudy fluid and little agglutination of the mucosal folds. The epithelium lining such a tube is low and flat; however, in the remaining tubal folds characteristic ciliated and secretory cells may be recognized. The distortion of the tubal architecture and thinning of the muscular wall prevent normal tubal function even though patency may be restored by salpingostomy. A rare finding with chronic salpingitis is hematosalpinx. However, until proven otherwise, the latter should be considered the result of tubal pregnancy with its associated intraluminal hemorrhage. Nevertheless, neoplasia, trauma, and endometriosis are potential etiologies. The tuboovarian inflammatory complex represents the most serious of the infectious processes in the adnexa. In the acute phase, appropriate antibiotic therapy, bed rest in a lithotomy position, and careful monitoring of the vital signs are necessary. In the chronic state with recurrent febrile episodes and pain, surgery is indicated, usually hysterectomy and bilateral salpingo-oophorectomy.

COMPLICATIONS OF PELVIC INFLAMMATORY DISEASE

Pelvic pain, unilateral or bilateral, is a common post-pelvic inflammatory disease problem. Rarely is this incapacitating; nevertheless, recurrent episodes impair performance of routine duties. Too often pelvic pain in the female is interpreted as an indication of inflammatory disease. The symptoms of recurrent midcycle pain with no history of infertility does not necessarily make the patient a candidate for the diagnosis of PID. Recent laparoscopic studies indicate that the clinical diagnosis of PID is erroneous in 35–40% of the cases.

On rare occasions, right upper quadrant pain may be the result of a more diffuse peritonitis originating in the pelvis. Formerly associated with gonococcal disease, the "violin string" adhesions between the liver and adjacent peritoneal surfaces can produce symptoms suggestive of gallbladder disease. The Curtis-Fitzhugh syndrome is a rare entity which indicates the extent of the peritonitis associated with salpingitis.

Rupture of an adnexal abscess may occur spontaneously; mortality approached 90% prior to the institution of definitive surgery, namely hysterectomy and bilateral salpingo-oophorectomy. Attempts at surgical drainage alone were routinely unsuccessful unless a cul-de-sac abscess could be defined, but this was successful only before rupture. With the advent of current antibiotic therapy, radical surgery is rarely necessary. Still, the threat of rupture is always present.

Infertility is the most common and troublesome complication of pelvic inflammatory disease. The results of early and appropriate antibiotic therapy were alluded to in the discussion of salpingitis. The disappointing results of tuboplastic procedures for the badly damaged tube are well known. Whether *in vitro* fertilization and embryo transplant will help these individuals remains to be seen, but with extensive adhesive disease the possibilities of success are limited.

GRANULOMATOUS SALPINGITIS

Such lesions are uncommon in the United States today. Whereas thirty or forty years ago approximately 2% to 3% of cases of salpingitis were caused by tuberculosis, currently only 0.1% to 0.2% of salpingitis lesions seen in this country are granulomatous. But people from diverse parts of the world may be represented in any society, and it is important to be aware of the diseases to which the

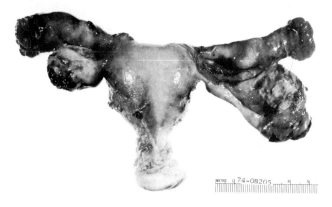

Figure 6–27. Tuberculous salpingitis. Note patent fimbria but thickened edematous tubal wall.

patient may have been exposed prior to her current residence. Tuberculosis is still common in some countries and other granulomatous diseases such as schistosomiasis are prevalent in many African countries.

Interestingly, the fimbria although edematous are patent in 50% of the cases of tuberculous salpingitis (Figure 6–27). Regardless of treatment, post-treatment pregnancies are rare. Furthermore, approximately 50% of subsequent gestations in patients with tuberculous salpingitis are tubal. The reproductive performance in such situations is poor.[18]

ECCYESIS (ECTOPIC PREGNANCY)

Eccyesis accounts for 10% to 12% of maternal deaths in the U.S. The incidence of tubal pregnancy is increasing in the United States, or perhaps it is being diagnosed more accurately. Whereas fifteen or twenty years ago the usual incidence figures were quoted as one extrauterine pregnancy per 150–200 intrauterine pregnancies, the current figure is one to 55–60.

The reasons for the increase in tubal pregnancy are multiple. Certainly the early treatment of salpingitis restores the tube to more or less normal function, but there still may be agglutination of folds and pockets formed in which the fertilized egg could be implanted.

As noted before, endometriosis may be a contributing factor to the production of tubal gestation. Since the delay in passage of the fertilized egg to the uterine cavity is the usual suspected cause for tubal gestation, the decidual reaction in the fallopian tube may not only present a fertile site for implantation but also reduce the caliber of the lumen. As noted, the common finding of salpingitis isthmica nodosa (more accurately, adenomyosis in the cornual region) is undoubtedly related to the development of pregnancy at the isthmus or ampullary isthmic junction.

The intrauterine device has been incriminated as a cause for increased extrauterine gestations. This is more apparent than real since there is an obvious decrease in intrauterine pregnancy and thus a seeming increase in extrauterine gestation. There is no evidence that the intrauterine device is in itself a cause of tubal pregnancy in the absence of inflammatory disease. Generally, tubal disease associated with the IUD has been perisalpingeal rather than endosalpingeal. Nevertheless, interruption of the passage of the fertilized egg, whether intrinsic or extrinsic, is a potential etiologic factor.

Tumors in the paraovarium, particularly the paraovarian cyst and uterine leiomyoma, or possibly even an ovarian cyst, may impinge on the tubal lumen and thus interrupt the passage of the fertilized egg. Although these problems are theoretically possible, the documented relationships are rare. The frequent delay in attempting to conceive, commonly seen in our society, may allow for the genesis of problems such as endometriosis, which contribute to the development of extrauterine pregnancy.

There is little question that extrauterine pregnancies are being diagnosed earlier.[20,21] The improvement in determination of human chorionic gonadotropin has allowed for the earlier demonstration of pregnancy. Ultrasound, used in appropriate fashion, when the level of hCG is 6500 IU or more, will identify the presence of an intrauterine sac and thus improve the differential diagnosis between early intrauterine and extrauterine pregnancy.[22] Certainly the laparoscope has offered a great opportunity for early diagnosis, although there still are problems in differentiating between an enlarged bleeding ovary, with a hemorrhagic corpus luteum and a small amount of blood in the abdominal cavity from the early tubal pregnancy. Culdocentesis has been a commonly accepted diagnostic technique to identify the presence of intraabdominal bleeding. The presence of non-clotting blood has become the diagnostic hallmark of ruptured extrauterine pregnancy. Recent studies suggest that there are many false positives in the interpretation of cul-de-sac blood.[23] Thus, careful history including specific past history of pelvic disease and treatment,[17,18] previous pregnancies and present illness are of major significance. Careful use of ultrasound, evaluation of hCG and careful pelvic examination remain the standards of diagnostic excellence. When uterine bleeding is present, the study of the endometrium for gestational endometriosis without fetal parts demands careful evaluation of pelvic contents (Figure 6–28).

The possibility of a recurrence of eccyesis in the contralateral tube is generally quoted at 12% to 15%. Subsequent fertility following surgical treatment of eccyesis has been reported as low as 25% to 30%; however, recent studies employing more conservative therapy report as high as 60% fertility rate.[24] Frequency of recurrence of eccyesis supports the thesis that such abnormalities as salpingitis isthmica nodosa and minimal distortion associated with follicular salpingitis play a major role in the genesis of tubal pregnancy, since this abnormality is classically noted bilaterally.

PATHOLOGY OF TUBAL PREGNANCY

Approximately 75% of tubal pregnancies are found in the ampullary-isthmic region (Figure 6–28). The site is logical since it is the site of the first major reduction in the diameter of the lumen in the passage of the fertilized egg from the fimbriated end of the tube to the uterus. And this area is in juxtaposition to the cornual portion, the common site of salpingitis isthmica nodosa (Figure 6–29). Being adjacent to the uterus, this site often demonstrates the presence of an endometrial-type stroma with its common decidual reaction during pregnancy. Eccyesis developing in the ampullary and infundibular areas is less common, accounting for 10% to 15% of tubal gestation. It is in these areas that the pregnancy is more frequently associated with follicular salpingitis or (rarely) the finding of accessory lumina or a paraovarian cyst. In a study of 250 cases of tubal pregnancy at the Johns Hopkins Hospital, Berger[26] found either salpingitis isth-

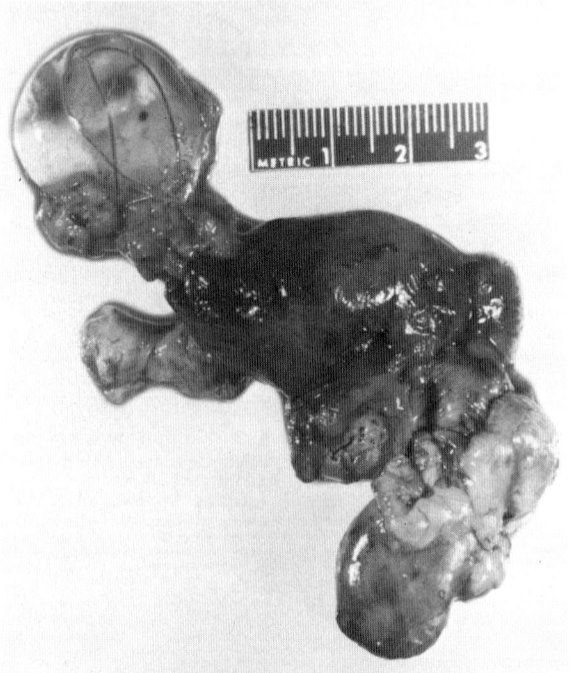

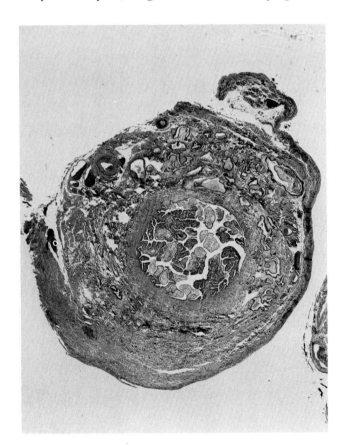

Figure 6–28. Tubal pregnancy with intact sac ruptured through tubal wall near ampullary-isthmic junction.

Figure 6–29. Salpingitis isthmica nodosa. Note gland-like structures throughout entire tubal wall.

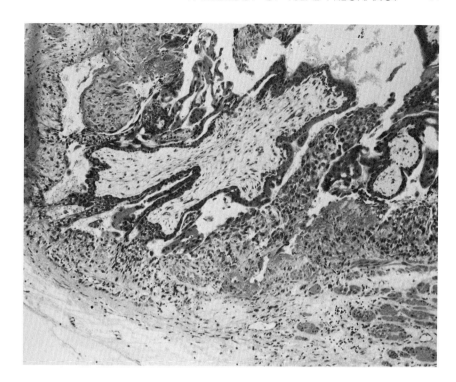

Figure 6–30. Tubal pregnancy. Implantation site showing penetration of trophoblast through tubal wall. Note the remaining muscle bundles in lower right and absence of decidua at implantation site.

mica nodosa or follicular salpingitis in the adjacent tube in the majority of cases.

Study of the implantation site reveals some interesting features[25]: Initially, in at least 50% of the cases, there is little or no definable decidua at this critical site. Thus, as in the uterus, the absence of this important barrier to direct invasion of the trophoblast produces a situation similar to that noted in the uterus with placenta accreta. This destruction of the adjacent muscularis results in hemorrhage into the tubal wall. The latter dissects be-

tween the muscle and serosa (Figure 6–30). Consequently, rupture into the peritoneal cavity would be the logical result of such hemorrhagic diathesis. In addition, the attempt to enucleate the pregnancy with immediate repair of the wall if fraught with hazard due to the dissection of the hemorrhage into the subserosal space. Thus rupture is *not* due to pressure of the blood-filled tube but rather to the destruction of the integrity of the tubal wall (Figure 6–31).

On rare occasions implantation may take place on the

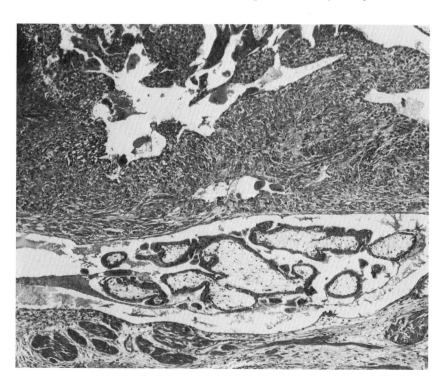

Figure 6–31. Implantation site (above) with absent decidua. Note trophoblast invading the myosalpinx and dissecting the muscle bundles.

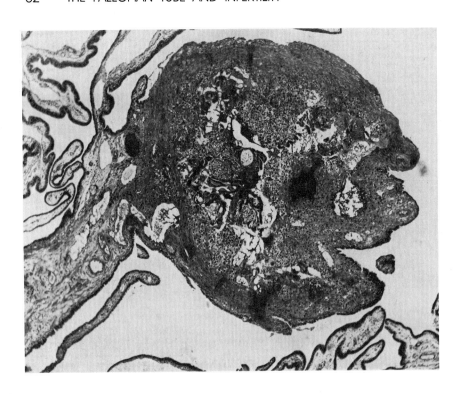

Figure 6–32. Tubal pregnancy with implantation in lumen on tips of tubal folds.

tips of the mucosal folds (Figure 6–32); tubal abortion may result with extension of the pregnancy into the abdominal cavity. In the past this was felt to be the common cause of abdominal pregnancy with secondary implantation on the peritoneum. Currently it is felt that only one implantation can take place and thus extruded pregnancies will die, but products of conception may be found floating in the pelvic cavity. Finally, it must be recognized that some 150–200 tubal pregnancies have attained viability.

The treatment of eccyesis depends on the findings at the time of exploration. Obviously, if the opposite adnexa have been removed for either inflammatory disease, benign neoplasm, or tubal pregnancy, when the patient is desirous of further reproduction, every effort should be made to preserve at least the ovary and, if possible, the tube. Conversely, with contralateral normal adnexa, it is important not to leave a seriously damaged tube only to have it turn out to be the site of another ectopic pregnancy or the cause of pelvic pain caused by adhesions. While it is important that the patient be involved in the final decision, the surgeon must do what is best for the patient.

References

1. Witschi E.: Embryology of the uterus. Ann NY Acad Sci 75:412, 1959.
2. Genadry R, Parmley T, Woodruff JD: The origin and clinical behavior of the paraovarian tumor. Am J Obstet Gynecol 129:873, 1977.
3. Gardner, GH, Greene RL, Peckham BM: Normal and cystic structures of the broad ligament. Am J Obstet Gynecol 55:917, 1948.
4. Samaha M, Woodruff JD: Paratubal cysts. Obstet Gynecol 65:691, 1985.
5. Adashi E, Rosenshein NB, Parmley TH, et al.: Histogenesis of the broad ligament adrenal rest. Int J Gynaecol Obstet 18:102–104, 1980.
6. Woodruff JD, Pauerstein CJ: The fallopian tube. Baltimore, Williams & Wilkins, 1969.
7. Pauerstein CJ: The fallopian tube, a reappraisal. Philadelphia, Lea & Febiger, 1974.
8. Woodruff JD, Solomon D, Sullivant H: Multifocal disease in the upper genital canal. Obstet Gynec 65:695, 1985.
9. Seminar on tubal physiology and biochemistry—Gynecologic Investigation 6:3–4, 1975. CJ Pauerstein (ed).
10. WHO Symposium: Ovum transport and fertility regulation. Copenhagen, Scriptor, 1976.
11. Rock JA, Parmley TH, King TM: Endometriosis and the development of tuboperitoneal fistula after tubal ligation. Fertil Steril 35:16, 1981.
12. Everett HS: Possible tubal origin of endometriosis. Am J Obstet Gynecol 22:1, 1931.
13. Barrett CW, Lash AF: Spontaneous amputation and subsequent acute torsion of the normal left fallopian tube and fibroma of the right ovary. West J SGO 51:135, 1943.
14. Savage JE: Twisted hematosalpinx complicating pregnancy. Am J Obstet Gynecol 32:1043, 1936.
15. Novak E, Woodruff JD: Novak's Obstetric and Gynecologic Pathology, 9th Edition. Philadelphia, WB Saunders, 1979.
16. Niebyl JR, Parmley TH, Spence MR, et al.: Unilateral ovarian abscess associated with the intrauterine device. Obstet Gynecol 52:165, 1978.
17. Westrom L: Effect of acute pelvic inflammatory disease on fertility. Am J Obstet Gynecol 121:707, 1975.
18. Sutherland AM: Genital tuberculosis in women. Am J Obstet Gynecol 79:486, 1960.
19. Curtis AH: Chronic pelvic infections. Surg Gynecol Obstet 42:6, 1926.

20. Thorneycroft IH: When you suspect ectopic pregnancy. Cont Ob/Gyn, pp 81, July, 1983.

21. Weckstein LN, *et al.*: Accurate diagnosis of early ectopic pregnancy. Obstet Gynecol 65:393, 1985.

22. Kadar N, DeVore G, Romero R: Discriminatory hCG zone. Obstet Gynecol 58:156, 1981.

23. Romero R, *et al.*: The value of culdocentesis in the diagnosis of ectopic pregnancy. Obstet Gynecol 65:519, 1985.

24. DeCherney AH, Minkin MJ, Spangler S: Contemporary management of ectopic pregnancy. J Reprod Med 26:519, 1981.

25. Budowick M, Johnson TRB, Genadry R, *et al.*: The histopathology of the developing tubal ectopic pregnancy. Fertil Steril 34:169, 1980.

26. Berger N, *et al.*: Pathologic findings of tubal pregnancy. Obstet Gynecol (to be published).

Color Plates

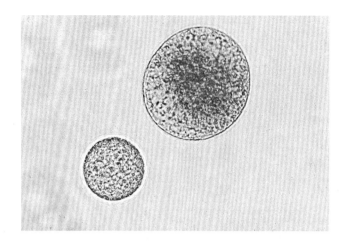

Figure 2–5. Two zona-free hamster eggs are compared, one of which has swollen and taken up trypan blue. Both eggs were exposed to the same heat-inactivated human serum from a woman with unexplained infertility. The large egg was exposed to guinea pig serum (1:32 dilution) as a source of active complement, while the smaller egg was exposed to heat-inactivated guinea pig serum.

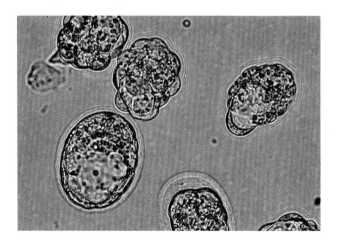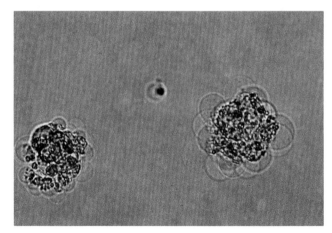

Figure 2–6. A. Zona-intact and zona-free blastocysts from oviducts of the mouse at the two-cell stage and cultured *in vitro* for 72 to 96 hours. B. Zona-free mouse blastocysts, following *in vitro* hatching, were exposed to heat-inactivated human serum from a woman with unexplained infertility, and guinea pig serum as a source of complement. Collapse of the blastocoele and cytoplasmic blebbing of trophectoderm were apparent in the presence of complement but not in its absence.

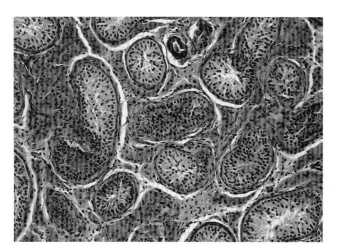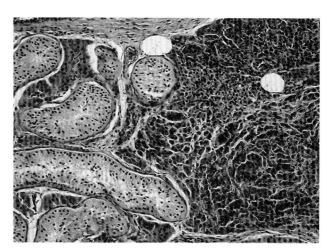

Figure 14–12. Appearance of Leydig cells in developmental disorders. A. 17-ketosteroid reductase deficiency. B. Complete androgen insensitivity syndrome.

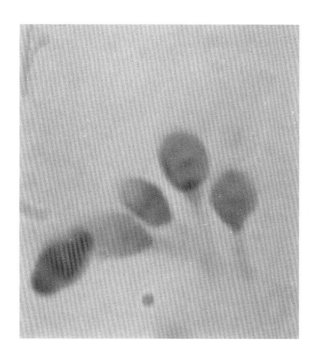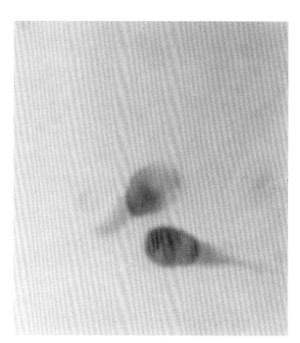

Figure 20–7. A. B. Acrosome reaction patterns with the triple stain showing living sperm that are acrosome intact (pink) and acrosome reacted (white). (Provided by Dr. P. Talbot).

7. Pelvic Endometriosis: Etiology and Pathology

A.F. Haney

Endometriosis remains an enigmatic disease despite intense study by pathologists and gynecologists since the turn of the century. Histologically and functionally it is linked to the uterine endometrium, but the basic issues of why and how it develops remain controversial. Endometriosis is defined as the presence of typical endometrial glands and stroma outside the uterus with evidence of menstrual cyclicity manifested by the presence of hemosiderin-laden macrophages. Endometrial tissue within the myometrium was initially thought to be a variant of the disease, but it is now apparent this is a distinct entity with a unique clinical population, a different pattern of disease, and a separate etiology.[1]

The purpose of this chapter is to give the reader an updated understanding of the etiology and pathology of endometriosis. This is of critical importance—not only in making an accurate pathologic diagnosis, but also in devising strategies for minimizing the likelihood of developing the disease, and for providing effective treatment of it. We need to do this to retain control over conception without jeopardizing the single most important biologic function of our or any species: safe and efficient reproduction.

CLINICAL FEATURES

The clinical presentation is highly variable, ranging from severe dysmenorrhea, chronic pelvic pain, an asymptomatic pelvic mass, severe dysmenorrhea, chronic pelvic pain, and infertility, to an incidental finding at the time of gynecologic surgery.[2–10] The disease is usually confined to the pelvis, but rarely it may be encountered in extrapelvic sites such as lungs,[11,12] brain,[13] lymph nodes,[14,15] and umbilicus.[16] Because of the rarity of extrapelvic endometriosis, it is almost always an unanticipated pathologic finding after excision of an unusual tumor. The natural history of this disease is likewise poorly understood, with many women experiencing no demonstrable change in the pattern of their disease over long intervals of time. There is, however, a significant minority in whom endometriosis is a progressively debilitating and destructive process necessitating radical measures such as surgical castration.

The true prevalence of the disease in the general population is difficult to estimate since endometriosis is found in 1% to 50% of patients undergoing gynecologic procedures.[3,17,18] Virtually all the available studies have inherent selection bias because women undergo pelvic operations only if there are significant symptoms, palpable disease, or for elective sterilization. The presenting clinical symptomatology has changed over the years with infertility being the most frequent current complaint. Thirty to 40% of infertile women in a referral setting are ultimately found to have endometriosis.[19,20] Previously, pelvic masses and debilitating pelvic pain were the most common antecedents to the diagnosis. The increasing use of laparoscopy for sterilization and diagnostic evaluation of the pelvis has provided a more realistic estimate of the prevalence of endometriosis than before, when direct visualization of the pelvis was limited to women with symptoms or physical findings severe enough to justify laparotomy. The best available data regarding the prevalence in the general population come from Strathy *et al.*[21] who found endometriosis in 2% of asymptomatic women undergoing laparoscopic tubal ligations. While there is some selection bias in this study as the women were asymptomatic and multiparous, it does tend to support the concept of an overall incidence of 5% or less in the general population.

The physical findings in endometriosis vary dramatically according to the character of the population under study. Nodularity or tenderness in the cul-de-sac is highly suggestive of endometriosis and is the most common physical feature identified, ranging from 34% to 76%.[2] Other frequent palpable findings include parametrial "thickening" and adnexal masses. A retrodisplaced uterus has been noted in 22% to 46% of patients, but it appears unrelated to the severity of the disease.[2,10] Extrapelvic sites such as the skin, vagina, perineum, umbilicus, muscle, and surgical scars are rarely encountered, usually presenting as soft tissue masses. Endometriosis at these distant sites may have no demonstrable cyclicity and provide no clue as to the nature of the process. Increased peritoneal fluid volume[22] as well as ascites[23] have been reported with intraperitoneal endometriosis, but the mechanism is unclear. Because of the high prevalence of the disease in infertile women without any other suggestive symptoms or physical findings, a normal pelvic examination cannot be relied upon to exclude this diagnosis.

EPIDEMIOLOGY

The initial step in attempting to unravel the character of any disease process is to evaluate carefully the population afflicted. While a thorough epidemiologic picture of endometriosis is lacking, certain features of the disease are apparent, the most important being that it is a disease of reproductive age women. Original reports suggested the typical patient was in her late 30's and early 40's, but these studies were limited to women with symptoms or palpable disease severe enough to warrant laparotomy.[6,9] Today's typical patient has her diagnosis made in her late 20's and early 30's, probably secondary to the increasing use of diagnostic laparoscopy for infertility.[20,24] Another distinction is the difference between the age at onset of symptomatology and the age at diagnosis. Currently, the mean age at onset of symptoms is 20, roughly five to ten years prior to the usual age of definitive diagnosis.[20] With the increasing appreciation of the widespread prevalence of this disorder and the near-universal availability of laparoscopy, a further drop in the average age at diagnosis may be anticipated.

It is not surprising that endometriosis has not been reported in the prepubertal years because there is need for gonadal hormone production for endometrial growth. The disease is not uncommon in teenagers with dysmenorrhea and pelvic pain sufficiently severe to justify laparoscopy. Two studies have demonstrated endometriosis in 47% and 65% of women under 20 years of age.[21,25] In the first few years after menarche, there is a disproportionately large number of cases related to müllerian anomalies with uterine outflow obstruction.[4,26–28]

Once endometriosis gets established, ectopically located endometrium can occasionally be maintained beyond the menopause and encountered many years after the cessation of menses. It is estimated that from 2% to 4% of all women requiring laparotomy for endometriosis are postmenopausal.[29–31] Those cases can be explained either by the use of postmenopausal estrogen replacement therapy[30] or by significant endogenous estrogen production, usually attributed to obesity. As the use of postmenopausal estrogen therapy increases, more reports of the disease in older women will undoubtedly be forthcoming.

The demography of endometriosis has been the subject of speculation by many authors—and remains highly controversial. It was originally thought that this disease had marked racial differences, and in 1949, Meigs reported endometriosis in 28% of white patients undergoing laparotomy, but only 5.8% of black women.[32] This study, however, was flawed; it did not control for potential confounding variables such as the availability of health care, access to contraception, cultural differences regarding childbearing patterns, and attitudes toward menses and pain.[32–34] Recent studies controlling for these factors have demonstrated that the higher rates of endometriosis in whites previously reported were a result of

socioeconomic factors rather than race.[8,35] Similarly, alleged links with education, occupation, and geographic location were probably dependent on cultural differences as well.

A genetic influence on the occurrence of endometriosis has long been suspected. Ranney in 1971 demonstrated what appeared to be hereditary tendencies to develop the disease in a relatively homogeneous population.[36] Recent studies have demonstrated endometriosis in 7% of close female relatives of affected women, suggesting a polygenic or multifactorial mode of inheritance.[37,38] No obvious relationship with the HLA-cell surface antigens has been detected.

PATHOGENESIS

Numerous theories of pathogenesis of endometriosis followed the description of the disease by von Rokitansky in 1860.[39] These early explanations for the development of endometriosis were grounded in the precepts of the morphologists at the turn of the century. Given the level of scientific development at that time, it is not surprising that the thinking centered around coelomic metaplasia. This was championed by Robert Meyer, the dean of gynecologic pathology at the time. He felt that endometriosis developed by metaplasia of the original coelomic membrane and that the process of tissue differentiation could occur in the adult in selected tissues. His views predominated despite the lack of any experimental evidence supporting this theory. Several features of the disease have raised serious doubt as to the validity of that concept:

1. The disease is present only in women. There are three case reports of endometriosis in men, each with prostatic carcinoma treated with high doses of estrogen. The endometriosis was noted in the tissue specimen at the time of prostatectomy.[40–43] A likely explanation in each case is hypertrophy of cell rests of the prostatic utricle, the remnant of the müllerian ducts in males.

2. The location of the implants of endometriosis follows no embryologic pattern. Maximov[44] and Filatow[45] have demonstrated that the coelomic membrane contributes to the thoracic lining as well as the peritoneal lining. Endometriosis is not noted at that site with equal frequency.

3. The development of endometriosis requires the presence of endometrium. The old maxim, "Endometriosis only comes from endometrium," is well supported in the literature, implying endometrial shedding is the sole source of implants. The occasional case of müllerian agenesis associated with endometriosis invariably includes remnants of müllerian ducts, typically a small blind uterine horn providing the source of endometrial cells.

4. If coelomic metaplasia occurs, one would anticipate an increasing incidence of endometriosis with age. This disease is confined to women of reproductive age and it is abruptly halted by the onset of menopause.

Thus it appears that coelomic metaplasia is a holdover from the days of descriptive morphology and, with the absence of experimental evidence, there is no justification for concluding it plays a role in the development of endometriosis.

Our current understanding of the pathophysiology of endometriosis began in 1921 with the pioneering observations of Dr. J.A. Sampson, a private practitioner in Albany, New York. Over the course of the next 25 years, he presented his theory of endometrial transplantation as the most reasonable explanation for the disease in a series of insightful publications.[46-62] The traditional dogma of the metaplastic etiology unfortunately continued to have its adherents and, to this day, a comprehensive understanding of the pathophysiology of the disease eludes most practicing physicians.

Sampson's observations of the anatomic pattern of clinical disease led him to postulate that retrograde menstruation was the primary mechanism of development. Other routes of transplanting endometrium originating from the uterine endometrium have also been demonstrated, including lymphatic, vascular, and iatrogenic dissemination.

Lymphatic Dissemination

The spread of endometrial tissue through lymphatics was first proposed by Halban in 1924 when he reported five cases of endometriosis thought to have occurred by lymphatic spread.[14] Javert demonstrated microscopic evidence of endometrial cells in lymphatics and in lymph nodes in 1949.[15] There have been reports of endometriosis in the umbilicus which have lymphatics draining the pelvis,[16] and a report of an endometriotic cyst with an adenoacanthoma in an obturator lymph node.[63] The paucity of reports suggest, this is a relatively rare route of dissemination of endometriosis.

Hematogenous Dissemination

Hematogenous dissemination was proposed by Sampson in 1925.[53] Javert later identified endometrial tissue in pelvic veins,[64] and there are now many reports of endometriosis in well vascularized organs such as the lungs, skin, muscles, and other distant sites.[39,65,66] The frequency of sloughing of endometrial cells in the pelvic veins is unknown, but in view of the rarity of the finding, it is either extremely unusual or the viability of the cells in the vascular system is limited.

Iatrogenic Dissemination

Iatrogenic transplantation of endometriosis has long been appreciated by gynecologists who have observed endometriotic nodules after hysterectomy in abdominal incisions.[39] This mode of transplantation has been utilized experimentally in subhuman primates to develop experimental models of endometriosis.

Retrograde Menstruation

In contrast to most mammals, women undergo menstrual rather than estrous cycles. The basic difference is the development of a spontaneous luteal phase with corpus luteum formation and specialized endometrial changes, i.e., secretory endometrium in the absence of coitus or conception. This requires reversion to proliferative endometrium in every cycle in which conception does not occur.[67] This process is termed menstruation and involves a reduction in the height of the endometrium, reversion of the secretory changes, both biochemically and morphologically, to a proliferative pattern, with a loss of extracellular fluid and endometrial cells. The cellular content of the menstrual debris is modest and is predominantly composed of small clusters of cells, not intact fragments of endometrium.[1]

Sampson surmised that regurgitation of endometrial cells through the fallopian tubes at the time of menstruation was the explanation of the disease. Little attention has been paid to the direction of menstrual flow in women other than in those with iatrogenic or congenital impediments to uterine outflow. When evaluated objectively, retrograde menstruation appears to be a near universal event in women undergoing ovulatory menstrual cycles. Evidence of this comes from several sources. First, peritoneal dialysis of women with kidney disease demonstrates bloody peritoneal dialysates during menses when they are metabolically healthy enough to ovulate.[68] Second, when laparoscopies are performed for sterilization during menses, bloody peritoneal fluid is encountered in approximately 90% of the women.[69] Third, there is a high incidence of endometriosis on the peritoneum adjacent to the site of partial salpingectomy, presumably secondary to the reflux of the menstrual effluent through transient tuboperitoneal fistulae.[70]

In trying to understand the pathophysiology of retrograde menstruation, one must consider the physiology of menstruation. In the absence of conception, progesterone production by the corpus luteum declines and prostaglandins are released by the endometrial decidua. The prostaglandins cause arterial vasospasm resulting in partial autolysis of the superficial layer of endometrium. Both clusters and individual cells are extruded into the uterine lumen along with blood and extracellular fluid. Simultaneous prostaglandin-mediated uterine contractions increase the pressure within the uterus, expelling the menstrual debris through the path of least resistance.[71]

There are three exits available for expulsion of menstrual debris—the cervix and both tubal ostia. Presumably, the cervix is the largest ostium with the lowest resistance to flow. Little is known of the physiology of the uterotubal junction, but the tubal caliber is small and presumably the resistance to flow is greater than in the cervix. A fraction of the menstrual debris, however, appears to be extruded from the uterine cavity via the oviducts in most women. The well-known association of endometriosis and impeded uterine outflow (cervical stenosis, cervical obstruction, etc.) is thus presumably explained by a greater proportion of the menstrual debris taking the path of least resistance through the oviducts and being regurgitated into the peritoneal cavity. A clearer understanding of the intraluminal pressure relationships between the cervix and fallopian tubes will be necessary to understand better the determinants of the direction of menstrual flow.

Supporting evidence for retrograde menstruation as the mechanism of entry of endometrial cells into the peritoneal cavity leading to the development of endometriosis is overwhelming. It includes the following:

1. Viable cells are present in menstrual debris. This has been demonstrated with culture of menstrual debris showing living endometrial cells.[72,73]

2. Endometrial cells have been found to pass through the fallopian tubes. This has been demonstrated by perfusion of human fallopian tubes *in vitro*.[74,75]

3. As outlined earlier, retrograde menstruation is a near universal event in ovulating women.

4. Endometrial tissue can implant and grow within the peritoneal cavity. This has been well demonstrated in both humans and animal species.[76] Women with a uterine fundus, but without a cervix for drainage, predictably develop endometriosis after the onset of puberty. There appears to be no requirement for gonadal hormones for the implantation of endometrial cells in the primate peritoneum, but continued growth and cyclicity is dependent upon the secretion of trophic sex steroids.[77]

5. Endometrial cells within the menstrual debris can be transplanted in the human. Ridley and Edwards demonstrated transplantation of endometrial cells from the menstrual effluent to the abdominal wall fascia.[39,78]

In summary, many other theories have been advanced to explain the presence of endometrial tissue at ectopic sites.[39] These include coelomic metaplasia mediated by gonadal hormones or a substance within menses, congenital embryonic rests of either the paramesonephric or mesonephric ducts, and the direct extension of the endometrium through the uterus to adjacent tissues. The above are listed here merely for historical interest, as they have virtually no scientific basis. While dissemination of viable endometrial cells may occur by lymphatic, hematogenous or iatrogenic routes, the clinical pattern most strongly supports retrograde menstruation as a cause of endometriosis in the vast majority of patients. Koch's postulates, as adapted for this disease, have been fulfilled, defining the nature of the disease as that of retrograde menstruation. First, ectopic glands and stroma are, by definition, seen in every case. Second, these cells can be identified as endometrial in origin in terms of functional status, i.e., menstrual cyclicity and hormone dependence. Third, the disease can be produced by transplanting endometrium. Lastly, the ectopic glands and stroma observed in experimentally created disease are indistinguishable from the naturally occurring condition.

It is unclear whether all women are equally susceptible to the development of endometriosis. The likelihood of developing the disease may be a quantitative phenomenon dependent upon the amount of endometrium delivered to the peritoneal cavity over time. Alternatively, there may be unique features in women who develop the disease, such as an altered immune response or an enhanced receptivity of the pelvic tissues to transplanted endometrial cells. A great deal more effort will be required to identify the critical factors involved in the development of endometriosis.

PATHOLOGY

Gross Appearance

Classically, clinicians have diagnosed endometriosis by the characteristic blue-gray "powderburn" lesions on the peritoneal surfaces in the pelvis and on other abdominal viscera. This distinctive discoloration is attributed to the encapsulated menstrual sloughing of the implant. The age of the implant is critical to its appearance. The earliest morphologic indication that retrograde menstruation is occurring is the presence of hemosiderin staining of the dependent areas of the pelvic peritoneum. This may be a transient phenomenon if an insufficient number of viable cells is present to establish implants and the likelihood of developing subsequent endometriosis is unknown. Freshly implanted disease may appear as any irregularity or discoloration of the peritoneal surface. Frequently, the lesions are bloody or tan in color. Older implants are encapsulated by collagen which traps the menstrual debris and gives the implant the classic blue-gray appearance, i.e., the "powderburn" (Figure 7–1).

The distinctive discoloration of implants is often lost during surgical dissection by inadvertently incising the surrounding scar, allowing the hemolyzed menstrual debris to escape. Routine histologic examination frequently does not reveal the widely scattered endometrial glands and scant stromal cells present within the background of extensive collagen deposition. For these reasons the diagnosis of endometriosis may be more apparent to the surgeon at the operating table than to the pathologist after specimen preparation. When the surgical diagnosis is endometriosis and this is not readily apparent on the initial histologic examination, the specimen should be recut and every effort made to identify the nature of the process as this will have great importance in therapeutic decision-making.

Anatomic Distribution

The location of peritoneal implants of endometriosis can be accounted for by the presence of endometrial cells within the peritoneal cavity coupled with the principle of transplantation biology. These include the following: 1. the site of entry, 2. the effects of gravity, 3. the mobility of the transplantation site, and 4. local factors affecting the suitability of that site for accepting transplants. Implants are frequent on the uterosacral ligaments adjacent to the fallopian tube ostia, the route of entry of endometrial cells. Endometriosis is typically found in the most dependent areas of the peritoneal cavity. Organ mobility seems to reduce the probability of implantation, as immobile structures are more often affected. This is indicated by the frequent involvement of the fixed portion of the sigmoid colon with substantially less disease on the

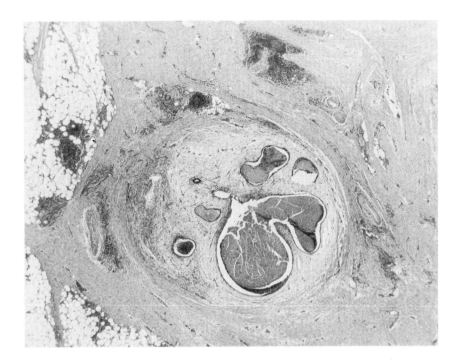

Figure 7–1. Peritoneal "powderburn" of endometriosis. The typical histologic appearance is shown in this photomicrograph. Many of the glands are cystic, and extensive scarring has entrapped the menstrual debris and is responsible for the distinctive color of the implants. Little endometrial stroma surrounding the glands is apparent. H & E (×25).

small intestine or fallopian tubes, both of which are present continuously in the pelvis. The receptivity of the surface epithelium covering an organ is of major importance, with implantation frequent on the peritoneum and ovarian capsule but relatively rare on the squamous epithelium of the cervix or vagina.

Table 7–1 characterizes the observed distribution of grossly visible endometriosis in the pelvis as seen at laparoscopy for infertility. The pattern of disease observed will depend upon the clinical population studied. This is apparent from the differences in distribution noted when the disease is encountered at laparotomy, presumably with more severe disease (Table 7–2). Endometriosis at distant sites is so rare as not to be represented.

The effect of gravity on the anatomic distribution of endometriosis can be demonstrated by considering compartmentalization of the pelvis, with the uterus as the dividing organ (Table 7–3). Anterior compartment endometriosis, i.e., in the uterovesical fold and on the anterior bladder peritoneum, is far more likely to be encountered when an anteflexed uterus is present. When a severely anteflexed uterus is present, exclusive anterior compartment disease is more common. With a retrodisplaced uterus, rarely are implants noted in the anterior compartment as there is no dependent cul-de-sac anterior to the uterus. Posterior compartment endometriosis is common with any uterine position as the posterior cul-de-sac is always a dependent site.

Peritoneal Scarring

Collagen deposition around ectopic endometrial implants is universally observed, both encapsulating the endometrial debris as well as deforming the surrounding peritoneum and adjacent pelvic viscera (Figure 7–1).

When scar contracture alters the normal relationship between the ovary and fallopian tube, the probability of conception is reduced proportional to the degree of anatomic distortion. Adhesions are common when endometriosis is present between two naturally apposed and relatively immobile peritoneal surfaces, and parallels the anatomic pattern of the disease (Table 7–4). Consequently, the scarring secondary to endometriosis is common between the posterior aspect of the uterus or vagina and the sigmoid colon, the undersurface of the ovary and

Table 7–1. Anatomic Distribution of Endometriosis in 182 Infertile Women[a]

Site	Occurrence (%)	
Anterior uterovesical fold	34.6	
Posterior cul-de-sac	34.0	
Sigmoid colon	3.8	
Uterus	11.5	
Small intestine	0.5	
Anterior bladder peritoneum	0.5	

	Left (%)	Right (%)
Round ligament	0.5	0.5
Anterior broad ligament	0.0	1.1
Fallopian tube	4.3	1.6
Posterior broad ligament	25.2	21.4
Ovary	44.0	31.3
Uterosacral ligament	20.8	15.3
Ureter	1.1	1.6

[a] As observed at laparoscopy.[79]

Table 7–2. Anatomic Distribution of Endometriosis in Women[a]

Site	Fallas[3] and Rosenblum	Haydon[5] (%)	Holmes[6] (%)	Scott[8] and TeLinde (%)	Ranney[7] (%)
Ovaries	32.3	60.6	72.5	79.8	100.0
Uterus	62.3	55.0	5.0	14.1	—
Fallopian tubes	2.3	2.8	2.5	15.3	—
Uterosacral ligaments	1.2	—	41.2	3.7	—
Anterior cul-de-sac	—	—	15.0	5.3	—
Posterior cul-de-sac	6.2	33.6	43.8	19.2	—
Posterior broad ligament	—	—	12.5	1.0	—

[a] As observed at laparotomy.[79]

the posterior broad ligament, and the uterine serosa and the visceral peritoneum of the bladder in the anterior uterovesical fold.

The degree of scarring is quite variable from patient to patient and ranges from encapsulated peritoneal implants without visceral adhesions to a virtually "frozen" pelvis with all the pelvic organs agglutinated together in a dense fibrotic mass. Indeed, some of the most challenging operations for the gynecologist involve the removal of severe endometriosis with marked visceral scarring. Whether this fibrotic reaction is due to the general irritating effect of menstrual sloughing by implants or a more specific effect of a secretory product of the implant is unclear. The necessity for continued menstrual cyclicity for eliciting collagen deposition or simply the presence of a non-cycling endometrial implant has not been established. Even in the same woman, the scarring is to some extent site-specific. For example, lesions within the stroma of the ovary are infrequently associated with collagen deposition (Figure 7–2), whereas implants on the ovarian capsule are typically associated with extensive scarring (Figure 7–3, Table 7–4). This often results in

severe adhesions between the ovary and the adjacent posterior leaf of the broad ligament or other pelvic viscera. Infertility is common when a significant proportion of the ovarian capsule is involved in the adhesive process, limiting the number of ovulations available to the fimbria of the fallopian tube.

Substantial collagen deposition around a peritoneal implant may yield a pale peritoneal scar without the distinctive discoloration characteristic of implants. These peritoneal defects are often described as "inactive" or "burnt-out" endometriosis. Despite the lack of longitudinal data about the fate of implants, these white lesions are probably the end result of the inflammatory reaction in which the viable endometrial tissue has been obliterated by the collagen. This issue remains controversial, as the natural history of peritoneal implants is difficult to study and animal models of endometriosis are inadequate to evaluate this question because of species differences.[80]

Abdominal viscera underlying implants may be involved either by direct extension of endometriosis or the associated scar. Endometrial implants on peritoneal surfaces generally do not compromise the function of the

Table 7–3. Uterine Position Related to Compartmentalization of Endometriosis[a] in 182 Infertile Women[b]

Uterine Position	Anterior Compartment Disease (%)	Exclusive Anterior Compartment Disease (%)	Posterior Compartment Disease (%)
Anteflexed n = 113	40.7	3.5	59.3
Extreme anteflexion n = 5	100.0	60.0	40.0
Mid-position n = 18	38.9	0.0	61.1
Posterior n = 51	11.8	0.0	88.2

[a] Anterior compartment endometriosis is defined as disease anterior to the uterus, i.e., the uterovesical fold and anterior bladder peritoneum. Posterior compartment endometriosis is defined as disease posterior to the uterine fundus, i.e., the posterior cul-de-sac, posterior broad ligaments, and the ovaries.

[b] As observed at laparoscopy.[79]

Table 7–4. Anatomic Distribution of Adhesions in 182 Infertile Women with Endometriosis[a]

Site	Occurrence (%)		
Anterior uterovesical fold	2.2		
Posterior cul-de-sac	11.0		
Sigmoid colon	12.1		
Uterus	3.3		
Small intestine	2.2		
Anterior bladder peritoneum	0.5		
Anterior abdominal wall	1.6		
Omentum	2.2		
		Left (%)	Right (%)
Round ligament		1.1	1.1
Anterior broad ligament		1.6	1.1
Fallopian tube		15.4	11.0
Posterior broad ligament		27.5	16.5
Ovary		24.7	14.3
Uterosacral ligament		4.4	2.7

[a] As observed at laparoscopy.[79]

larger viscera such as the bladder, colon, and small intestine (Figure 7–4). By contrast, the ureter, due to its small caliber and location immediately under the peritoneal surface, is uniquely vulnerable to obstruction when overlying implants elicit a retroperitoneal scarring reaction.[81] The cellular composition of the implant is important, because, when the ureter is distorted by scar contracture and not by the growth of endometrial cells within the implant, hormonal manipulations designed to shrink endometrium are ineffective in reversing the compromise of the ureter. If the implant is largely composed of endometrial cells, the suppression of the glands and stroma by hormonal manipulation may provide a dramatic response to therapy.

The Ovary

The ovary is a unique organ in terms of susceptibility to the implantation of ectopic endometrium. It is the most common site of endometriosis either by surface "powderburns" or cystic intraovarian endometrioma formation (Table 7–1). These cysts contain a viscous chocolate-brown fluid representing the remnants of menstrual sloughing. These may reach impressive size and be completely enclosed within the ovary, thus making the nature of the process only discoverable at the time of surgery; they illustrate the effect of reproductive steroids on endometrial tissue. This is not surprising as the thecal, granulosal, and stromal compartments all secrete significant amounts of sex steroids.

Typically, the lining of the cyst can be mechanically separated from the underlying stroma allowing complete excision of the endometrioma with reconstruction of the ovary and minimal loss of normal ovarian tissue. Since most of the follicles are located near the surface of the ovary, excision of endometriomas usually results in a minimal loss of germ cells. The mechanism by which endometrial cells enter the ovarian parenchyma probably involves the ovulatory stigma. This break in the ovarian capsule with its excellent vascularity and trophic hormone production by the corpus luteum provides an optimal transplantation site. Rapid re-epithelization of the ovulatory site accounts for the intact overlying ovarian capsule.

Superficial implants on the ovary are common and have the same characteristics as implants elsewhere on

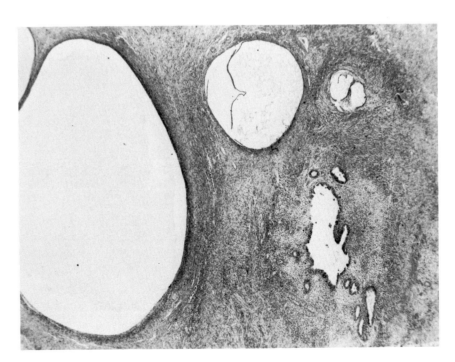

Figure 7–2. Endometriosis within the ovarian stroma. Typical endometrial glands and stroma are present within the parenchyma of the ovary. There is a noticeable lack of surrounding inflammation or scarring. Several of the glands are cystic, and adjacent follicular activity is undisturbed. H & E (×25).

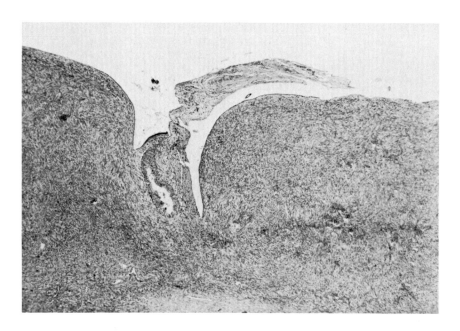

Figure 7–3. Adhesive disease associated with ovarian endometriosis. A surface implant of endometriosis is present within a furrow of the ovarian capsule. The fibrotic reaction is confined to the ovarian surface overlying the implant with no comparable reaction in the adjacent ovarian stroma. H & E (×52).

peritoneal surfaces (Figure 7–5). The reason for the high rate of ovarian involvement is unknown but may be related to the proximity to the fallopian tube ostia, the convoluted surface, the intrinsic properties of the surface epithelium, or the effects of gonadal steroids produced in the ovary.

The Fallopian Tube

The fallopian tube is infrequently the site of endometriosis despite often being involved in adnexal scarring (Table 7–1). Obviously, the regurgitation of menstrual de-

bris through the oviducts provides ample opportunity for endometrial cell transplantation. The lack of involvement of the oviduct is curious. Possible explanations include the motility of the oviduct, the presence of cilitated epithelium constantly transporting the regurgitated endometrial cells, or an endosalpingial epithelium intrinsically less receptive to transplantation. Interestingly, in uterotubal junction obstruction, intraluminal endometriosis in the proximal segment (Figure 7–6) has been reported in about a third of the women with this unusual pattern of tubal obstruction.[82] The presence of endometriosis in the obstructed isthmic portion of one tube has also been observed with obliterative fibrosis in the con-

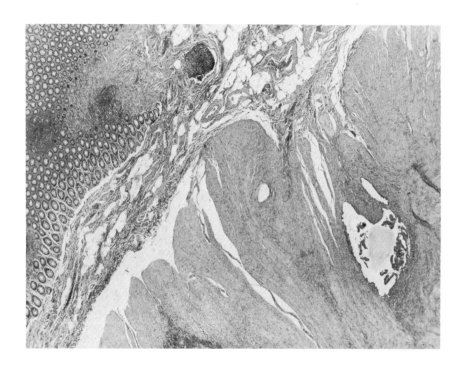

Figure 7–4. Endometriosis of the appendix. Typical mucosa of the appendix is present with endometriotic involvement of the muscular wall. Note the cystic glands with scant adjacent stroma. H & E (×32).

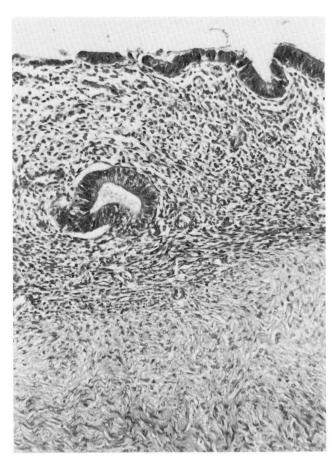

Figure 7–5. Superficial endometrial implant on the ovary. An implant of endometriosis on the ovarian capsule is present with a substantial amount of ovarian stroma surrounding the gland. H & E (×170).

tralateral obstructed isthmic segment.[82] This suggests that fibrosis is the end result of the irritation caused by intraluminal shedding of the explanted endometrium.

Microscopic Appearance

The original guidelines for the microscopic diagnosis of endometriosis were not based on a thorough understanding of the pathophysiology of the disease, but were rather an attempt to establish histologic criteria which could unequivocally confirm the presence of ectopic endometrium. These included the presence of typical endometrial glands and stroma, as well as the presence of hemosiderin-laden macrophages (Figure 7–7), thought to reflect bleeding by the lesion and thus proving menstrual cyclicity. These criteria were considered definitive regardless of the gross appearance, location, or clinical course of the disease. While this approach may have been appropriate when endometriosis was first being described to insure the reliability of the diagnosis, it is inadequate given our current understanding of the disease process. A substantial number of implants do not meet these overly-stringent histologic criteria which have never been validated. Endometriosis will be substantially under-diagnosed if only the traditional histologic criteria are utilized and clinical corroboration is helpful.

Endometriotic implants infrequently have the histologic appearance of endometrium *in situ*. The reasons are several-fold. First, the pattern of cell loss during menstruation is that of shedding small clusters of cells rather than intact fragments of endometrium.[1] Consequently, it is now appreciated that isolated glands, with a variable amount of attached stroma (Figures 7–8, 7–9), are far

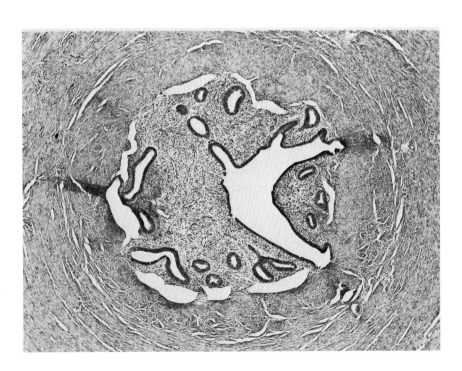

Figure 7–6. Intraluminal endometriosis causing uterotubal junction obstruction. Typical endometrial glands and stroma have completely replaced the lumen of the fallopian tube. The process is confined within the normal layers of tubal muscle, and the separation between the inner muscle layer and the endometrium is distinct. H & E (×40).

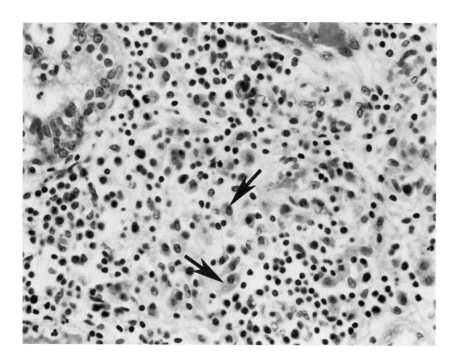

Figure 7–7. Hemosiderin-laden macrophages in an endometrial implant. A large number are present in the endometrial stroma of this implant. Inflammatory cells are present throughout the stroma and vacuolization is apparent in the gland epithelium. H & E (×400).

more common than the typical appearance of normal endometrium, i.e., glands within a stromal background. Second, identification of isolated stromal cells without glands has not been reported. Perhaps this occurs but is overlooked without the more characteristic and easily identifiable glandular component. Third, the isolated glands are often cystic in appearance with the individual epithelial cells not possessing the typical appearance of endometrial glands (See Figures 7–1, 7–2, 7–4, 7–8). This is likely due to the absence of the appropriate architecture. Without a pathway for expulsion of the luminal secretions, the glands become dilated and pressure atro-

phy distorts the features of the individual epithelial cells, making their identification as endometrial cells difficult. The implants are typically confused with peritoneal occlusion cysts and mesonephric remnants. Connective tissue stains are occasionally helpful in distinguishing the mesonephric remnants which are surrounded by smooth muscle.

Endometrial implants on the ovary usually have a closer resemblance to normal endometrium than implants at other sites. The probable explanation is the excellent vascularity and the local production of sex steroids required for growth of the endometrium. When

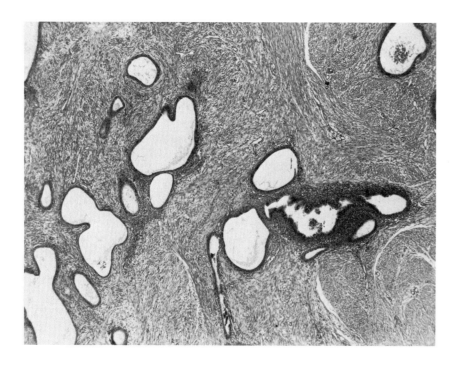

Figure 7–8. Peritoneal implant of endometriosis. The endometrial glands in this implant appear quite variable, with several showing cystic changes. The amount of adjacent stroma also varies, with some glands having no identifiable attached stroma and others being virtually surrounded by a well-defined stromal component. H & E (×32).

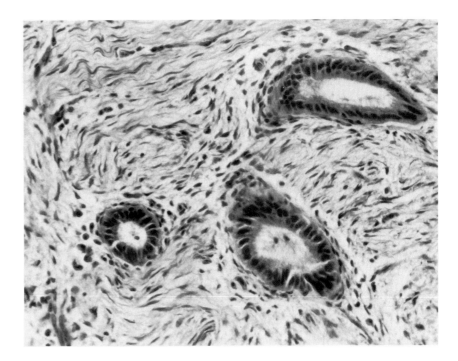

Figure 7–9. Peritoneal implant of endometriosis. This high-magnification view of isolated endometrial glands shows a minimal amount of adjacent stroma with intervening collagenous connective tissue. H & E (×325).

endometrial cells are within the ovary, endometrioma formation occurs. In contrast to surface implants, the cells lining the cyst wall are typically rather nondescript, with a simple cuboidal epithelium and little histologic evidence of menstrual cyclicity except for occasional hemosiderin-laden macrophages in the surrounding stroma. This histologic appearance is undoubtedly due to pressure atrophy and not a lack of hormonal responsiveness as the entrapped "chocolate" material obviously represents evidence of continued menstrual cyclicity. In the absence of characteristic histology of endometrial tissue, the diagnosis of endometriosis is most reliably made by the operating surgeon who describes the "chocolate" material within the cyst. Since other ovarian neoplasms can have old blood within cystic spaces, careful microscopic evaluation is mandatory to exclude a malignant neoplasm.

Hormonal Responsiveness of Ectopic Endometrium

The response of ectopic endometrial implants to gonadal hormones is difficult to assess. Certainly, the hemosiderin-laden macrophages surrounding many implants (Figure 7–7), the gross color of implants, and the presence of chocolate-colored menstrual debris within ovarian endometriomas provide ample evidence of previous menstrual cyclicity. Ectopically implanted endometrium has been observed to undergo cyclic histologic changes in synchrony with normal endometrium as predicted by cyclic hormone fluctuations (Figures 7–10 and 7–11). When objectively evaluated, however, the vast majority of implants do not demonstrate the typical microscopic changes observed within the uterus.[83] If histologic cyclicity is observed, it is frequently asynchronous with the uterine endometrium. Whether this abnormal hormonal responsiveness is due to altered steroid receptor populations, an altered epithelial-stromal relationship or the presence of an associated inflammatory reaction is unknown.

Despite their variable cyclic status, endometrial implants appear to depend upon gonadal hormones as the disease regresses after menopause, commensurate with the decline in circulating gonadal hormones. Similarly, castration results in rapid atrophy of endometriosis unless endogenous nongonadal estrogen production is significant. This suggests that ectopic implants are maintained by sex steroids, if not in a fully functional state. Pregnancy has also been associated with regression of endometriosis, but the histologic pattern is markedly different.[84,85] The high levels of estrogen and progesterone circulating in early pregnancy cause initial hypersecretory decidualization, and only later is progestational atrophy evident.

Several therapeutic regimens have been devised in an attempt to mimic the effects of these naturally occurring hormonal states. The use of continuous oral contraceptives provides a high estrogen/progesterone milieu similar to pregnancy and results in regression by decidual atrophy comparable to that observed in pregnancy, i.e., "pseudopregnancy".[86] Cyclic oral contraceptives may provide a similar effect, as many patients experience progestational atrophy of the endometrium while on oral contraceptives with minimal vaginal withdrawal bleeding. Danazol, a 17-ethinylated derivative of testosterone, alters gonadotropin secretion, creating a state of chronic anovulation. Without normal menstrual cyclicity, the endometrium tends to regress.[87] Significant estrogen production is still present and consequently regression is variable. Progestins, such as medroxyprogesterone acetate, when used continuously, also suppress gonadotro-

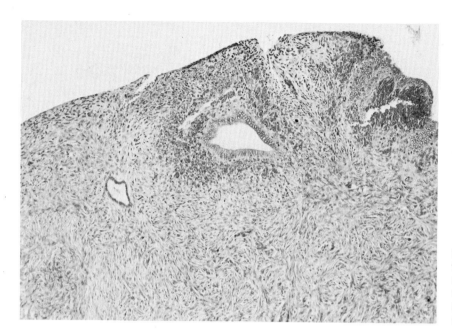

Figure 7–10. Hemorrhage in an endometrial implant. This ovarian implant of endometriosis demonstrates areas of hemorrhage, and it is such bleeding that forms the basis for postulating hormonal responsiveness. H & E (×100).

pin secretion and have been used in treating endometriosis.[88,89] The endometrium is initially progestationalized but, without continuous estrogen support, the endometrial tissue becomes atrophic. This is attributed to the fact that estrogen is required to induce progesterone receptors, and without receptors the progestins cannot bind, reducing trophic hormonal support of the endometrium. When evaluating the histologic appearance of peritoneal lesions, the hormonal milieu just prior to surgery should be kept in mind.

Ultrastructural Appearance

The ultrastructural appearance of normal endometrium changes all throughout the menstrual cycle, paralleling the well-described light microscopic changes.[90,91] Giant mitochondria are observed, as well as the development of nuclear channel systems coinciding with ovulation. By contrast, ectopically implanted endometrium does not demonstrate these characteristic ultrastructural changes but, rather, is composed of bizarre cells.[92] Collagen fibrils are readily apparent around implants confirming the character of the scarring process.[92] The ultrastructural appearance of individual endometrial cells within a background of collagen may be the only means of identifying the tissue as endometrial in origin. High-resolution scanning electron micrographs of the peritoneal surfaces have identified small implants of endometrial cells without the typical "powderburn" appearance.[93] The clinically obvious implants may represent a fraction of the

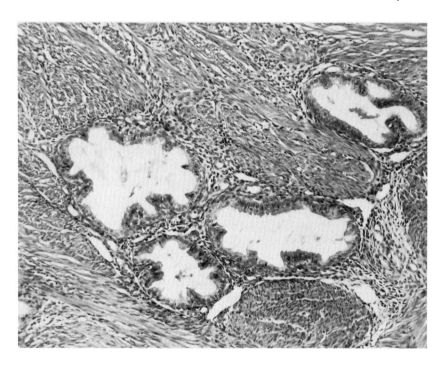

Figure 7–11. Secretory activity in an endometriotic implant. This cluster of endometrial glands has clearly identifiable adjacent stroma in a background of dense collagen. The epithelium of the glands demonstrates vacuolization; secretory material is present in the lumen similar to the histologic changes of luteal phase endometrium. The serrated architecture of the glands further suggests a response to cycling ovarian sex steroids. H & E (×250).

total number of endometrial cells attached to pelvic peritoneum.

BIOCHEMISTRY OF ENDOMETRIAL IMPLANTS

Biochemical changes in normal endometrium are directed toward the secretion of uterine luminal proteins thought to be important for early embryo development and, in the absence of pregnancy, prostaglandins necessary for menstruation. Histochemical studies of endometriotic implants demonstrate that they may display the same enzymatic changes as cyclic endometrium.[94] While prostaglandins have been detected in ectopic endometrial implants,[95] controversy still exists as to whether prostanoids are increased in the peritoneal fluid of women with endometriosis. There have been studies demonstrating increases in the prostanoid content of the peritoneal fluid of women with endometriosis,[96–100] while others have been unable to confirm these observations.[101–103] Prostaglandins are less than optimal markers of the secretory capability of ectopic endometrial implants because they have a rapid half-life, are cycle-dependent, and are secreted by another cell present in the abdominal cavity, the peritoneal macrophage. Another protein, prolactin, is a secretory product of luteal phase endometrium, has a much longer half-life, and is not secreted by other cells in the peritoneal cavity. Prolactin has not been found to be elevated in the peritoneal fluid in women with endometriosis.[104] These data argue against a quantitatively significant secretory capability of endometrial implants and add further controversy to the question of the functionality of ectopic endometrium.

There seems little doubt that at some point endometriotic implants respond to gonadal sex hormones and hence steroid receptor populations should be identifiable. While most endometrial implants possess progesterone receptors, only 30% have estrogen receptors,[105] and ovarian implants have fewer of both estrogen and progesterone receptors than normal endometrium.[106,107] Because the quantities of endometrial glands and stroma in implants are limited, receptor populations are difficult to quantify. Qualitative assessment of estrogen receptors by preparing autoradiograms with labeled hormones reveals a substantial difference in the stromal-epithelial distribution of receptors in ectopic implants compared to normal endometrium.[108] As hormones are likely to act via stromal binding and, in turn, influence the epithelial cells, the observed alteration in the normal stromal-epithelial interaction may explain the variability of hormone-responsiveness observed in ectopic endometrium.

PERITONEAL CYTOLOGY IN ENDOMETRIOSIS

Pelvic endometriosis is associated with an intraperitoneal inflammatory exudate. This is manifested by an increase in the peritoneal fluid volume[22] and the number of leukocytes[109] in women with endometriosis. Differential cell counts reveal that approximately 90% of the cells are macrophages with a small number of lymphocytes and polymorphonuclear leukocytes.[109] The macrophages possess all the characteristics of mononuclear phagocytes, such as phagocytosis, staining for nonspecific esterase and peroxidase, and tumor cell killing. Interestingly, few, if any, cells in the peritoneal fluid can be designated as mesothelial in origin based on functional characteristics such as phagocytosis, etc. Further evidence of the inflammatory nature of the exudate is the finding of increased concentrations or proteolytic enzymes associated with states of inflammation.[110] Macrophages appear to enter the abdominal cavity by migration across the peritoneum, as when the fallopian tubes are obstructed at the fimbriated end; aspiration of the resultant hydrosalpinx yields an extremely small number of cells.[111] Intratubal macrophage counts are elevated in endometriosis suggesting that these cells enter the genital tract through the fimbrial ostia.[111] This is a local inflammatory reaction since no alterations in the peripheral leukocyte populations have been identified.[112]

It seems likely that the inflammatory cells are elicited by the presence of menstrual debris from retrograde menstruation rather than by sloughing by the implants. The number of endometrial cells within ectopic implants is modest and most are completely encapsulated by scar. Secretion of an unidentified factor or factors responsible for eliciting the macrophages by the endometrial implants is also unlikely since other endometrial-specific secretory products, such as prolactin,[104] are not elevated in the peritoneal fluid of women with endometriosis.

IMMUNOLOGICAL CONSIDERATIONS

Several investigators have suggested subtle differences in the immune system of women with endometriosis. An autoimmune phenomenon has been suggested by several lines of experimental evidence, but few clinical data are available. Complement deposition has been observed around the intrauterine endometrial glands of women with endometriosis at midcycle.[113] No pregnancies were observed in a group of women with endometriosis when complement was identified in the endometrium.[114] Similarly, Ouchterlony immunodiffusion has been shown to produce precipitation lines between autologous endometrial cell homogenates and serum in two of three women with endometriosis but not in three controls.[115] Autoantibodies to endometrial antigens were found by the hemagglutination technique in 11 of 13 women with endometriosis, but not in controls.[116] The two women lacking antibodies to endometrium were the only ones in this study without ovarian involvement, suggesting the necessity for direct interaction between the inflammatory cells elicited by endometriosis and ovarian tissue. Interestingly, autoantibodies to ovarian antigens in the thecal and granulosa cells were also noted. A recent report using a monoclonal antibody to the membrane antigen CA-125 noted elevated CA-125 levels in 80% of women with epithelial cancer of the ovary, in <2% of normal women, and in 49% of women with advanced stages of endometriosis.[117]

While there is no evidence for an alteration in the general immune status or the peripheral leukocyte subsets in women with endometriosis,[112] T-lymphocyte-mediated cytotoxicity to autologous endometrial cells *in vitro* has been shown to be reduced.[118] This was found to be inversely correlated with the stage of the disease. Similarly, concentrations of the complement components C_3c and C_4 were elevated in the serum and peritoneal fluid of women with endometriosis.[115]

While interesting, these observations on the autoimmune status of women with endometriosis are of unknown significance. Only with clinical corroboration will a uniform picture of the immune status of the woman with endometriosis emerge.

References

1. Flowers CE Jr, Wilborn WH: New observations in the physiology of menstruation. Obstet Gynecol 51:16, 1978.
2. Buttram VC Jr: Conservative surgery for endometriosis in the infertile female: a study of 206 patients with implications for both medical and surgical therapy. Fertil Steril 31:117, 1979.
3. Fallus R, Rosenblum G: Endometriosis: a study of 260 private hospital cases. Am J Obstet Gynecol 39:964, 1940.
4. Hanton EM, Malkasian GD Jr, Dockerty MB, *et al.*: Endometriosis in young women. Am J Obstet Gynecol 98:116, 1967.
5. Haydon GB: A study of 569 cases of endometriosis. Am J Obstet Gynecol 43:704, 1941.
6. Holmes WR: Endometriosis. Am J Obstet Gynecol 43:255, 1942.
7. Ranney B: Endometriosis III. Complete operations: reasons, sequelae, treatment. Am J Obstet Gynecol 109, 1137, 1971.
8. Scott RB, TeLinde RW: External endometriosis—scourge of private patient. Ann Surg 131:697, 1950.
9. Sensky TE, Liu DTY: Endometriosis: associations with menorrhagia, infertility, and oral contraceptives. Int J Gynecol Obstet 17:573, 1980.
10. Smith GVS: Endometrioma. Am J Obstet Gynecol 17:806, 1929.
11. Lattes R, Shepard F, Tovell H, *et al.*: A clinical and pathologic study of endometriosis of the lung. Surg Gynecol Obstet 103, 552:1956.
12. Rodman MH, Jones CW: Catamenial hemoptysis due to bronchial endometriosis. NEJM 266:805, 1962.
13. Kitchin JD: Endometriosis, p. 1. *In* JJ Sciarra (ed): Gynecology and Obstetrics. Vol. 1. Chapter 20. Philadelphia, Harper and Row, 1982.
14. Halban J: Hysteroadenosis metastatica. Die lymphogere Genese der sog. Adenofibromatosis heterotopica. Arch Gynaekol 124:457, 1925.
15. Javert CT: Pathogenesis of endometriosis based on endometrial homeoplasia direct extension, exfoliation and implantation, lymphomatic and hematogeneous metastasis. Cancer 2:399, 1949.
16. Scott RB, Nowak RJ, Tindale RM: Umbilical endometriosis and Cullen's sign: study of lymphatic transport from pelvis to umbilicus in monkeys. Obstet Gynecol 11:556, 1958.
17. Jeffcoate TA: Principles of Gynaecology. London, Butterworth, 1975.
18. Williams TJ, Pratt JH: Endometriosis in 1,000 consecutive celiotomies: incidence and management. Am J Obstet Gynecol 129:245, 1977.
19. Dmowski WP: Current concepts in the management of endometriosis. Obstet Gynecol Annu 10:279, 1981.
20. Norwood GE: Sterility and fertility in women with pelvic endometriosis. Clin Obstet Gynecol 3:456, 1960.
21. Strathy JH, Molgaard CA, Coulam CG, *et al.*: Endometriosis and infertility: a laparoscopic study of endometriosis among fertile and infertile women. Fertil Steril 38:667, 1982.
22. Drake T, O'Brien W, Grunert G, *et al.*: Peritoneal fluid volume in endometriosis. Fertil Steril 34:280, 1980.
23. Jenks, JE, Artman LE, Hoskins, WJ, *et al.*: Endometriosis with ascites. Obstet Gynecol 63:75S, 1984.
24. Olive DL, Franklin RR, Gratkins LV: Association between endometriosis and spontaneous abortions: a retrospective clinical study. J Reprod Med 27:333, 1982.
25. Chatman DL, Ward AB: Endometriosis in adolescents. J Reprod Med 27:156, 1982.
26. Huffman W: Endometriosis in young teenage girls. Pediatr Ann 10:44, 1981.
27. Baker ER, Horger EO, Williamson HO: Congenital atresia of the uterine cervix: two cases. J Reprod Med 27:156, 1982.
28. Schifrin BS, Erez S, Moore JG: Teenage endometriosis. Am J Obstet Gynecol 116:973, 1973.
29. Kempers RD, Dockerty MB, Hunt AB, *et al.*: Significant postmenopausal endometriosis. Surg Gynecol Obstet 111:348, 1960.
30. Punnonen R, Klemi P, Nikkanen V: Postmenopausal endometriosis. Eur J Obstet Gynecol Reprod Biol 11:195, 1980.
31. Djursing H, Peterson K, Weberg E: Symptomatic postmenopausal endometriosis. Acta Obstet Gynecol Scand 60:529, 1981.
32. Meigs JV: Medical treatment of endometriosis and significance of endometriosis. Surg Gynecol Obstet 89:317, 1949.
33. Chatman DL: Endometriosis and the black woman. J Reprod Med 16:303, 1976.
34. Miyazawa K: Incidence of endometriosis among Japanese women. Obstet Gynecol 48:407, 1976.
35. Lloyd FP: Endometriosis in the Negro woman. Am J Obstet Gynecol 89:468, 1964.
36. Ranney B: Endometriosis IV. Hereditary tendencies. Obstet Gynecol 37:734, 1971.
37. Malinak LR, Buttram VC Jr, Elias S, *et al.*: Heritable aspects of endometriosis II. Clinical characteristics of familial endometriosis. Am J Obstet Gynecol 137:332, 1980.
38. Simpson JL, Elias S, Malinak LR, *et al.*: Heritable aspects of endometriosis I. Genetic studies. Am J Obstet Gynecol 137:327, 1980.
39. Ridley JH: The histiogenesis of endometriosis: a review of facts and fancies. Obstet Gynecol Surv 23:1, 1968.
40. Melicow MM, Pachter MR: Endometrial carcinoma of the prostatic utricle (uterus masculinus). Cancer 20:1715, 1967.

41. Oliker AF, Harns AE: Endometriosis of the bladder in a male patient. J Urol 106:858, 1971.

42. Pinkert TC, Catlow CE, Straus R: Endometriosis of the urinary bladder in a man with prostatic carcinoma. Cancer 43:1562, 1979.

43. Schrodt GR, Alcorn MD, Ibanez J: Endometriosis of the male urinary system: a case report. J Urol 124:722, 1980.

44. Maximow A: Über der Mesothel (Deckzellen der serosen Haute) und die Zellen der serosen Exsudate. Untersuchungen an entzündetem Gewebe und an Gewebskulturen. Arch Exp Zellforsch 4:1, 1927.

45. Filatow D: Über die Bildung des Anfangsstadiums bei der Extremitatenentwicklung. Arch Entwicklungsmech Organ 127:776, 1933.

46. Sampson JA: Perforating hemorrhagic (chocolate) cysts of the ovary. Arch Surg 3:245, 1921.

47. Sampson JA: Ovarian hematomas of endometrial type (perforating hemorrhagic cysts of the ovary) and implantation adenomas of endometrial type. Boston Med Surg J 186:445, 1922.

48. Sampson JA: Life history of ovarian hematomas. Am J Obstet Gynecol 4:451, 1922.

49. Sampson JA: Intestinal adenomas of endometrial type, their importance, and their relation to ovarian hematomas of endometrial type (perforating hemorrhagic cysts of the ovary). Arch Surg 5:217, 1922.

50. Sampson JA: Benign and malignant endometrial implants in the peritoneal cavity and their relation to certain ovarian tumors. Surg Gynecol Obstet 38:287, 1924.

51. Sampson JA: Endometrial carcinoma of the ovary arising in endometrial tissue in that organ. Arch Surg 10:1, 1925.

52. Sampson JA: Inguinal endometriosis (often reported as endometrial tissue in the groin, adenomyoma in the groin, and adenomyoma of the round ligament). Am J Obstet Gynecol 10:462, 1925.

53. Sampson JA: Heterotopic or misplaced endometrial tissue. Am J Obstet Gynecol 10:649, 1925.

54. Sampson JA: Endometriosis of the sac of the right inguinal hernia associated with pelvic peritoneal endometriosis and endometrial cyst of the ovary. Am J Obstet Gynecol 12:459, 1926.

55. Sampson JA: Metastatic or embolic endometriosis due to menstrual dissemination of endometrial tissue into the venous circulation. Am J Pathol 3:93, 1927.

56. Sampson JA: Peritoneal endometriosis due to the menstrual dissemination of endometrial tissue into the peritoneal cavity. Am J Obstet Gynecol 14:422, 1927.

57. Sampson JA: Endometriosis following salpingectomy. Am J Obstet Gynecol 16:461, 1928.

58. Sampson JA: Infected endometrial cysts of the ovaries: a report of three cases, two of which were bilateral. Am J Obstet Gynecol 18:1, 1929.

59. Sampson JA: Postsalpingectomy endometriosis (endosalpingiosis). Am J Obstet Gynecol 20:443, 1930.

60. Sampson JA: Pelvic endometriosis and tubal fimbriae. Am J Obstet Gynecol 24:497, 1932.

61. Sampson JA: The development of the implantation theory for the origin of peritoneal endometriosis. Am J Obstet Gynecol 40:549, 1940.

62. Sampson JA: Pathogenesis of postsalpingectomy endometriosis in laparotomy scars. Am J Obstet Gynecol 50:597, 1945.

63. Koss LG: Miniature adenocanthoma arising in an endometriotic cyst in an obturator lymph node. Cancer 16:1369, 1963.

64. Javert CT: The spread of benign and malignant endometrium in the lymphatic system with a note of coexisting vascular involvement. Am J Obstet Gynecol 64:780, 1952.

65. Duncan C, Pitney WR: Endometrial tumors in the extremities. Med J Aust 2:715, 1949.

66. Nunn LL: Endometrioma of the thigh. Northwest Med 48:474, 1949.

67. Markee JE: Morphological basis for menstrual bleeding. Bull N.Y. Acad Med 24:253, 1948.

68. Blumenkrantz MJ, Gallagher N, Bashore RA, et al.: Retrograde menstruation in women undergoing chronic peritoneal dialysis. Obstet Gynecol 57:667, 1981.

69. Halme J, Hammond MG, Hulka JF, et al.: Retrograde menstruation in healthy women and in patients with endometriosis. Obstet Gynecol 64:151, 1984.

70. Rock JA, Parmley TH, King TM, et al.: Endometriosis and the development of tuboperitoneal fistulas after tubal ligation. Fertil Steril 35:16, 1981.

71. Vijayakumar R, Walters WAW: Myometrial prostaglandins during the human menstrual cycle. Am J Obstet Gynecol 141:313, 1981.

72. Cron RS, Gey G: The viability of the cast-off menstrual endometrium. Am J Obstet Gynecol 43:645, 1927.

73. Kistner, RW, Wiegler, AM, Behrman SJ: Suggested classification for endometriosis: relationship to infertility. Fertil Steril 28:1008, 1977.

74. Geist SH: The viability of fragments of menstrual endometrium. Am J Obstet Gynecol 25:751, 1979.

75. Manning JO, Shaver EF Jr: The demonstration of endometrial cells by Papanicolaou, and supravital techniques obtained by culdocentesis. Bull. Tulane Univ. Med. Fac. 18:193, 1959.

76. Allen E, Peterson LF, Campbell ZB: Clinical and experimental endometriosis. Am J Obstet Gynecol 68:356, 1954.

77. DiZerega GS, Barber DL, Hodgen GD: Endometriosis: role of ovarian steroids in initiation, maintenance, and suppression. Fertil Steril 33:649, 1980.

78. Ridley JH, Edwards IK: Experimental endometriosis in the human. Am J Obstet Gynecol 76:783, 1958.

79. Jenkins S, Olive DL, Haney AF: The location of endometriosis lesions in an infertile patient population. Obstet Gynecol (to be published).

80. McCann TO, Myers RE: Endometriosis in rhesus monkeys. Am J Obstet Gynecol 106:516, 1970.

81. Bates JS, Beecham CT: Retroperitoneal endometriosis with ureteral obstruction. Obstet Gynecol 34:242, 1969.

82. Fortier KJ, Haney AF: The pathologic spectrum of uterotubal junction obstruction. Obstet Gynecol 65:93, 1985.

83. Roddick JW, Conkey G, Jacobs EJ: The hormonal response of endometriotic implants and its relationship to symptomatology. Am J Obstet Gynecol 79:1173, 1960.

84. McArthur JW, Ulfelder H: The effect of pregnancy upon endometriosis. Obstet Gynecol Surv 20:709, 1965.

85. Walton LA: A reexamination of endometriosis after pregnancy. J Reprod Med 19:341, 1977.

86. Andrews MC, Andrews WC, Strauss AF: Effects of progestin-induced pseudopregnancy on endometriosis: clinical and microscopic studies. Am J Obstet Gynecol 78:776, 1959.

87. Floyd WS: Danazol: endocrine and endometrial effects. Int J Fertil 25:75, 1980.

88. Johnston WIH: Dydrogesterone and endometriosis. Br J Obstet Gynaecol 83:77, 1976.

89. Moghissi KS, Boyce CR: Management of endometriosis with oral medroxyprogesterone acetate. Obstet Gynecol 47:265, 1976.

90. Ferenczy A: Studies on the cytodynamics of human endometrial regeneration. I. Scanning electron microscopy. Am J Obstet Gynecol 124:64, 1976.

91. Ferenczy A: Studies on the cytodynamics of human endometrial regeneration. II. Transmission electron microscopy and histochemistry. Am J Obstet Gynecol 124:582, 1976.

92. Lox CD, Word L, Heine MW, et al.: Ultrastructural evaluation of endometriosis. Fertil Steril 41:755, 1984.

93. Brosens I, Vasquez G, Gordts S: Scanning electron microscopic study of the pelvic peritoneum in unexplained infertility and endometriosis. Fertil Steril 41:215, 1984.

94. Prakash S, Ulfelder H, Cohen RB: Enzyme-histochemical observations on endometriosis. Am J Obstet Gynecol 91:990, 1965.

95. Moon YS, Leung PCS, Yuen BH, et al.: Prostaglandin F in human endometriotic tissue. Am J Obstet Gynecol 141:344, 1981.

96. Meldrum D, Shamonki I, Clark K: Prostaglandin content of ascitic fluid in endometriosis: a preliminary report. Presented at the 25th annual meeting of the Pacific Coast Fertility Society, Palm Springs, CA, 1977, Abstract 17.

97. Drake TS, O'Brien WF, Ramwell PW, et al.: Peritoneal fluid thromboxane B2 and 6-keto-prostaglandin Fla in endometriosis. Am J Obstet Gynecol 140:401, 1981.

98. Soundheimer SJ, Flickinger G: Prostaglandin F2a in the peritoneal fluid of patients with endometriosis. Int J Fertil 27:73, 1982.

99. Badawy SZA, Marshall L, Gabal AA, et al.: The concentration of 13,14-dihydro-15-keto-prostaglandin F2a and prostaglandin E2 in peritoneal fluid of infertile patients with and without endometriosis. Fertil Steril 38:166, 1982.

100. Ylikorkala O, Koskimies A, Laatkainen T, et al.: Peritoneal fluid prostaglandins in endometriosis, tubal disorders, and unexplained infertility. Obstet Gynecol 63:616, 1984.

101. Rock JA, Dubin NH, Ghodgaonkar RB, et al: Cul-de-sac fluid in women with endometriosis: fluid volume and prostanoid concentration during the proliferative phase of the cycle—Days 8 to 12. Fertil Steril 37:747, 1982.

102. Sgarlata CS, Hertelendy F, Mikhail G: The prostanoid content in peritoneal fluid and plasma of women with endometriosis. Am J Obstet Gynecol 147:563, 1983.

103. Dawood MY, Kahn-Dawood FS, Wilson L Jr: Peritoneal fluid prostaglandins and prostanoids in women with endometriosis, chronic pelvic inflammatory disease, and pelvic pain. Am J Obstet Gynecol 148:391, 1984.

104. Haney AF, Handwerger S, Weinberg JB: Peritoneal fluid prolactin in infertile women with endometriosis: lack of evidence of secretory activity by endometriotic implants. Fertil Steril 42:935, 1984.

105. Janne O, Kauppila A, Kokko E, et al.: Estrogen and progestin receptors in endometriosis lesions: comparison with endometrial tissue. Am J Obstet Gynecol 141:562, 1981.

106. Bergguist A, Rannevik G, Thorell J: Estrogen and progesterone cytosol receptor concentration in endometriotic tissue and intrauterine endometrium. Acta Obstet Gynecol Scand Suppl 101:53, 1981.

107. Tamaya T, Motoyaha T, Ohono Y, et al.: Steroid receptor levels and histology of endometriosis and adenomyosis. Fertil Steril 31:396, 1979.

108. Gould SF, Shannon JM, Cunha GR: Nuclear estrogen binding sites in human endometriosis. Fertil Steril 39:520, 1983.

109. Haney, AF, Muscato JJ, Weinberg JB: Peritoneal fluid cell populations in infertile patients. Fertil Steril 35:696, 1981.

110. Halme J, Becker S, Hammond MG, et al.: Increased activation of pelvic macrophages in infertile women with mild endometriosis. Am J Obstet Gynecol 145:333, 1983.

111. Haney AF, Misukonis MA, Weinberg JB: Macrophages and infertility: oviductal macrophages as potential mediators of infertility. Fertil Steril 39:310, 1983.

112. Gleicher N, Dmowski WP, Siegel I, et al.: Lymphocyte subsets in endometriosis. Obstet Gynecol 63:463, 1984.

113. Weed JC, Arquembourg PC: Endometriosis: Can it produce an autoimmune response resulting in infertility? Clinical Obstet Gynecol 23:885, 1980.

114. Bartosik D, Viscarello RR, Damjanov I: Endometriosis as an autoimmune disease. Fertil Steril 41:21S, 1984.

115. Badawy SZA, Guenca V, Stitzel A, et al.: Autoimmune phenomena in infertile patients with endometriosis. Obstet Gynecol 63:271, 1984.

116. Mathur S, Peress MR, Williamson HO, et al: Autoimmunity to endometrium and ovary in endometriosis. Clin Exp Immunol 50:259, 1982.

117. Barbieri RL, Bast RC, Niloff JM, et al.: Evaluation of a serological test for the diagnosis of endometriosis using a monoclonal antibody OC-125. Presented at the annual meeting of the Society for Gynecologic Investigation, March 1985. Abstract 33/P.

118. Steele RW, Dmowski WP, Marmar DJ: Immunologic aspects of human endometriosis. Am J Reprod Immunol 6:33, 1984.

8. Disorders of Ovarian Development

Bernard Gondos

Establishment and maintenance of normal ovarian function result from a series of developmental events beginning early in fetal development and continuing into the postnatal period. Oocyte maturation is initiated in the fetus during the first trimester and oogenesis proceeds throughout the later stages of gestation. Follicle formation begins shortly after oocyte differentiation at midgestation. By the time of birth, the definitive population of oocytes is present and follicle growth is well established. Endocrine differentiation, while relatively limited during fetal development, involves profound changes in the prepubertal and adolescent ovary.

In the succeeding chapters abnormalities of ovarian function affecting fertility are considered. The critical role of the ovary in reproductive function involves two principal aspects: oocyte maturation and sex hormone production. The pathophysiologic mechanisms in the different types of ovarian disorders are related to problems in oocyte maturation or sex steroid production, or a combination of the two. In dealing with these disorders, it is necessary to recognize that understanding of pathologic changes in the ovary requires thorough understanding of normal developmental events. For this reason, special emphasis in this chapter will be given to a review of normal ovarian development. The major changes occurring in the fetal ovary are summarized in Table 8–1.

Developmental disorders will be considered in terms of alterations in specific maturational events. Since oogenesis is established during fetal development, dysgenetic changes in the ovaries are produced during this time. The mechanisms involved relate to intrinsic genetic and chromosomal abnormalities which produce their effects early in development. A variety of extrinsic factors, such as radiation and chemotherapy, can also affect the ovary during the fetal and postnatal periods. These effects may be on the oocyte or the sex-steroid producing cells. Regardless of the timing and specific effects, the impact on later reproductive function may be significant and will depend on the type and extent of damage produced.

OVARIAN DEVELOPMENT

Development of the mammalian ovary can be divided into prefollicular, follicular, and ovulatory stages. In the human ovary the stage of prefollicular development extends from the time of gonadal differentiation in the second month of gestation to midgestation (Figure 8–1). During this period, germ cells and granulosa cells are arranged in cords and sheets within the ovarian cortex. Follicle formation begins at the end of the fifth month and continues through the second half of gestation. The process starts with the encirclement of individual oocytes by surrounding granulosa cells. Growth of follicles is evident in the prenatal and postnatal ovary. During childhood small follicles enter the growth phase at all times and develop into preantral and antral follicles. Ovulatory cycles are first established at the time of puberty, when the ovary includes follicles at all stages of development and corpus luteum formation is evident.

Prefollicular Stage

The changes involved in maturation of the fetal ovary begin with modification of the general structure of the genital ridge which develops early in the second month of gestation as a thickening on the medial aspect of the coelomic cavity. The gonadal outgrowth which arises from the genital ridge is composed of coelomic epithelium and underlying mesenchyme.

Primitive germ cells (Figure 8–2) complete their migration to the presumptive gonad from the yolk sac endoderm at this time.[1] Shortly thereafter, cells from the coelomic or surface epithelium and from adjacent mesonephric tissue move into the gonadal mesenchyme. During this period the term indifferent gonad is used since neither ovarian nor testicular differentiation is evident. Seminiferous cords begin to form in the male gonad at six weeks as the first morphologic indication of gonadal sex differentiation.[2] The female gonad shows no evidence of sex differentiation for another few weeks and can only be recognized as an ovary by exclusion.

Under normal circumstances there is direct correlation of the presence of a Y chromosome (46,XY) with testicular differentiation and absence of a Y (46,XX) with ovarian differentiation. However, information derived from developmental disorders indicates that the situation may be somewhat more complicated, particularly in the presence of chromosome anomalies. (See Chapter 15). It has been proposed that H-Y antigen, a histocompatibility antigen linked to sex chromosome function, is the key sex-

Table 8–1. Development of Fetal Ovary

Developmental Stage	Fetal Age	Appearance of Ovary
Sexual indifference	4–6 wk	Germ cells migrate to genital ridge Gonadal primordia project into coelomic cavity
Gonadal sex differentiation	6–9 wk	Testicular differentiation evident Ovary appears undifferentiated, contains primitive germ cells
Oogonial proliferation	9–11 wk	Oogonia in interphase and mitosis, interspersed with granulosa cells
Initiation of oogenesis	11–12 wk	Meiosis begins in inner cortex, oogonial mitosis continues
Oocyte differentiation	12–18 wk	Oocytes progress through meiotic prophase, oogonia also present, as well as degenerating germ cells
Follicle formation	18–20 wk	Follicle formation begins in inner cortex, oogonia and oocytes in all stages meiotic prophase present
Follicle growth	20 wk–term	Follicle formation continues, oocyte differentiation to diplotene reaches completion, follicle growth begins

determining factor,[3] but problems in documenting this association have cast some doubt on its significance.[4]

Normal ovarian differentiation evidently requires the presence of two X chromosomes in addition to absence of a Y chromosome. One of the X chromosomes becomes inactivated early in embryogenesis, well before gonadal differentiation takes place.[5] The sex chromatin mass (Barr body) which results from the inactivation appears as early as the third week of gestation.[6] Barr bodies, however, are not seen in oocytes and it has been shown that two functional X chromosomes are present in fetal germ cells.[7]

The first recognizable structural change in the presumptive ovary is the active proliferation of germ cells during the third month. The cells undergoing mitosis, referred to as oogonia (Figure 8–3), proceed through a series of divisions characterized by incomplete cytokinesis and persistence of intercellular bridges between adjacent cells.[8] This results in formation of syncytial groups of cells which develop in synchrony. Somatic cells associ-

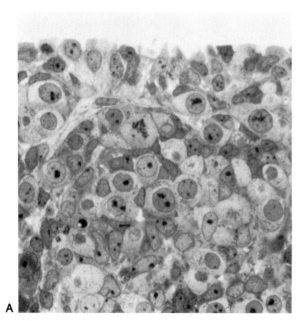
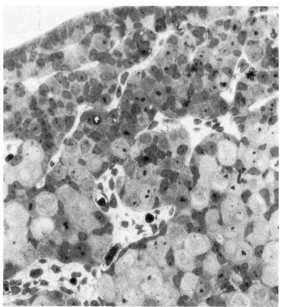

A
B

Figure 8–1. Appearance of ovary during prefollicular stage of fetal development. A. Primitive germ cells and oogonia fill cortex beneath surface epithelium, 10 weeks gestation. B. Cords of oocytes in meiosis, 16 weeks gestation. Toluidine blue (×400).

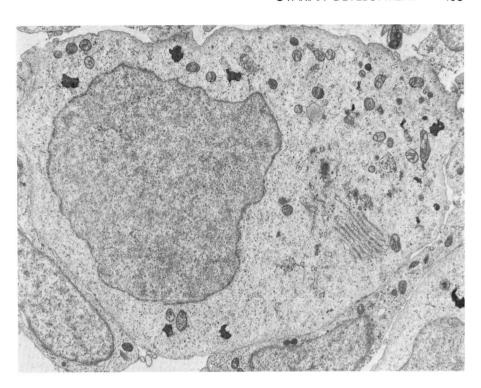

Figure 8–2. Electron micrograph, primitive germ cell, 9 weeks gestation. Note eccentric nucleus and ameboid appearance. (×6,000).

ated with the germ cells have the general morphologic and ultrastructural features of granulosa cells.

Transformation of oogonia into oocytes, indicated by the onset of meiosis, begins at 11 to 12 weeks.[2,9] This is preceded by a preleptotene stage of DNA synthesis. The entry into meiosis progresses from the innermost cortex to more peripheral regions in a locally synchronized manner. Initiation of meiosis is considered to be regulated by a meiosis-inducing substance produced by the fetal rete ovarii.[10]

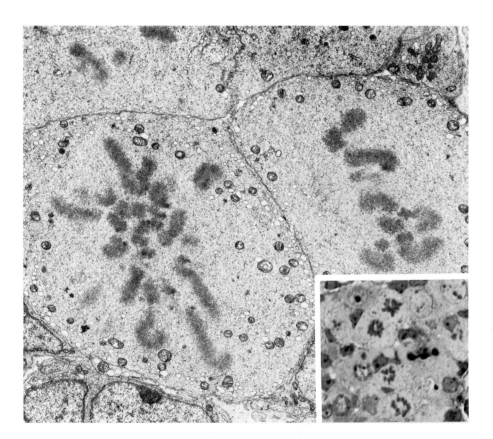

Figure 8–3. Oogonia in mitosis, fetal ovarian cortex. (×5,500). Inset, light microscopic appearance. Toluidine blue (×400).

Oocytes undergo two meiotic divisions, but only a portion of the first occurs in the prefollicular stage of development. Leptotene, zygotene, pachytene, and diplotene stages of the first meiotic prophase are seen in the ovary at this time (Figure 8–4). There is a shift to more mature forms with advancing age and, by midgestation, a predominance of later stages is present.

Many of the germ cells undergo degeneration during the prefollicular period. Degeneration occurs in three distinct waves, affecting oogonia in mitosis, oocytes in pachytene, and oocytes in diplotene.[11] Surviving oocytes are separated from their neighbors by elongated extensions of granulosa cells as the process of follicle formation begins.

Electron microscopic studies have demonstrated that the cytoplasm of fetal granulosa cells contains abundant lipid but lacks the large mitochondria and smooth endoplasmic reticulum characteristic of steroid-producing cells. Such structures are found in fetal interstitial cells.[12] The latter are present at the corticomedullary junction in the prefollicular stage (Figure 8–5) and have been shown to contain steroidogenic enzymes.[13,14] Although significant amounts of estradiol have not been detected in extracts of fetal ovaries, the human fetal ovary is evidently able to synthesize some progesterone and androgens *in vitro*.[15] Estrogen synthesis by conversion of testosterone to estradiol has been described in prefollicular human ovaries;[16] however, endocrine activity in the fetal ovary is minimal and the prevailing view at present is that, in contrast to the fetal testis, the ovary does not play a major role in reproductive tract differentiation.

Similarly, a role for gonadotropins in prefollicular ovarian development remains to be demonstrated. The human fetal pituitary can synthesize gonadotropins as early as 10 to 11 weeks gestation, prior to the onset of oogenesis.[17] The follicle-stimulating hormone (FSH) content in females greatly exceeds that in males and serum FSH and luteinizing hormone (LH) levels are significantly higher in the prefollicular stage than at term.[18,19] However, *in vitro* investigations in human fetal ovarian explants indicate that gonadotropins do not have an influence on oogenesis.[20] Studies of ovaries from anencephalic fetuses have shown an effect on follicle growth but not follicle formation.[21] In monkeys fetal hypophysectomy does result in reduction in the number of oocytes and follicles,[22] suggesting a possible role of gonadotropins in early ovarian development.

Follicular Stage

The stage of follicular development is prolonged, extending from early development into the adult period. Follicle formation begins during the fifth month of gestation.[1,2,9] As with the onset of meiosis, follicle formation progresses from the innermost cortex peripherally.[23] This process continues throughout the second half of gestation and is completed by the early neonatal period when all of the surviving oocytes have become incorporated in follicles.

Formation of the follicle involves separation of the oocytes, enclosure of individual oocytes by granulosa cells, and development of a basement membrane around this unit (Figure 8–6). Initially, each oocyte is surrounded by a single layer of granulosa cells. With the proliferation of granulosa cells, there is progressive follicular enlarge-

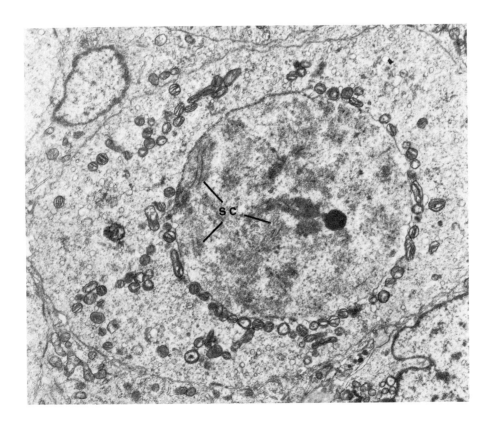

Figure 8–4. Oocyte in meiotic prophase, characterized by synaptinemal complexes (sc) and perinuclear arrangement of mitochondria. (×7,000).

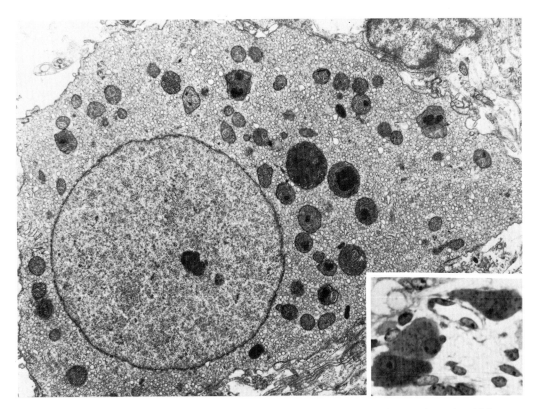

Figure 8–5. Fetal interstitial cell with abundant smooth endoplasmic reticulum and prominent tubulovesicular mitochondria. (×3,800). Inset, light microscopic appearance. Toluidine blue (×400).

ment. The oocyte also undergoes extensive changes, including increase in size, formation of microvilli on the cell surface, and changes in the differentiation and distribution of cytoplasmic organelles.[24] The oocyte nucleus remains arrested in the diplotene stage of meiotic prophase during the growth phase, apparently under the influence of surrounding granulosa cells.[25]

With increase in follicular size, a zona pellucida forms between the oocyte and granulosa cells, and theca cells differentiate from surrounding mesenchymal cells to become incorporated in the envelope of the growing follicle. Theca cells begin to appear at mid- to late gestation as increasing numbers of follicles enter the growth phase. The theca interna portion of the follicle remains separated from the inner granulosa cell layers by the membrana granulosa and, in contrast to the granulosa cell compartment, becomes well vascularized. In general there is relatively sparse vascularization in the fetal and neonatal ovary, but, with increasing age, conspicuous spiral arteries and tortuous veins appear in the ovarian stroma.

Follicle growth is associated with changes in the size of the oocyte, the number of cells in the envelope, and formation of a fluid-filled antrum. Follicles can be classified as: 1. small, nongrowing follicles, in which the oocyte is enclosed by a single layer of granulosa cells, 2. preantral follicles, in which the growing oocyte is surrounded by multiple layers of proliferating granulosa and theca cells, and 3. antral follicles, in which the oocyte has terminated its growth while the envelope continues to enlarge and a fluid-filled antrum is present. The descriptive indi-

cation of morphologic appearance and physiologic state illustrated in Figure 8–7 has been found to be particularly useful in classifying developing follicles.[26]

Follicle growth and degeneration occur simultaneously and continuously, with extensive follicular atresia evident in the fetal and postnatal periods. Atresia is a physiologic process whereby follicles undergo degenerative changes resulting in their shrinkage and eventual resorption. Follicular atresia is an ongoing process, with the greatest number of follicles being lost during the developmental period (Figure 8–8). The result is a marked reduction in the number of oocytes from a peak of seven million at midgestation to approximately two million at the time of birth.[11]

In contrast to earlier views, it is now well established that the ovary is not quiescent during early childhood. Small follicles enter the growth phase at all times during childhood and develop to preantral and antral follicles.[27,28] More follicles enter the growth phase early, rather than late, in childhood, but more follicles reach larger antral size as the child grows older.[29] Increase in the number of follicles and stromal connective tissue results in progressive ovarian enlargement with advancing age.

Follicular development and oocyte growth are not associated with significant steroid hormone production by the ovary during the late fetal and early childhood periods. High circulating estradiol levels present in the first few days after birth are of placental origin.[30] There is also a slight transient increase in ovarian estradiol production between 2 and 4 months of age, associated with a compa-

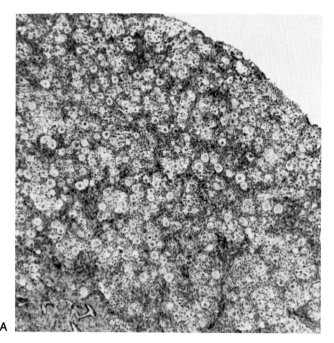

A

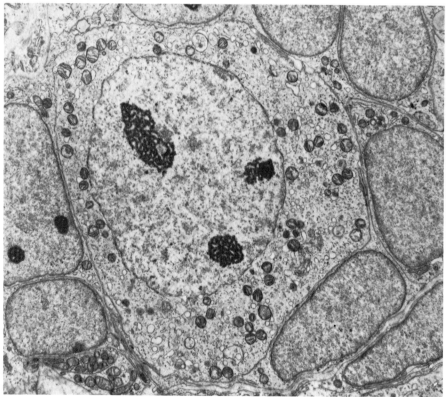

B

Figure 8–6. Early follicular stage. A. Light micrograph. H & E (×150). B. Electron micrograph. (×3,500).

rable elevation in gonadotropins, which exceeds that in male infants.[30,31] Estradiol levels are low in both sexes between 2 and 8 years of age, after which the level in girls exceeds that in boys.[32,33] Progesterone levels change little until after menarche. Testosterone, androstenedione, and estrone levels rise in a pattern similar to that of estradiol, but without as sharp an increase as at the time of puberty. Estradiol levels undergo an approximately six-fold in-

crease in the four years preceding the development of ovulatory cycles. It is likely that rising levels of gonadotropins have a direct influence on the development of the prepubertal ovary and the stimulation of estradiol production (Figure 8–9).

Except for the transient rise in the neonatal period, gonadotropin levels remain low during early childhood.[30,31,33,34] There is a gradual rise after the age of 6

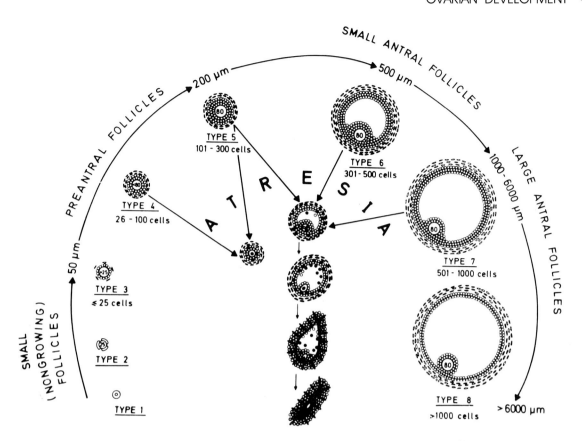

Figure 8–7. Classification of follicles in the human ovary. (From Peters and McNatty,[26] with permission.)

years, concomitant with an increase in the number and size of antral follicles. Serum LH levels start to increase later than FSH levels.[30,31,35,36] Prolactin levels, which increase gradually in the prepubertal period, show a slight dip at the time of the initial FSH rise and then continue to rise.[30] The sharpest rise around menarche is that of LH, characterized by episodic release particularly in relation to sleep, apparently under the influence of modulations in gonadotropin-releasing hormone pulse frequency.[35] The evidence supports the view that gonadotropins may

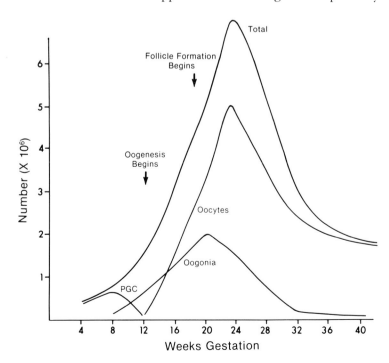

Figure 8–8. Numbers of germ cells in human fetal ovary at different ages. Peak occurs at midgestation, followed by progressive and extensive loss during late gestation. PGC, primitive germ cells. (Modified from Baker[11]).

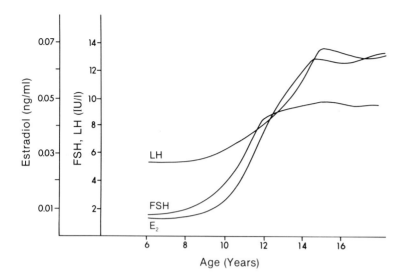

Figure 8–9. Estradiol, FSH, and LH levels in girls during childhood and pubertal development. (Data from Refs. 34 and 36.)

not be required for follicle formation and early development, but have their major influence in promoting growth of follicles to the antral stage, proliferation of granulosa cells, theca cell differentiation, secretion of follicular fluid, and, eventually, induction of ovulatory cycles.

Ovulatory Stage

Following the gonadotropin increments that occur during late childhood, a major event in the process of ovarian maturation is the appearance of ovulatory potential whereby a gonadal signal causes a surge release of LH. This positive feedback process, which does not exist in the prepubertal or early pubertal period, allows rising estrogen levels to stimulate LH and produce ovulation.[37] Ovulation does not occur prior to menarche, although even before menarche gonadotropins are already secreted in a cyclic pattern of irregular duration.[38]

Morphological changes associated with ovulation and corpus luteum formation are known to be induced by LH. Accumulation of smooth endoplasmic reticulum, large tubulovesicular mitochondria, and other organelles involved in steroid hormone production (Figure 8–10) is under the direct influence of this hormone.[39,40]

At the time that ovulatory capacity is established, the structure of the ovary is not substantially different from that in childhood, with the exception of corpus luteum formation. With development of the cyclic ovulatory pattern, fresh corpora lutea and those of previous cycles can be recognized. Specific morphologic changes in the pubertal ovary that might account for ovulatory capacity have not been identified, and it is likely that the transition from the follicular to the ovulatory stage is based primarily on functional changes.

An interesting change does occur in the appearance of the ovaries. While the two ovaries have a relatively similar appearance throughout the early juvenile period, with approaching maturity there is increasing dissimilarity.[29] The observation of increasing bilateral dissimilarity has possible functional implications. It has been suggested

that asymmetric estradiol secretion in premenarchial individuals and local variations in intraovarian gonadotropins and sex steroids may contribute significantly to the development of pubertal changes.[41,42]

CHROMOSOMAL AND GENETIC DISORDERS

A major group of developmental abnormalities of the ovary includes those related to chromosomal and genetic defects. The most important in relation to effects on fertility are sex chromosome and related anomalies leading to defective ovarian differentiation. These conditions are associated with characteristic clinical and endocrine abnormalities. They are classified here according to the pathologic changes in the gonads, the underlying pathogenesis, and karyotypic findings. In addition to disorders with primary effects on gonadal differentiation, autosomal abnormalities with secondary effects on ovarian development are briefly considered.

GONADAL DYSGENESIS

In gonadal dysgenesis the principal defect is the presence of streak gonads. The disorders are generally a result of sex chromosome abnormalities, although a variety of genetic disturbances may be involved. Affected individuals generally have a female phenotype. Since phenotype is related to the presence or absence of androgenic influences, failure of normal ovarian differentiation does not alter the basic pattern of female phenotypic development. The pathogenesis of gonadal dysgenesis is typically related to oocyte loss and ovarian involution occurring during fetal development. This is the common pathway for a variety of conditions ranging from the absence or structural alterations of an X chromosome, as in Turner's syndrome, to gene mutations in individuals with apparently normal female or male chromosomal complements

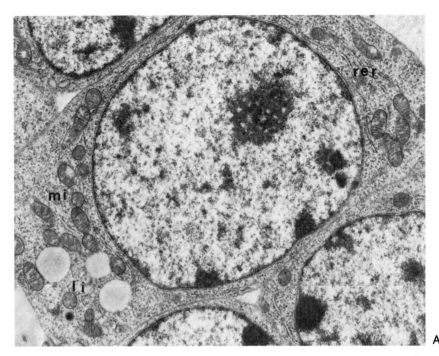

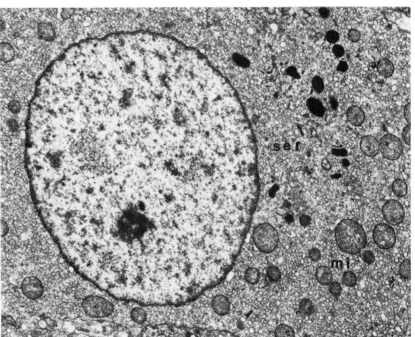

Figure 8–10. Ultrastructural appearance of granulosa cells in preovulatory follicle (A) and corpus luteum (B). Note proliferation of smooth endoplasmic reticulum (ser) and prominence of mitochondria (mi) in luteinized granulosa cell. li, lipid. rer, rough endoplasmic reticulum. (×6,500).

to various forms of sex chromosome mosaicism. The characteristic findings in the different types of gonadal dysgenesis are summarized in Table 8–2.

Turner's Syndrome

The classical components of the syndrome are streak ovaries, primary amenorrhea, failure of secondary sex development, and a number of somatic abnormalities including short stature, webbing of the neck, and low posterior hairline.[43,44] Many other anomalies have also been de-

scribed. In general the occurrence of congenital malformations of various types is greater in patients with this disorder than in the general population.

The condition is typically associated with absence of one X chromosome (45,X), but may also occur with various X chromosome defects in 46,XX individuals. These include primary or secondary losses of portions of the X chromosome. Patients with Y chromosome defects and those with mosaicism may also exhibit features of the syndrome. The latter constitute about 10% of the cases of Turner's syndrome.[45]

The incidence of 45,X newborns is about 1 per 10,000

Table 8–2. Pathogenesis and Appearance of Gonads in Different Forms of Gonadal Dysgenesis

Type	Etiology	Pathogenesis	Gonads	Typical Findings
Turner's syndrome (45,X, mosaicism or X chromosome defect)	Chromosome loss or nondisjunction, defects of X short and long arms	Oocyte degeneration, failure of follicle development	Fibrous streaks lacking follicles in most cases; follicles may be present, particularly with mosaicism	Short stature, numerous somatic abnormalities, low estradiol, elevated gonadotropins, diagnosis by karyotype studies
46,XX Gonadal dysgenesis[a]	Autosomal recessive gene defect in familial cases	Unknown; may be similar to Turner's syndrome	Fibrous streaks lacking follicles or hypoplastic ovaries	Normal stature, primary amenorrhea associated with normal karyotype, elevated gonadotropins, neurologic abnormalities, positive family history
46,XY Gonadal dysgenesis[a]	X-linked recessive or male-limited autosomal dominant gene defect in familial cases	May be defect in either ovarian or testicular differentiation	Variable; usually bilateral streak gonads	Female phenotype associated with 46,XY karyotype, elevated gonadotropins, high incidence of gonadoblastoma
45,X/46,XY Gonadal dysgenesis	Translocation, deletion or other abnormality of Y chromosome, mitotic loss of Y chromosome	Partial or complete failure of testicular differentiation	Variable; streak or dysgenetic testis[b]	Ambiguous genitalia and/or secondary sex characteristic abnormalities, mosaicism on karyotype, elevated gonadotropins, high incidence of gonadoblastoma

[a] May be referred to as pure gonadal dysgenesis.

[b] Presence of streak on one side and dysgenetic testis on other side referred to as mixed gonadal dysgenesis.

females. It has been estimated that the frequency of zygotes lacking an X chromosome is 0.8%, probably the commonest chromosome anomaly in man, but less than 3% of 45,X conceptuses survive to term.[46,47]

The condition may arise from a variety of chromosome errors. Nondisjunction or chromosome loss during gametogenesis in either parent, leading to a sperm or oocyte lacking a sex chromosome, could account for the 45, X condition. It could also result from a mitotic error at the first cleavage. In those individuals with X chromosome defects, translocation is a likely cause.

Diagnosis is established by karyotype analysis of blood, skin, or gonadal tissue. Buccal smear evaluation demonstrating absence of Barr bodies and determination of elevated plasma and urinary gonadotropins, particularly FSH, are useful as screening methods. Barr body analysis should be interpreted with caution, since in cases of mosaicism the presence of Barr bodies could be misleading. Karyotype studies represent the only reliable approach to provide a definitive diagnosis. Thorough karyotypic analysis, utilizing multiple tissues and evaluating an adequate number of cells, is of critical importance in this condition.

The pathologic changes, while usually characteristic, can be variable. Typically, the reproductive ducts and external genitalia are normal female, but immature. The gonads are elongated pale white structures located in the mesosalpinges. These streak-like structures are composed of fibrous connective tissue and bands of basophilic stroma resembling theca externa (Figure 8–11). Follicles are sparse or absent. As discussed below, persistence of follicles may occur in some cases, particularly

those with mosaicism. Mesonephric remnants and aggregates of hilus cells are often seen (Figure 8–12).

The pathogenesis is related to extensive oocyte degeneration and failure of follicle formation. Observations on fetal ovaries from abortuses with a 45,X karyotype have indicated that migration of germ cells to the developing gonad and oogonial proliferation occur in a normal manner.[48] It is only when meiosis begins at the end of the third month that germ cell loss starts to take place. Although oocyte degeneration is widespread during the subsequent period, it is not unusual to find a few small follicles in 45,X infants at birth.[49] This is an unusual finding by late childhood and adolescence[50]; however, the rate of oocyte degeneration varies and it is evident that some individuals retain sufficient numbers of oocytes to develop cyclic ovulatory function.

This is indicated by the reports of conceptions in women with extensive karyotypic studies revealing only a 45,X line in multiple tissues.[51,52] It is evident therefore that lack of an X chromosome does not always imply complete impairment of fertility. However, fertility is a rare occurrence in 45,X individuals—approximately 3% of these patients menstruate—while, when mosaicism is present, menstruation occurs in 12%,[45] and fertility has been reported in a number of cases.[53] Patients with X chromosome abnormalities, rather than monosomy, may also be fertile.[54] So it is important for purposes of counseling to make every effort to perform thorough cytogenetic analysis. In addition, young patients with this condition who develop menstrual function should be made aware that they have a shorter reproductive life period than normal because of accelerated oocyte loss and that

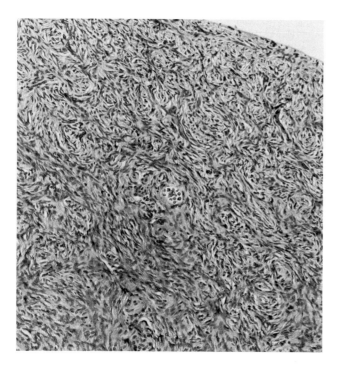

Figure 8–11. Ovary in Turner's syndrome, with dense collagenous tissue in outer cortex and underlying bands of interweaving stroma. Follicles are absent. H & E (×250).

there is an increased incidence of abortion and abnormal offspring.[55]

Since there does not appear to be an increased risk of gonadal neoplasia in this condition as in other types of developmental disorders (see below), gonadal preserva-

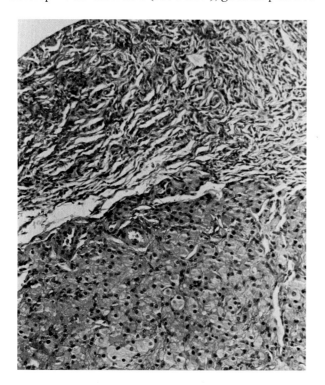

Figure 8–12. Prominent hilus cell aggregate in streak gonad. H & E (×250).

tion and therapy directed toward induction of secondary sex characteristics and menstrual function should be considered. Possible exceptions are cases with mosaicism, including the presence of a Y chromosome, which could indicate a risk for tumor development. Reports of endometrial carcinoma in patients receiving estrogen replacement therapy suggest that there is a potential risk of neoplasia not related to the condition itself but to its treatment.[56,57] It has been recommended therefore that patients receive estrogen therapy at the lowest possible level.[58]

46,XX Gonadal Dysgenesis

XX gonadal dysgenesis is characterized by normal stature, bilateral streak gonads, sexual infantilism, female internal and external genitalia, primary amenorrhea, elevated gonadotropins, and absence of the somatic stigmata of Turner's syndrome. The available data suggest autosomal recessive inheritance in most cases.[59] Families with multiple affected siblings have been described.[60] Some cases have had a few somatic abnormalities, but not the classical manifestations of Turner's syndrome; neurologic abnormalities, including neurosensory deafness, microcephaly, and mental retardation, have been associated in several families.[61]

Diagnosis is made by finding a normal karyotype in a phenotypic female with sexual infantilism and hypergonadotropic hypogonadism consistent with streak gonads. A positive family history is usually obtainable.

The pathogenesis may be similar to that of Turner's syndrome, but studies of the gonads of fetuses with XX gonadal dysgenesis are lacking. The mechanism of gene action in this condition could involve a variety of possible effects on the development of the ovary. Whether the abnormality is one of excessive germ cell attrition, as in 45,X dysgenesis, or failure of germ cell formation, migration, or proliferation is unclear, but the end result is the formation of streak gonads and the corresponding clinical and endocrine findings.

46,XY Gonadal Dysgenesis

XY gonadal dysgenesis is characterized by a female phenotype, sexual infantilism, normal stature, streak gonads, primary amenorrhea, and presence of tubes, uterus, and vagina. Familial aggregates as well as sporadic cases have been described.[62] At least 20 familial aggregates exist in which it has been established that the disorder results from an X-linked recessive or male-limited autosomal dominant gene.[59]

Diagnosis is made by finding an XY karyotype in an individual with female phenotype, sexual infantilism, and elevated gonadotropins. A positive family history may be present.

The pathogenesis of this condition is unclear. Data can be cited in support of either ovarian or testicular origin in XY gonadal dysgenesis. In some instances follicular structures are found[62,63] and in others rudimentary seminiferous cords consistent with dysgenetic testes are present.[64] Studies with H-Y antigen have provided conflicting evidence and have failed to clarify the nature of this condition. It may be that this is a heterogeneous group of disorders based upon different modes of inheritance.

There is a high incidence of gonadoblastoma, estimated at 20% to 30%, in this syndrome.[65,66] Gonadoblastoma is a complex tumor composed of germ cells, Sertoli cells, and occasionally Leydig cells, with frequent calcification (Figure 8–13). Although originally considered to be a germ cell tumor, it is now classified separately.[67] The pattern of gonadoblastoma has not been reported in a metastasis, but mitotic activity is usually present in germ cells in the tumor, and there is invasion of the surrounding tissue in half the patients. Progression to a malignant germinoma (dysgerminoma) or other form of germ cell tumor with metastatic potential occurs in about 30% of gonadoblastomas.[68] The risk for tumor development in this and other forms of gonadal dysgenesis appears to correlate with the presence of a Y chromosome.[69] Therefore, bilateral gonadectomy is indicated in patients with gonadal dysgenesis whenever a Y component is present.

45,X/46,XY Gonadal Dysgenesis

Individuals with sex chromosome mosaicism may appear as phenotypic females or males or, most commonly, have ambiguous genitalia.[70] Short stature and other somatic

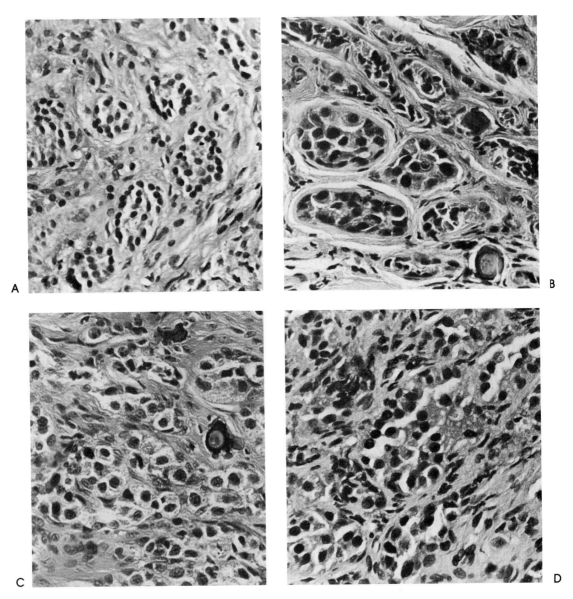

Figure 8–13. Gonadoblastoma in 17-year-old phenotypic female with 46,XY karyotype, streak gonad on left and tumor on right. A. Dysgenetic right gonad with primitive testicular cords. B. Section showing gonadoblastoma with nests of germ cells and Sertoli cells and foci of calcification. C. Cords of abnormal germ cells in area of transition to dysgerminoma. D. Section of tumor with area of diffuse infiltration. H & E (×350).

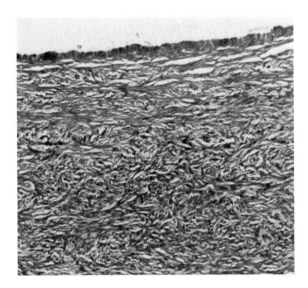

Figure 8–14. Streak gonad in 45,X/46,XY gonadal dysgenesis. Note prominent surface epithelium and dense underlying stroma. H & E (×450).

abnormalities are inconstant features. Most individuals are reared as females.

Diagnosis is made by karyotype studies demonstrating mosaicism in an individual with ambiguous genitalia and/or secondary sex and somatic anomalies. Structural abnormalities of the Y chromosome are typically present and absence of bright fluorescence is often noted.

The cause of this condition may relate to translocation or deletion of the Y chromosome. In some patients, abnormal banding and alteration of the Y chromosome are seen. The defects could also result from mitotic loss of the Y producing a 45,X cell line and mosaicism. The condition has been observed in various other forms of mosaicism, such as 45,X/47,XYY and 45,X/46,XY/47,XYY.

The pathologic changes are variable, with the gonads appearing as dysgenetic testes or streaks (Figure 8–14) which may be similar or dissimilar bilaterally.[68] The finding of a streak or absent gonadal tissue on one side and a dysgenetic testis on the other is referred to as mixed gonadal dysgenesis. In some cases the gonad is completely replaced by tumor. Internal genital structures typically include both müllerian elements, such as tubes and uterus, and mesonephric elements, such as vas deferens.

The propensity to develop gonadoblastoma is high since a Y chromosome is present. A risk of about 20% to 25% overall has been estimated.[66,69] Ultrastructural studies have suggested that dysgenetic testicular elements are the source of gonadoblastomas.[71] Because of the possibility for progression to tumors with metastatic potential, bilateral gonadectomy is imperative.

TRUE HERMAPHRODITISM

Presence of both ovarian and testicular tissue in the same or opposite gonads is required for the diagnosis of true hermaphroditism. This is an uncommon disorder. Clini-

cal presentation and hormonal findings are variable, as is the karyotype pattern, the most common being 46,XX followed by 46,XX/46,XY mosaicism.[72] Most cases described have been sporadic rather than familial.

Diagnosis of true hermaphroditism should be considered in all patients with ambiguous genitalia, particularly those with XX/XY mosaicism; however, other more common types of developmental abnormalities should be ruled out first by appropriate studies. Establishing a diagnosis of true hermaphroditism depends on histologic demonstration of ovarian and testicular elements.

This condition may result from sex chromosome mosaicism, chimerism, translocation, or an autosomal mutant gene. There is evidence in support of all of these possibilities in different cases studied.[6,73] It is therefore evident that the condition represents a heterogeneous group of disorders.

The pathologic changes are also variable (Figure 8–15). There may be an ovary on one side and a testis on the other, bilateral ovotestes, or an ovotestis on one side and an ovary or testis on the other. When an ovotestis is present, the ovarian follicular structures may be present in the outer cortical region and the testicular cords in the inner medullary portion, following the normal pattern of differentiation, or the distribution may be irregular. In patients with an ovary on one side and a testis on the other, the development of the internal genitalia is consistent with the homolateral gonad. An ovotestis is usually associated with predominantly müllerian duct development.

The tendency for tumor development in this condition is difficult to assess because of the small number of cases. In accordance with the general approach to developmentally abnormal gonads, those individuals with a Y chromosome would be at special risk. However, the finding of a gonadoblastoma in a true hermaphrodite with a 46,XX karyotype[74] suggests that the presence of testicular elements may be the key factor, in which case all patients with this condition would be at risk.

POLYSOMY X

47,XXX individuals may experience delayed menarche or premature ovarian failure. It has been postulated that the increased number of X chromosomes results from failure of meiotic disjunction.[45] Fertility is commonly present in 47,XXX women and most offspring have been found to be chromosomally normal.[54]

AUTOSOMAL DISORDERS

Certain autosomal abnormalities are associated with defective ovarian development as a secondary effect. Although the changes may not be as severe as in primary disorders, clinical evidence of disturbance of ovarian function is often evident. A number of chromosomal abnormalities can be shown to influence gonadal function. Those conditions in which specific information on ovarian development is available are discussed here.

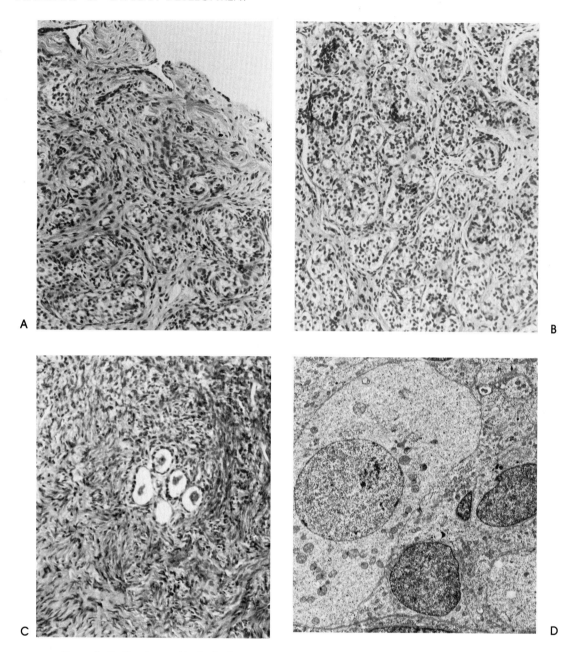

Figure 8–15. Ovarian and testicular tissue in same gonad, indicating true hermaphroditism. A. Ovarian cortical stroma and underlying testicular cords. B. Dense arrangement of testicular cords in medullary region. C. Group of small ovarian follicles. H & E (×150). D. Electron micrograph of testicular cord showing germ cell at left. (×1,500).

Trisomy 18

Ovarian abnormalities have been described as relatively frequent in trisomy 18,[75] which is characteristically associated with facial, skeletal, and cardiovascular anomalies. The ovaries show a reduction in the number of follicles and increased atresia. In some cases severe depletion of oocytes has been noted,[23] while in others only minimal changes are evident (Figure 8–16). The findings could be secondary to defects in hypothalamic-pituitary regulation.

Trisomy 21 (Down Syndrome)

In Down syndrome, late menarche and delayed sexual development are often evident. A study of the development of the ovaries in this condition indicated that the number of small follicles was reduced and follicle growth was partially or totally inhibited (Figure 8–17).[76] These findings would be consistent with a disturbance in gonadotropin production, which is supported by the observation of abnormalities in the anterior pituitary.[77]

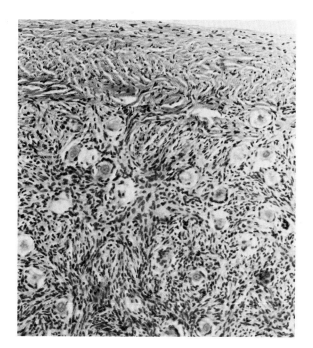

Figure 8–16. Ovary from stillborn fetus with trisomy 18. Follicle development is present, but reduction in the number of oocytes is evident. H & E (×250).

Ataxia Telangiectasia

Ataxia telangiectasia is a single gene autosomal recessive disorder associated with multiple neurologic, immunologic, and endocrine abnormalities. The ovaries of girls with this disease are characterized by a paucity of small and antral follicles and in some cases marked gonadal atrophy (Figure 8–18).[78] Although the pathogenesis of ataxia telangiectasia is not known, autoimmune effects associated with thymic and neuronal degeneration have been described.[79] Since neonatal thymectomy in animals is known to result in profound developmental changes in the ovary,[80] an immunologic basis for the defective ovarian development in this condition is a possible consideration. The role of autoimmune factors in ovarian failure is discussed further in Chapter 9.

RADIATION EFFECTS

Radiation to the developing ovaries may result in primary amenorrhea, hypogonadism, and elevated gonadotropins.[81,82] The effects of radiation on the developing ovary relate to the marked radiosensitivity of differentiating germ cells. The damaging effects can be critical since there is not a pool of surviving stem cells as there is in the testis and, therefore, oocyte loss is permanent.

The sensitivity of germ cells to radiation is maximal during oogonial differentiation and then decreases with the transformation to oocytes. Studies on ovarian tissue removed from aborted fetuses and subjected to irradiation indicated greatest sensitivity in oogonia undergoing mitosis.[83] It has been suggested that oocytes in diplotene in which the chromosome loops are condensed and surrounded by a dense sheath of ribonucleoprotein are likely to be resistant to radiation effects.[84] From these observations the greatest sensitivity of the developing ovary would be during midgestation when the highest proportion of germ cells are in the oogonial stage (Figure 8–8).

Although effects on oocytes in the follicular stage are probably limited, radiation may affect granulosa cells, particularly during follicular growth when they undergo active proliferation. Stage of follicular development and local environmental factors probably play an important

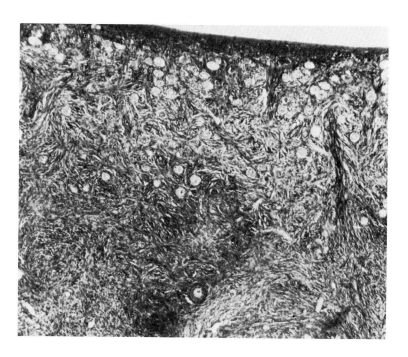

Figure 8–17. Ovary from child with Down syndrome, showing limited follicle growth. H & E (×150). (From Højager, et al.,[76] with permission).

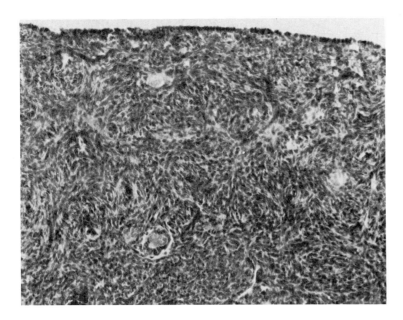

Figure 8–18. Ovary in ataxia telangiectasia. Marked oocyte loss is evident. H & E. (×250). (Provided by Dr. J. Chatten).

part in determining the effects of radiation. Data from postmortem studies on changes in the childhood ovary following radiotherapy for abdominal tumors indicate that follicle growth is inhibited and the number of small follicles markedly reduced.[23] Clinical studies in patients who have survived have shown markedly elevated FSH levels and low estradiol levels consistent with ovarian failure.[85,86] The presence of primary amenorrhea in some of these individuals suggests that the effects may be permanent, although in others menarche and conception have been reported. (See Chapter 9.)

The pathologic changes in the ovary consist of cortical atrophy and follicle depletion (Figure 8–19). The extent of damage undoubtedly relates to the dosage, duration, and manner of administration. Because many of the cases

studied have received both radiation and chemotherapy, the specific effects related to radiation damage are difficult to evaluate and there could be an additive effect.

Differential diagnosis includes a variety of other conditions causing similar changes such as Turner's syndrome, drug effects, and idiopathic ovarian failure. A history of radiation exposure would explain the findings.

DRUG EFFECTS

Women treated with cytotoxic drugs may have impaired fertility or ovarian dysfunction manifested by irregular or absent menses for substantial periods of time.[87,88] Cytotoxic drugs have the capacity to produce a picture similar to that following radiation. As in the latter, it might be expected that actively proliferating cells would be particularly vulnerable to toxic effects. Chemical agents can produce chromosomal aberrations in developing germ cells, including structural and numerical changes. The incidence of structural anomalies in germ cells induced by methotrexate and cyclophosphamide is highest during the oogonial stage of differentiation,[89] a finding similar to that induced by radiation.

Treatment of prepubertal girls with cytotoxic chemotherapeutic agents has in most cases not resulted in subsequent ovarian dysfunction.[86,90] Postpubertal evaluation of ovarian function following cyclophosphamide treatment for nephrotic syndrome before and during puberty indicated no menstrual disorders or gonadotropin abnormalities.[91] Ovaries of girls dying after treatment for acute leukemia have shown decreased numbers of follicles and inhibition of follicle maturation, but general destruction of oocytes was lacking.[92] There does, however, appear to be an increased risk of injury when chemotherapy is initiated during puberty. (See Chapter 9.)

Studies on the effects of a variety of chemotherapeutic agents have indicated an association with oocyte destruction and ovulatory dysfunction when administered to

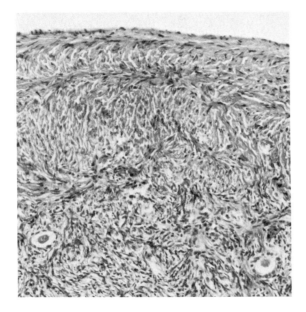

Figure 8–19. Cortical atrophy and follicle depletion, post-radiation therapy. H & E (×250).

adults, but minimal to absent changes when used in the childhood period.[86,88] While effects on the oocyte are the most obvious result, it is likely that changes are also induced in proliferating granulosa cells and theca cells. Therefore, even without significant oocyte loss, effects on follicular maturation and steroidogenesis could be present.

The effect of busulfan on ovarian morphogenesis has been the subject of a number of experimental studies.[93,94] If administered at the time of gonadal differentiation, marked germ cell depletion results without impairment of general structural differentiation. However, the absence of oocytes is associated with severe defects in steroidogenic activity at later stages of development. This implies that germ cell destruction can have a secondary effect on ovarian endocrine function.

The pathologic changes induced by cytotoxic agents are similar to other conditions associated with oocyte loss; however, the extent of damage to the childhood ovary appears to be relatively limited. As a rule, the greater the number of chemotherapeutic agents, the more intensive the therapy, and the older the individual, the higher the likelihood of ovarian injury and of permanent loss of reproductive function.[88]

PREMATURE DEVELOPMENT

Premature onset of ovarian function is associated with development of estrogen-dependent secondary sex characteristics and reproductive capability prior to the normal time of expected puberty. In general, occurrence of such changes in girls under 9 years implies an aberration in ovarian function.

True precocious puberty results from premature activation of cyclic hypothalamic-pituitary function, which induces sex steroid secretion and ovulatory function in a manner identical to that occurring in the reproductive years. The changes are of extrinsic origin, secondary to central nervous system disease, or idiopathic in nature. Pathologic effects in the ovary are not present, other than the evidence of premature ovulation and luteinization. Differential diagnosis is directed toward determining the source of the premature stimulation of ovarian function.

Much less frequently, intrinsic ovarian changes are responsible for premature development. Since the mechanisms involved here are not directly analogous to the normal regulation of pubertal development, this condition is referred to as precocious pseudopuberty.[95] Adrenal as well as ovarian diseases may be involved or the changes may result from exogenous estrogens.

Among the primary ovarian lesions, tumors or non-neoplastic cysts may be encountered (Table 8–3). The tumors are typically of sex cord-stromal type, that is, neoplasms derived from steroid hormone secreting cells. The most common of these is the granulosa cell tumor. Such tumors are capable of producing estrogens and eliciting corresponding endocrine changes. The tumors generally found in young girls (Figure 8–20) differ somewhat from the adult form and have been referred to as juvenile granulosa cell tumors.[96] Among granulosa cell tumors occurring in girls under 9 years approximately 80% are associated with evidence of isosexual precocity.[97] However, less than 25% are seen primarily because of endocrine-associated symptoms, abdominal pain, and distention representing the usual complaints.[93]

Other tumors of sex cord-stromal type associated with endocrine changes are the Sertoli-Leydig cell tumor, also known as arrhenoblastoma, and lipoid cell tumors. The latter two groups typically produce androgens and therefore may be associated with hirsutism and clitoromegaly in addition to signs of isosexual precocity.[99] Germ cell tumors, such as dysgerminomas and endodermal sinus tumors, may also produce endocrine changes of virilizing type.[100,101] These changes result from stimulation of stromal cells around the tumor to luteinize and produce androgens (Figure 8–21).

In general, removal of steroid-producing ovarian tumors associated with precocious developmental changes will result in regression of these changes and menarche will occur at a normal age.[102] Follow-up studies available indicate that there is no effect on subsequent fertility.[103]

Non-neoplastic cysts have also been associated with

Table 8–3. Ovarian Tumors in Children and Sexual Precocity

Type	% of Total	Association with Endocrine Changes
Germ cell	80	Rare; if present, virilization
Teratoma, dysgerminoma, choriocarcinoma, endodermal sinus tumor		
Sex cord-stromal	10	Frequent; changes depend on cell type
Granulosa cell tumor		isosexual precocity
Sertoli-Leydig cell tumor		virilization or isosexual precocity
Lipoid cell tumors		virilization or isosexual precocity
Epithelial	10	Rare; if present, virilization
Serous, mucinous, endometrioid, clear cell tumors		

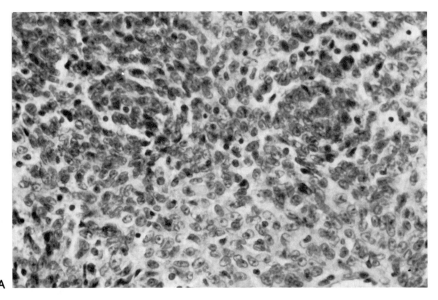

A

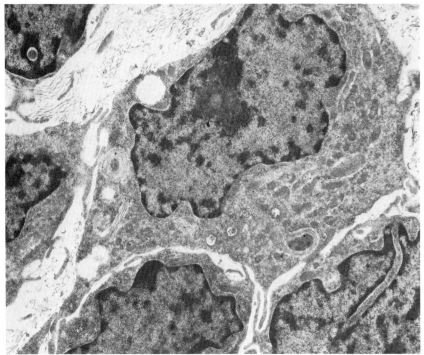

B

Figure 8–20. Juvenile granulosa cell tumor, 12 year-old-patient. A. Light micrograph, showing diffuse sheets of oval to elongated cells and evidence of luteinization. H & E (×250). B. Electron micrograph of neoplastic granulosa cells. (×5,500).

precocious maturation, but their removal results in regression of findings in only a limited number of cases. This suggests lack of an etiologic relationship. Follicle cysts are commonly encountered in childhood and the association is therefore likely to be coincidental. Some of the cysts may show evidence of luteinization on histologic examination, suggesting a basis for the endocrine activity, but this finding is probably of a secondary nature. Since there is limited likelihood that removal of a nonneoplastic cyst will alter the clinical course, cysts should be distinguished from sex cord-stromal tumors, which are usually solid. However, some of the latter are cystic and therefore the distinction between a non-neoplastic cyst and hormone-secreting tumor may require removal and microscopic examination.

DELAYED MATURATION

Delayed initiation and progression of puberty are indicated by absent or delayed development of secondary sex characteristics and primary amenorrhea. Intrinsic ovarian disorders may be involved, including a number of the conditions already discussed. Consequently, pathologic effects of various types can be associated with delayed

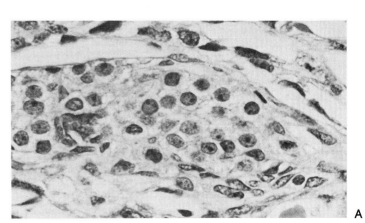

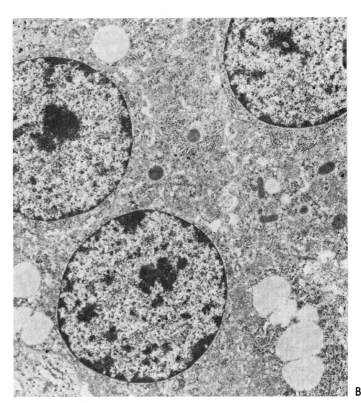

Figure 8–21. Stromal luteinization associated with endodermal sinus tumor. A. Light micrograph. H & E (×350). B. Electron micrograph. (×5,000).

ovarian maturation. In those conditions in which the disorder is of extrinsic origin, the changes in the ovaries will depend on the type and severity of the disorder. Diagnosis will depend on identifying the specific source of the abnormality.

References

1. Witschi E: Embryology of the ovary. *In* HG Grady, DE Smith (eds) The Ovary. Baltimore, Williams & Wilkins, 1963.

2. van Wagenen G, Simpson ME: Embryology of the Ovary and Testis: *Homo sapiens* and *Macaca mulatta*. New Haven, Yale University Press, 1965.

3. Wachtel SS, Ohno S, Koo GC, *et al.*: Possible role for H-Y antigen in the primary determination of sex. Nature 257:235-236, 1975.

4. Gore-Langton RE, Tung PS, Fritz IB: The absence of specific interactions of Sertoli-cell-secreted proteins with antibodies directed against H-Y antigen. Cell 32:289–301, 1983.

5. Lyon MF: Mechanism and evolutionary origins of variable X-chromosome activity in mammals. Proc R Soc Lond (Biol) 187:243–268, 1974.

6. Grumbach MM, Conte FA: Disorders of sex differentiation. *In* RH Williams (ed) Textbook of Endocrinology (6th ed.). Philadelphia, WB Saunders, 1981.

7. Gartler SM, Andina RJ, Gant N: Ontogeny of X-chromosome inactivation in the female germ line. Exp Cell Res 91:454–457, 1975.

8. Gondos B: Germ cell differentiation and intercellular

bridges. *In* J van Blerkom, PM Motta (eds) Ultrastructure of Reproduction. Boston, Martinus Nijhoff, 1984.

9. Gondos B, Bhiraleus P, Hobel CJ: Ultrastructural observations on germ cells in human fetal ovaries. Am J Obstet Gynecol 110:644–652, 1971.

10. Byskov AG: Regulation of meiosis in mammals. Ann Biol Anim Biochim Biophys 19:1251–1261, 1979.

11. Baker TG: A quantitative and cytological study of germ cells in human ovaries. Proc R Soc London (Biol) 158:417–433, 1963.

12. Gondos B, Hobel CJ: Interstitial cells in the human fetal ovary. Endocrinology 93:736–739, 1973.

13. Brandau H, Lehmann V: Histoenzymatische Untersuchungen an menschlichen Gonaden während der intrauterinen Entwicklung. Z Geburtshilfe Gynäk 173:233–249, 1970.

14. Høyer PE: Histoenzymology of the human ovary. *In* PM Motta, ESE Hafez (eds) Biology of the Ovary. Boston, Martinus Nijhoff, 1980.

15. Payne AH, Jaffe RB: Androgen formation from pregnenolone sulfate by the human fetal ovary. J Clin Endocrinol Metab 39:300–304, 1974.

16. George FW, Wilson JD: Conversion of androgen to estrogen by the human fetal ovary. J Clin Endocrinol Metab 47:550–555, 1978.

17. Kaplan SL, Grumbach MM: The ontogenesis of human fetal hormones: II. Luteinizing hormone (LH) and follicle stimulating hormone (FSH). Acta Endocrinol (Copenh) 81:808–829, 1976.

18. Clements JA, Reyes FI, Winter JSD, *et al.*: Studies on human sexual development. III. Fetal pituitary and serum and amniotic fluid concentrations of LH, CG, and FSH. J Clin Endocrinol Metab 42:9–19, 1974.

19. Takagi S, Yoshida T, Tsubata, K, *et al.*: Sex differences in fetal gonadotropins and androgens. J Steroid Biochem 8:609–620, 1977.

20. Baker TG, Neal P: Oogenesis in human fetal ovaries maintained in organ culture. J Anat 117:591–604, 1974.

21. Ch'in KY: The endocrine glands of anencephalic foetuses. A quantitative and morphologic study of 15 cases. Chinese Med J (Engl) 2:63–90, 1938.

22. Gulyas BJ, Hodgen GD, Tullner WW, *et al.*: Effects of fetal or maternal hypophysectomy on endocrine organs and body weight in infant rhesus monkeys (*Macaca mulatta*): with particular emphasis on oogenesis. Biol Reprod 16:216–227, 1977.

23. Peters H, Byskov AG, Grinsted J: Follicular growth in fetal and prepubertal ovaries of humans and other primates. Clin Endocrinol Metab 7:469–485, 1978.

24. Zamboni L: Comparative studies on the ultrastructure of mammalian oocytes. *In* JD Biggers, AW Schuetz (eds) Oogenesis. Baltimore, University Park Press, 1972.

25. Baker TG, O WS: Development of the ovary and oogenesis. Clin Obstet Gynecol 3:3–26, 1976.

26. Peters H, McNatty KP: The Ovary. London, Granada, 1980.

27. Valdes-Dapena M: The normal ovary of childhood. Ann NY Acad Sci 142:597–613, 1967.

28. Peters H, Himelstein-Braw R, Faber M: The normal development of the ovary in childhood. Acta Endocrinol (Copenh) 82:617–630, 1976.

29. Peters H: The human ovary in childhood and early maturity. Europ J Obstet Gynecol Reprod Biol 9:137–144, 1979.

30. Lee PA: Ovarian function from conception to puberty: physiology and disorders. In GB Serra (ed) The Ovary. New York, Raven Press, 1983.

31. Winter JSD, Faiman C, Hobson WC, *et al.*: Pituitary-gonadal relations in infancy. I. Patterns of serum gonadotropin concentrations from birth to 4 years of age in man and chimpanzee. J Clin Endocrinol Metab 40:545–551, 1975.

32. Bidlingmaier F, Wagner-Barnack M, Butenandt O, *et al.*: Plasma estrogens in childhood and puberty under physiologic and pathologic conditions. Pediatr Res 7:901–907, 1973.

33. Lee PA, Xenakis T, Winer J, *et al.*: Puberty in girls: correlation of serum levels of gonadotropins, prolactin, androgens, estrogens, and progestins with physical changes. J Clin Endocrinol Metab 43:775–784, 1976.

34. Apter D, Pakarinen A, Vikho R: Serum prolactin, FSH, and LH during puberty in girls and boys. Acta Paediatr Scand 67:417–423, 1978.

35. Bohnet HG: Gonadotropins, prolactin, and sex steroid secretion in pubertal maturation of normal girls and agonadal subjects. *In* C Flamigni, S Venturoli, JR Givens (eds) Adolescence in Females. Chicago, Year Book Medical Publishers, 1985.

36. Apter D: Serum steroids and pituitary hormones in female puberty: a partly longitudinal study. Clin Endocrinol 12:107–120, 1980.

37. Reiter EO, Kulin HE, Hamwood SM: The absence of positive feedback between estrogen and luteinizing hormone in sexually immature girls. Pediatr Res 8:740–745, 1974.

38. Hansen JW, Hoffman HJ, Ross, GT: Monthly gonadotropin cycles in premenarcheal girls. Science 190:161–163, 1975.

39. Blanchette EJ: Ovarian steroid cells: I. Differentiation of the lutein cell from the granulosa follicle cell during the preovulatory stage and under the influence of exogenous gonadotrophins. J Cell Biol 31:501–516, 1966.

40. Bjersing L: Maturation, morphology, and endocrine function of the follicular wall in mammals. *In* RE Jones (ed) The Vertebrate Ovary. New York, Plenum Press, 1978.

41. Williams RF, Turner CK, Hodgen GD: The late pubertal cascade in perimenarcheal monkeys: onset of asymmetrical ovarian estradiol secretion and bioassayable luteinizing hormone release. J Clin Endocrinol Metab 55:660–665, 1982.

42. Hillier SG, van den Boogaard AMJ, Reichert LE, *et al.*: The intraovarian hormonal milieu and follicle growth and development in the human ovary. *In* E Cacciari, A Prader (eds) Pathophysiology of Puberty. New York, Academic Press, 1980.

43. Simpson JL: Disorders of Sexual Differentiation: Etiology and Clinical Delineation. New York, Academic Press, 1976.

44. Palmer CG, Reichman A: Chromosomal and clinical findings in 110 females with Turner syndrome. Hum Genet 35:35–49, 1976.

45. Simpson JL: Gonadal dysgenesis and sex chromosome abnormalities: phenotypic-karyotypic correlations. *In* HL Vallet, IH Porter (eds) Genetic Mechanisms of Sexual Development. New York, Academic Press, 1979.

46. Jacobs PA: The incidence and etiology of sex chromosome abnormalities in man. Birth Defects 15(1):3–14, 1979.

47. Carr DH: Chromosomes and abortion. *In* H Harris, K Hirschhorn (eds) Advances in Human Genetics (Vol. 2). New York, Plenum Press, 1971.

48. Singh RP, Carr DH: The anatomy and histology of XO human embryos and fetuses. Anat Rec 155:369–384, 1966.

49. Carr DH, Haggar RA, Hart AG: Germ cells in the ovaries of XO female infants. Am J Clin Pathol 49:521–526, 1968.

50. Weiss L: Additional evidence of gradual loss of germ cells in the pathogenesis of streak ovaries in Turner's syndrome. J Med Genet 8:540–544, 1971.

51. Philip J, Sele V: 45,XO Turner's syndrome without evidence of mosaicism in a patient with two pregnancies. Acta Obstet Gynecol Scand 55:283–286, 1976.

52. Wray HL, Freeman MVR, Ming PL: Pregnancy in the Turner syndrome with only 45,X chromosomal constitution. Fertil Steril 35:509–514, 1981.

53. McCorquodale MM, Bowdle FC: Two pregnancies and the loss of the 46,XX cell line in a 45,X/46,XX Turner mosaic patient. Fertil Steril 43:229–233, 1985.

54. Maraschio P, Fraccaro M: X chromosome abnormalities and female fertility. In PG Crosignani, BL Rubin, M Fraccaro (eds) Genetic Control of Gamete Production and Function. London, Academic Press, 1982.

55. Reyes FI, Koh KS, Faiman C: Fertility in women with gonadal dysgenesis. Am J Obstet Gynecol 126:668–670, 1976.

56. Cutler BS, Forbes AP, Ingersoll FM, et al.: Endometrial carcinoma after stilbestrol therapy in gonadal dysgenesis. N Engl J Med 287:628–631, 1972.

57. Wilkinson EJ, Friedrich EG, Mattingly RF, et al.: Turner's syndrome with endometrial adenocarcinoma and stilbestrol therapy. Obstet Gynecol 42:193–200, 1973.

58. Rosenwaks Z, Urban MD, Wentz AC, et al.: Endometrial pathology and its relation to estrogen therapy in patients with hypogonadism. Pediatr 62:1184–1188, 1979.

59. Simpson JL: Genetic disorders of gonadal development in humans. In PG Crosignani, BL Rubin, M Fraccaro (eds) Genetic Control of Gamete Production and Function. London, Academic Press, 1982.

60. Smith A, Fraser IS, Noel M: Three siblings with premature gonadal failure. Fertil Steril 32:528–530, 1979.

61. Pallister PD, Opitz JM: The Perrault syndrome: autosomal recessive ovarian dysgenesis with facultative, non-sex-limited sensorineural deafness. Am J Med Genet 4:239–246, 1979.

62. German J, Simpson JL, Chaganti RSK, et al.: Genetically determined sex reversal in 46,XY humans. Science 202:53–56, 1978.

63. Bernstein R, Koo GC, Wachtel SS: Abnormality of the X chromosome in human 46,XY female siblings with dysgenetic ovaries. Science 207:768–769, 1980.

64. Wolman SR, McMorrow LE, Roy S, et al.: Aberrant testicular differentiation in 46,XY gonadal dysgenesis: morphology, endocrinology, serology. Hum Genet 55:321–325, 1980.

65. Scully RE: Gonadoblastoma: a review of 74 cases. Cancer 25:1340–1356, 1970.

66. Simpson JL, Photopulos G: The relationship of neoplasia to disorders of abnormal sexual differentiation. Birth Defects 12(1):15–50, 1976.

67. Scully RE: Ovarian tumors. Am J Pathol 87:686–720, 1977.

68. Robboy SJ, Miller T, Donahoe PK, et al.: Dysgenesis of testicular and streak gonads in the syndrome of mixed gonadal dysgenesis. Hum Pathol 13:700–716, 1982.

69. Schellhas HF: Malignant potential of the dysgenetic gonad. Obstet Gynecol 44:298–309; 455–462, 1974.

70. Zäh W, Kalderon RE, Tucci JR: Mixed gonadal dysgenesis: a case report and review of the world literature. Acta Endocrinol 79(Suppl. 197):3–39, 1975.

71. Ishida T, Tagatz GE, Okagaki T: Gonadoblastoma: ultrastructural evidence for testicular origin. Cancer 37:1770–1781, 1976.

72. van Niekerk WA: True hermaphroditism: an analytic review with a report of 3 new cases. Am J Obstet Gynecol 126:890–905, 1976.

73. Simpson JL: True hermaphroditism: etiology and phenotypic considerations. Birth Defects 14(6C):9–35, 1978.

74. McDonough PG, Byrd JR, Tho PT, et al.: Gonadoblastoma in a true hermaphrodite with a 46,XX karyotype. Obstet Gynecol 47:355–358, 1976.

75. Russell P, Altshuler G: The ovarian dysgenesis of trisomy 18. Pathology 7:149–155, 1975.

76. Højager B, Peters H, Byskov AG, et al.: Follicular development in ovaries of children with Down's syndrome. Acta Paediatr Scand 67:637–643, 1978.

77. Benda CE: Down's Syndrome. New York, Grune and Stratton, 1969.

78. Miller ME, Chatten J: Ovarian changes in ataxia telangiectasia. Acta Paediatr Scand 56:559–561, 1967.

79. Teplitz RL: Ataxia telangiectasia. Arch Neurol 35:553–554, 1978.

80. Nishizuka Y, Taguchi O, Sakaguchi S, et al.: Ovarian and testicular dysgenesis in immunodeficient mice: its genesis and autoimmune nature. In AG Byskov, H Peters (eds) Development and Function of Reproductive Organs. Amsterdam, Excerpta Medica, 1981.

81. Shalet SM, Beardwell CG, Morris Jones PH, et al.: Ovarian failure following abdominal irradiation in childhood. Br J Cancer 33:655–658, 1976.

82. Himelstein-Braw R, Peters H, Faber M: Influence of irradiation and chemotherapy on the ovaries of children with abdominal tumors. Br J Cancer 36:269–275, 1977.

83. Baker TG, Neal P: The effects of X-irradiation on mammalian oocytes in organ culture. Biophysik 6:39–45, 1969.

84. Baker TG: Radiosensitivity of mammalian oocytes with particular reference to the human female. Am J Obstet Gynecol 110:746–761, 1971.

85. Stillman RJ, Schinfield JS, Schiff I, et al.: Ovarian failure in long-term survivors of childhood malignancy. Am J Obstet Gynecol 139:62–66, 1981.

86. Shalet SM: The effects of cancer treatment on growth and sexual development. In A Aynsley-Green (ed) Paediatric Endocrinology in Clinical Practice. Boston, MTP Press, 1984.

87. Chapman RM, Sutcliffe SB, Malpas JS: Cytotoxic-induced ovarian failure in women with Hodgkin's disease: I. Hormone function. JAMA 245:1877–1881, 1981.

88. Haney AF: Effects of toxic agents on ovarian function. In JA Thomas, KS Korach, JA McLachlan (eds) Endocrine Toxicology. New York, Raven Press, 1985.

89. Hansmann I: Chromosome aberrations in metaphase II-oocytes: stage sensitivity in the mouse oogenesis to amethopterin and cyclophosphamide. Mutat Res 22:175–191, 1974.

90. Siris ES, Leventhal BG, Vaitukaitis JL: Effects of childhood leukemia and chemotherapy on puberty and reproductive function in girls. N Engl J Med 294:1143–1146, 1976.

91. Lentz RD, Berstein J, Steffes MW, et al.: Postpuberal evaluation of gonadal function following cyclophosphamide

therapy before and during puberty. J Pediatr 91:385–394, 1977.

92. Himelstein-Braw R, Peters H, Faber M: Morphological study of the ovaries of leukaemic children. Br J Cancer 38:82–87, 1978.

93. Merchant-Larios H: Rat gonadal and ovarian organogenesis with and without germ cells: an ultrastructural study. Dev Biol 44:1–21, 1975.

94. Reddoch RB, Pelletier RM, Armstrong DT: Lack of ovarian responsiveness to gonadotropic stimulation in neonatal rats sterilized with busulfan. Biol Reprod 32(Suppl. 1):60, 1985.

95. Ross GT, Vande Wiele RL: The ovaries. *In* RH Williams (ed) Textbook of Endocrinology (6th ed.). Philadelphia, WB Saunders, 1981.

96. Scully RE: Sex cord-stromal tumors. *In* A Blaustein (ed) Pathology of the Female Genital Tract (2nd ed.). New York, Springer-Verlag, 1982.

97. Young RH, Dickersin GR, Scully RE: Juvenile granulosa cell tumor of the ovary: a clinicopathological analysis of 125 cases. Am J Surg Pathol 8:575–596, 1984.

98. Zaloudek C, Norris HJ: Granulosa cell tumors of the ovary in children: a clinical and pathologic study of 32 cases. Am J Surg Pathol 6:503–512, 1982.

99. Teilum G: Special Tumors of Ovary and Testis and Related Extragonadal Lesions: comparative Pathology and Histological Identification (2nd ed.). Philadelphia, JB Lippincott, 1976.

100. Ueda G, Hamanaka N, Hayakawa K, *et al.:* Clinical, histochemical, and biochemical studies of an ovarian dysgerminoma with trophoblasts and Leydig cells. Am J Obstet Gynecol 114:748–754, 1972.

101. Stewart KR, Casey MJ, Gondos B: Endodermal sinus tumor of the ovary with virilization: light- and electron-microscopic study. Am J Surg Pathol 5:385–391, 1981.

102. Lack EE, Perez-Atayde AR, Murthy ASR, *et al.:* Granulosa theca cell tumors in premenarchal girls: a clinical and pathologic study of ten cases. Cancer 48:1846–1854, 1981.

103. Grant DB, Murram D, Dewhurst J: Precocious puberty: implications on adult reproductive function. *In* C Flamigni, S Venturoli, JR Givens (eds) Adolescence in Females. Chicago, Year Book Medical Publishers, 1985.

9. Premature Ovarian Failure

Robert W. Rebar, Gregory F. Erickson, and
Carolyn B. Coulam

Premature ovarian failure (POF) has been recognized as an entity for several years. The term itself has generally been applied to women who have hypergonadotropic amenorrhea and hypoestrogenism prior to the age of 40.[1] Since elevated levels of both luteinizing hormone (LH) and, especially, follicle-stimulating hormone (FSH) were thought to exist only when the ovaries had ceased functioning because of an absence of follicles (or following castration), the term ovarian "failure" seemed appropriate. The report of Goldenberg et al.,[2] documented that no ovarian follicles were present in amenorrheic women with elevated circulating concentrations of LH and FSH of greater than 40 milliInternational Units per milliliter of the Second International Reference Preparation of human Menopausal Gonadotropin (2nd IRP-hMG), and served to confirm this designation of ovarian failure as appropriate. However, several years ago, isolated case reports began to appear documenting the initiation or resumption of cyclic menses and/or pregnancy.[3–5] These reports, as well as observations about the association of autoimmune disease with early ovarian failure,[6–8] led investigators to reconsider the disorder. Reports of large series of women with POF led to the conclusion that POF must be a heterogeneous disorder.

THE CLINICAL SPECTRUM

In 1982 Coulam[9] summarized the clinical findings in 81 women with POF who had 46,XX karyotypes (Table 9–1). Eighteen percent had associated autoimmune diseases. Of the patients, 11 had primary amenorrhea and 70, secondary amenorrhea. The age at the last menstrual period ranged from 11 to 34 years in those women with secondary amenorrhea. In 2 women, many primordial follicles were present on ovarian biopsy. In the others, only a few or no follicles were found on biopsy. In neither patient who had primordial follicles was failure of other endocrine organs demonstrated. Thus, these observations implicate an autoimmune mechanism in some patients with POF.

Rebar, Erickson, and Yen[10] summarized the clinical and endocrine characteristics of 32 women with presumptive POF seen sequentially over a three-year period. The initial diagnosis was based upon the following criteria: age less than 35 years, amenorrhea or oligomenorrhea, and serum FSH greater than 40 mIU/ml on initial screening. Six patients had karyotypic abnormalities. One woman had the stigmata of Turner's syndrome and a 45,X karyotype. Three others had mosaic gonadal dysgenesis (45,X/46,XX). Two individuals presented with 47,XXX karyotypes and were reported separately.[11]

Even the 26 women with normal karyotypes were quite heterogeneous. Four had primary amenorrhea and two others had only a single menstrual period. Ten individuals failed to undergo complete sexual development as determined by Tanner staging.[12] Eleven women achieved complete sexual development and had regular menses for some years before amenorrhea began, between the ages of 11 and 27 years. Five women had hormonal evidence of at least sporadic ovulation, and one of these patients conceived following estrogen replacement. Five had conceived prior to being treated. Eighteen of the 26 women with normal karyotype had hot flushes. One individual resumed ovulatory cycles after 8 years of hypergonadotropic amenorrhea associated with signs and symptoms of hypoestrogenism. Three of the women had documented thyroiditis, suggesting autoimmune involvement.

Blood samples were obtained daily, for approximately 30 days, from 18 of the 26 women with 46,XX karyotypes for measurement of gonadotropins and gonadal steroids. In nine, gonadotropin levels were very high (>40 mIU/ml) and estradiol levels were very low (Figure 9–1). However, in the other nine women sampled there was evidence of follicular function based on increased estradiol concentrations (Figure 9–2). Two women had presumptive evidence of ovulation, with elevated serum progesterone levels during the sampling period, and two others had evidence of ovulation after completion of frequent sampling (Figures 9–3, 9–4).

Nine of these women underwent ovarian biopsy. In specimens from 4 of the 9 there were a few typical, apparently healthy, primordial follicles, but no evidence of follicular development.

More recently, Aiman and Smentek[13] have added a series of 35 patients to the published literature and summarized the results of several surveys, including those of Coulam[9] and Rebar, Erickson, and Yen[10] just discussed. Of a total of 236 reported patients with POF, 18% (28) of

Table 9–1. Pathological Findings in Women with Premature Ovarian Failure[a]

No. of Patients	Appearance of Gonads	Age at Last Menstrual Period (yr)
11	No gonads or hypoplastic without follicles	Primary amenorrhea
65	Hypoplastic without follicles	11–34
1	Diminished number of primordial follicles	22
1	Follicles present with lymphocytic infiltration	19
1	Secondary follicles and hemosiderin present	15
2	Many primordial follicles	14,31

[a] Modified from Coulam CB: Autoimmune ovarian failure. Semin Reprod Endocrinol 1:161–167, 1983.

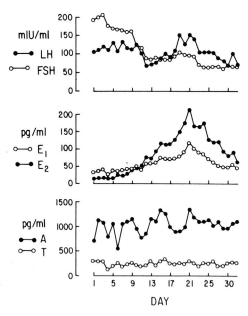

Figure 9–2. Patterns of daily concentrations of circulating LH, FSH, E_1, E_2, A, and T in a young woman with POF and evidence of follicular activity. Although both LH and FSH levels are greater than 40 mIU/ml, the ratio of LH to FSH changes as the circulating concentrations of E_1 and E_2 rise. Levels of estradiol of the magnitude depicted must come from functional granulosa cells within the ovaries. The levels of A and T did not show any consistent pattern of change over the sampling period.

the 157 women undergoing ovarian biopsy had ovarian follicles present. Twenty-seven women (11%) had evidence of associated autoimmune disorders. Fourteen of the women conceived after the diagnosis was established, and two of those had no oocytes on biopsy.

These data emphasize the heterogeneity of the syndrome. In addition, it is apparent that ovulation and even pregnancy seem possible in some women with ovarian "failure." Some of the women studied may have been

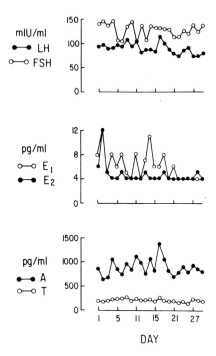

Figure 9–1. Representative patterns of circulating LH, FSH, estrone (E_1), estradiol (E_2), androstenedione (A), and testosterone (T) in daily blood samples obtained from a young woman with premature ovarian failure (POF) and no evidence of follicular function. LH and FSH levels are markedly elevated (>40 mIU/ml) with FSH greater than LH, E_1 and E_2 are very low and indicative of virtually no gonadal secretion (values in agonadal women: E_1 = 37 ± 14 SD pg/ml, E_2 = 14 ± 11 pg/ml), and the androgens A and T are also low (agonadal women: A = 754 ± 696 pg/ml, T = 198 ± 108 pg/ml).

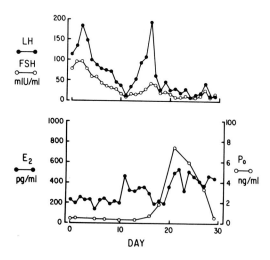

Figure 9–3. Patterns of daily concentrations of LH, FSH, E_2 and progesterone (Po) in a patient with POF and presumptive ovulation on the basis of increased levels of Po. A preovulatory increase in E_2 levels occurred prior to an obvious LH surge.

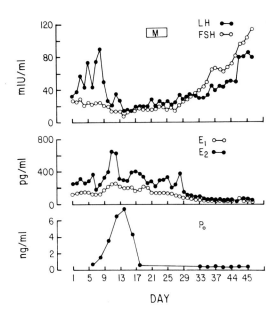

Figure 9–4. Patterns of daily concentration of LH, FSH, E₁, E₂, and Po in a patient with POF, luteal activity, and presumptive ovulation. Menses (M) followed the increase in Po levels. E₁ and E₂ levels decreased, and LH and FSH increased markedly following menses.

merely "perimenopausal," with circulating hormone levels elevated similar to those described by Sherman and Korenman.[14] What is clear is that permanent, irreversible ovarian failure cannot be diagnosed just because circulating FSH levels are elevated, or even because no oocytes are present on ovarian biopsy. Each affected individual must be assessed individually, thus requiring a consideration of the possible disorders exhibiting hypergonado-

tropic amenorrhea and presumptive "premature ovarian failure."

CLASSIFICATION

Gonadal failure may occur at any time during embryonic or postnatal development. Coulam[15] has proposed that disorders resulting in gonadal failure before birth and caused by gonadal abnormalities should be distinguished from premature ovarian failure. A modification of her classification of those disorders she distinguishes from POF is shown in Table 9–2. This classification scheme emphasizes the need to consider genetic abnormalities in individuals who have hypergonadotropic amenorrhea. Since individuals with ovarian dysgenesis have the normal complement of oocytes at 20 weeks of fetal age[16] but then have accelerated atresia until birth, some of these girls may undergo sexual development, ovulate for a time, and even conceive if some oocytes remain.[17] Thus the classification proposed is not ideal. It should be viewed as an artificial separation of what, in reality, represents a continuum.

Excluding the gonadal disorders just discussed, premature ovarian failure still consists of several distinct disorders as delineated in Table 9–3.

Inherited Characteristics

Theoretically, premature loss of oocytes could result from failure of all germ cells to migrate to the genital ridges, from a reduced complement of oogonia, or accelerated loss of oocytes (atresia) arising on a genetic basis.

Table 9–2. Proposed Classification of Gonadal Failure Arising Before Birth[a]

Disorder	Previous Nomenclature	Karyotype	Müllerian Duct	Wolffian Duct	External Genitalia	Days After Fertilization
Defective germ cell migration	Pure gonadal dysgenesis Swyer's syndrome Familial 46,XX dysgenesis Familial 46,XY dysgenesis 46,XX dysgenesis 46,XY dysgenesis	46,XX or 46,XY	Present	Absent	Female	Before 43
Testicular regression	True agonadism Testicular dysgenesis Embryonic testicular regression Testicular regression syndrome	46,XY	Present to absent	Absent to present	Female to ambiguous to male	43–120
Testicular dysgenesis	Dysgenetic gonads Mixed gonadal dysgenesis	45,X or mosaic (commonly 45,X/46,XY)	Present to absent	Absent to present	Female to ambiguous	43–84
Ovarian dysgenesis	Gonadal agenesis Gonadal dysgenesis Turner's syndrome Ovarian agenesis Ovarian dysgenesis Streak gonad	45,X or mosaic (commonly 45,X/46,XX)	Present	Absent	Female	After 80

[a] Modified from Coulam, CB: Editor's formulation. Semin Reprod Endocrinol 1:177–178, 1983.

Table 9–3. Tentative Classification of Premature Ovarian Failure

- I. Inherited characteristics
  - A. Reduced germ cell number
  - B. Accelerated atresia (?)
  - C. Trisomy X with or without mosaicism
- II. Enzymatic defects
  - A. 17α-hydroxylase deficiency
  - B. Galactosemia
- III. Defects in gonadotropin secretion
  - A. Secretion of biologically inactive forms
  - B. α or β subunit defects
- IV. Gonadotropin receptor and/or post-receptor defects (Resistant ovary or Savage syndrome)
- V. Autoimmune disorders
  - A. Associated with other endocrine disorders
  - B. Isolated
- VI. Congenital thymic aplasia
- VII. Physical causes
  - A. Irradiation
  - B. Chemotherapeutic agents
  - C. Viral agents
  - D. Cigarette smoking
  - E. Surgical extirpation
- VIII. Idiopathic

Accelerated loss of oocytes theoretically may result from an increased rate of atresia or from recruitment of an increased number of oocytes within each cohort which then undergo atresia at the normal rate. Since each cohort is larger, the oocytes are depleted more quickly. Decreased migration has never been demonstrated in humans. Studies of oocyte number in different strains of mice have indicated that the genetic complement varies tremendously among strains, as does the rate of oocyte atresia.[18] Similarly, the data of Block[19,20] suggest that there may be marked differences in oocyte endowment and rates of follicular atresia among women. In addition, the etiology of the premature ovarian failure which coexists with the neurological disorder myotonia dystrophica[21] is unknown, but may well be on the basis of decreased germ cell number or accelerated atresia. Apparently an excess of X chromosomes may also be associated with decreased germ cell number or accelerated atresia as well.[11,22,23]

Several reports[24–27] have described the familial occurrence of premature ovarian failure with vertical transmission of the trait, suggesting the possible mode of inheritance to be consistent with autosomal-dominant, sex-linked inheritance. Because affected women had regular menses and apparently normal fertility before cessation of menses and because inheritance is compatible with an autosomal-dominant pattern, heritability of premature ovarian failure has significant implications for reproductive counseling in affected families.

Enzymatic Defects

Sexual infantilism and primary amenorrhea in association with increased circulating gonadotropin concentrations, hypertension with hypokalemic alkalosis, and increased circulating deoxycorticosterone and progesterone levels are present in girls with 17α-hydroxylase deficiency who survive until the expected age of puberty.[28-30] Ovarian biopsy of affected individuals has revealed numerous large cysts and primordial follicles with complete failure of orderly follicular maturation.[30]

Galactosemia is an inherited disorder involving decreased galactose 1-phosphate uridyltransferase activity. As a result, galactose 1-phosphate, galactose, and galactitol are increased throughout the body. Galactosemia is characterized by mental retardation, cataracts, hepatosplenomegaly, and renal tubular dysfunction. It has only recently been recognized that affected individuals may also have premature ovarian failure with elevated gonadotropin levels, even when a galactose-restricted diet is introduced early in infancy.[31,32] The etiology of the ovarian failure in galactosemia is unknown. However, it is tempting to speculate that the carbohydrate moieties on gonadotropin molecules are altered, rendering the LH and FSH biologically inactive. On the other hand, a direct effect of the sugars on the oocyte is also a possibility. Pregnant rats fed a 50% galactose diet delivered offspring with markedly reduced oocyte number, apparently as a result of decreased germ cell migration to the genital ridges.[33]

Defects in Gonadotropin Secretion

Abnormal forms of gonadotropin with reduced biological activity may lead to accelerated follicular atresia and premature ovarian failure early in human development. Support for this possibility is provided by the observation that fetal removal of the pituitary gland in monkeys, leading to reduced gonadotropin secretion, results in ovaries devoid of oocytes at birth (i.e., accelerated atresia).[34] In fact, cases of male pseudohermaphroditism with immunologically active but biologically inactive LH have been documented.[35,36] Although no such documented cases exist for women with premature ovarian failure, we have noted differences in either immunoreactive LH or FSH in urinary extracts from women with POF compared to those from castrate and postmenopausal women.[37] Whether the immunologically altered gonadotropin is also biologically altered remains to be determined. However, these data suggest that metabolism and/or excretion of gonadotropins and possibly their subunits are altered in some cases of POF and may be important in the development of the ovarian failure by causing accelerated atresia prior to birth. Since such individuals with remaining ovarian follicles should ovulate in response to exogenous biologically active gonadotropin, it is important to identify them.

Gonadotropin Receptor and/or Post-receptor Defects

As originally characterized, the "resistant ovary" or "Savage syndrome" consisted of young amenorrheic women with (1) elevated peripheral gonadotropin concentrations, (2) normal but immature follicles in the ovaries on biopsy, (3) 46,XX karyotype, (4) complete sexual development, and (5) hyposensitivity to exogenous gonadotropin stimulation.[38] The pathogenesis of this disorder remains obscure, but a gonadotropin receptor or post-receptor defect is certainly possible, as is an isolated autoimmune disorder. Until the etiology is established, it seems reasonable to consider these women as distinct from those with autoimmune disturbances. Failure of gonadotropin to bind to its receptor, failure of the gonadotropin-receptor complex to activate adenylate cyclase, or failure to stimulate any other postreceptor step might lead to accelerated atresia and premature ovarian failure.

Maxson and Wentz[39] recently found only 14 cases in the literature that fulfilled strict criteria for this rare syndrome. Six had primary amenorrhea (suggesting that "complete" sexual development was not present). In the eight with secondary amenorrhea, the average age of cessation of menses was 21.4 years, with a range of 13 to 30 years.

Netter and colleagues[40] have suggested that the resistant ovary syndrome represents pure 46,XX ovarian dysgenesis prior to astresia of all primordial follicles, and that the ovaries of these patients may evolve from small hypoplastic gonads to true streak gonads.

Ovarian Failure and Autoimmune Disorders

Premature ovarian failure has been observed to occur in women with a number of other autoimmune disorders[9,10,13,41-49] (Table 9–4). Most commonly, ovarian failure has been noted in patients with polyglandular failure including hypoparathyroidism, hypoadrenalism, and mucocutaneous candidiasis.[42-44] That the autoimmune ovarian failure is also heterogeneous is suggested by the numerous endocrinopathies with which it is associated. In addition, it seems reasonable to surmise that autoimmune ovarian failure may occur independently of any other autoimmune disorder.

Antireceptor antibodies have been implicated in the pathogenesis of several autoimmune disorders. For example, individuals with myasthenia gravis have circulating antibodies to acetylcholine receptors present in muscle.[50] Antibodies in the circulation of patients with Graves' disease compete with TSH for binding sites on thyroid membranes, activate adenylate cyclase, and cause hyperthyroidism.[51] Thus, antibodies to ovarian gonadotropin receptors could block gonadotropin action and follicular maturation in some women with POF. The intermittent nature of autoimmune disorders and fluctuating antibody levels could result in sporadic ovulation and occasional pregnancies.

Table 9–4. Other Conditions Found in Various Combinations in Association with Premature Ovarian Failure

Alopecia
Anemia, both acquired hemolytic and pernicious
Crohn's disease
Chronic active hepatitis
Diabetes mellitus
Hypoadrenalism (Addison's disease)
Hypoparathyroidism
Hypophysitis
Idiopathic thrombocytopenia purpura
Juvenile rheumatoid arthritis
Keratoconjunctivitis and Sjögren's syndrome
Malabsorption syndrome
Myasthenia gravis
Primary biliary cirrhosis
Quantitative immunoglobulin abnormalities
Systemic lupus erythematosis
Thyroid disorders, including Graves' disease and thyroiditis
Vitiligo

Several investigators have detected circulating antibodies to human ovarian tissue in the sera of patients with POF.[6,46,49,52] The cytotoxic effects of serum from a few such patients on human granulosa cells in culture has been noted.[53] Austin, Coulam, and Ryan[27] failed to detect any antibodies to LH receptors in a study of 14 women with POF. However, Chiauzzi and colleagues[54] recently demonstrated apparent FSH receptor antibodies in two women with myasthenia gravis and hypergonadotropic amenorrhea. Clearly, additional efforts to determine the autoimmune basis for hypergonadotropic amenorrhea are warranted in POF.

The importance of identifying and understanding autoimmune POF lies in the fact that it should be reversible in the early stages. That this is the case is suggested by sequential studies in one teenage patient whose gonadotropin levels decreased when corticosteroids prescribed for adrenal insufficiency were taken regularly.[4] In addition, ovulation returned temporarily following plasmapheresis in a woman with myasthenia gravis,[55] and with glucocorticoid therapy in a woman with a perifollicular lymphocytic infiltrate.[8]

Unfortunately, however, the diagnosis of ovarian failure arising on an autoimmune basis is in most cases only presumptive. The presence of another autoimmune disorder, circulating antibodies to tissues other than ovary, or even a lymphocytic infiltrate of the follicles on ovarian biopsy provide only indirect evidence that the ovarian failure is due to ovarian autoimmunity. More specific evidence requires at least the presence of humoral antiovarian antibodies or preferably documentation that a circulating immunoglobulin interferes with ovarian function.

Congenital Thymic Aplasia

Only recently has a relationship between the thymus gland and reproductive function become apparent. Evidence is accumulating to suggest that the presence of the thymus is necessary for normal gonadotropin secretion and to prevent accelerated follicular atresia. Congenitally athymic mice, which develop premature ovarian failure[56], have lower gonadotropin concentrations than their normal heterozygous littermates prior to maturation.[57] Furthermore, both the hormonal alterations and the accelerated loss of oocytes which occur in the athymic mice can be prevented by thymic transplantation at birth.[58-60]

In comparing rodents to primates, it is important to remember that the stages of ovarian development that occur in the mouse in the first few weeks after birth occur *in utero* in monkeys and in humans. Thus, in primates the thymus should play a role in regulating oocyte number prior to birth. Data for both monkeys and humans support this premise. Healy and colleagues[61] have recently reported that thymic extirpation in rhesus monkeys *in utero* results in a marked reduction in oocyte number at birth. Miller and Chatten[62] have demonstrated that congenitally athymic girls who died before puberty had ovaries devoid of oocytes on autopsy. Since Rebar and colleagues[63] have demonstrated that a synthetic thymic peptide, thymosin β_4, can stimulate the secretion of gonadotropin-releasing hormone (GnRH) and thus LH and FSH, it would seem that gonadotropin secretion early in development is required to prevent accelerated atresia. These data are also consistent with the observation, discussed earlier, that fetal hypophysectomy in monkeys results in accelerated atresia.[34]

Physical Causes

In 1939 Jacox[64] reported that irradiation of the ovaries with 800 rads over 3 days is generally sufficient to induce ovarian failure. Permanent ovarian failure has occurred in somewhat less than 50% of the women subjected to radiation and who received 400 to 500 rads to the ovaries over 4 to 6 weeks as partial treatment for Hodgkin's disease; in others only temporary hypergonadotropic amenorrhea occurred.[65,66]

Alkylating agents, especially cyclophosphamide, are also capable of inducing ovarian failure.[67] Interestingly, the "failure" that results is sometimes reversible.[68] A number of studies have concluded that the ovaries of younger women are more resistant to the deleterious effects of chemotherapeutic agents than are those of older women.[68] In addition, Koyama and colleagues[69] found that a larger total dose of cyclophosphamide was necessary to produce permanent amenorrhea in younger women than in older women. Ovaries of prepubertal girls seem less sensitive than those of pubertal girls and those of adults. Studies in rodents suggest that treatment with long-acting GnRH analogs may protect the ovaries from the effects of alkylating agents[70]; human trials, however, remain to be reported.

Mumps virus has been implicated as the cause of premature ovarian failure and/or infertility.[71,72] At present there is no evidence that other viruses can cause POF, although diagnosis of viral oophoritis is obviously difficult.

On the basis of epidemiologic studies it now appears that there is an inverse dose-response relationship between the number of cigarettes smoked per day and the age of menopause.[73-75] At any given age between 44 and 53 years, a woman who smokes one pack per day is more likely to have undergone menopause than a woman who smokes one-half per day or less. The effect of smoking is apparently independent of body mass and other confounding factors.[73,75] Although the agent responsible for this effect is unknown, polycyclic aromatic hydrocarbons are toxic to oocytes in several animal test systems.[76] Since cigarette smoking is so prevalent and POF so uncommon, it is difficult to believe that smoking plays any significant role in inducing early ovarian failure. However, the possibility should not be dismissed in the absence of data.

It appears that relatively few cases of POF are due to environmental factors. In an affected woman with no history of systemic disease, radiation therapy, or chemotherapy, an etiology distinct from an environmental cause should be sought.

Idiopathic POF

At present the diagnosis of idiopathic POF must be regarded as a diagnosis of exclusion. Unfortunately no obvious cause for POF is found in the majority of cases. In their review of 236 cases Aiman and Smentek[13] classified 24% of the patients as having POF of undetermined etiology. However, they classified separately those patients with no follicles on biopsy (54%) and those with follicles present (18%). These groups may really be considered together as a single group for the present. It is also possible that some women classified as having "resistant ovaries" (11%) may have neither gonadotropin receptor nor postreceptor defects, but have ovarian failure of as yet undetermined (i.e., idiopathic) etiology. No doubt other causes of POF will be identified in the future.

PATHOLOGY

To understand the pathology of the POF ovary, one needs to consider first some events that occur in the normal ovary between the time of birth and the menopause.

The very essence of a menstrual cycle is continuous change and this phenomenon depends completely upon the cyclic production of cohorts of ovarian follicles.[77,78] In the reproductive years, normally, one follicle from each cohort is selected to differentiate as a dominant follicle which produces increasing amounts of estradiol. At midcycle, this follicle expels its oocyte into the peritoneal cavity and the granulosa and theca cells differentiate into a corpus luteum which secretes, primarily, progesterone. The evolution of the structural and functional organization of a dominant follicle is a clearly ordered process which becomes progressively expressed. During normal development, puberty is marked by the first ovulatory cycle and menopause by the complete cessation of this phenomenon.

All dominant follicles arise from a preexisting pool of primordial follicles. There is no other way for a preovulatory follicle (and thus a menstrual cycle) to be produced. Histologically, a primordial follicle possesses an elegantly simple organization. As seen in Figure 9–5, each primordial follicle is bounded on its outer surface by a basal lamina which is composed of noncellular material. Inside the basal lamina, two very different types of cells are found: a small (approximately 25 μm in diameter) oocyte which is arrested in dictyotene of meiosis and one layer of flattened epithelial cells from which future granulosa cells will originate.

In women, the primordial follicles are set aside very early in embryonic development. This important event occurs in the cortical regions of the fetal ovaries between the fifth and the ninth months of gestation[79]. One of the fundamental consequences of this differentiation process is that all potential future eggs have entered meiosis by birth and no reserve oogonia remain. In other words, all oocytes capable of participating in reproduction during a woman's life are present by the time of birth.

Once the primordial follicles are formed, some are recruited or stimulated to initiate growth.[80–83] Most important, this phenomenon is controlled by intraovarian mechanisms.[78] As a consequence of recruitment, the size of the pool of primordial follicles becomes progressively smaller. Between the time of birth and the onset of menarche, the number of primordial follicles decreases from several million to several hundred thousand.[84] As a woman ages, the number of primordial follicles (and thus oocytes) continues to decline until at the menopause there are few, if any, left.[84,85] This basic principle in ovarian physiology is clearly illustrated in Figure 9–6. If one considers that gametogenesis is not a continuous process in the female, then it is evident that, once the pool of primordial follicles is depleted, menstrual cycles will cease. This is true regardless of the age of the individual.

Along with the primordial follicles, any given biopsy of a normal premenopausal ovary will exhibit numerous preantral and antral follicles. After a primordial follicle is recruited, it grows and develops to the primary and secondary preantral stages (Figure 9–7A). When a secondary follicle reaches approximately 400 μm in diameter, follicular fluid begins to accumulate in the antrum and the unit undergoes its differentiation as a tertiary (or Graafian) follicle. This developmental event is completely dependent upon bioactive FSH and LH.[78] All Graafian follicles are composed of multiple layers of granulosa cells, theca cells, and a fully grown oocyte (Figure 9–7B).

Developmentally, a Graafian follicle will either grow and develop into a dominant preovulatory follicle or it will die by atresia. Although the oocyte and granulosa die during atresia,[86] the cells in the theca interna undergo hypertrophy and survive as clusters of highly differentiated secondary interstitial cells (Figure 9–7B). The presence of islands of secondary interstitial cells is a characteristic feature of the normal human ovary.[87] Physi-

ologically, the secondary interstitial cells contain LH receptor and respond to LH by secreting C_{19} androgens, most notably androstenedione.[86,87]

Finally, examination of a cross-section of a normal ovary during the reproductive years might reveal a corpus luteum (Figure 9–8A). If a functional corpus luteum is found, it will typically contain an outer layer of relatively small theca luteal cells and an inner layer of very large granulosa luteal cells (Figure 9–8B). In their differentiated state (Figure 9–8C), both the theca and granulosa luteal cells exist as highly differentiated endocrine cells whose fine structural features are typical of those found in active steroid-secreting cells.[88]

So much for the structures in the normal ovary. What of the histological organization of ovaries in a woman with POF? Typically, a biopsy of a POF ovary reveals a dense network of connective tissue with no evidence of oocytes, follicles, or corpora lutea (Figure 9–9A). When examined with the electron microscope, such a cross-section reveals a mass of dense connective tissue composed of collagenous fibers and fibroblasts (Figure 9–10). Occasionally, small blood vessels are seen, thus demonstrating that gonadotropins and other factors are being delivered to the POF ovaries (Figure 9–10). When one examines the ultrastructure of a POF ovary, no secondary interstitial cells are visible (Figures 9–9, 9–10). This structural aspect is supported by the fact that circulating androgens in POF patients are low and typical of those present in other agonadal women (Figure 9–1). Findings of this type support the conclusion that the POF ovary is essentially the same (structurally and functionally) as in the postmenopausal state.[88,89]

One of the most interesting and important aspects of the premature ovarian failure syndrome concerns the manner in which some patients generate a spontaneous, fertile menstrual cycle.[10] As discussed earlier, the basis of a menstrual cycle is causally connected to the presence of a pool of primordial follicles. In this regard, evidence has been obtained that some ovarian biopsies of POF patients actually contain a few primordial follicles. As shown in Figure 9–9B, the primordial follicles in POF appear indistinguishable from their counterparts in a normal ovary. (Compare Figures 9–5 and 9–9B). Moreover, if one looks closely at the POF primordial follicle in Figure 9–9B, it is clear that it is undergoing recruitment, as some granulosa cells are becoming cuboidal in shape. On rare occasions a biopsy of a POF ovary will reveal developing secondary and Graafian follicles. This is clearly shown in Figure 9–11. Importantly, the granulosa and theca cells are marked by hypertrophy in these tertiary follicles (Figure 9–11B). This histologic evidence is important because it indicates that the granulosa and theca cells in these POF follicles are responding to high levels of bioactive FSH and LH, respectively.[78,86,87]

In this connection, we have obtained some rather striking morphological evidence to further support this concept. The analysis of one biopsy of a POF ovary clearly revealed the presence of luteal cells with a high level of organization. As seen in Figure 9–12, fully differentiated granulosa lutein and theca lutein cells are found in great numbers packaged in what appears to be a more or less

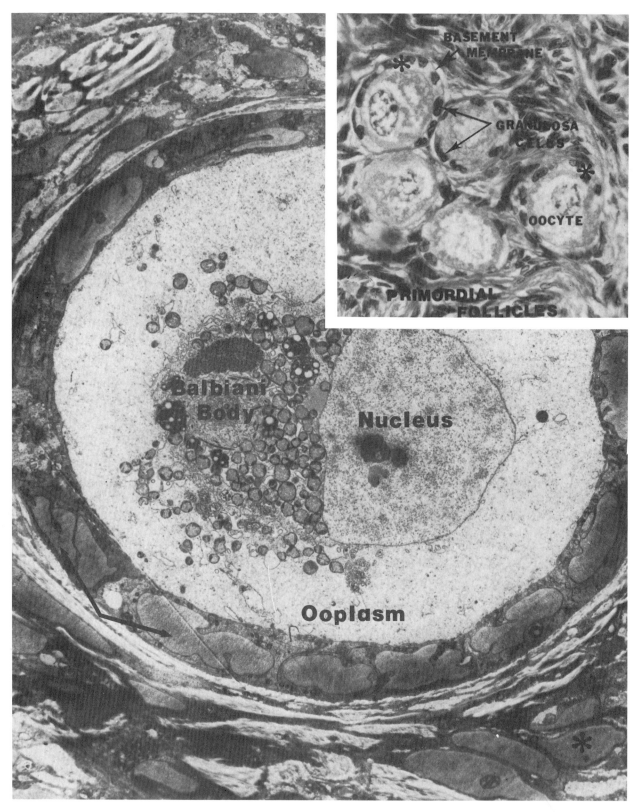

Figure 9–5. Photomicrographs of human ovaries. Inset: Light micrograph showing a group of primordial follicles. Each is composed of a nongrowing oocyte (arrested in dictyotene of meiosis), a single layer of highly flattened granulosa cells, and a basal lamina. Note the transition of some granulosa cells to a cuboidal shape (arrows). This change in shape is a hallmark of recruitment.[94] Electron micrograph of a typical primordial follicle located in the dense connective tissue (*) of the ovarian cortex. In the oocyte, note the characteristic aggregation of the cytoplasmic organelles into the so-called Balbiani body; flattened granulosa cells (arrows). (Electron micrograph, courtesy of A. Hertig.[95])

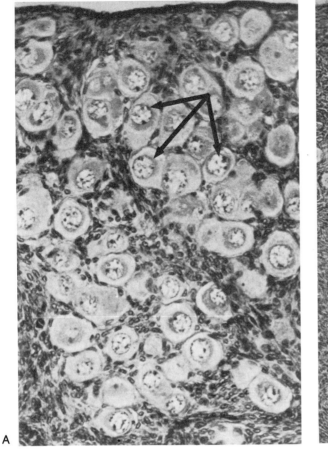

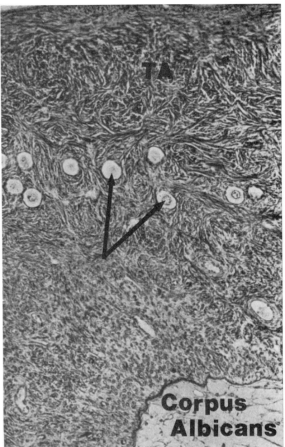

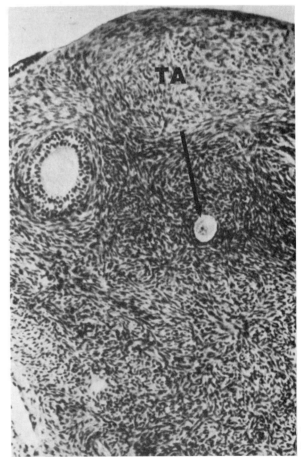

Figure 9–6. Normal ovaries: A. Birth. B. 25 years old. C. 50 years old. Photomicrographs of sections through the cortex of human ovaries at different periods of life showing the progressive decrease in the size of the nongrowing pool of primordial follicles and oocytes (arrows). Tunica albuginea (TA).

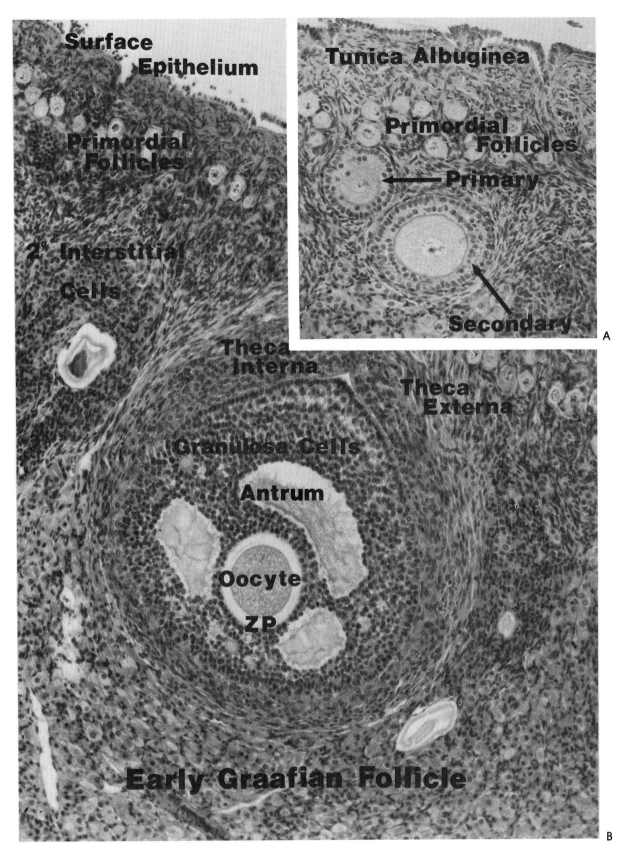

Figure 9–7. Photomicrographs of a normal ovary during the reproductive years. A. The pool of nongrowing primordial follicles is distributed as a band just beneath the tunica albuginea. Here some follicles have been recruited and appear at the primary and secondary stages. B. Once recruited, the follicle migrates deep into the ovarian medulla where it forms an antrum and develops the thecal layers. Such antral or Graafian follicles are characteristic features of the normal ovary in the reproductive years. Note clusters of large secondary interstitial cells in the cortical stroma.

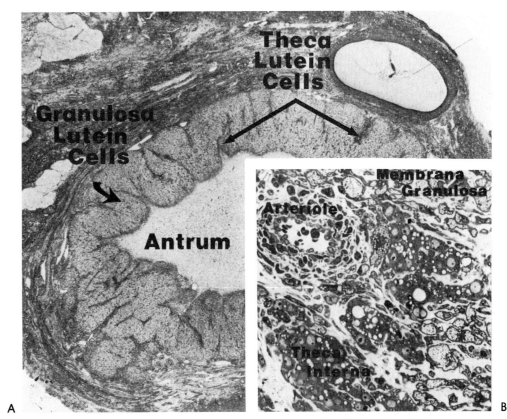

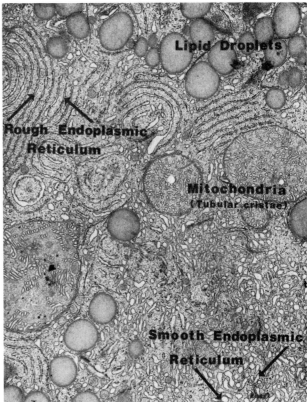

Figure 9–8. Photomicrographs of a normal human corpus luteum. A. Light micrograph showing a fibrin clot in the antral cavity surrounded by granulosa and theca lutein cells. B. Higher magnification showing the large, lipid-filled granulosa lutein cells and the smaller, more darkly stained theca lutein cells. C. Electron micrograph of luteal cell showing the organelles typically found in active steroidogenic cells. (Photomicrographs, courtesy of T. Crisp.)

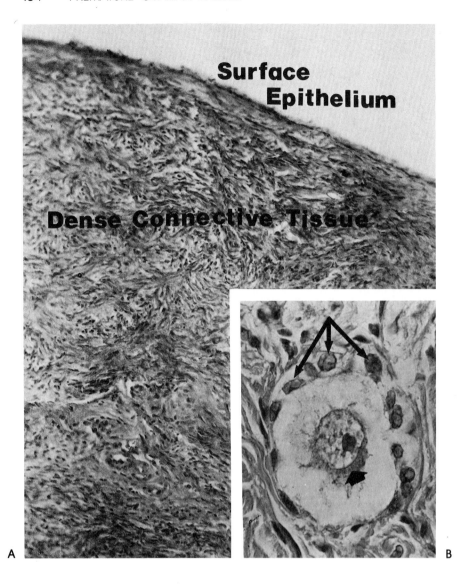

Surface Epithelium

Dense Connective Tissue

A

B

Figure 9–9. Light micrograph of an ovary from a POF patient. A. Low magnification illustrating dense connective tissue with no follicles or oocytes. B. Another POF ovary showing a typical primordial follicle. Note the Balbiani body (thick arrow). Also, some granulosa cells are transforming from a flattened to cuboidal shape (thin arrows). This change is a hallmark of recruitment.[94]

typical corpus luteum. (Compare Figures 9–8, 9–12) Examination with the electron microscope (Figure 9–13) reveals a highly differentiated ultrastructure in the POF luteal cells typical of that found in a normal corpus luteum.[89] Although biochemical analysis was not performed, this distinct ultrastructural morphology would be consistent with progestin synthesis by the POF corpus luteum. If one considers that a corpus luteum is formed from a dominant preovulatory follicle, then one is led to the conclusion that a primordial follicle in the POF ovary has shifted along a path of specialized differentiation to a dominant follicle, expelled its oocyte, and then expressed its terminal steps in the differentiation process and evolved as a progestin-secreting tissue.

It is also worthy of note that histopathologic analysis of rare POF ovaries has revealed lymphocytes in and around follicular structures.[8] This supports the hypothesis that destruction of developing follicles in this syndrome might be causally linked to autoimmune mechanisms in some individuals.

In conclusion, it is apparent from this discussion that much of what we know about the POF ovary has come from studies conducted on biopsy specimens. Certainly, considerable insight into a pathologic process can be gained by histological analysis of a tissue biopsy; however, there is great danger in the case of POF of drawing erroneous conclusions about the reproductive potential of a POF patient based upon an ovarian biopsy because of the rarity and nonuniform distribution of follicular structures in the ovaries. It is obvious from this discussion that follicles, oocytes, and luteal cells can exist in POF ovaries. Therefore, based on all the available evidence, it seems clinically sound to assume that many POF patients may indeed have some remaining primordial follicles, and that these follicles are capable of naturally transforming from the undifferentiated to the fully differentiated state at any given moment.

DIAGNOSTIC CONSIDERATIONS

To eliminate potentially treatable causes of hypergonadotropic amenorrhea in young women and to identify other

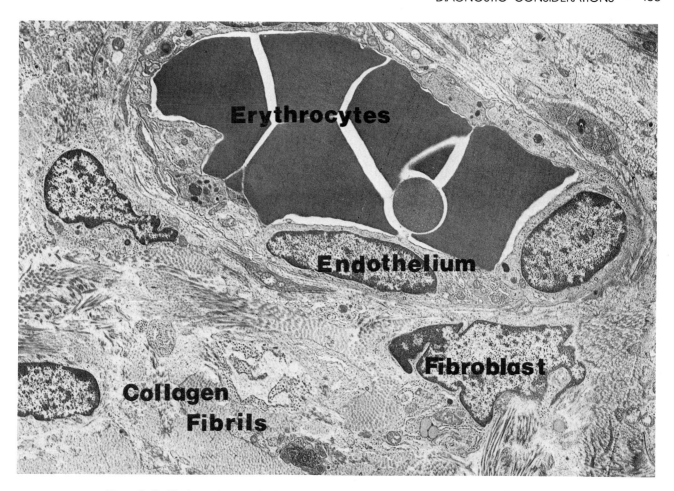

Figure 9–10. Electron micrograph of a portion of a typical POF ovary illustrating a small blood vessel within a network of dense connective tissue. No follicles or oocytes are seen.

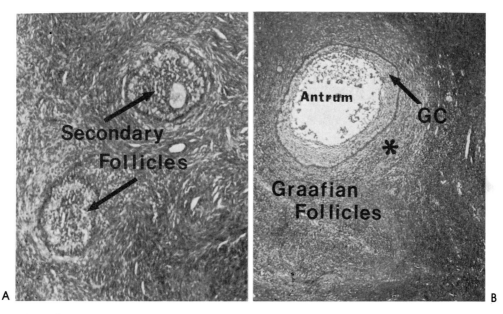

Figure 9–11. Light micrographs of a POF ovary. A. Two secondary follicles, each packed with healthy granulosa cells. B. A large Graafian follicle with multiple layers of healthy granulosa cells (GC) and a very thick theca interna (*) not unlike that seen in a patient with polycystic ovary disease.[94]

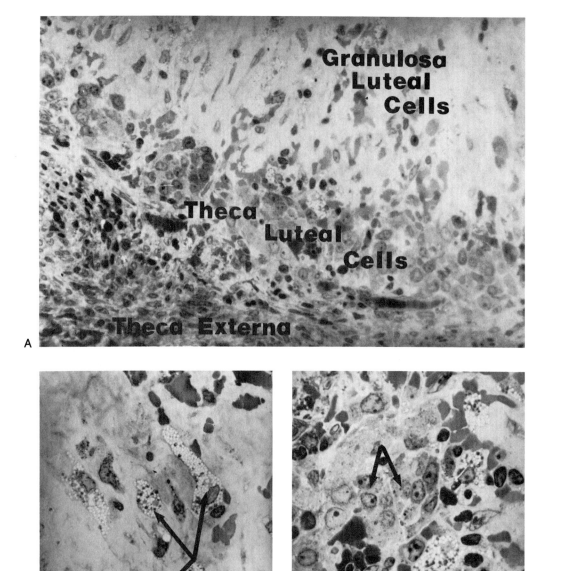

Figure 9–12. Photomicrograph of a corpus luteum in an ovary of a POF patient. A. Large, lipid-filled cells in the fibrin clot are granulosa lutein cells, and the smaller, darker ones below are the theca lutein cells. B. Higher magnification of granulosa lutein cells. C. Higher magnification of theca lutein cells.

associated disorders which may require treatment, it seems reasonable to evaluate affected patients as depicted in Table 9–5 and adapted from Rebar.[90] A complete history and thorough physical examination should be conducted first. Together with the maturation index, a simple clinical assessment of the estrogen status can be made. Chromosomal studies should be performed in affected women under age 35 to identify those with forms of gonadal dysgenesis without the stigmata of Turner's syndrome, individuals with mosaicism, and those with

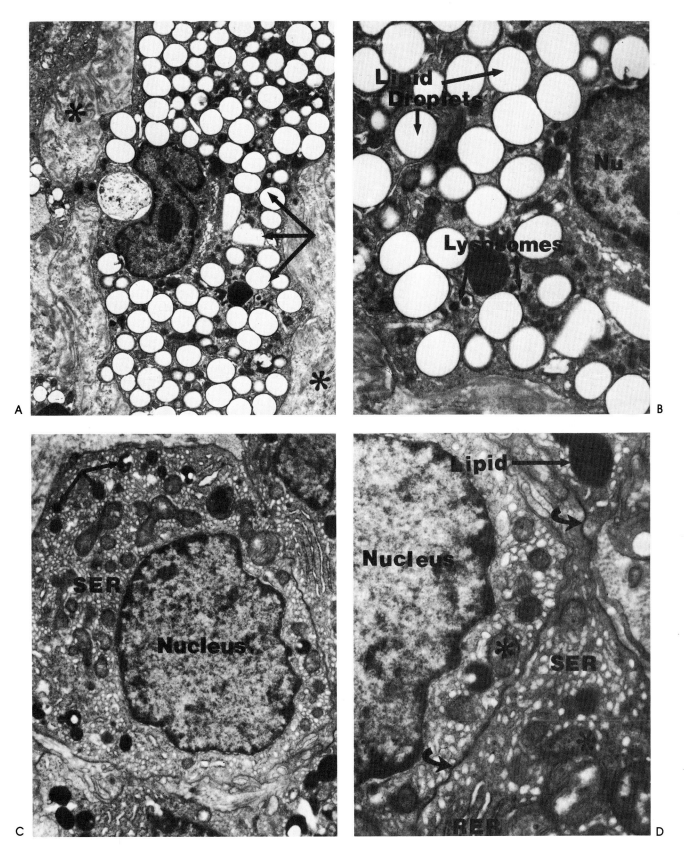

Figure 9–13. Electron micrographs of the POF corpus luteum. A,B. Portion of a granulosa lutein cell showing large numbers of lipid droplets (arrows), lysosomes, and some rough endoplasmic reticulum. C,D. Portion of a theca lutein cell showing well-developed smooth endoplasmic reticulum (SER), some mitochondria with tubular cristae, lysosomes (arrows) and lipid droplets. Note prominent gap junctions (curved arrows) between adjacent cells.

Table 9–5. Evaluation of Hypergonadotropic Amenorrhea in Young Women (Presumptive Premature Ovarian Failure)

1. Complete history and physical examination
2. Maturation index
3. Karyotype
4. Complete blood count with differential, sedimentation rate, total serum protein and albumin/globulin ratio, rheumatoid factor, antinuclear antibody
5. Fasting blood sugar, a.m. cortisol, serum calcium, and phosphorus
6. T4, TSH, anti-thyroglobulin, and anti-microsomal antibodies
7. LH, FSH, and estradiol, on at least 2 occasions

trisomy X or a Y chromosome. If karyotypic abnormalities exist, then indicated additional studies should be carried out and appropriate therapy provided. A few simple laboratory tests should be performed to rule out thyroid disease, hypoparathyroidism, hypoadrenalism, diabetes mellitus, and other evidence of autoimmune dysfunction. The tests include (but need not be limited to) those delineated in Table 9–5, which are those most commonly abnormal in affected women with autoimmune disorders. If available, testing of the patient's serum for antibodies to endocrine tissues, including ovary, may be of value.

Once the etiology of autoimmune ovarian dysfunction is established, other tests may be developed to identify women with autoimmune POF. Testing to determine if the gonadotropins are biologically active may also be informative. Measurement of circulating LH, FSH, and estradiol concentrations on more than one occasion may help to determine if any functional oocytes remain in the ovary. If the estradiol concentration is greater than 50 pg/ml or if the LH level is significantly greater than the FSH in terms of mIU/ml in any sample, then the probability of viable oocytes is considerable. Irregular uterine bleeding, indicative of continuing estrogen production, also provides good evidence of remaining functional ovarian follicles. In fact, amenorrhea and permanent estrogen deficiency need not be present in women with this syndrome. Intermittent menstruation may occur and signs and symptoms of estrogen deficiency may appear sporadically in women with hypergonadotropinism.[9,10,13] The evaluation of such women should be no different from that just delineated.

Ovarian biopsy no longer appears justified in women with POF with a normal karyotype. Aiman and Smentek[13] reported that one of their two patients who eventually conceived had no oocytes present on biopsy by laparotomy. Similarly, one of the women in the series reported by Rebar, Erickson, and Yen[10] who subsequently conceived (following publication of the study) had no oocytes on biopsy (unpublished). As noted by Aiman and Smentek,[13] if five sections of an ovarian biopsy are examined and each is 6 μm thick, then the presence of follicles is sought from a sample representing less than 0.15% of a $2 \times 3 \times 4$ cm ovary. Thus an ovarian biopsy, even if obtained by laparotomy, can provide misleading information. Furthermore, affected patients generally require estrogen replacement regardless of the results of the biopsy.

THERAPEUTIC CONSIDERATIONS

Currently, women with POF should be treated identically, whether or not they desire pregnancy. Estrogen replacement is indicated to prevent the accelerated bone loss which has been documented in affected women.[91] The estrogen should always be given sequentially with a progestin to prevent endometrial hyperplasia. Furthermore, as documented by Aiman and Smentek,[13] pregnancy was reported as occurring in 14 women between 1964 and 1984. At least 11 of these women conceived while taking estrogen for replacement therapy. Since the one patient reported by Rebar, Erickson, and Yen[10] included in the series of 14 was also on estrogen at the time of conception (unpublished), the number was actually 12. However, the possibility of pregnancy for affected women is still extremely low, even while on estrogen. In fact, it has been estimated that the probability of pregnancy is less than 1 per 9200 affected women.[13] Since one of the authors (R.W.R.) has seen 6% of affected women conceive after the diagnosis was made (unpublished), this estimate seems too low. Despite these considerations, probably no other contraceptive agent is required for those patients who do not wish pregnancy but who are sexually active. However, women on estrogen should be warned to contact their physician if they develop any signs or symptoms of pregnancy or do not withdraw to progestin. One of the authors (R.W.R.) has had three women not desiring pregnancy conceive while taking estrogen. Recently, Check and Chase[92] reported two pregnancies in five women with POF in whom gonadotropin levels were suppressed with estrogen and then treated with human menopausal gonadotropin. Thus, ovulation induction with either clomiphene citrate or human menopausal gonadotropin may be considered in women failing to conceive while on estrogen replacement. Why women with POF conceive while taking estrogen is enigmatic. Pregnancy may occur because follicular development can begin once FSH receptors are induced by the exogenous estrogen or because gonadotropin receptors become unoccupied once circulating levels are reduced. However, these are merely speculations.

As noted previously, women with evidence of autoimmune ovarian failure may ovulate following therapy with corticosteroids and/or plasmapheresis as a result of a reduction in circulating autoantibodies.[8,55] But effective treatment regimens remain to be established. The use of such agents as azathioprine, which has been used in treating other autoimmune disorders, seems contraindicated in patients in whom the only reason for therapy is ovulation induction. Individuals with biologically inactive forms of gonadotropin should respond to induction of ovulation with human menopausal and chorionic gonadotropins. Routine use of such therapeutic modalities will require more knowledge about the pathophysiologic bases of the various disorders that result in POF. Similarly, the treatment of women with POF by hormone replacement to mimic the normal menstrual cycle and embryo transfer, as has been successfully reported,[93] must be considered only a research procedure at the present time.

SUMMARY

What is clear is that POF occurs much more frequently than appreciated heretofore. Unfortunately, specific treatment must await better understanding of the etiologies of ovarian failure. Even biopsy of the ovaries has not proven to be of much help in determining the etiology or in assessing the possibility of conception in individual patients.

It would seem rational to hypothesize that POF results from disturbances in the recruitment and selection of oocytes. For any of several reasons, the follicles undergo accelerated atresia or atresia at the normal rate in a smaller than normal pool of follicles that eventually results in depletion of all oocytes. Since FSH appears to be the principal regulator of folliculogenesis, it would seem that most causes of POF must somehow involve FSH secretion or action. The pituitary gland might secrete aberrant forms of FSH of LH. Peripheral tissues, including the ovary, may process FSH or LH abnormally. Circulating autoantibodies to FSH or to ovarian FSH receptors or other circulating factors might prevent stimulation of follicular cells by FSH. A defect could also develop in the follicular cells themselves, preventing them from responding to gonadotropin appropriately. These possibilities are testable. Undoubtedly future biochemical studies will be of great value in helping us to understand—then successfully to treat—this complex disorder.

References

1. de Moraes M, Jones GS: Premature ovarian failure. Fertil Steril 18:440–461, 1967.
2. Goldenberg RL, Grodin JM, Rodbard D, *et al.*: Gonadotropins in women with amenorrhea. Am J Obstet Gynecol 116:1003–1012, 1973.
3. Johnson TR Jr., Peterson EP: Gonadotropin-induced pregnancy following "premature ovarian failure." Fertil Steril 31:351–352, 1979.
4. Lucky AW, Rebar RW, Blizzard RM, *et al.*: Pubertal progression in the presence of elevated serum gonadotropins in girls with multiple endocrine deficiencies. J Clin Endocrinol Metab 45:673–678, 1977.
5. Schreiber JR, Davajan V, Kletzy OA: A case of intermittent ovarian failure. Am J Obstet Gynecol 132:698–699, 1978.
6. Irvine WJ, Chan MMW, Scarth L, *et al.*: Immunological aspects of premature ovarian failure associated with idiopathic Addison's disease. Lancet 2:883–887, 1968.
7. Turkington, RW, Lebovitz HE: Extra-adrenal endocrine deficiencies in Addison's disease. Am J Med 43:499–507, 1967.
8. Coulam CB, Kempers RD, Randall RV: Premature ovarian failure: evidence for the autoimmune mechanism. Fertil Steril 36:238–240, 1981.
9. Coulam CB: Premature gonadal failure. Fertil Steril 38:645–665, 1982.
10. Rebar R, Erickson GF, Yen, SSC: "Idiopathic premature ovarian failure": clinical and endocrine characteristics. Fertil Steril 37:35–41, 1982.
11. Villanueva AL, Rebar RW: The triple X syndrome and premature ovarian failure. Obstet Gynecol 62:70S–73S, 1983.
12. Marshall WA, Tanner JM: Variations in patterns of pubertal changes in girls. Arch Dis Child 44:291, 1969.
13. Aiman J, Smentek, C: Premature ovarian failure. Obstet Gynecol 66:9–14, 1985.
14. Sherman BM, Korenman SG: Hormonal characteristics of the human menstrual cycle throughout reproductive life. J Clin Invest 55:699–706, 1975.
15. Coulam CB: Editor's formulation: classification and treatment of premature gonadal failure. Semin Reprod Endocrinol 1:177–178, 1983.
16. Singh RP, Carr DH: The anatomy and histology of XO human embryos and fetuses. Anat Rec 155:369–381, 1966.
17. Reyes FI, Koh KS, Faiman C: Fertility in women with gonadal dysgenesis. Am J Obstet Gynecol 126:668, 1976.
18. Jones EC, Krohn PL: The relationship between age, numbers of oocytes, and fertility in virgin and multiparous mice. J Endocrinol 21:469–495, 1961.
19. Block E: Quantitative morphological investigations of the follicular system in women. Variations at different ages. Acta Anat 14:108–123, 1952.
20. Block E: A quantitative morphological investigation of the follicular system in newborn female infants. Acta Anat 17:201–206, 1953.
21. Harper PS, Dyken PR: Early onset dystrophia myotonica. Lancet 2:53–55, 1972.
22. Day RW, Larson W, Wright SW: Clinical and cytogenetic studies on a group of females with XXX sex chromosome complements. J Pediatr 64:24–33, 1964.
23. Gordon DL, Paulsen CA: Premature menopause in XO/XX/XXX/XXXX mosaicism. Am J Obstet Gynecol 97:85–90, 1967.
24. Mattison DR, Evans MI, Schwimmer WB, *et al.*: Familial premature ovarian failure. Am J Hum Genet 36:1341–1348, 1984.
25. Starup J, Sele V: Premature ovarian failure. Acta Obstet Gynecol Scand 52:259, 1973.
26. Coulam CB, Stringfellow S, Hoefnagel D: Evidence for a genetic factor in the etiology of premature ovarian failure. Fertil Steril 40:693, 1983.
27. Austin GE, Coulam CB, Ryan RJ: A search for antibodies to luteinizing hormone receptors in premature ovarian failure. Mayo Clin Proc 54:394–400, 1979.
28. Biglieri EG, Herron MA, Brust N: 17-hydroxylation deficiency in man. J Clin Invest 45:1946–1954, 1966.
29. Goldsmith O, Solomon DH, Horton R: Hypogonadism and mineralocorticoid excess. The 17-hydroxylase deficiency syndrome. N Engl J Med 277:673–677, 1967.
30. Mallin SR: Congenital adrenal hyperplasia secondary to 17-hydroxylase deficiency. Two sisters with amenorrhea, hypokalemia, hypertension, and cystic ovaries. Ann Int Med 70:69–75, 1969.
31. Hoefnagel D, Wurser-Hili D, Child EL: Ovarian failure in galactosaemia. Lancet 2:1197, 1979.
32. Kaufman F, Kogut MD, Donnell GN, *et al.*: Ovarian failure in galactosaemia. Lancet 11:737–738, 1979.

33. Chen Y-T, Mattison DR, Feigenbaum L, *et al.*: Reduction in oocyte number following prenatal exposure to a diet high in galactose. Science 214:1145–1147, 1981.

34. Gulyas, BJ, Hodgen GD, Tullner WW, *et al.*: Effects of fetal or maternal hypophysectomy on endocrine organs and body weight in infant rhesus monkeys (*Macaca mulatta*): with particular emphasis on oogenesis. Biol Reprod 16:216–227, 1977.

35. Axelrod L, Neer RM, Kliman B: Hypogonadism in a male with immunologically active, biologically inactive luteinizing hormone: an exception to a venerable rule. J Clin Endocrinol Metab 48:279–287, 1979.

36. Park IJ, Burnett LS, Jones HW Jr., *et al.*: A case of male pseudohermaphroditism associated with elevated LH, normal FSH, and low testosterone possibly due to the secretion of an abnormal LH molecule. Acta Endocrinol 83:173–181, 1976.

37. Rebar RW, Silva de Sa MF: The reproductive age: premature ovarian failure. *In* G Serra (ed) Comprehensive Endocrinology. The Ovary, Chapter 13. New York, Raven Press, pp 241–256, 1983.

38. Jones GS, de Moraes-Ruehsen M: A new syndrome of amenorrhea in association with hypergonadotropism and apparently normal ovarian follicular apparatus. Am J Obstet Gynecol 104:597–600, 1969.

39. Maxson WS, Wentz AC: The gonadotropin-resistant ovary syndrome. Semin Reprod Endocrinol 1:147–160, 1983.

40. Netter A, Cahen G, Rozenbaum H: Le syndrome des ovaires résistants aux gonadotropines. Actual Gynecol (Paris) 8:29–35, 1977.

41. Collen RJ, Lippen BM, Kaplan SA: Primary ovarian failure, juvenile rheumatoid arthritis, and vitiligo. Am J Dis Child 133:598–600, 1979.

42. Drury MI, Keelan DM, Timoney FJ, *et al.*: Juvenile familial endocrinopathy. Clin Exp Immunol 7:125–132, 1970.

43. Golonka JE, Goodman AD: Coexistence of primary ovarian insufficiency, primary adrenocortical insufficiency, and idiopathic hypoparathyroidism. J Clin Endocrinol Metab 28:79–82, 1968.

44. Kleerekoper M, Basten A, Penny R, *et al.*: Idiopathic hypoparathyroidism with primary ovarian failure. Report of a case with detailed immunological studies. Arch Intern Med 134:944–947, 1974.

45. Lundberg PO, Persson B-H: Disappearance of amenorrhea after thymectomy. A case report. Acta Soc Med Upsal 74:206–208, 1969.

46. Vazquez AM, Kenny FM: Ovarian failure and antiovarian antibodies in association with hypoparathyroidism, moniliasis, and Addison's and Hashimoto's diseases. Obstet Gynecol 41:414–418, 1973.

47. Williamson HO, Phansey SA, Mathur S, *et al.*: Myasthenia gravis, premature menopause, and thyroid autoimmunity. Am J Obstet Gynecol 137:893–901, 1980.

48. Christy NP, Holub DA, Tomasi TB: Primary ovarian, thyroidal, and adrenocortical deficiencies simulating pituitary insufficiency, associated with diabetes mellitus. J Clin Endocrinol Metab 22:155–160, 1962.

49. de Moraes-Ruehsen M, Blizzard RM, Garcia-Bunvel R, *et al.*: Autoimmunity and ovarian failure. Am J Obstet Gynecol 112:693–703, 1972.

50. Patrick J, Lindstrom J: Autoimmune response to acetylcholine receptor. Science 180:871–872, 1973.

51. Manley SW, Bourke JR, Hawker RW: The thyrotropin receptor in guinea pig thyroid homogenate: Interaction with the long-acting thyroid stimulator. J Endocrinol 61:437–445, 1974.

52. Coulam CB, Ryan RJ: Premature menopause. I. Etiology. Am J Obstet Gynecol 133:639–643, 1979.

53. McNatty KP, Short RV, Barnes EW, *et al.*: The cytotoxic effect of serum from patients with Addison's disease and autoimmune ovarian failure on human granulosa cells in culture. Clin Exp Immunol 22:373–384, 1975.

54. Chiauzzi V, Cigorraga S, Escobar ME, *et al.*: Inhibition of follicle-stimulating hormone receptor binding by circulating immunoglobulins. J Clin Endocrinol Metab 54:1221–1228, 1982.

55. Bateman BG, Nunley WC, Kitchin JD III: Reversal of apparent premature ovarian failure in a patient with myasthenia gravis. Fertil Steril 39:108, 1983.

56. Lintern-Moore S, Pantelouris EM: Ovarian development in athymic nude mice. I. The size and composition of the follicle population. Mech Ageing Dev 4:385–390, 1975.

57. Rebar RW, Morandini IC, Erickson GF, *et al.*: The hormonal basis of reproductive defects in athymic mice: diminished gonadotropins in prepubertal females. Endocrinology 108:120–126, 1981.

58. Rebar RW, Morandini IC, Benirschke K, *et al.*: Reduced gonadotropins in athymic mice: Prevention by thymic transplantation. Endocrinology 107:2130–2132, 1980.

59. Pierpaoli W, Besedovsky HO: Role of the thymus in programming of neuroendocrine functions. Clin Exp Immunol 20:323–338, 1975.

60. Sakakura T, Nishizuka Y: Thymic control mechanism in ovarian development: reconstitution of ovarian dysgenesis in thymectomized mice by replacement with thymic and other lymphoid tissues. Endocrinology 90:431–437, 1972.

61. Healy DL, Bacher J, Hodgen GD: Thymic regulation of primate fetal ovarian-adrenal differentiation. Biol Reprod 32:1127–1133, 1985.

62. Miller ME, Chatten J: Ovarian changes in ataxia telangiectasia. Acta Paediatr Scand 56:559–561, 1967.

63. Rebar RW, Miyake A, Low TLK, *et al.*: Thymosin stimulates secretion of luteinizing hormone-releasing factor. Science 214:669–671, 1981.

64. Jacox HW: Recovery following human ovarian irradiation. Radiology 32:538–545, 1939.

65. Baker JW, Morgan RL, Peckham MJ, *et al.*: Preservation of ovarian function in patients requiring radiotherapy for para-aortic and pelvic Hodgkin's disease. Lancet 1:1307–1308, 1972.

66. Ray GR, Trueblood HW, Enright LP, *et al.*: Oophoropexy: A means of preserving ovarian function following pelvic megavoltage radiotherapy for Hodgkin's disease. Radiology 96:175–180, 1970.

67. Koyama H, Wada J, Nishizawa Y, *et al.*: Cyclophosphamide-induced ovarian failure and its therapeutic significance in patients with breast cancer. Cancer 39:1403–1409, 1977.

68. Siris ES, Leventhal BG, Vaitukaitis JL: Effects of childhood leukemia and chemotherapy on puberty and reproductive function in girls. N Engl J Med 294:1143–1146, 1976.

69. Lentz RD, Bergstein J, Steffes MW, *et al.*: Postpubertal evaluation of gonadal function following cyclophosphamide therapy before and during puberty. J Pediatr 91:385–394, 1977.

70. Ataya KM, McKanna JA, Weintraub AM, *et al.:* Treatment with LHRH agonist prevents chemotherapy-induced follicular loss in rats. 32nd Annual Meeting of the Society for Gynecologic Investigation, 1985, (March 20–23); Phoenix, Arizona, Abstract No. 464, p. 260.

71. Morrison JC, Givens JR, Wiser WL, *et al.:* Mumps oophoritis: a cause of premature menopause. Fertil Steril 26:655–659, 1975.

72. Prinz W, Taubert H-D: Mumps in pubescent females and its effect on later reproductive function. Gynaekologia 167:23–27, 1968.

73. Jick H, Porter J, Morrison AS: Relation between smoking and age of natural menopause. Lancet 1:1354–1355, 1977.

74. Bailey A, Robinson D, Vessey M: Smoking and age of natural menopause. Lancet 2:722, 1977.

75. Daniell HW: Smoking, obesity, and the menopause. Lancet 2:373, 1978.

76. Mattison DR: How xenobiotic compounds can destroy oocytes. Contemp Obstet Gynecol 15:157–169, 1980.

77. Erickson GF: Normal ovarian function. Clin Obstet Gynecol 21:31–52, 1978.

78. Erickson GF: Follicular growth and development: *In* JJ Sciarra, L Speroff (eds) Reproductive Endocrinology, Infertility, and Genetics: gynecology and obstetrics. Harper and Row, Hagerstown, MD, pp. 1–16, 1981.

79. Ohno S, Klinger HP, Atkin NB: Human oogenesis. Cytogenetics I: 42–51, 1962.

80. Peters H, Byskov AG, Faber M: Intraovarian regulation of follicle growth in the immature mouse. *In* The Development and Maturation of the Ovary and its Functions. Excerpta Medica, Int Cong (Ser No) 269:20–23, 1973.

81. Lintern-Moore S, Peters H, Moore GPM, *et al.:* Follicular development in the infant human ovary. J Reprod Fertil 39:53–64, 1974.

82. Peters H, Byskov AG, Himelstein-Braw R, *et al.:* Follicular growth: the basic event in the mouse and human ovary. J Reprod Fertil 45:559–566, 1975.

83. Peters H, Himelstein-Braw R, Faber M: The normal development of the ovary in childhood. Acta Endocrinol 82:617–630, 1976.

84. Baker TG: A quantitative and cytological study of germ cells in human ovaries. Proc R Soc B 158:417–433, 1963.

85. Baker TG, O WS: Development of the ovary and oogenesis. Clin Obstet Gynecol 3:3–18, 1976.

86. Erickson GF, Magoffin DA, Dyer CA, *et al.:* The ovarian androgen producing cells: a review of structure/function relationships. Endo Rev 6:371–399, 1985.

87. Erickson GF, Yen SSC: New data on follicle cells in polycystic ovaries: a proposed mechanism for the genesis of cystic follicles. Semin Reprod Endocrinol 2:231–243, 1984.

88. Longcope C, Hunter R, Franz C: Steroid secretion by the postmenopausal ovary. Am J Obstet Gynecol 138:564–568, 1980.

89. Fawcett DW, Long JA, Jones AL: The ultrastructure of endocrine glands. Recent Prog Horm Res 25:315–379, 1969.

90. Rebar RW: Hypergonadotropic hypogonadism and premature ovarian failure: a review. J Reprod Med 27:179–186, 1982.

91. Cann CE, Martin MC, Genant HK, *et al.:* Decreased spinal mineral content in amenorrheic women. JAMA 251:626–629, 1984.

92. Check JH, Chase JS: Ovulation induction in hypergonadotropic amenorrhea with estrogen and human menopausal gonadotropin therapy. Fertil Steril 42:919–922, 1984.

93. Lutjen P, Trunson A, Leston J, *et al.:* The establishment and maintenance of pregnancy using *in vitro* fertilization and embryo donation in a patient with primary ovarian failure. Nature 307:174–175, 1984.

94. Pedersen T: Follicle growth in the immature mouse ovary. Acta Endocrinol 62:117–132, 1969.

95. Hertig AT: The primary human oocyte: Some observations on the fine structure of Balbiani's vitelline body and the origin of annulate lamellae. AM J Anat 122:107–138, 1968.

10. Polycystic Ovary Syndrome and Related Abnormalities

R. Jeffrey Chang and Dominique de Ziegler

The term polycystic ovary syndrome (PCO) is best reserved for describing a clinical but not a specific pathophysiologic entity since the cause of this disorder encompasses several different abnormalities with similar clinical presentations. It has been estimated that approximately 3% of women experience this problem, making it the most common reproductive endocrinologic disorder among women during their years of menstruation.[1,2] Patients with the syndrome present a triad of symptoms.[3,4] First, there is evidence of chronic anovulation. This is reflected by menstrual disorders including amenorrhea, oligomenorrhea, and irregular anovulatory bleeding. Second, there is androgen excess manifested by hirsutism and occasionally mild virilization. Lastly, approximately 40% of patients exhibit exogenous obesity. These clinical symptoms and signs are usually associated with bilaterally enlarged and cystic ovaries with no evidence of recent ovulation. The clinical course of the disease is characterized by the appearance of symptoms during or shortly after the onset of puberty.[3] In general, patients seek medical attention for this problem during their late teens and twenties. For unknown reasons it is less common to see patients during their fourth decade or later.

The impact of PCO in women during their reproductive years is substantial. Infertility has been estimated to afflict approximately 10%-15% of married couples. Ovulatory problems account for about 10% of these cases, and PCO is responsible for most (70%-85%) of these ovulatory problems.[5,6] Hirsutism is one of the most common endocrine problems in women, with PCO being the leading ovarian cause of this disorder. Although cancer of the endometrium is uncommon in premenopausal women, these patients often exhibit the classical findings of PCO.[7,8]

In some cases the etiology appears to be familial and an X-linked dominant inheritance has been suggested;[9,11] however, many patients clearly have no family history. That this syndrome is associated with a variety of clearly defined diseases suggests multiple etiologies which lead to a final common pathophysiologic process. If these diseases are corrected, the syndrome usually resolves. Diseases which are known to be associated with PCO include androgen-secreting tumors of the adrenal glands and ovaries, late-onset or acquired adrenal hyperplasia, Cushing's disease, luteinizing hormone secreting pitui-

tary tumor, and the syndromes of insulin resistance.[3,12,13] This suggests that underlying defects of the hypothalamic-pituitary system, ovaries, adrenal glands and/or insulin action could result in the presentation of this symptom complex.

PATHOPHYSIOLOGY

PCO represents a disorder of abnormal hypothalamic-pituitary-ovarian/adrenal interaction. The specific alterations of hormone secretion have been well described previously.[14,15] Characteristically, there are increases of circulating androgens which arise primarily from the ovaries and adrenal glands. Through peripheral conversion mechanisms these androgens are metabolized to estrogens. In the absence of ovulation progesterone levels remain low. Gonadotropin secretion is marked by suppressed FSH secretion and increased serum LH. Circulating ACTH levels are normal. It is apparent that a major endocrinologic disruption in PCO is abnormal steroid production.

Excess Androgen Production

A hallmark of abnormal steroid metabolism in PCO is hyperandrogenism. Specifically, there are significant elevations of the major androgens, androstenedione, and testosterone. In addition, at least 50% of patients exhibit an increase of circulating DHEA-S concentrations.[16] In PCO the derivation of these androgens has not been firmly established. It has been proposed that androstenedione and testosterone originate from the abnormal polycystic ovary stimulated by increased LH secretion. On the other hand, in one half of the patients DHEA-S levels are elevated, implying excess adrenal androgen production which includes significant amounts of androstenedione and testosterone. Much of this concept is extrapolated from adrenal suppression studies conducted in normal women showing that approximately 50% of androstenedione and testosterone were of adrenal origin.[17]

In the past, the source of excess androgen production in PCO has been studied extensively. Both the ovary and adrenal glands have been shown to contribute to the increased androgen pool. Still, the principal site of production remains controversial. Efforts to elucidate the role of the ovary and adrenal gland have been limited by methodologic variation and technical difficulty. Identification of the source of hyperandrogenism in PCO is important for at least two reasons. First, it may serve to clarify the mechanism of excess androgen production and potentially shed light on the pathogenesis of PCO. Second, it will influence the choice of therapy in patients suffering from this disorder.

In the earliest accounts of PCO, clinical observations strongly suggested a primary adrenal disease rather than a disorder of ovarian function.[18–28] However, the utilization of in vitro studies of ovarian tissue clearly indicated a defect of ovarian androgen metabolism. Incubation of polycystic ovarian tissues with radiolabeled progesterone or acetate induced androstenedione and testosterone production in amounts significantly greater than those derived from normal ovaries.[29–35] In addition, the androstenedione level in the cyst fluid of follicles from polycystic ovaries was increased compared to that found in the follicular fluid of normal ovaries.[36]

With the recognition that polycystic ovaries in vitro had the capacity to produce excess androgen, several attempts were made in vivo to substantiate this observation. The most common method has been to use oral contraceptives and assess circulating androgens before and after treatment.[37–43] While a marked reduction of androstenedione and testosterone in PCO has been demonstrated, it also has been shown that norethindrone, 1 mg, and mestranol, 80 μgm, significantly lowered circulating ACTH and DHEA-S levels in normal women.[44] This latter result was attributed to decreased clearance of free cortisol, leading to a negative feedback effect on ACTH. Attempts to define the role of the ovary by stimulation with hCG have been limited by apparent nonselectivity as well as inconsistent results.[8,45,46] Furthermore, it has been documented that hCG may stimulate androgen secretion from adrenal tumors, which raises the issue of ovarian specificity.[47,48]

Estimation of ovarian androgen secretion in PCO has been studied indirectly by suppression of adrenal function using glucocorticoids. This approach has appeared to provide more consistent findings compared to ovarian suppression. Most reports have demonstrated that at least 50% of hirsute patients show evidence of adrenal androgen excess.[38–42,49–54] The major problem with this technique has been the overlap effect on pituitary-ovarian function. In animal studies dexamethasone administration has been associated with reduced serum LH levels.[55] In humans similar treatment with corticosteroid has produced mixed results. In one instance women with elevated LH levels exhibited a reduction of LH, FSH, androstenedione, and testosterone,[56,57] whereas in another study women with normal circulating LH displayed increases of LH, androstenedione, and testosterone, and a decrease of FSH.[50] In addition, selective ovarian vein catheterization performed in some PCO patients revealed a lowering of androgen levels in the ovarian venous effluent following dexamethasone.[58] Adrenal gland stimulation has been encumbered by the lack of consistency and

specificity. That ACTH may influence theca cell function has been suggested by results from in vitro studies of normal and polycystic ovaries.[59] Evidence also exists which shows that ACTH may alter serum LH concentrations.[50,60]

In the past selective ovarian and adrenal vein catheterization has proved useful in localizing androgen-producing tumors, but its benefit in defining the primary source of androgen excess in PCO has not been successful.[58,60,61] Methodologic and technical errors have been cited as reasons for inconsistency.[52,62] In a large series of patients with nonneoplastic hyperandrogenism, selective catheterization confirmed the lack of reliability of this method.[63]

The recent development of long-acting GnRH agonists has provided a means of achieving complete ovarian suppression in a variety of physiologic and pathologic conditions including PCO.[64–66] These potent compounds inhibit ovarian steroid secretion by desensitizing the pituitary gonadotropes to further GnRH stimulation and effectively eliminate the release of bioactive LH (Figure 10–1).[67] When administered to PCO patients at a dose of 100 μg daily for four weeks, there were reductions of elevated androstenedione and testosterone as well as estrone and estradiol levels to values found in castrate women of comparable age (Figures 10–2, 10–3).[68] The decrease of these androgens was dramatic and uniform, as all subjects demonstrated post-treatment concentrations within the range of oophorectomized women (Figure 10–4). In contrast, adrenal androgen secretion, DHEA, DHEA-S, and cortisol were unaffected throughout the course of GnRH-a treatment (Figure 10–5). Further studies of adrenal function confirmed this finding, as 24-hour secretion patterns and responses to ACTH infusion were similar before and after therapy (Figures 10–6, 10–7). That circulating estrone, estradiol, androstenedione,

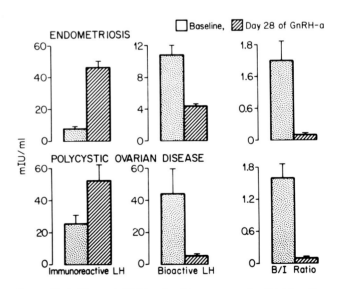

Figure 10–1. Mean ± SEM levels of immunoreactive LH, bioactive LH, and the LH bioactive/immunoreactive (B/I) ratio in women with endometriosis (upper panel) and polycystic ovarian disease (lower panel) before treatment (stippled bars) and on the 28th day of GnRH agonist administration (hatched bars).

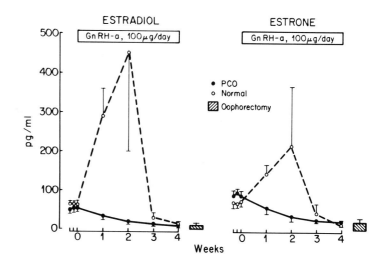

Figure 10–2. Mean serum estradiol and estrone concentrations in PCO patients and normal ovulatory women with endometriosis before and during GnRH-a treatment and in oophorectomized women.

and testosterone levels were similar to values found in oophorectomized women suggested complete eradication of ovarian steroid secretion. From these data it was concluded that in PCO the exclusive source of excess androstenedione and testosterone was ovarian and not adrenal in origin.

That the polycystic ovary is the principal site of androgen excess should not be surprising. Since the ovary is the target organ for gonadotropin action, it is understandable that increased androgen production results from chronic stimulation by increased pituitary LH secretion. Moreover, it has been shown that bio-active LH concen-

trations are significantly elevated in patients with the PCO syndrome.[69]

As much as ovarian androgen excess appears to be central to the pathophysiology of PCO, increased adrenal androgen production has also been implicated as a contributor to the maintenance and possible genesis of this disorder for the following reasons: First, circulating adrenal androgens, DHEA and DHEA-S, are elevated in adult patients with PCO.[70,71] Second, historically the onset of symptoms usually occurs at puberty. Since increases in adrenal androgens mark the initial endocrine changes at this time, it has been proposed that PCO may result from an exaggerated adrenarche.[15] Third, studies in pubertal patients between the ages of 13 and 16 [with PCO] have shown that adrenal androgens are elevated.[72] Fourth, adrenal disorders which lead to an increase of circulating

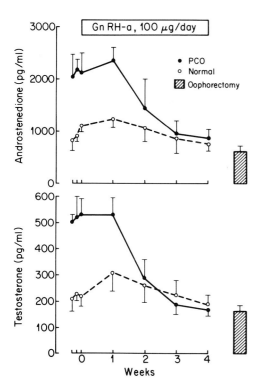

Figure 10–3. Mean serum androstenedione and testosterone concentrations in PCO patients and normal ovulatory women with endometriosis before and after GnRH-a treatment and in oophorectomized women.

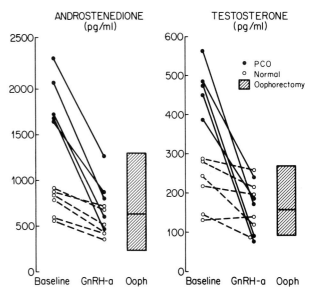

Figure 10–4. Individual androstenedione and testosterone concentrations in PCO patients and normal ovulatory women with endometriosis before (baseline) and after GnRH-a treatment compared to the mean and ranges of values in oophorectomized women.

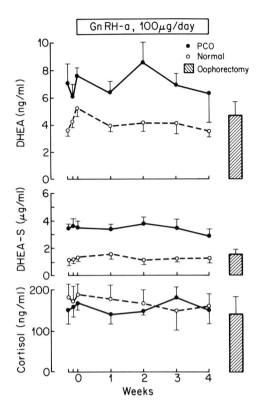

Figure 10–5. Mean serum DHEA, DHEA-S, and cortisol concentrations in PCO patients and normal ovulatory women with endometriosis before and during GnRH-a treatment and in oophorectomized women.

androgens often mimic the symptoms of PCO and can be clinically indistinguishable.[73,74]

The mechanisms responsible for the adrenal androgen excess are unknown. There are several possibilities which may explain this abnormality, including excess

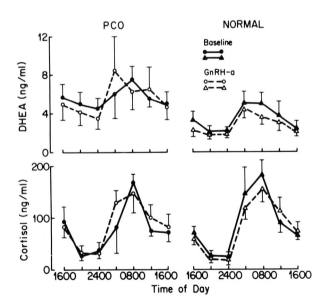

Figure 10–6. Mean serum DHEA and cortisol concentrations throughout 24 hours in PCO patients and normal ovulatory women before (baseline) and after GnRH-a treatment.

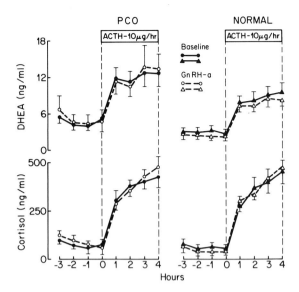

Figure 10–7. Mean serum DHEA and cortisol concentrations before and during ACTH infusion in PCO patients and normal ovulatory women with endometriosis before (baseline) and after GnRH-a treatment.

ACTH secretion, presence of a specific stimulator of the zona reticularis, adrenal enzyme deficiency, and disruption of normal adrenal secretion by abnormal ovarian steroidogenesis.

Available evidence suggests that the ACTH-adrenal axis is intact and functioning normally, since plasma ACTH and corresponding serum cortisol levels are equivalent to those of normal women (Figure 10–8).[75] The 24-hour secretion pattern of ACTH has not been studied, although the circadian rhythm of cortisol is normal.[68] In addition, urinary free cortisol concentrations, the most accurate measure of cortisol production, also were shown to be normal.[76] In spite of a normal ACTH-cortisol relationship, provocative stimulation by ACTH has resulted in small and significant increases of 17-hydroxyprogesterone, 17-

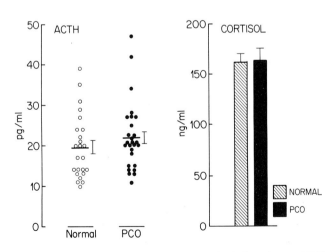

Figure 10–8. Mean (± SE) basal levels of circulating plasma ACTH and serum cortisol in PCO patients and normal subjects. Individual ACTH values are shown for PCO patients (solid circles) and normal women (open circles).

hydroxypregnenolone, and DHEA levels. This was interpreted as possibly representing a compensated subtle adrenal enzyme defect of 21- or 11β-hydroxylase.[77] The findings suggest that factors other than ACTH are responsible for adrenal androgen production or that there is a specific alteration of response by the zone reticularis to ACTH.

A pituitary factor, other than ACTH, has been proposed which contributes to stimulation of adrenal steroidogenesis, in particular adrenal androgens. *In vitro* studies have demonstrated that incubation of minced adrenal tissue with whole pituitary extract resulted in greater production of DHEA compared to that of cortisol (Figure 10–9).[78] Incubation with ACTH, 1-24 or 1-39, produced equivalent amounts of DHEA and cortisol. These findings, together with physiologic and clinical conditions which have demonstrated discordance between ACTH secretion and adrenal androgen production, such as adrenarche, imply existence of a separate cortical adrenal stimulating hormone (CASH). This putative hormone has not as yet been identified. Recent studies have indicated that the molecular weight of CASH is about 40,000 to 60,000.[78] A functional relationship between CASH and ACTH has not been established.

Structurally ACTH is derived from a large parent molecule, proopiomelanocortin, which also gives rise to melanocyte-stimulating hormone, lipotropins, and endorphins. It has been shown in PCO that beta-endorphin

levels are elevated compared to those of control subjects.[79] However, some reports have suggested that there is no direct stimulating role of beta-endorphin on adrenal androgens.[80] This finding may result from the possibility that the pathophysiologic alterations that are responsible for increased pituitary beta-endorphin secretion may also directly influence adrenal androgen secretion.

A role of prolactin in the excess production of DHEA-S has been suggested, based on treatment of PCO patients with either dopamine or its potent agonist, bromocriptine.[81] Consideration of bromocriptine administration in this disorder evolved from the finding of elevated prolactin levels in about 20% to 30% of patients (Figure 10–10). Moreover, the prolactin increase has been correlated with concentrations of DHEA-S in this syndrome.[82] Significant reduction of both hormones was achieved following treatment with bromocriptine. The coincident fall of prolactin and DHEA-S, together with unchanged cortisol levels, suggests a direct action of prolactin on adrenal androgen production. In addition, prolactin receptors have been demonstrated in adrenal tissue.[83] If prolactin is to exert an action on adrenal androgen, then it appears to be mediated by an increased production rate of DHEA-S rather than a change in its metabolic clearance rate.[84]

Specific alterations of adrenal responsiveness to ACTH may explain the increased androgen production. Recent studies have demonstrated that there is increased DHEA response to ACTH in approximately one-third of PCO patients, whereas the remaining patients had responses similar to those of normal women.[85] Intrinsic defects within the adrenal gland, such as enzyme deficiencies, have been suggested as a mechanism for increased androgens.[73,74] The evidence for this is not convincing. In a prospective study of 83 hirsute patients, most of whom had PCO, measurement of 17-hydroxyprogesterone before and after ACTH administration revealed only one patient with an enzyme deficiency—21-hydroxylase (Figure 10–11).[86] In addition, in families with 21-hydroxylase deficiency the expression of disease is HLA-linked. Since PCO may also exhibit a familial occurrence, patients and

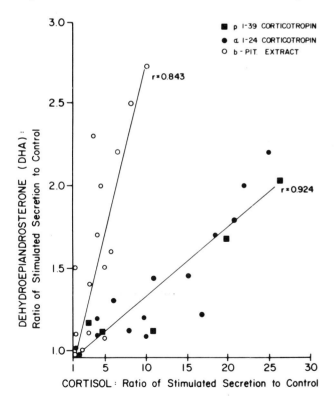

Figure 10–9. Ratio of *in vivo* stimulated DHA: cortisol secretion in dexamethasone-suppressed castrated dogs during infusions of porcine corticotropin (1-39), cosyntropin, and bovine pituitary extract. Bovine pituitary extract is more potent than either form of ACTH in stimulating DHA per unit amount of cortisol produced. (Reproduced with permission from Parker and Odell.[78])

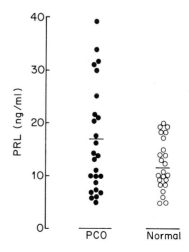

Figure 10–10. Circulating levels of serum prolactin in PCO patients and normal ovulatory women.

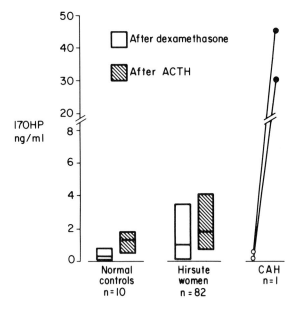

Figure 10–11. Means and ranges of 17-hydroxyprogesterone (17-OHP) after overnight dexamethasone suppression and 1 hour after ACTH injection in normal women, hirsute women, and one woman with suspected CAH who was tested on two occasions.

their families have been subjected to HLA genotyping.[87] The results failed to show a consistent HLA pattern in affected and unaffected siblings and their parents. These findings suggested that a close genetic linkage between HLA and a postulated gene carrying PCO could be excluded for either a simple dominant or recessive mode of inheritance of an HLA-linked gene. Whether PCO truly exists as an inherited disorder remains to be established. An HLA-linkage has not been found for 11β-hydroxylase and 3β-hydroxysteroid dehydrogenase deficiencies, both of which can simulate the features of PCO.[88]

The influence of ovarian steroids on adrenal androgen production has been considered previously, but clarification of this relationship, particularly in PCO, has not been definitely established. Studies performed in postmenopausal women indicated that administration of conjugated estrogens resulted in a significant increase of adrenal androgens, DHEA, and DHEA-sulfate.[89] A decrease of these androgens (but not cortisol) has been reported in premenopausal women following surgical castration, suggesting a specific effect of the ovary on adrenal androgen production.[90] *In vitro,* estrogen has been shown to non-competitively inhibit 3β-hydroxysteroid dehydrogenase, which may explain the results of the above clinical studies.[91] However, in a study of premenopausal women who had undergone previous ovariectomy, alterations in adrenal androgen levels in response to high dose estrogen could not be detected.[92]

Chronic Estrogen Secretion

In PCO estrogen secretion is primarily a direct result of excess androgen production. The ovarian androgens, androstenedione and testosterone, undergo aromatization

in extraglandular tissues to produce estrone and estradiol, respectively. Since androstenedione is the predominant androgen in PCO, the formation of estrone usually exceeds that of estradiol. Measurement of circulating estrogens reveals that estrone concentrations are equivalent to the highest levels observed in normal ovulatory women whereas estradiol levels are similar to the lowest levels.[4] So there is a reversal of the normal serum estrone to estradiol ratio in PCO.

The major extraglandular tissues which participate in the peripheral conversion of androgens to estrogens are the skin, muscle, brain, and fat. Interestingly, only 14% of aromatase enzyme is found within adipocytes whereas the remaining 86% is located in the stromal and vascular tissues.[93] Moreover, the percent conversion of androstenedione to estrone is not influenced by weight loss. These results are particularly relevant to PCO because some patients are not obese and yet manifest the typical hormonal profile similar to that seen in obese patients. Thus a biochemical basis exists for the occurrence of PCO in non-obese women.

Direct glandular secretion of estrogen by the polycystic ovary appears to be negligible, although a thorough study of this subject has not been done. In early studies, when androstenedione was utilized as precursor substrate, minimal estrogen was derived from the *in vitro* incubation of polycystic ovarian tissue, whereas normal ovaries produced substantial amounts of estrogen.[31,32] This led investigators to speculate that aromatase enzyme activity within the polycystic ovary was deficient or absent. Subsequently it was shown that in these patients the capacity for aromatization was maintained by the ovary and that the apparent enzyme defect was secondary.[94] It was shown that using granulosa cells from follicles obtained from normal and polycystic ovaries, estrogen production was minimal in PCO tissues compared to the large amounts produced by normal ovaries despite increasing concentrations of androstenedione substrate. With the

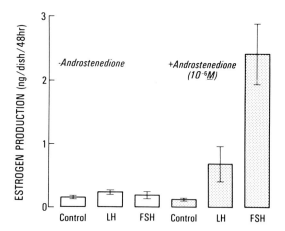

Figure 10–12. Effects of gonadotropins on estrogen production by cultured granulosa cells isolated from 4- to 6-mm follicles of a patient with PCO. Granulosa cells (2×10^5 viable cells/dish) were cultured for 2 days in 2 ml culture medium containing one or a combination of the following hormones: human LH (100 ng/ml), human FSH (100 ng/ml), and 10^{-7} M androstenedione. Data points indicate the mean ± SE of four separate culture dishes.

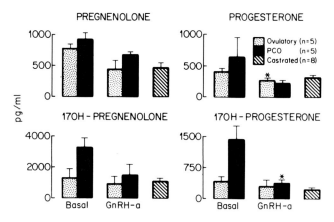

PREGNENOLONE   PROGESTERONE

170H - PREGNENOLONE   170H - PROGESTERONE

Figure 10–13. Mean ± SE levels of serum progestins in normal ovulatory women with endometriosis and PCO patients before and after GnRH-a as compared to values observed in castrate women. The asterisk denotes a statistically significant (p < 0.05) change from baseline values in each group of subjects.

addition of LH, a small increment of estrogen production was noted. With the addition of FSH, a huge increase of estrogen occurred (Figure 10–12). Since FSH secretion is known to stimulate aromatase and is decreased in PCO, a lack of ovarian estrogen production in this syndrome appears to be principally due to diminished FSH secretion.

The clinical impact of chronic estrogen secretion is magnified by the anovulatory status of these patients since serum progesterone levels are low. In the absence of progesterone, the chronic secretion of estrogen is unopposed and susceptible target tissues, i.e., endometrium, are subject to hyperstimulation. This is particularly true considering that obesity and hyperandrogenism are known to lower sex-hormone binding globulin, which increases the circulating levels of free estradiol. These patients are thus more disposed to develop endometrial hyperplasia and adenocarcinoma.

Progestin Secretion

It has been previously noted that serum 17-hydroxyprogesterone concentrations are significantly increased in PCO compared to those of normal women. The unique suppressive properties of GnRH-a have provided a method to determine whether this hormone is derived from the ovary or adrenal gland. In response to GnRH-a, elevated 17-hydroxyprogesterone levels fell 73% from baseline compared to a decrement of 26% and 56% for pregnenolone and 17-hydroxypregnenolone, respectively (Figure 10–13).[95] These results were supported by lack of the 17-hydroxyprogesterone response to dexamethasone suppression compared to the other progestins. Collectively the data indicated that in PCO 17-hydroxyprogesterone is principally derived from the ovary, whereas pregnenolone and 17-hydroxypregnenolone are of mixed ovarian and adrenal origin.

Inappropriate Gonadotropin Release

In PCO pituitary gonadotropin secretion is characterized by increased LH secretion and decreased FSH release.[96] In approximately two-thirds of patients, serum LH concentrations are increased, while the remaining one-third is normal compared to ovulatory women studied during the early follicular phase of their menstrual cycles. That all PCO patients do not exhibit increased circulating concentrations of LH may be attributed to sporadic and spontaneous follicular activity which results in an increase of ovarian estrogen in amounts sufficient to exert a negative feedback effect on LH (Figure 10–14).[97] Further studies of LH secretion in PCO have revealed that the magnitude and, commonly, the frequency of LH pulsations are also increased.[98] Similarly LH responses to GnRH are greater than those of normal women during the early follicular phase. In contrast to LH, serum FSH release is marked by lower mean levels, attenuated pulsatile activity, and

Figure 10–14. Long-term daily fluctuations of LH, FSH, estrone (E₁), estradiol (E₂) and progesterone (shaded areas) in a patient with PCO studied for three consecutive months. Presumptive ovulation apparently occurred twice during the sampling period on the basis of LH surges and increased progesterone levels. Such increases in LH need not be indicative of ovulation in patients with PCO. (Reproduced with permission from Yen, as published in Rebar.[97])

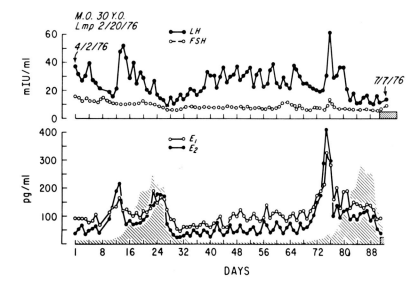

blunted or normal responses to GnRH. Thus, the ratio of LH to FSH, which normally approaches unity, is usually increased in this disorder.

The mechanism for this inappropriate release of gonadotropins has not been totally clarified. It has been well established that there is increased sensitivity of pituitary LH to exogenously administered GnRH. Previous studies conducted in normal women have demonstrated that the LH response to GnRH may be augmented by estradiol depending on the dose and duration of exposure.[99,100] These findings led to the concept that chronic, unopposed estrogen secretion in PCO could amplify GnRH-stimulated LH release. Support for this concept is provided by the LH response to GnRH, which is significantly increased compared to that of normal women in spite of equivalent estradiol levels (Figure 10–15). Increased pituitary sensitivity to GnRH may also be engendered by GnRH itself. The ability of GnRH to "prime" the pituitary and result in enhanced responses to subsequent GnRH administration has been demonstrated previously in both animals and human subjects (Figure 10–16).[101] The apparent requirements of this self-priming effect are those of increased GnRH pulse frequency and magnitude. If this is the case, then increased GnRH activity in PCO as reflected by increased LH secretion could be responsible for increased pituitary sensitivity. In animals LH pulses have been correlated to pulses of GnRH as measured in portal blood vessels.[102]

It has been proposed that increased GnRH neuronal activity may be due to a reduction of the inhibitory effect

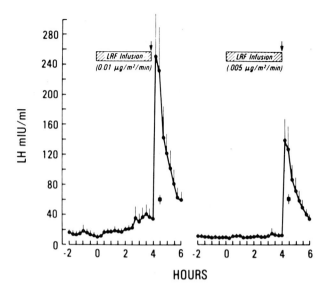

Figure 10–16. The patterns of serum LH responses (mean ± SE) to LRF infusions (0.01 and 0.005 μg/m² · min) followed immediately by a pulse of LRF (10 μg) during the midluteal phase. The peak mean (± SE) LH level (solid square) in response to a pulse of LRF (10 μg) in noninfused controls in the midluteal phase is shown for comparison (with permission from Lasley[100]).

of hypothalamic dopamine.[103] This possibility is supported by the observation that elevated LH levels in PCO were substantially lowered by the intravenous administration of dopamine (Figure 10–17). Conversely, treatment with a dopamine antagonist, metoclopromide, failed to alter serum LH in these patients.[104] Opioid peptides also have been implicated as inhibitors of GnRH secretion in humans. That a lack of an opioid influence on GnRH exists in PCO does not appear plausible since administration of beta-endorphin failed to suppress LH concentrations.[104] In this study serum prolactin levels increased, which prompted the investigators to suggest that

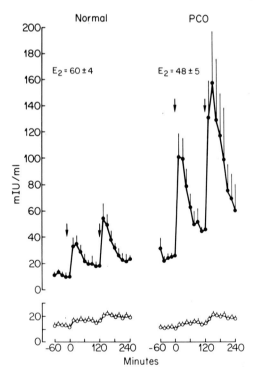

Figure 10–15. Responses of LH (solid circles) and FSH (open circles) to two consecutive bolus injections of GnRH, 10 μg iv (arrows) in normal ovulatory women during the early follicular phase of the menstrual cycle and in patients with PCO. Note equivalent levels of estradiol (E₂).

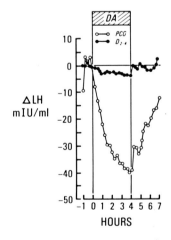

Figure 10–17. Mean net (Δ) decrement in serum LH levels before, during, and after dopamine (DA) infusion (4 μg/kg/min) for 4 hours in eight patients with PCO (open circles) and six normal women studied on day 2-4 of the menstrual cycle (solid circles) (with permission from Quigley[102]).

a complete uncoupling of normal opioid inhibitory influences in GnRH neurons may be operative in PCO. Furthermore, patients given an intravenous infusion of naloxone, an opioid antagonist, failed to show any change in serum LH.[104]

The suppression of FSH release in this syndrome has been largely attributed to the negative feedback effects of acyclic estrogen secretion. The negative feedback mechanism in PCO has been shown to be intact as judged by gonadotropin responses during administration of estradiol.[98] In addition, patients treated with the predominant estrogen of PCO, estrone, as the benzoate conjugate, displayed a reduction of FSH without alteration of LH thereby enhancing the disparity in gonadotropin secretion (Figure 10–18).[105] This finding is consistent with the hypothesis that diminished FSH release resulting from the extraglandular aromatization of androgens could lead to the anovulation commonly encountered in this disorder.

Another consideration in the mechanism of FSH suppression is that of ovarian proteins, a variety of which are present in follicular fluid and appear to participate in the regulation of ovarian activity. Of particular note is the protein, inhibin, which has been shown to suppress selectively FSH secretion.[106] Recent studies have indicated that inhibin levels in the follicular fluid of polycystic ovaries are significantly higher than the levels found in the follicular fluid of normal women during all stages of the ovarian cycle.[107] However, the significance of this difference was reduced when comparisons were made between inhibin levels in follicular fluid of PCO ovaries and normal women in the late follicular phase of the cycle, that portion of the cycle which is most similar to that of PCO. It is hoped that future studies will clarify the role of inhibin and that of other ovarian proteins in the regulation of FSH and the pathogenesis of PCO.

Thus, the interactions of hypothalamus, pituitary, and ovary in PCO combined to provide a convenient hypothesis of altered physiology (Figure 10–19). Elevated LH levels stimulate the ovary to synthesize and release excess quantities of androgens, in particular, androstenedione and testosterone. Through peripheral conversion mechanisms the ovarian androgens are metabolized to estrogens, particularly, androstenedione to estrone. These chronically elevated levels of estrogen, particularly, estrone and free estradiol, enhance the sensitivity of the pituitary to gonadotropin-releasing hormone stimulation in regard to LH release. This results in increased pulsatile release of LH and contributes to elevated LH levels. At the same time the chronically elevated levels of estrogen suppress FSH release resulting in inadequate folliculogenesis and anovulation.

Insulin Resistance

An association between abnormal androgen secretion and increased insulin secretion or insulin resistance has been established in several published studies.[108–111] Patients with PCO constitute a large portion of these study subjects, all of whom were obese or exhibited dermatologic features of acanthosis nigricans.[13,112,113] Both conditions are known to predispose to the development of insulin resistance in the absence of hyperandrogenism. Recently, it has been shown that nonobese PCO patients without evidence of acanthosis nigricans also exhibit insulin resistance.[114] Basal insulin levels and insulin responses to oral glucose administration were increased, compared to those of height- and weight-matched controls (Figure 10–20). In addition a positive linear rela-

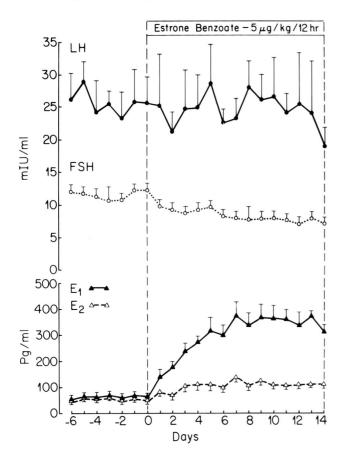

Figure 10–18. Mean (± SE) daily concentrations of LH, FSH, E₁, and E₂ in PCO subjects before and during estrone benzoate administration.

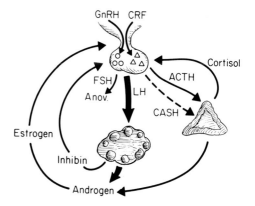

Figure 10–19. Proposed hypothesis of altered physiology in PCO. CRF, Corticotropin releasing factor. CASH, cortical adrenal stimulating hormone.

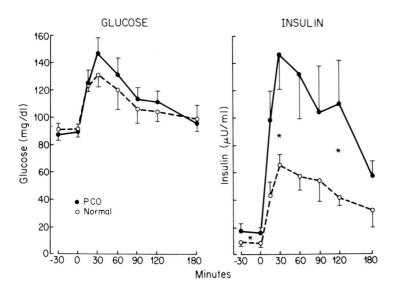

Figure 10–20. Circulating levels of glucose and insulin in PCO patients and normal control subjects in response to oral glucose administration.

tionship was found between insulin and both androstenedione and testosterone (Figures 10–21, 10–22). More extensive investigation into this relationship has demonstrated *in vivo* evidence of decreased insulin sensitivity and increased insulin secretion.[115] The insulin resistance of PCO does not appear to be limited to glucose metabolism. *In vitro* assessment of the anabolic property of insulin has revealed that in PCO certain cells known to respond to insulin fail to grow and propagate in the presence of insulin. Finally, receptor studies in the nonobese PCO have been normal with regard to number and binding. These data suggest that insulin resistance in PCO is a postreceptor phenomenon, or at least a defect beyond that of insulin binding.

The clinical significance of hyperinsulinemia and hyperandrogenism has not yet been established. The suggestion that androgen excess induces insulin resistance suffers from several inconsistencies. First, hyperinsulinemia has only been documented in humans following administration of synthetic anabolic steroids, but not native testosterone.[116,117] Second, the effect of anabolic steroids may be indirect due to the increased weight associated with their use.[118] Third, testosterone levels in PCO do not exceed those of normal men who have no evidence of

insulin resistance. Fourth, it has recently been shown that women with hyperthecosis treated by bilateral oophorectomy failed to exhibit changes in their insulin secretion despite marked reduction of ovarian androgens.[119] Fifth, preliminary data from our laboratory indicate that in nonobese PCO administration of GnRH-a for six months resulted in complete suppression of ovarian androgen production and a persistence of insulin resistance. Conversely, there are suggestions that hyperinsulinemia may play a role in the pathogenesis of PCO. First, *in vitro* studies using anterior pituitary cell cultures show that insulin enhances the gonadotropin response to GnRH.[120] Second, gonadal tissues of both sexes are sensitive to insulin as reflected in an increase of steroidogenesis. For instance, insulin augments the synthesis and release of progesterone in cultured swine granulosa cells.[121] In hyperandrogenized women, it has been reported that insulin stimulated the *in vitro* accumulation of androstenedione and testosterone from both thecal and stromal tissues.[122] Moreover, insulin receptors have been identified in ovarian tissue of normal women and in patients with PCO.[123,124] To relate these findings to PCO it has been proposed that in the presence of insulin resistance, gonadal tissues selectively retain their sensitivity to insu-

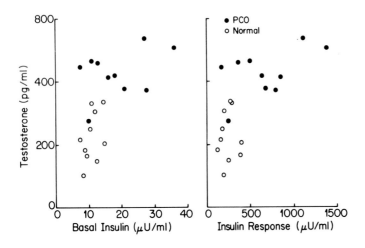

Figure 10–21. Correlation of serum testosterone with basal insulin levels and sums of insulin concentrations during oral glucose administration.

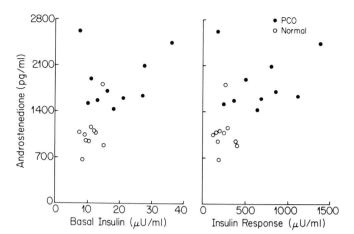

Figure 10–22. Correlation of serum androstenedione with basal insulin levels and sums of insulin concentrations during oral glucose administration.

lin action.[125] Alternatively, excess ovarian androgen production in PCO may be an indirect result of insulin binding to structurally related peptides such as insulin-like growth factors, nerve growth factor, relaxin, and multiplication stimulating activity. Obviously, more work is required to delineate the role of insulin in PCO.

PATHOLOGY OF THE POLYCYSTIC OVARY

The gross pathology of the polycystic ovary is manifested by bilateral enlargement, a thickened sclerotic capsule, and multiple subcapsular cysts (Figures 10–23, 10–24). It should be pointed out that not all these features are necessary for the diagnosis of PCO. In fact, uncommonly, the ovaries may be normal-sized or enlargement may occur unilaterally.[126]

The clinical significance of the sclerotic coat of the ovary has not been established (Figure 10–25). A mean capsular thickness was reported to be 0.2-0.4 mm in 65% of patients undergoing wedge resection.[127] Immediately below the epithelial layer, there are thickened collagen

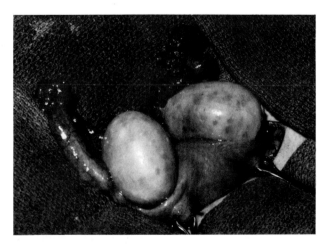

Figure 10–23. Bilaterally enlarged cystic ovaries from a patient with PCO.

fibers which extend into and merge with the cellular outer cortical stroma. It is within this collagenous stroma that many primordial follicles appear shrunken and atretic. Clearly there is no credence to the theory that the capsule acts as a mechanical obstruction to ovulation since successful induction of ovulation can be achieved with medical treatment including the administration of clomiphene citrate and human chorionic gonadotropin.[128] It has also been shown that in PCO patients unilateral ovarian wedge resection resulted in cyclic ovulation from the contralateral ovary.[129] No correlation has been found between the thickness of the capsule and the morphology of ovarian structures. More important, thickness may vary considerably between ovaries as well as within an individual ovary from the same patient.[130] In fact, the sclerotic changes may merely reflect the disease process rather than contribute to it, since testosterone administration to animals results in a thickened ovarian capsule.[131] On the other hand, it has been suggested that the thickening process occurs in response to chronic ovarian distention.[132]

Formation of multiple follicle cysts within the cortex of the polycystic ovary is characteristic of this disorder. The primordial follicles are located in the outer cortex and appear degenerative, particularly when this region is dense with collagen fibers. Primary and secondary follicles are found deeper in the cortex and are increased in number (Figure 10–24). Commonly, follicle growth is arrested in the mid-antral stage of development or the follicles are atretic. Nevertheless, there may, infrequently, be normal maturation followed by ovulation and corpus luteum development as indicated by spontaneous menstruation and the occasional pregnancy in these patients. The precise mechanism which leads to cyst formation and follicular arrest remains unknown. Whether the process is related to steroid or protein hormone concentrations within the cyst fluid is not clear. As previously described, in the antral fluid of normal follicles greater than 8 mm there is a predominance of estrogen compared to androgen,[133] but in non-healthy, degenerative follicles the ratio decreases and favors the presence of androgen.[134] There is little if any evidence of estradiol formation in the follicular fluid of polycystic ovaries.[135] This fact, combined with the enormous amount of intraovar-

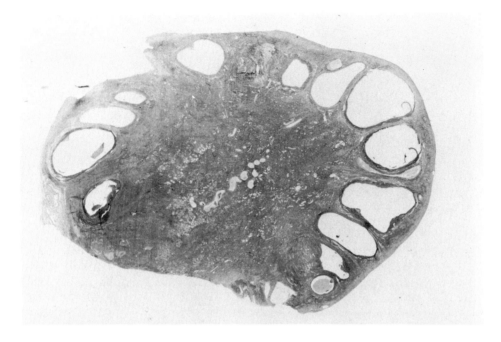

Figure 10–24. Histologic appearance of a polycystic ovary. Note the thickened capsule and multiple subcapsular cysts. H & E (× 4.32).

ian androgen, may account in part for poor follicular development. Another consideration is the presence of an aromatase inhibitor such as dihydrotestosterone. Nonetheless, measurement of this hormone in the follicular fluid of polycystic ovaries reveals significantly lower concentrations than those found in the fluid of normal follicles and physiologic amounts of DHT fail to inhibit aromatization of androstenedione.[134,136]

Lining the antrum of the cystic follicle are the granulosa cells, which differ from those of normal antral follicles in that there are fewer layers. In addition, there is decreased mitotic activity in these cells compared to that in normal follicles. The diminished population of granulosa cells results in a corresponding reduction of FSH receptors which are found exclusively on the membranes

of these cells. A plausible explanation for decreased numbers of granulosa cells is provided by the lack of FSH stimulation and consequent absence of aromatase enzyme activity. As a result intraovarian androgens are incapable of conversion to estrogens and the granulosa cells are deprived of an essential mitogenic factor. Examination of granulosa cells by electron microscopy indicates that the cytoplasm is filled with rough-surfaced endoplasmic reticulum, large numbers of polyribosomes, a well-developed Golgi apparatus, and mitochondria with lamellar cristae (Figure 10–26).[137] These findings are consistent with active protein production rather than steroidogenesis by the granulosa cell. The potential clinical significance is apparent when one considers follicular fluid proteins, one of which is inhibin, a specific inhibitor

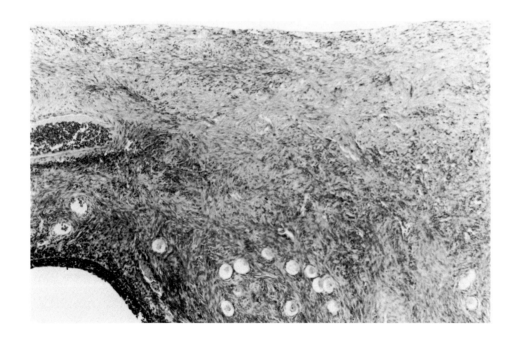

Figure 10–25. Microscopic appearance of the thickened sclerotic coat of the polycystic ovary. The fibrous capsule consists of densely packed collagen fibers which merge into the outer cortical stroma. Note the primordial follicles, many of which will become degenerative and atretic. H & E (× 75).

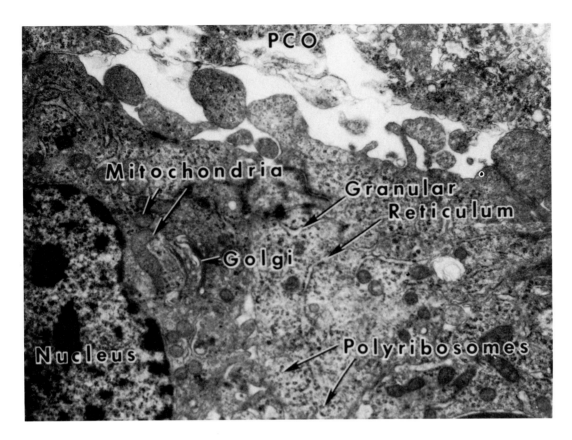

Figure 10–26. Electron micrograph of a portion of human granulosa cell in a 6-mm PCO follicle. There is considerable heterochromatin associated with the inner nuclear membrane, a well-developed Golgi apparatus, large numbers of free polyribosomes scattered throughout the cytoplasm, abundant granular endoplasmic reticulum, little or no smooth endoplasmic reticulum and lamellar cristae in the mitochondria. (With permission, from Erickson.[136])

of FSH release. Whether the granulosa cell production of inhibin is sufficient to make an impact on pituitary FSH release and interfere with follicle development remains to be clarified. Clinically, the reduction of granulosa cell number may account for the poor ovarian response to gonadotropin stimulation in PCO. Standard doses of clomiphene citrate administered to normal subjects and PCO patients resulted in comparable elevations of serum LH and FSH but much greater increases of estradiol in the normal group.[98] Administration of similar doses of human menopausal gonadotropins to normal and PCO women produced equivalent elevations of circulating gonadotropins, but significantly increased serum estradiol responses were observed in normal women (Figure 10–27).[138]

Surrounding the granulosa cells and separated from them by a basal lamina are cells of the theca interna. In PCO the dominant elements of the follicular unit are the theca cells, which are dense, multilayered, and always thicker than the corresponding granulosa cell layer (Figure 10–28).[139] It has been noted that the theca interna may not always be thickened, but the relative proportion of the granulosa cell layer is uniformly maintained.[139] Luteinization is also evident in theca cells of most PCO patients, which is a reflection of constant LH stimulation.

It has been reported that the degree of theca luteinization in PCO is not different from that observed in ovaries of normal women;[140] however, since there are many more follicles in the polycystic ovary, there is an absolute increase in this process. Electron microscopic analysis of theca cells demonstrates abundant smooth-surfaced endoplasmic reticulum, numerous lipid droplets, and mitochondria with tubular cristae.[137] These cytoplasmic features are typical of the steroid-producing cell. The steroidogenic potential of these cells is governed by the high intracellular concentrations of 17α-hydroxylase and C_{17-20} lyase, which are stimulated by LH.[137] The presence of these enzymes allows for the metabolism of progesterone to androgens, in particular androstenedione, which is the major ovarian androgen in PCO. This fact is supported by the predominant production of androstenedione during incubation of thecal tissue from polycystic ovaries in the presence or absence of LH.[137,141] These studies also showed that in PCO androstenedione production is considerably greater than that by an equivalent number of normal thecal cells, whether occurring spontaneously or LH-induced. The increased sensitivity of the theca cell is undoubtedly a result of increased LH secretion inherent in this syndrome. Thus, the role of the theca cell in PCO is characterized by 1. hyperplasia, 2. lutein-

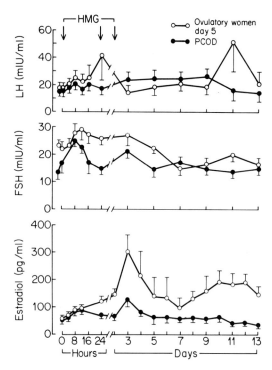

Figure 10–27. Mean (± SE) serum LH, FSH, and estradiol levels in response to administration of human menopausal gonadotropin (HMG), 150 IU/day for three consecutive days to PCO and ovulatory women commencing on day 5 of the menstrual cycle.

ization, 3. increased 17α-hydroxylase and C_{17-20} lyase concentrations, and 4. androstenedione production, all of which are stimulated by LH. These actions of LH are mediated by specific membrane receptors located on theca cells.

A relationship between increased thecal production of androgens and arrested follicular maturation has been proposed previously as an alternative or associative factor to decreased FSH stimulation. Studies performed in animals indicate that, within the ovary, disruption of follicular activity may result from local production of excess androgen. In hypophysectomized immature female rats the ovarian weight response to diethylstilbestrol is inhibited by human chorionic gonadotropin.[142] This effect is reversed by administration of anti-androgens. In another study employing the same rat model, dihydrotestosterone or HCG treatment accelerated granulosa cell death and follicular attrition in medium-sized follicles.[143] These findings suggest that follicular atresia may be induced by intraovarian androgens. In humans, hyperandrogenic ovaries are often associated with multiple follicular cysts, most of which are degenerative and devoid of healthy looking oocytes.[134] Thus, the chronic anovulation of PCO may reflect a direct inhibitory action of excess ovarian androgen on follicular maturation as well as a lack of pituitary FSH stimulation.

CLINICAL FEATURES

The foregoing material indicates that in PCO the ovary is ultimately responsible for anovulation and excess androgen production. These fundamental alterations lead to several clinical features of the disorder. Perhaps the most significant of these is the effect of chronic unopposed estrogen secretion on the endometrium. Previous reports have established an association between PCO and endometrial hyperplasia and adenocarcinoma.[7,8,144] In most instances of adenocarcinoma the lesion is well-differentiated, although in some patients the histologic dis-

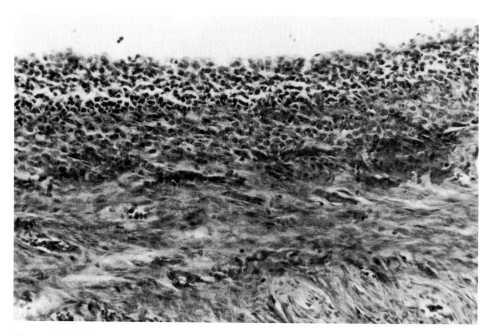

Figure 10–28. Granulosa and theca cells in a follicle from a polycystic ovary. Note the greater thickness of the theca cell layer compared to the granulosa cell layer. H & E (×290).

tinction between atypical adenomatous hyperplasia (Figure 10–29 and adenocarcinoma has not been clear.[7,145] A progression of endometrial hyperplasia to carcinoma was suggested by a 14-year follow-up study of 97 young women, 14% of whom developed endometrial cancer.[146] In 25% of these patients a diagnosis of PCO had been made. In chronic anovulatory women, the relative risk of developing endometrial carcinoma has been reported as 3.1.[8] Interestingly enough, poorly differentiated or metastatic cancer is found infrequently and most patients responded successfully to surgical management. The less aggressive nature of these cancers appears to be related to the presence of endogenous and unopposed estrogen secretion in young women since older women with typical disease seem to be at greater risk for poor outcome.

The microscopic appearance of endometrial carcinoma in women with PCO does not appear to differ from that of older women. In most instances the lesion is well-differentiated and, occasionally, distinction from endometrial hyperplasia may be difficult. The prognosis is usually good and rarely will there be metastatic spread.[7] Thus, histologic features do not account for the less morbid neoplastic behavior in PCO. The possibility that the course of the disease may be dictated by endogenous unopposed estrogen secretion has prompted the use of progestins as a therapeutic deterrent to carcinomatous change.[7,146] This approach has appeared to reduce the risk of progressive disease, although appropriate studies have not been performed.

A second aspect of estrogen secretion in PCO is irregular anovulatory bleeding. The likely explanation may relate to the degree of endometrial proliferation prior to sudden and sporadic decreases of estrogen. As a result the frequency and amount of vaginal bleeding is highly variable. In the absence of progesterone secretion, the usual premenstrual symptoms are lacking, which suggests anovulation.

The most prominent and cosmetically troublesome manifestation of androgen excess is the effect on the pilosebaceous unit: approximately 70% of patients exhibit hirsutism and a lesser percentage experience acne.[3] The primary affected areas are the facial and suprapubic regions of the body. Other common sites include the breasts and areola, chest, and perineum. The mechanism principally responsible for hair growth in PCO is overproduction of ovarian androgens. In this regard hirsutism correlates with the testosterone production rate.[147] Of the circulating hormones, free testosterone appears to have the best correlation.[148] While most increased hair growth can be attributed to ovarian androgen production, target organ responsiveness to androgen may be enhanced. Within the hair follicle, androstenedione and testosterone are metabolized to 5α-androstane-3α,17β-diol (3α-diol) via dihydrotestosterone. A majority of 3α-diol is conjugated in the skin to 3α-diol glucuronide (3α-diol G). Recent studies have suggested that 3α-diol G may be a useful marker of peripheral androgen action. In a study of hirsute and non-hirsute PCO patients, serum levels of androstenedione and testosterone were equivocal whereas 3α-diol G was markedly elevated in the hirsute group.[149] For unexplained reasons, this hormone does not distinguish between hirsute women with functional disorders and those with androgen-producing tumors.[150] The findings indicate that enhanced target organ responsiveness to androgen action may contribute significantly to excessive hair growth in PCO. Occasionally the impact of hyperandrogenism may be so great in the individual patient that virilizing signs are present. Fortunately, virilization is uncommon in this disorder.

Other clinical features of PCO include obesity, galac-

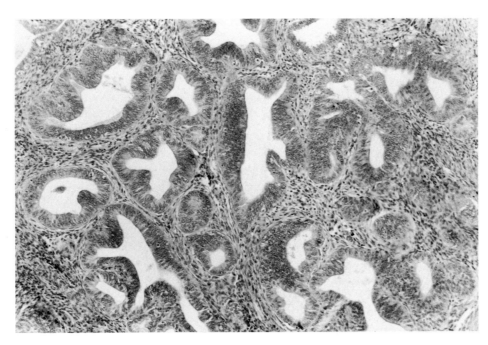

Figure 10–29. Microscopic appearance of endometrial adenomatous hyperplasia in a patient with PCO. H & E (×90).

torrhea, ovarian tumors, and acanthosis nigricans. Obesity is present in approximately one-half of all patients.[3] The nature of this weight gain has not been carefully studied but may relate to the anabolic property of androgens and possibly insulin. Galactorrhea should not be surprising, since 30% of PCO patients have hyperprolactinemia.[151,152] In addition, once the breasts have been previously exposed to excessive amounts of either endogenous or exogenous estrogen, the patient appears predisposed to galactorrhea. Ovarian tumors have been reported to occur with increased frequency, 5% to 17%, in PCO.[153–155] The most common neoplasm is a dermoid cyst, which is consistent with the age of the patient population. Recent studies suggest that acanthosis is a distinct but uncommon accompaniment of PCO in less than 5% of the cases.[156] A mechanism for this dermatologic lesion has not been established but may relate to severe hyperinsulinemia as found in the syndromes of insulin resistance.

HETEROGENEITY OF THE POLYCYSTIC OVARY

As previously mentioned, the syndrome of PCO is a symptom complex which is usually associated with bilat-

erally enlarged cystic ovaries. Over the years it has been recognized that the appearance of the ovaries in this disorder occasionally varies; they may be normal-sized or enlarged unilaterally. Paradoxically, polycystic ovaries may accompany a variety of functional disorders which are closely related to PCO or have a distinctly separate etiology.

Hyperthecosis was a term introduced in 1943 to describe theca cell hyperplasia of the ovarian stroma, which invariably was luteinized.[157] In 1949 the syndrome of hyperthecosis was established, relating the recognized pathological findings with clinical symptoms of hyperandrogenism.[158] The close similarity between hyperthecosis and PCO has led to the idea that the former represents merely an extension of the latter. Grossly, the ovaries may be normal-sized or enlarged. The texture is very firm and, upon sectioning, the cut surface is yellow and coarse. In general, multiple cyst formation is not found, although in individual cases the gross appearance may be indistinguishable from that of PCO. The major histologic feature of hyperthecosis is the densely packed ovarian stroma which often contains nests of large, clear luteinized cells (Figure 10–30). While stromal hyperthecosis is characteristic for this disorder, the follicles may also be surrounded by hyperplastic theca cells. Interestingly, the degree of hyperthecotic transformation in the ovary is not correlated to the severity of disease.[159] Rather, it is the

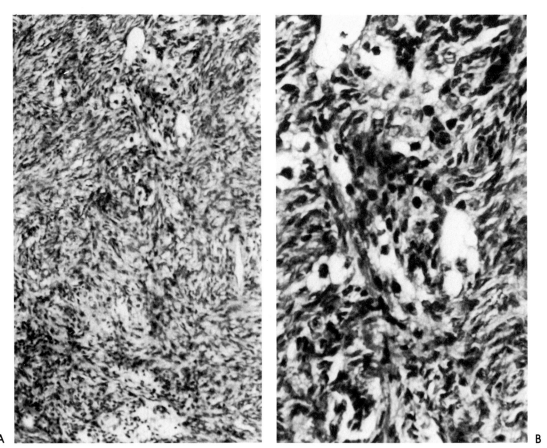

Figure 10–30. Histologic appearance of hyperthecosis. A. The ovarian stroma is dense and hyperplastic. H & E (×290). B. Within the stroma are nests of luteinized theca cells which characterize this condition. H & E (×510).

amount of androgen production which determines the clinical manifestations. In contrast to PCO, most patients have severe hirsutism, and a significant percent exhibit virilizing signs such as clitoromegaly, temporal balding, and deepening of the voice. Obesity is common and some patients will show evidence of acanthosis nigricans. Marked insulin resistance has also been reported. Menstrual irregularity is frequent, but normal menses do exist. Similar to PCO these patients have an increased incidence of endometrial cancer, presumably due to the amount of estrogen formed from the peripheral conversion of excess circulating androgens.[160]

In hyperthecosis circulating levels of ovarian androgens, androstenedione and testosterone, usually exceed those seen in PCO and not infrequently are in the range of values observed with functional neoplasms. In addition, metabolic clearance and production rates of androstenedione and testosterone are increased.[160] Selective venous catheterization studies have confirmed the ovarian origin of these androgens. This accounts for the normal serum DHEA-S concentrations seen in these patients.[161] Ovarian androgen production is in part a result of LH stimulation, although normal-to-low LH levels have generally been found in hyperthecosis.[159,161] Measurement of LH bioactivity has not been performed in this disorder and should be considered, since bioactive LH levels are definitely increased in PCO.[69] An alternative explanation to account for normal LH secretion has been increased ovarian responsiveness to LH stimulation. Further studies are necessary to elucidate the mechanism of this disease.

Functional disorders of the adrenal gland may also mimic the clinical features and in some instances the pathologic findings of PCO. Congenital adrenal hyperplasia (CAH) is a term used to describe an assortment of clinical entities which arise from inborn errors in steroid synthesis. Symptomatology associated with each entity is due to steroid overproduction or underproduction or both, secondary to an enzyme deficiency.

Within the adrenal gland normal steroidogenesis involves a series of enzymatic reactions which begin with the metabolism of cholesterol and result in the production of glucocorticoids, mineralocorticoids, and adrenal androgens. The multiple presentations of CAH relate to the abnormal secretion of particular steroids, or their precursors, as a result of a specific enzyme defect. The enzyme defects which bear resemblance to PCO are those of 21-hydroxylase, 11β-hydroxylase, and 3β-hydroxysteroid dehydrogenase. By far the most common of these is 21-hydroxylase deficiency. This inherited condition has an autosomal recessive mode of transmission and is linked genetically to the HLA system.[162]

In 80% of cases the defect is partial whereas the remainder exhibit complete absence of 21-hydroxylase. The complete form of the disease is commonly found in the newborn with ambiguous genitalia (virilization in females), salt-wasting, and peripheral vascular collapse. If not diagnosed immediately the condition may be fatal. The incomplete form has variable clinical expression in that the enzyme block may be extremely subtle and only 50% will manifest life-threatening situations. This fact and the recognition that androgen production by the zona reticularis is physiologically stimulated in early puberty may account for the emergence of late-onset or acquired 21-hydroxylase deficiency after puberty.

These patients can exhibit increases of serum androstenedione, testosterone, and DHEA-S, much like those associated with PCO.[73] In addition, the LH to FSH ratio may be increased. Accordingly, most patients are hirsute and many have evidence of virilization, and menstrual function is frequently normal. Despite hyperandrogenism in this disorder, the biochemical hallmark is increased secretion of 17-hydroxyprogesterone, an immediate substrate for 21-hydroxylation. In PCO, serum 17-hydroxyprogesterone concentrations are also elevated and derived from an ovarian source.[95] The two conditions are distinguished by administering the ACTH stimulation test. In 21-hydroxylase deficiency there is an obvious exaggerated 17-hydroxyprogesterone response to ACTH which is significantly greater than that found in PCO patients (Figure 10–11).[163] Morphologically the ovaries have been reported to appear similar to PCO. Examination of ovaries during subtotal adrenalectomies for adrenogenital syndrome revealed enlargement and diffuse thickening of the capsule.[164] Recently, polycystic ovaries were noted in patients with late-onset 21-hydroxylase deficiency,[165] but other investigators have been unable to demonstrate typical polycystic ovaries in these patients.[166,167]

Clinical, hormonal, and morphologic changes consistent with PCO have also been described for deficiencies of 11β-hydroxylase and 3β-hydroxysteroid dehydrogenase.[168,169] Both disorders are rare and not linked to HLA genotyping. Hirsutism and virilization are usually present, their extent depending upon the degree of excess androgen production. Inherent in a deficiency of 11β-hydroxylase are increases of desoxycorticosterone which lead to salt retention and hypertension. The marker hormone for this enzyme block is increased desoxycortisol or compound S. It has been pointed out, however, that hyperandrogenism may induce a relative deficiency of 11β-hydroxylase, thereby raising the issue of whether the mechanism of altered steroidogenesis occurs primarily or secondarily in hirsute women.[170] In a defect of 3β-hydroxysteroid dehydrogenase, there is accumulation of Δ^5 steroids over their paired Δ^4 steroid metabolites. As a result serum DHEA-S and androstenediol levels are markedly elevated and responsible for hyperandrogenic signs. It has been proposed that 3β-hydroxysteroid dehydrogenase deficiency may arise from a mechanism comparable to the inhibitory effect of androgen on 11β-hydroxylase. However, it has been observed that in these patients estrogen levels do not exceed physiologic concentrations, and potent androgens such as androstenedione and testosterone are not elevated but, rather, quite low.[92,171] The functional relationship of polycystic ovaries to these enzyme defects which mimic POC is not clear and difficult to explain. In one respect the morphologic appearance may be integrated with the pathophysiology of resultant androgen excess. On the other hand, it may be that the presence of polycystic ovaries is coincidental and separate, implying concomitant disease processes.

Cushing's disease refers to excessive pituitary ACTH production and results in clinical features of adrenal steroid overproduction, in particular hypercortisolism and hyperandrogenism; consequently, the preponderant findings are obesity, hirsutism, acne, and menstrual irregularity. These suggest the diagnosis of PCO. But additional evidence of moon-like facies, buffalo hump, hypertension, muscle wasting, abdominal striae, and osteoporosis should indicate a primary problem of cortisol excess. While circulating androgen levels are elevated, there is also abnormal cortisol secretion characterized by increased basal levels, loss of circadian rhythmicity, and failure of suppression in response to dexamethasone. In contrast to congenital adrenal hyperplasia, careful examination of the ovaries does not reveal changes typical of PCO in the vast majority of cases.[172]

ANDROGEN-PRODUCING TUMORS AND OTHER HYPERANDROGENIC DISORDERS

The most important clinical consideration in hyperandrogenic women is the possible existence of an androgen-producing neoplasm. As a group, functional ovarian tumors comprise about 5%-10% of all ovarian neoplasms.[173] Tumors in this category are referred to as sex cord-stromal tumors.[174] The malignant potential of these lesions is significant since they make up 10% of all solid ovarian cancers. Androgen-producing tumors are usually distinguished from functional disorders by the rapid onset of symptoms, in particular hirsutism. In addition, virilizing signs such as clitoromegaly, temporal balding, deepending of the voice, and a male body habitus are commonly present. Despite the severity of androgenic manifestations, the early stages of development of these tumors can mimic PCO or other functional hyperandrogenic syndromes.

Granulosa-theca Cell Tumors

These tumors are typically associated with excess estrogen secretion whether the predominant cell type is granulosa or theca;[175,176] consequently, the most common symptom is irregular bleeding, with hirsutism uncommon, and virilization rare. However, it has also been established that primary excess androgen production may be associated with all forms of these tumors, including pure granulosa or pure theca cell types.[177-180] In these patients the presenting symptoms may be hirsutism or virilization, with or without endometrial hyperplasia and irregular bleeding. The major androgen produced appears to be testosterone as determined from basal hormone concentrations, provocative stimulation and suppression tests, and in vitro hormone production by tumor tissue.[178-180] With the large amount of androgen available there is substantial peripheral conversion to estrogen. This accounts for the coexistence of both androgenizing and estrogenizing signs in some patients. The clinical presentation of granulosa-theca cell tumors includes a unilateral mass which is usually solid, but occasionally cystic. Since the lesions tend to grow insidiously, a mass may be palpated abdominally or on pelvic examination. Classification of graunlosa cell tumors has been based on microscopic appearance. Granulosa cells grow in a wide variety of patterns which are commonly admixed. Microfollicular, macrofollicular, trabecular, insular, and solid tubular arrangements are characteristic of the more highly differentiated tumors. The microfollicular pattern, which is the most distinctive, features multiple small cavities known as Call-Exner bodies (Figure 10–31). Occasionally the granulosa cells are divided into sheets giving the appearance of columns or trabeculae (Figure 10–32).

The risk of malignancy is greatest in lesions containing granulosa cells, while thecomas tend to follow a benign course. The granulosa cell tumor in general is of low-grade malignancy, reflected in its indolent growth and

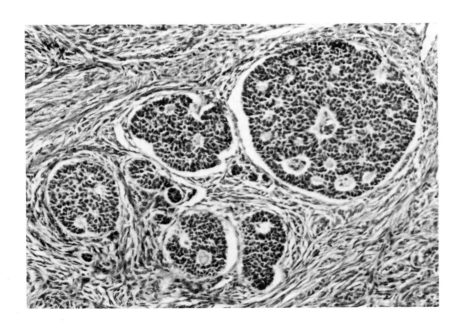

Figure 10–31. Microfollicular form of granulosa-theca cell tumor, with numerous Call-Exner bodies. H & E (×125).

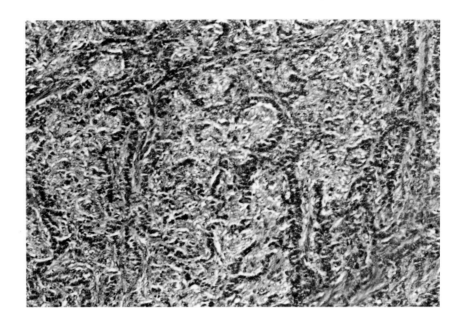

Figure 10–32. Trabecular form of granulosa-theca cell tumor. Large islands of granulosa cells interspersed among theca cells are often divided, giving the appearance of columns. H & E (×125).

infrequent recurrence. Treatment may vary, depending on the nature and extent of the tumor and the desires of the patient. In young women wishing to preserve childbearing, a unilateral oophorectomy is adequate. In postmenopausal women or those with lesions of stage II or more, a total abdominal hysterectomy and bilateral salpingo-oophorectomy is required.

Sertoli-Leydig Cell Tumors

Sertoli-Leydig cell tumors, also known as arrhenoblastomas or androblastomas are sex cord tumors which generally produce marked androgen excess. These neoplasms account for less than 0.5% of all ovarian tumors but are among the more fascinating from both clinical and pathologic viewpoints. Characteristically, they tend to occur in young women between 20 to 30 years of age.[181] In addition to virilization, menstrual abnormalities are frequently encountered. The size of these lesions may be substantial, and often they can be palpated during pelvic examination. Suspicion of an adnexal mass may be confirmed by ultrasonography. The tumor is usually solid, although cystic degeneration may occur. Microscopically, Sertoli-Leydig tumors have a wide range of appearances, depending on the degree of differentiation and whether Sertoli or Leydig cells predominate. In the highly differentiated form, the resemblance to seminiferous tubules is striking, whereas Leydig cells are not prominent. In these patients virilizing signs are not common. In the intermediate form attempts at tubule formation are recognizable but incomplete. Occasionally, there are cords of cells with nuclei arranged perpendicularly to the long axis of the cords. Leydig cells may be found in focal nests or islands, and stain positive for lipid. With the increasing presence of these cells, signs of hyperandrogenism become more evident. An undifferentiated tumor may appear almost sarcomatoid. However, incomplete tubule formation, cord-like structures, and lipid-containing cellular elements can be identified. The abundance of lipid-containing cells relates to the virilizing nature of this undifferentiated form. Reinke crystals are frequently found. Functionally the major androgen produced is testosterone, although *in vitro* studies have demonstrated androstenedione formation from tissue incubated with pregnenolone and progesterone.[182] In tumors composed only of Sertoli cells there may be demonstrable estrogen production.[173] Typically these patients are at risk for endometrial carcinoma because of peripheral conversion of androgens to estrogens. Since the tumor is unilateral in 90% of cases, and the malignant potential is low, conservative surgical management may be instituted. If a cancer is discovered, the prognosis correlates poorly with the histologic pattern. The five-year recurrence rate is estimated to be about 22% to 33%.[183] The survival rate is generally favorable in the better-differentiated tumors which are limited to one ovary.[184]

Lipid Cell Tumors

This category includes hilus cell tumors, lipoid cell tumors, and adrenal rest tumors. On cut section the tissue is usually yellow or tan in color. Microscopically the cells are large and contain clear cytoplasm, giving them a foamy appearance. These tumors receive their name from the lipid-staining property of the cellular elements. Lipid tumor cells are responsible for high amounts of androgen production, namely testosterone and androstenedione. Clinically, the patients exhibit the rapid onset of severe hirsutism and virilization. Amenorrhea is common. Uterine enlargement and endometrial hyperplasia may result from increased estrogen secretion due to peripheral aromatization of excess androgen. Distinction of specific tumor cell type from physical signs and clinical symptoms is generally impossible. Hilus cell tumors frequently arise within or near the hilum of the ovary. A primary histologic feature is the presence of Reinke crystals, which are found in about 50% of cases (Figure 10–33).[174,185] The principal hormone product of these tumors

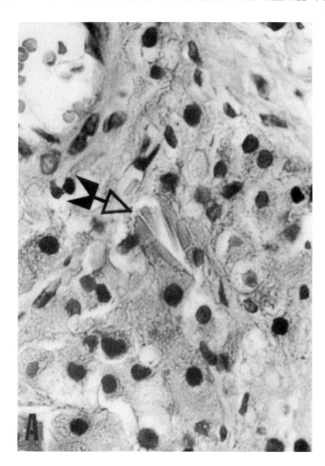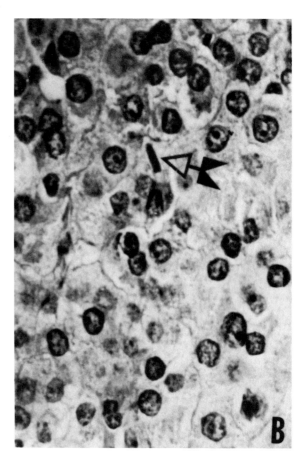

Figure 10–33. Microscopic sections of hilus cell tumors from two patients. Note that the cells contain abundant cytoplasm and lipid droplets. Reinke crystals are indicated by the arrows. A, ×625. B, ×800. (With permission, from Mandel.[185])

is testosterone.[186] Lipoid cell tumors may exhibit a clinical picture identical to that of hilus cell tumors. The lipid-producing cells of this tumor are indistinguishable from those of hilus cell tumors except that Reinke crystals are rarely found. The major androgen produced is androstenedione.[186] These neoplasms must be distinguished from adrenal rests. All lipid cell tumors retain the potential for cortisol production. Interestingly, Cushing's syndrome arising from these lesions is usually not associated with elevated serum cortisol levels, although the typical circadian pattern is lost.[187,188] Accordingly, the clinical manifestation of cortisol excess is mild. In general, lipid cell tumors are small at the time of discovery and often escape detection by pelvic examination. Ultrasound may be useful. The malignant potential of these lesions has been estimated at 20%.[183] Management of these neoplasms may be accomplished by unilateral oophorectomy. However, careful inspection of the lesion and abdomen is warranted to verify the extent of the disease.

Pregnancy-associated Hyperandrogenic Disorders

The luteoma of pregnancy is rare and suspected when signs of rapid androgenization occur in the gravid pa-

tient. The lesion is large, solid, and fleshy, with a yellowish color. The histologic pattern is one of scattered nodules of hyperplastic rather than neoplastic cells.[189] These cells appear large and polygonal with sparse stroma. Bilaterality is common. Approximately 10%-50% of patients have exhibited evidence of severe hyperandrogenism with clitoromegaly and frank virilization.[190] Correspondingly, more than 50% of female infants born during affected pregnancies have demonstrated some masculinization.[189] The maternal virilization is self-limited and regresses during the postpartum period along with a decrease in androgen production. These lesions are not related to excessive HCG levels and it has not been possible to induce their development experimentally by increasing gonadotropins.[192] While clearly functional in nature, the pathogenesis is not known.

In contrast to the luteoma of pregnancy, theca lutein cysts have a well-known association with conditions of increased HCG, including molar pregnancies and multiple gestations.[190] Patients with a prior history of oligoanovulation and cystic ovaries seem predisposed to develop theca lutein cysts. It may be that lutein cysts result from an increased intrinsic ability of the ovary for androgen production once stimulated by excessive gonadotropin. As implied in the name, the ovaries are grossly cystic. Microscopically, they show evidence of thickening and luteinization of the theca interna of large follicular cysts. There is abundant reticulum with argyrophilic fibers.[190] Approximately 25% of cases have evidence of maternal virilization. Interestingly, fetal masculinization is not seen.[191] In fact, studies seem to indicate that the placenta plays a protective role by aromatization of maternal androgens, exposing the fetus to increased estrogen rather than androgen.[191,192] The differences in fetal effects between theca lutein cysts and pregnancy luteomas cannot be explained by either the degree of hyperandrogenism or by timing during the pregnancy.[190] Again, as with the pregnancy luteoma, theca lutein cysts and their manifestations are self-limited and regress with the termination of pregnancy.

Reactive Stromal Luteinization

Occasionally, non-functional tumors of the ovary are associated with excess androgen or estrogen production by surrounding stroma which results in clinical masculinization or feminization.[173] The neoplasms may be primary, including Brenner tumors, dermoid cysts, cystadenomas, and cystadenocarcinomas, or they may be metastatic. The mechanism which stimulates luteinization of adjacent stroma is unclear. A mechanical induction of stromal steroidogenesis by the enlarging mass has been proposed but remains to be verified.[193,194] A few tumors may produce human chorionic gonadotropin, which could explain local stromal luteinization, but most cases in this group do not demonstrate measurable levels of chorionic gonadotropin.[195–198] In addition, reactive ovarian stroma is not seen when carcinoma has not spread to the ovary. The microscopic appearance of the stromal tissue reveals clusters of plump, spindle-shaped, or polygonal cells, which often stain for lipid. These cells are essentially indistinguishable from luteinized stroma associated with other non-neoplastic stromal proliferative conditions such as hyperthecosis and luteoma of pregnancy. In most instances signs of hyperandrogenism are encountered, although significant estrogen and progesterone effects may occur concomitantly or separately.[199–202] Removal of the ovarian lesions usually resolves the clinical features or hormone excess.

EVALUATION OF ANDROGEN EXCESS

The evaluation of hyperandrogenic disorders is focused primarily upon detection of an androgen-producing tumor. Both clinical history and physical examination provide valuable information regarding functional versus neoplastic diseases. The former are distinguished by slow and gradual progression of symptoms, whereas the latter are noted for their rapid onset. Usually a mild to moderate degree of hirsutism suggests a functional problem. For instance, the development of excess hair growth in women with PCO is commonly mild to moderate, but may be severe after many years of the disease. The hallmark of PCO is the irregular and infrequent menstrual bleeding pattern arising from chronic anovulation. In hyperthecosis symptoms of androgen excess are more severe because of the large amount of androgen produced. Virilization and amenorrhea are common. In contrast, patients suffering from congenital adrenal hyperplasia due to 21-hydroxylase deficiency tend to have regular menstrual cycles that accompany severe hirsutism and clitoromegaly. Cushing's syndrome may be suspected by symptoms arising from hypercortisolemia.

Fundamental screening laboratory tests are recommended to exclude a neoplasm and consist of measuring circulating total testosterone and DHEA-sulfate. A total testosterone level greater than 200 ng/dl as determined by radioimmunoassay with chromatographic separation suggests an androgen-producing tumor of either the ovary or adrenal gland.[203] DHEA-sulfate is a marker for adrenal androgen production, and a tumor is suspected when values exceed 8,000 ng/ml. Discriminatory tests for congenital adrenal hyperplasia due to 21-hydroxylase deficiency or Cushing's syndrome are ACTH stimulation and dexamethasone suppression, respectively. Once a tumor has been suggested, localization of the lesion may be achieved by either pelvic examination or ultrasonography (ovary) and CT scanning (adrenal). If these methods fail to localize the tumor, selective venous catheterization may be necessary.[204]

References

1. Vara P, Niemineva K: Small cystic degeneration of ovaries as incidental finding in gynecological laparotomies. Acta Obstet Gynecol Scand 31:94–107, 1951.
2. Sommer SC, Wadman PJ: Pathogenesis of polycystic ovaries. Am J Obstet Gynecol 72:160–169, 1956.
3. Goldzieher JW: Polycystic ovarian disease. Fertil Steril 35:371–394, 1981.
4. Judd HL: Endocrinology of polycystic ovarian disease. Clin Obstet Gynecol 21:99–144, 1978.
5. MacGregor AH, Johnson JE, Bunde CA: Further clinical experience with clomiphene citrate. Fertil Steril 19:616–620, 1968.
6. Rust LA, Israel R, Mishell DR: An individualized graduated therapeutic regimen for clomiphene citrate. Am J Obstet Gynecol 120:785–790, 1974.
7. Fechner RE, Kaufman RH: Endometrial adenocarcinoma in Stein-Leventhal syndrome. 34:444–452, 1974.
8. Coulam CB, Annegers JF, Kranz JS: Chronic anovulation syndrome and associated neoplasia. Obstet Gynecol 61:403–407, 1983.
9. Cooper HE, Spellacy WN, Prem KA, et al.: Hereditary factors in the Stein-Leventhal syndrome. Am J Obstet Gynecol 100:371–387, 1968.
10. Givens JR, Wiser WL, Coleman SA, et al.: Familial ovarian hyperthecosis: a study of two families. Am J Obstet Gynecol 110:959–972, 1971.
11. McDonough PG, Mahesh VB, Ellegood JO: Steroid, follicle-stimulating hormone, and luteinizing hormone profiles in identical twins with polycystic ovaries. Am J Obstet Gynecol 113:1072–1078, 1972.
12. Yen SSC: The polycystic ovary syndrome. Clin Endocrinol 12:177–207, 1980.
13. Kahn CR, Flier JS, Bar RS, et al.: The syndromes of insulin resistance and acanthosis nigricans. Insulin receptor studies in man. N Engl J Med 294:739–745, 1976.

14. Yen SSC, Vela P, Rankin J: Inappropriate secretion of follicle-stimulating hormone and luteinizing hormone in polycystic ovarian disease. J Clin Endocrinol Metab 30:435–442, 1970.

15. Yen SSC, Chaney C, Judd HL: Functional aberrations of the hypothalamicpituitary system in polycystic ovary syndrome: a consideration of the pathogenesis. In VHT James, M Serio, G Giusti (eds) The Endocrine Function of the Human Ovary. New York, Academic Press, 1976.

16. Hoffman D, Lobo RA: The prevalence and significance of elevated DHEA-S levels in anovulatory women. Fertil Steril 39:404–405, 1983.

17. Abraham GE: Ovarian and adrenal contribution to peripheral androgens during the normal menstrual cycle. J Clin Endocrinol Metab 39:340–346, 1974.

18. Lipsett MB, Riter B: Urinary ketosteroids and pregnanetriol in hirsutism. J Clin Endocrinol Metab 20:180–186, 1960.

19. Brooks RV, Prunty FTG: Patterns of steroid excretion in three types of post-pubertal hirsutism. J Endocrinol 21:263–276, 1960.

20. Gallagher TF, Kappas A, Hellman L, et al.: Adrenocorticol hyperfunction in "idiopathic" hirsutism and the Stein-Leventhal syndrome. J Clin Invest 37:794–799, 1958.

21. Goldzieher JW, Green JA: The polycystic ovary. I. Clinical and histologic features. J Clin Endocrinol Metab 22:325–337, 1962.

22. Lanthier A: Urinary 17-ketosteroids in the syndrome of polycystic ovaries and hyperthecosis. J Clin Endocrinol Metab 20:1587–1591, 1960.

23. Mellinger RC, Smith RW, Patti AA: Adrenocorticol function in the polycystic ovary syndrome. J Clin Endocrinol Metab 16:967–970, 1956.

24. DuToit DAH: Polycystic Ovaries, Menstrual Disturbances, and Hirsutism Hyperthecosis. Leiden, Kroese, 1951.

25. Kovacic N: Congenital adrenal hyperplasia and precocious gonadotropin secretion in a six-year-old girl. J Clin Endocrinol Metab 19:844–848, 1959.

26. Gold JJ, Frank R: The borderline adrenogenital syndrome: an intermediate entity. Am J Obstet Gynecol 75:1034–1042, 1958.

27. Perloff WH, Channick BJ, Suplick B, et al.: Clinical management of idiopathic hirsutism (adrenal virilism). JAMA 167:2041–2043, 1958.

28. Perloff WH, Hadd HE, Channick BJ, et al.: Hirsutism. Arch Intern Med 100:981–983, 1957.

29. O'Donnell V, McCraig J: Biosynthesis of steroids by human ovaries. Biochem J 71:9P, 1959.

30. Goldzieher JW, Axelrod LR: Adrenal and ovarian steroidogenesis in the sclerocystic ovary syndrome. Acta Endocrinol 51:617–624, 1960.

31. Axelrod LR, Goldzieher JW: The polycystic ovary. III. Steroid biosynthesis in normal and polycystic ovarian tissue. J Clin Endocrinol 22:431–438, 1962.

32. Axelrod LR, Goldzieher JW: Enzymic inadequacies of human polycystic ovaries. Arch Biochem Biophys 95:547–551, 1961.

33. Leon N, Castro MN, Dorfman RI: Biosynthesis of testosterone by a Stein-Leventhal ovary. Acta Endocrinol 39:411–419, 1962.

34. Kase N, Kowal J, Soffer LJ: In vitro production of testosterone and androstenedione in normal and Stein-Leventhal ovaries. Acta Endocrinol 44:8–13, 1963.

35. Sandor T, Lanthier A: The in vitro transformation of 4-androstene-3,17-dione to testosterone by surviving human ovarian slices. Rev Can Biol 19:445–447, 1960.

36. Short RV, London DR: Defective biosynthesis of ovarian steroids in the Stein-Leventhal syndrome. Br Med J 1:1724–1725, 1961.

37. Givens JR, Andersen RN, Wiser WL, et al.: Dynamics of suppression and recovery of plasma FSH, LH, androstenedione and testosterone in polycystic ovarian disease using an oral contraceptive. J Clin Endocrinol 38:727–735, 1974.

38. Benjamin F, Cohen M, Romney SL: Sequential adrenal and ovarian suppression tests in the differential diagnosis of the polycystic ovary syndrome. Fertil Steril 21:854–859, 1970.

39. Ettinger B, Goldfield EB, Burrill KC, et al.: Plasma testosterone stimulation suppression dynamics in hirsute women: correlation with long-term therapy. Am J Med 54:195–202, 1973.

40. Sciarra F, Toscano V, Concolino G, et al.: Simultaneous estimation of four plasma androgens before and after dynamic tests in women with hirsutism: correlation with long-term therapy. Horm Res 7:16–22, 1976.

41. Kim MH, Rosenfield RL, Hosseinian AH, et al.: Ovarian hyperandrogenism with normal and abnormal histologic findings of the ovaries. Am J Obstet Gynecol 134:445–452, 1979.

42. Pugeat M, Forest MG, Nisula BC, et al.: Evidence of excessive androgen secretion by both the ovary and the adrenal in patients with idiopathic hirsutism. Obstet Gynecol 59:46–51, 1982.

43. Wild RA, Umstot ES, Andersen RN, et al.: Adrenal function in hirsutism. II. Effect of an oral contraceptive. J Clin Endocrinol Metab 54:676–681, 1982.

44. Carr BR, Parker CR, Madden JD, et al.: Plasma levels of adrenocorticotropin and cortisol in women receiving oral contraceptive steroid treatment. J Clin Endocrinol Metab 49:346–349, 1979.

45. Abraham GE, Chakmakjian ZH, Buster JE, et al.: Ovarian and adrenal contributions to peripheral androgens in hirsute women. Obstet Gynecol 46:169–173, 1975.

46. Goldzieher JW: The interplay of adrenocortical and ovarian function. In HC Mack (ed) The Ovary. Springfield, Ill., CC Thomas, 1968.

47. Werk EE, Sholiton LH, Kalejs L: Testosterone-secreting adrenal adenoma under gonadotropin control. N Engl J Med 189:767–772, 1973.

48. Givens JR, Anderson RN, Wiser WL, et al.: A gonadotropin-responsive adrenocortical adenoma. J Clin Endocrinol Metab 38:126–133, 1974.

49. Cooke CW, McEvoy D, Bulaschenko H, et al.: Adrenocortical and ovarian function in hirsute women. Am J Obstet Gynecol 114:65–77, 1972.

50. Givens JR, Andersen RN, Ragland JB, et al.: Adrenal function in hirsutism. I. Diurnal change and response of plasma androstenedione, testosterone, 17-hydroxyprogesterone, cortisol, LH, and GSH to dexamethasone and ½ unit of ACTH. J Clin Endocrinol Metab 40:988–1000, 1975.

51. Abraham GE, Maroulis GB, Buster JE, et al.: Effect of dexamethasone on serum cortisol and androgen levels in hirsute patients. Obstet Gynecol 47:395–401, 1976.

52. Judd HL, McPherson RA, Rakoff JS, et al.: Correlation of the effect of dexamethasone administration on urinary 17-ketosteroids and serum androgen levels in patients with hirsutism. Am J Obstet Gynecol 128:408–417, 1977.

53. Cortes-Gallegos V, Alonso-Uriarte ME, Said LE, *et al.:* Effect of paramethasone acetate on women with secondary amenorrhea: a preliminary report. Fertil Steril 29:402–406, 1978.

54. Abraham GE, Maroulis GB, Boyers SP, *et al.:* Dexamethasone suppression test in the management of hyperandrogenized patients. Obstet Gynecol 57:158–165, 1981.

55. Baldwin DM, Sawyer CH: Effects of dexamethasone on LH release and ovulation in the rat. Endocrinol 94:1397–1401, 1974.

56. Gonzales-Barcena D, Kastin AJ, Shalk DS, *et al.:* Response to LH-RH in women before and after treatment with prednisone. Int J Fertil 19:107–110, 1974.

57. Sakakura M, Takebe K, Nakagawa S: Inhibition of luteinizing hormone secretion induced by synthetic LRH by long-term treatment with glucocorticoids in human subjects. J Clin Endocrinol Metab 40:774–779, 1975.

58. Kirschner MA, Jacobs JB: Combined ovarian and adrenal vein catheterization to determine the site(s) of androgen overproduction in hirsute women. J Clin Endocrinol Metab 33:199–209, 1971.

59. Wilson EA, Erickson GF, Zarutski P, *et al.:* Endocrine studies of normal and polycystic ovarian tissues *in vitro.* Am J Obstet Gynecol 134:56–63, 1979.

60. Kirschner MA, Zucker IR, Jespersen D: Idiopathic hirsutism—an ovarian abnormality. N Engl J Med 294:637–641, 1976.

61. Milewic A, Silber D, Mielecki T: The origin of androgen synthesis in polycystic ovary syndrome. Obstet Gynecol 62:601–604, 1983.

62. Rosenfield RL: Letter to the Editor. N Engl J Med 295:232–233, 1976.

63. Moltz L, Schwartz U, Sörenson R, *et al.:* Ovarian and adrenal vein steroids in patients with non-neoplastic hyperandrogenism: selective catheterization findings. Fertil Steril 42:69–75, 1984.

64. Meldrum DR, Chang RJ, Lu J, *et al.:* "Medical oophorectomy" using a long-acting GnRH agonist—a possible new approach to the treatment of endometriosis. J Clin Endocrinol Metab 54:1081–1083, 1982.

65. Crowley WF, Comite F, Vale W, *et al.:* Therapeutic use of pituitary desensitization with a long-acting LHRH agonist: a potential new treatment for idiopathic precocious puberty. J Clin Endocrinol Metab 52:370–373, 1981.

66. Nillius SJ, Bergquist C, Wide L: Inhibition of ovulation in women by chronic treatment with a stimulatory LRH analogue—a new approach to birth control. Contraception 17:537–545, 1978.

67. Meldrum DR, Tsao Z, Monroe SE, *et al.:* Stimulation of LH with reduced bioactivity following GnRH agonist administration in women. J Clin Endocrinol Metab 58:755–757, 1984.

68. Chang RJ, Laufer LR, Meldrum DR, *et al.:* Steroid secretion in polycystic ovarian disease after ovarian suppression by a long-acting gonadotropin-releasing agonist. J Clin Endocrinol Metab 56:897–904, 1983.

69. Lobo RA, Kletzky OA, diZerega GS: Elevated bioactive lutenizing hormone in women with the polycystic ovary syndrome. Fertil Steril 39:674–678, 1983.

70. DeVane GW, Czekala NM, Judd HL, *et al.:* Circulating gonadotropins, estrogens, and androgens in polycystic ovarian disease. Am J Obstet Gynecol 121:496–500, 1975.

71. Horton R, Neisler J: Plasma androgens in patient with polycystic ovary syndrome. J Clin Endocrinol Metab 28:479–484, 1968.

72. Lachelin GCL, Judd HL, Swanson SC, *et al.:* Long-term effects of nightly dexamethasone administration in patients with polycystic ovarian disease. J Clin Endocrinol Metab 55:768–773, 1982.

73. Lobo RA, Goebelsmann U: Adult manifestation of congenital adrenal hyperplasia due to incomplete 21-hydroxylase deficiency mimicking polycystic ovarian disease. Am J Obstet Gynecol 138:720–726, 1980.

74. Lobo RA, Goebelsmann U: Evidence for reduced 3β-ol-hydroxysteroid dehydrogenase activity in some hirsute women thought to have polycystic ovary syndrome. J Clin Endocrinol Metab 53:394–400, 1981.

75. Chang RJ, Mandel FP, Wolfsen AR, *et al.:* Circulating levels of plasma adrenocorticotropin in polycystic ovary disease. J Clin Endocrinol Metab 54:1265–1267, 1982.

76. Raj SG, Thompson IE, Berger MJ, *et al.:* Clinical aspects of the polycystic ovary syndrome. Obstet Gynecol 49:552–556, 1977.

77. Lachelin GCL, Barnett M, Hopper BR, *et al.:* Adrenal function in normal women and women with the polycystic ovary syndrome. J Clin Endocrinol Metab 49:892–898, 1979.

78. Parker LN, Odell WD: Control of adrenal androgen secretion. Endocrine Reviews 1:392–410, 1980.

79. Givens JR, Weidenmann E, Anderson RN, *et al.:* β-endorphin and β-lipotropin plasma levels in hirsute women: correlation with body weight. J Clin Endocrinol Metab 50:975–976, 1980.

80. Fujieda K, Faiman C, Reyes F, *et al.:* The control of steroidogenesis by human fetal adrenal cells in tissue culture. III. the effects of various hormonal peptides. J Clin Endocrinol Metab 53:690–695, 1981.

81. Lobo RA, Kletzky OA, Kaptein EM, *et al.:* Prolactin modulation of dehydroepiandrosterone sulfate secretion. Am J Obstet Gynecol 138:632–636, 1980.

82. Lobo RA, Paul WL, Goebelsmann U: Dehydroepiandrosterone sulfate as an indicator of adrenal androgen function. Obstet Gynecol 57:69–73, 1981.

83. Marshall S, Kledzik BS, Gelato M, *et al.:* Effects of estrogen and testosterone on specific prolactin binding in the kidneys and adrenals of rats. Steroids 27:187–191, 1976.

84. Vermeulen A, Ando S, Verdonck L: Prolactinomas testosterone-binding globulin, and androgen metabolism. J Clin Endocrinol Metab 54:409–412, 1982.

85. Hoffman D, Lobo RA: Exaggerated responses of adrenal androgens after ACTH infusion in some anovulatory women. (To be published.)

86. Chetkowski RJ, DeFazio J, Shamonki I, *et al.:* The incidence of late-onset congenital adrenal hyperplasia due to 21-hydroxylase deficiency among hirsute women. J Clin Endocrinol Metab 58:595–598, 1984.

87. Mandel FP, Chang RJ, Dupont B, *et al.:* HLA genotyping in family members and patients with familial polycystic ovarian disease. J Clin Endocrinol Metab 56:862–867, 1983.

88. Pang S, Levine LS, Lorenzen F, *et al.:* Hormonal studies in obligate heterozygotes and siblings of patients with 11β-hydroxylase deficiency congenital adrenal hyperplasia. J Clin Endocrinol Metab 50:586–589, 1980.

89. Abraham GE, Maroulis GB: Effect of exogenous estrogen on serum pregnenolone, cortisol, and androgens in postmenopausal women. Obstet Gynecol 45:271–274, 1975.

90. Barmach de Niepomniszsze AJ, Rosenfield RL, Hosseinian AH, *et al.*: Adrenal androgen production: dependence on ACTH and gonadal function. Proceedings of the 55th Annual Meeting of the Endocrine Society. p. A-194, 1973.

91. Yates J, Deshpande N: Kinetic studies on the enzyme catalyzing the conversion of 17α-hydroxyprogesterone and dehydroepiandrosterone in the human adrenal gland *in vitro.* J Endocrinol 60:27–35, 1974.

92. Anderson DC, Yen SSC: Effect of estrogens on adrenal 3β-hydroxysteroid dehydrogenase in ovariectomized women. J Clin Endocrinol Metab 43:561–570, 1976.

93. Ackerman GE, Smith ME, Mendelson CR, *et al.*: Aromatization of androstenedione by human adipose tissue stromal cells in monolayer culture. J Clin Endocrinol Metab 53:412–417, 1981.

94. Erickson GF, Hsueh AJW, Quigley ME, *et al.*: Functional studies of aromatase activity in human granulosa cells from normal and polycystic ovaries. J Clin Endocrinol Metab 49:514–519, 1979.

95. Chetkowski RJ, Chang RJ, DeFazio J, *et al.*: The origin of serum progestins in polycystic ovarian disease. Obstet Gynecol 64:27–31, 1984.

96. Yen SSC, Vela P, Rankin J: Inappropriate secretion of follicle-stimulating hormone and luteinizing hormone in polycystic ovarian disease. J Clin Endocrinol Metab 30:435–442, 1970.

97. Rebar RW: Gonadotropin secretion in polycystic ovarian disease. Semin Reprod Endocrinol 2:223–230, 1984.

98. Rebar RW, Judd HL, Yen SSC, *et al.*: Characterization of the inappropriate gonadotropin secretion in polycystic ovary syndrome. J Clin Invest 57:1320–1329, 1976.

99. Keye WR, Jaffe RB: Modulation of pituitary gonadotropin response to gonadotropin-releasing hormone by estradiol. J Clin Endocrinol Metab 38:805–810, 1974.

100. Jaffe RB, Keye WR Jr: Estradiol augmentation of pituitary responsiveness to gonadotropin-releasing hormone in women. J Clin Endocrinol Metab 39:850–855, 1974.

101. Hoff JD, Lasley BL, Yen SSC: The functional relationship between priming and releasing actions of luteinizing hormone-releasing hormone. J Clin Endocrinol Metab 49:8–11, 1979.

102. Clarke IJ, Cummins JT: The temporal relationship between gonadotropin releasing hormone (GnRH) and luteinizing hormone (LH) secretion in ovariectomized ewes. Endocrinol 111:1737–9, 1982.

103. Quigley ME, Rakoff JS, Yen SSC: Increased luteinizing hormone sensitivity to dopamine inhibition in polycystic ovary syndrome. J Clin Endocrinol Metab 52:231–234, 1981.

104. Cumming DC, Reid RL, Quigley ME, *et al.*: Evidence for decreased endogenous dopamine and opioid inhibitory influences on LH secretion in polycystic ovary syndrome. Clin Endocrinol 20:643–648, 1984.

105. Chang RJ, Mandel FP, Lu JKH, *et al.*: Enhanced disparity of gonadotropin secretion by estrone in women with polycystic ovarian disease. J Clin Endocrinol Metab 54:490–494, 1982.

106. Channing CP, Schaerf FW, Anderson LD, *et al.*: Ovarian follicular and luteal physiology. *In* RO Greep (ed) Reproductive Physiology III, International Review of Physiology, Vol 22, Chap 3. Baltimore, University Park Press, 1980.

107. Tanabe K, Gagliano P, Channing CP, *et al.*: Levels of inhibin-F activity and steroids in human follicular fluid from normal women and women with polycystic ovarian disease. J Clin Endocrinol Metab 57:24–31, 1983.

108. Imperato-McGinley J, Peterson RE, Sturla E, *et al.*: Primary amenorrhea associated with hirsutism, acanthosis nigricans, dermoid cysts of the ovaries, and a new type of insulin resistance. Am J Med 65:389–395, 1978.

109. Annos T, Taymor ML: Ovarian pathology associated with insulin resistance and acanthosis nigricans. Obstet Gynecol 58:662–XXX, 1981.

110. Taylor SI, Dons RF, Hernandez E, *et al.*: Insulin resistance associated with androgen excess in women with autoantibodies to the insulin receptor. Ann Int Med 97:851–855, 1982.

111. Flier JS, Young JB, Landsberg L: Familial insulin resistance with acanthosis nigricans, acral hypertrophy, and muscle cramps. N Engl J Med 303:970–973, 1980.

112. Burghen GA, Givens JK, Kitabchi AE: Correlation of hyperandrogenism with hyperinsulinism in polycystic ovarian disease. J Clin Endocrinol Metab 50:113–116, 1980.

113. Shoupe D, Lobo RA: Insulin resistance in polycystic ovary syndrome. Fertil Steril 41:385–389, 1984.

114. Chang RJ, Nakamura R, Judd HL, *et al.*: Insulin resistance in nonobese patients with polycystic ovarian disease. J Clin Endocrinol Metab 57:356–359, 1983.

115. Chang RJ, Geffner M, Golde D, *et al.*: Characterization of insulin resistance in polycystic ovarian disease (PCO). Proceedings of the 31st Annual Meeting of the Society for Gynecologic Investigation. p 232, Abstr. no 394, 1984.

116. McCullagh EP, Lewis LA: Carbohydrate metabolism of patients treated with methyl testosterone. J Clin Endocrinol Metab 2:507–514, 1942.

117. Woodard TL, Burghen GA, Kitabchi AE, *et al.*: Glucose intolerance and insulin resistance in aplastic anemia treated with oxymethalone. J Clin Endocrinol Metab 53:905–910, 1981.

118. Barbieri RL, Ryan KJ: Hyperandrogenism, insulin resistance, and acanthosis nigricans: A common endocrinopathy with distinct pathophysiologic features. Am J Obstet Gynecol 147:90–101, 1983.

119. Nagamani M, Dinh TV, Kelver ME: Hyperinsulinemia in hyperthecosis of the ovaries. Proceedings of the 32nd Annual Meeting of the Society for Gynecologic Investigation. p 42, Abstr. no. 74, 1985.

120. Adashi EY, Hsueh AJW, Yen SSC: Insulin enhancement of luteinizing hormone release by cultured pituitary cells. Endocrinol 108:1441–1449, 1981.

121. Veldhuis JD, Kolp LA, Toaff ME, *et al.*: Mechanisms subserving the trophic actions of insulin on ovarian cells. J Clin Invest 72:1046–1057, 1983.

122. Barbieri RL, Makris A, Ryan KJ: Insulin stimulates androgen accumulation in incubations of human ovarian stroma and theca. Obstet Gynecol 64:73–80, 1984.

123. Jarrett JC, Ballejo G, Tsibris JCM, *et al.*: Insulin binding to human ovaries. Proceedings of the 31st Annual Meeting of the Society for Gynecologic Investigation. p 99, Abstr. no 168P, 1984.

124. Poretsky L, Smith D, Seibel M, *et al.*: Specific binding sites in human ovary. J Clin Endocrinol Metab 59:809–811, 1984.

125. Harrankora J, Roth J, Brownstein MJ: Concentrations of insulin and insulin receptors in the brain are independent of peripheral insulin levels. J Clin Invest 64:636–642, 1979.

126. Dignam WJ, Pion RJ, Lamb EJ, et al.: Plasma androgens in women. II. Patients with polycystic ovaries and hirsutism. Acta Endocrinol (Kbh) 45:254–271, 1964.

127. Taymor ML, Clark BJ, Sturgis SH: The polycystic ovary. a clinical and laboratory study. Am J Obstet Gynecol 86:188–196, 1963.

128. Goldzieher JW, Green JA: The polycystic ovary. I. Clinical and histological features. J Clin Endocrinol Metab 22:325–338, 1962.

129. Greenblatt RB: The polycystic ovary syndrome of Stein-Leventhal. In CC Thomas (ed) The Hirsute Female. Springfield, Ill, 1963.

130. Gyves MT: The significance of peripheral sclerosis in the Stein-Leventhal syndrome. Fertil Steril 21:502–507, 1970.

131. Scott RB, Wharton LR: The effect of testosterone in experimental endometriosis in rhesus monkeys. Am J Obstet Gynecol 78:1020–1026, 1959.

132. Hughesdon PE: Morphology and morphogenesis of the Stein-Leventhal ovary and so-called "hyperthecosis." Obstet Gynecol Surv 37:59–77, 1982.

133. McNatty KP, Smith DM, Makris A, et al.: The microenvironment of the human antral follicle: interrelationships among the steroid levels in antral fluid, the population of granulosa cells, and the status of the oocyte in vivo and in vitro. J Clin Endocrinol Metab 49:851–860, 1979.

134. McNatty KP, Moore-Smith D, Makris A, et al.: The intraovarian sites of androgen and estrogen formation in women with normal and hyperandrogenic ovaries as judged by in vitro experiments. J Clin Endocrinol Metab 50:755–766, 1980.

135. Short RV, London DR: Defective biosynthesis of ovarian steroids in the Stein-Leventhal syndrome. Br Med J 1:1724–1727, 1961.

136. Hillier SG, van den Boogard AMJ, Reichert LE, et al.: Intraovarian sex steroid hormone interactions and the control of follicular maturation: aromatization of androgens by human granulosa cells in vitro. J Clin Endocrinol Metab 50:640–647, 1980.

137. Erickson GF, Yen SSC: New data on follicle cells in polycystic ovaries: a proposed mechanism for the genesis of cystic follicles. Semin Reprod Endocrinol 2:231–243, 1984.

138. DeFazio J, Meldrum DR, Lu JKH, et al.: Acute ovarian responses to a long-acting agonist of GnRH in ovulatory women and women with polycystic ovarian disease. Fertil Steril (To be published.)

139. Govan ADT, Black WP: Some observations on the histology of polycystic ovarian disease. In JRT Coutts (ed) Functional Morphology of the Human Ovary. Baltimore, University Park Press, 1981.

140. Green JA, Goldzieher JW: The polycystic ovary: IV. Light and electron microscope studies. Am J Obstet Gynecol 91:173–181, 1965.

141. Goldzieher JW, Axelrod LR: Clinical and biochemical features of polycystic ovarian disease. Fertil Steril 14:631–653, 1963.

142. Louvet JP, Harman SM, Schreiber JR, et al.: Evidence for a role of androgens in follicular maturation. Endocrinol 97:366–372, 1975.

143. Febres F, Gondos B, Siiteri P: Androgen-induced ovarian follicular atresia in the rat. Gynecol Invest 7:52, 1976.

144. Jackson RL, Dockerty MD: The Stein-Leventhal syndrome: analysis of 43 cases with special reference to association with endometrial carcinoma. Am J Obstet Gynecol 73:161–173, 1957.

145. Grattarola R: Misdiagnosis of endometrial adenocarcinoma in young women with polycystic ovarian disease. Am J Obstet Gynecol 105:498–502, 1969.

146. Chamlian DL, Taylor HB: Endometrial hyperplasia in young women. Obstet Gynecol 36:659–666, 1970.

147. Kirschner MA, Zucker IR, Jesperson DL: Ovarian and adrenal vein catheterization studies in women with idiopathic hirsutism. In VHT James, M Serio, G Guisti (eds) The Endocrine Function of the Ovary. New York, Academic Press, 1976.

148. Lucky AW, McGuire J, Rosenfield RL, et al.: Plasma androgens in women with acne vulgaris. J Invest Dermatol 81:70–75, 1983.

149. Horton R, Hawks D, Lobo R: 3α,17β-androstanediol glucuronide in plasma. A marker of androgen action in idiopathic hirsutism. J Clin Invest 69:1203–1205, 1982.

150. de Ziegler D, Chang J, Meldrum D, et al.: 3α,17β androstanediol glucuronide (AG) in androgenized women. Proceedings of the 32nd Annual Meeting of the Society for Gynecologic Investigation. p 24, Abstr. no. 42P, 1985.

151. del Pozo E, Falaschi P: Prolactin and cyclicity in polycystic ovary syndrome. In M L'Hermite, SJ Judd (eds) Progess in Reproductive Biology. Basel, S Karger, 1980.

152. White MC, Ginsburg J: The hirsute female. In PG Crosignani, BL Rubin (eds), Endocrinology of Human Infertility: New Aspects. London, Academic Press, 1981.

153. Hutchinson JR, Taylor HB, Zimmerman EA: The Stein-Leventhal syndrome and coincident ovarian neoplasms. Obstet Gynecol 28:700–703, 1966.

154. Moore JG, Schifrin BS, Erez S: Ovarian tumors in infancy, childhood, and adolescence. Am J Obstet Gynecol 99:913–922, 1967.

155. Babknia A, Calfopoulos P, Jones HW Jr: The Stein-Leventhal syndrome and coincidental ovarian tumors. Obstet Gynecol 47:223–224, 1976.

156. Case Records of the Massachusetts General Hospital (Case 25-1982). N Engl J Med 306:1537–1544, 1982.

157. Fraenkel L: Thecoma and hyperthecosis of the ovary. J Clin Endocrinol Metab 3:557–559, 1943.

158. Culiner A, Shippel S: Virilism and theca cell hyperplasia of the ovary syndrome. J Obstet Gynecol Br Com 56:439–445, 1949.

159. Judd HL, Scully RE, Herbst AL, et al.: Familial hyperthecosis: comparison of endocrinologic findings with polycystic ovarian disease. Am J Obstet Gynecol 117:976–982, 1973.

160. Aiman J, Edman CD, Worley RJ, et al.: Androgen and estrogen formation in women with ovarian hyperthecosis. Obstet Gynecol 51:1–9, 1978.

161. Steingold KA, Judd HL, Lu JHK, et al.: Treatment of severe ovarian hyperthecosis with a long-acting GnRH agonist. Am J Obstet Gynecol 154:1241–1248, 1986.

162. Levine LS, Zachmann M, New MI, et al.: Genetic mapping of the 21-hydroxylase deficiency gene within the HLA linkage group. Engl J Med 299:911–915, 1978.

163. Chetkowski RJ, DeFazio J, Shamonki I, et al.: The incidence of late-onset congenital adrenal hyperplasia due to 21-hydroxylase deficiency among hirsute women. J Clin Endocrinol Metab 58:595–599, 1984.

164. Broster LR: Eight years' experience with adrenal glands. Arch Surg 34:761–772, 1937.

165. Chrousos GP, Loriaux DL, Mann DL, *et al.*: Late-onset 21-hydroxylase deficiency mimicking idiopathic hirsutism or polycystic ovarian disease. Ann Intern Med 96:143–148, 1982.

166. Blackman SS, Jr: Concerning function and origin of reticularis zone of adrenal cortex: Hyperplasia in adrenogenital syndrome. Bull Johns Hopkins Hosp 78:180–188, 1946.

167. Jones HW, Jr, Jones GES: Gynecologic aspects of adrenal hyperplasia and allied disorders. Am J Obstet Gynecol 68:1330–1365, 1954.

168. Gabrilove JL, Sharma DC, Dorman RI: Adrenocortical 11β-hydroxylase deficiency and virilism first manifest in the adult woman. N Engl J Med 272:1189–1194, 1965.

169. Axelrod LR, Goldzieher JW, Ross SD: Concurrent 3β-hydroxysteroid dehydrogenase deficiency in adrenal and sclerocystic ovary. Acta Endocrinol 48:392–412, 1965.

170. Sharma DC, Forehielli E, Dorman RI: Inhibition of enzymatic steroid 11β-hydroxylation by androgens. J Biol Chem 238:572–577, 1963.

171. Munobi AK, Cassorla FG, Pfeiffer DG, *et al.*: The effects of testosterone on rat ovarian 17-hydroxylase and 3β-hydroxysteroid dehydrogenase enzyme activities. Proceedings of the 30th Annual Meeting of the Society for Gynecologic Investigation. p 41, Abstr. no. 75, 1983.

172. Iannaccone A, Gabrilove JL, Sohval AR, *et al*: The ovaries in Cushing's syndrome. N Engl J Med 261:775–780, 1959.

173. Norris HJ, Charlton I: Functioning tumors of the ovary. Clin Obstet Gynecol 17:189–228, 1974.

174. Scully RE: Sex cord-stromal tumors. In A Blaustein (ed) Pathology of the Female Genital Tract, *2nd* edition. New York, Springer-Verlag, 1982.

175. Novak ER, Kutchmeshgi J, Mupas RS, *et al.*: Feminizing gonadal stromal tumors: analysis of the granulosa-theca cell tumors of the ovarian tumor registry. Obstet Gynecol 38:701–713, 1971.

176. Malkasian GD, Jr Dockerty MB, Wilson RB, *et al.*: Functioning tumors of the ovary in women under 40. Obstet Gynecol 26:669–675, 1965.

177. Norris HJ, Taylor HB: Virilization associated with cystic granulosa cell tumors. Obstet Gynecol 34:629–635, 1969.

178. Giuntoli RL, Celebre JA, Wu CH, *et al.*: Androgenic function of a granulosa cell tumor. Obstet Gynecol 47:77–79, 1976.

179. Givens JR, Andersen RN, Wiser WL, *et al.*: A testosterone-secreting, gonadotropin-responsive pure thecoma and polycystic ovarian disease. J Clin Endocrinol Metab 41:845–853, 1975.

180. Hatjis CG, Polin JI, Wheeler JE, *et al.*: Amenorrhea-galactorrhea associated with a testosterone-producing, solid granulosa cell tumor. Am J Obstet Gynecol 131:226–227, 1978.

181. Teilum G: Special Tumors of Ovary and Testis and Related Extragonadal Lesions: Comparative Pathology and Histological Identification, *2nd* edition. Philadelphia, JB Lippincott, 1978.

182. Scully RE: Ovarian tumors: A review. Am J Pathol 87:686–720, 1977.

183. Novak ER, Woodruff JD (eds): Novak's Gynecologic and Obstetric Pathology. Philadelphia, WB Saunders Company, 1974.

184. Roth LM, Anderson MC, Govan ADT: Sertoli-Leydig cell tumors. Cancer 48:187–197, 1981.

185. Mandel FP, Voet RL, Weiland AJ, *et al.*: Steroid secretion by masculinizing and "feminizing" hilus cell tumors. J Clin Endocrinol Metab 52:779–784, 1981.

186. Bonaventura LM, Judd H, Roth LM, *et al.*: Androgen, estrogen, and progestogen production by a lipid cell tumor of the ovary. Am J Obstet Gynecol 131:403–409, 1978.

187. Chetkowski RJ, Judd HL, Jagger PI, *et al.*: Autonomous cortisol secretion by a lipoid cell tumor of the ovary. JAMA 254:2628–2631, 1985.

188. Imperato-McGinley J, Peterson RE, Dawood MY, *et al.*: Steroid hormone secretion from a virilizing lipoid cell tumor of the ovary. Obstet Gynecol 57:525–531, 1981.

189. Garcia-Bunel, Berek JS, Woodruff JD: Luteomas of pregnancy. Obstet Gynecol 45:407–414, 1975.

190. Hensleigh PA, Woodruff JD: Differential maternal-fetal response to androgenizing luteoma or hyperreactive luteinates. Obstet Gynecol Surv 33:262–270, 1978.

191. Hensleigh PA, Carter RP, Grotja HE: Fetal protection against masculinization. J Clin Endocrinol Metab 40:816–823, 1975.

192. White CA, Bradbury JT: Ovarian theca-lutein cysts. Am J Obstet Gynecol 92:976–980, 1965.

193. Woodruff JD, Williams TJ, Goldberg B: Hormone activity of the common ovarian neoplasm. Am J Obstet Gynecol 87:679–698, 1963.

194. Koudstaal J, Bossenbroek B Hardonk MJ: Ovarian tumors investigated by histochemical and enzyme histochemical methods. Am J Obstet Gynecol 102:1004–1017, 1968.

195. Pedowitz P, Felmus LB, Grayzel DM: Dysgerminoma of ovary. Am J Obstet Gynecol 70:1284–1297, 1956.

196. Usizima H: Ovarian dysgerminoma associated with masculinization. Cancer 9:736–739, 1956.

197. Scully RE: Gonadoblastoma. Cancer 6:455–463, 1953.

198. Scott JS, Lumsden CE, Levell MJ: Ovarian endocrine activity in association with hormonally inactive neoplasia. Am J Obstet Gynecol 97:161–170, 1967.

199. Novak ER, Goldberg B, Jones GS, *et al.*: Enzyme histochemistry of the menopausal ovary associated with normal and abnormal endometrium. Am J Obstet Gynecol 93:669–682, 1966.

200. Ober WB, Pollak A, Gerstmann KE, *et al.*: Krukenberg tumor with androgenic and progestational activity. Am J Obstet Gynecol 84:739–744, 1962.

201. Plotz EJ, Wiener M, Stein AA: Steroid synthesis in cystadenocarcinoma of the ovaries. Am J Obstet Gynecol 94:189–194, 1966.

202. Scully RE, Richardson GS: Luteinization of the stroma of metastatic cancer involving the ovary and its endocrine significance. Cancer 14:827–832, 1961.

203. Meldrum DR, Abraham GE: Peripheral and ovarian venous concentrations of various steroid hormones in virilizing ovarian tumors. Obstet Gynecol 53:36–43, 1979.

204. Weiland AJ, Bookstein JJ, Cleary RE, *et al.*: Preoperative localization of virilizing tumors by selective venous sampling. Am J Obstet Gynecol 131:797–802, 1978.

11. Luteal Phase Defects

Douglas C. Daly

Since its description by Jones[1] in 1949 the existence, techniques for diagnosis, and the methods of treatment of corpus luteal defects have been a subject of controversy.[2] In part this is due to the unfortunate designation—luteal phase defect (LPD)—of this group of clinical abnormalities. Since the cause of the inadequacy is frequently in the quality of folliculogenesis, a better designation might be dysfunctional ovulation. This would more accurately identify the abnormality as a defect in cyclic hypothalamic-pituitary-ovarian function in which significant progesterone is synthesized, thus separating it from anovulation, but with the quality of ovulation being abnormal. This terminology would accurately imply that any abnormality that could cause anovulation could also cause dysfunctional ovulation. Also like anovulation, the treatment of dysfunctional ovulation is dependent on the cause of the dysfunction rather than the presenting symptoms.

Unlike anovulation, the focus of diagnosis and treatment of LPD has been the endometrium, that is, how the cyclic changes in sex steroids affect its growth and maturation and presumably its relationship to the blastocyst. In this chapter on the pathology of luteal phase defect, or dysfunctional ovulation, the theoretical causes of LPD will be explored, the evidence for their existence examined and the methods of diagnosis reviewed. The chapter will conclude with a recommended protocol for diagnosing and treating LPD (dysfunctional ovulation) based on the specific underlying abnormality.

PATHOPHYSIOLOGY

Luteal phase defect is the result of abnormal physiologic changes and is only rarely caused by inherent anatomic or genetic abnormalities. Therefore, to understand the pathophysiology of LPD, it is necessary to understand normal ovulation. While the existence of the hypothalamic-pituitary-ovarian-uterine axis has been known since the work of Green,[3] the details of this relationship were not appreciated until the work of Knobil and colleagues.[4] Aspects of this relationship are discussed in detail in other chapters. For the purpose of understanding dysfunctional ovulation, a brief review is presented here, with emphasis on potential abnormalities that could cause luteal phase defects.

The hypothalamus acts as a pulse generator for GnRH.[4] It is known that variations in the rate of the pulsatile pattern will result in anovulation if this variation exceeds tolerances inherent in the pituitary and ovary[5] (Figure 11–1). Theoretically, less severe variations in pulsatile GnRH could result in dysfunctional ovulation with an inadequate luteal phase. While much of the initial work with pulsatile GnRH was done at constant pulse intervals, it is unclear whether the hypothalamus functions in this manner. It is probable that during the follicular phase there is a variation in pulsatile frequency, with an increase in GnRH secretion and/or pulse frequency as estradiol levels increase.[6] Therefore, individuals with excess extraovarian estrogen synthesis (such as in obesity) might have an inappropriately frequent pulsatile pattern that could result in dysfunctional ovulation. Other factors known to affect the pulsatile GnRH pattern and which could cause LPD are aberrations in thyroid metabolism and, particularly, an elevation in prolactin levels.[7] Individuals with decreased weight and perhaps those undergoing exercise-induced physical stress or excessive emotional stress have a decrease in frequency of GnRH pulse generation.[8] In the normal luteal phase the pulse generator is apparently slowed by progesterone.[9] These pulses are necessary for the continued synthesis of progesterone from the corpus luteum.

The pituitary functions as integrator-amplifier in the system, with the release of FSH and LH being dependent on the input of GnRH from the hypothalmic pulse generator and steroid hormones from the peripheral circulation. The pituitary has no method of determining the source of these inputs, so the pulsatile delivery of GnRH from a peripheral site may substitute for the hypothalamus.[10] Similarly, an excessive non-ovarian source of estradiol, such as occurs in obesity, or adrenal androgen excess (with peripheral conversion to estrone and estradiol) may be interpreted as representing ovarian activity. This may result in an inappropriate release of FSH and LH relative to the state of maturation of the ovarian follicle(s)[11], thereby resulting in dysfunctional ovulation (see Chapter 10).

The ovary is the transducer in the system, changing the primarily protein hormone messages of the hypothalamic-pituitary axis into steroidal messages which prime the endometrium and the endocervical mucus. These ste-

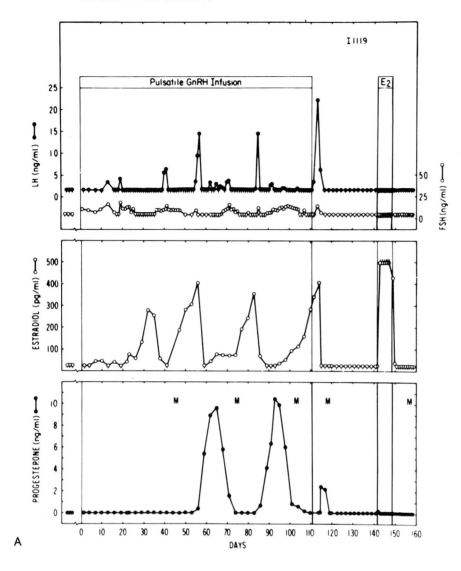

Figure 11–1. A. The pulsatile frequency and amplitude of the hypothalamic GnRH pulse generator are critical in the establishment of a normal FSH-LH pattern from the pituitary and the stimulation of the ovary through a normal ovulatory cycle. (Reproduced with permission from Wildt L, Marshall G, Knobil E: Experimental induction of puberty in the fertile female rhesus monkey. Sci 207:1373, 1981.)

roids also influence both the pulse generator of the hypothalamus and the integrator-amplifier activity of the pituitary. Estradiol appears to increase pulse frequency while progesterone decreases pulse frequency from the hypothalamus.[9] Similarly, estradiol augments the effect of GnRH on LH-FSH synthesis and storage while progesterone has the opposite effect.[12] The ovary accomplishes this function by developing and maturing a dominant follicle. The failure to develop such a follicle results in anovulation. The failure to adequately mature a dominant follicle would result in dysfunctional ovulation. Suppression of FSH in the early follicular phase due to inappropriate GnRH pulsation or by ovarian follicular proteins, such as inhibin, may result in this pattern[13] (Figure 11–2). Persistently low FSH in the early and mid-follicular phase has been documented in some patients with dysfunctional ovulation although the etiology has not been determined. It is probable that low FSH is the final common pathway in abnormal folliculogenesis in many patients with dysfunctional ovulation. Since it is the dominant follicle that determines the timing of the LH surge and subsequent

ovulation, it is possible that an inadequate dominant follicle would induce an aberrant LH surge. Since the LH surge, and the ability of the dominant follicle to respond to it by having acquired LH receptors, results in ovulation and final maturation of the ovum, an inadequately matured follicle could result in a lack of ovulation or an ovum incapable of normal fertilization and growth.

The uterus is not a static organ. The endometrium is highly active and each cycle undergoes transformation from a rapidly dividing proliferating tissue to a differentiated organ capable of synthezising new proteins, such as endometrial prolactin,[14] and thereby supporting an implanting pregnancy. Specifically, estradiol in the proliferative phase of the cycle primes the endometrium for progesterone stimulation in the luteal phase. Estradiol induces both its own receptor and the progesterone receptor (Table 11–1). As estradiol increases, its receptors increase, resulting in an exponential effect (Figure 11–3). This, in turn, results in an accelerating increase in progesterone receptors during the follicular phase that is exponential related to the rising estradiol levels present dur-

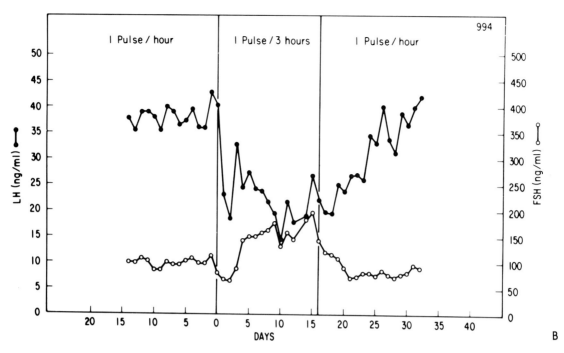

Figure 11–1. B. Pulse generation by a mechanical GnRH infusion at an acceptable pulse interval (1 pulse/hr) results in the establishment of an ovulatory cycle with normal estradiol-progesterone patterns in a prepubertal monkey. The decrease in pulse frequency (1 pulse/3 hours) results in suppression of an elevation of FSH and suppression of LH and anovulation. (Reproduced with permission from Knobil E: The neuroendocrine control of the menstrual cycle. Rec. Prog. in Hormone Research 36:53–88, 1981.)

ing the late follicular phase.[15] These receptors are then stimulated by the progesterone synthesized in the corpus luteum during the luteal phase (Figure 11–3). If the endometrial progesterone receptor level is inadequate, or the synthesis of progesterone in the luteal phase is inade-

quate, decidualization will not occur in a timely fashion and implantation may, therefore, be inadequate. The degree of histologic maturation of the late luteal phase endometrium is a bioassay for the entire ovarian steroid cycle, both the follicular and the luteal phase.

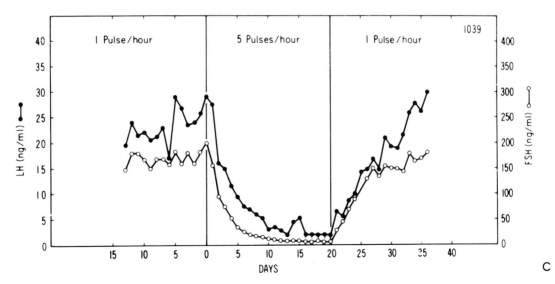

Figure 11–1. C. An increase in pulse frequency (5 pulse/hr) results in suppression of FSH and LH, which would lead to anovulation. It is likely that less extreme alterations in pulse generator frequency or amplitude would result in dysfunctional ovulation and luteal phase defect. (Reproduced with permission from Knobil, et al.[4])

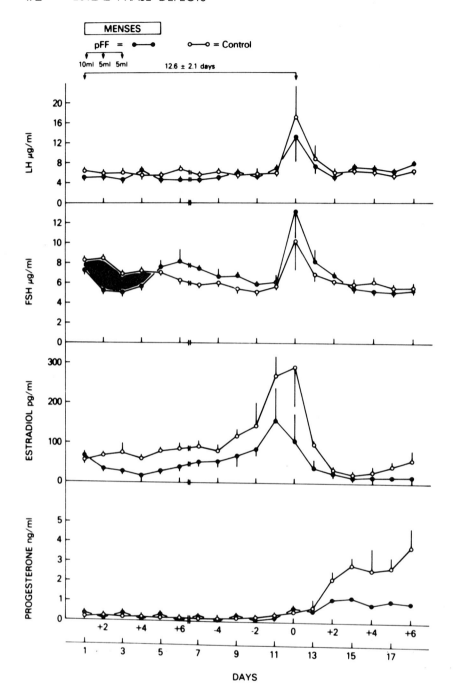

Figure 11-2. The infusion of steroid-free follicular proteins into a rhesus monkey during the early follicular phase results in suppression of FSH levels with the resultant induction of dysfunctional ovulation-LPD. (Reproduced with permission from DiZerega GS, Hodgen GD: Luteal phase dysfunction infertility: a sequel to aberrant folliculogenesis. Fertil Steril 35:489–499, 1981.)

METHODS OF DIAGNOSIS

Basal body temperature (BBT) charting is inadequate for making the diagnosis of dysfunctional ovulation in most circumstances; however, when the temperature elevation is 10 days or less, the quality of ovulation is nearly always inadequate. Even though implantation begins on day 6 postovulation, it is unlikely that human chorionic gonadotropin from implanting syncytiotrophoblast could rescue a corpus luteum already undergoing luteolysis. While an 11-day or 12-day luteal phase is suspicious for dysfunctional ovulation, this should not be used for diagnosis.

Progesterone levels in the luteal phase have been proposed as a method to diagnose LPD and have been used for this purpose ever since progesterone radioimmunoassay became available. Prior to that, total urinary pregnanediol (a metabolite of progesterone) excretion was used. Total urinary pregnanediol would seem to be an ideal diagnostic tool, except for the inconvenience of collection, since it presumably reflects ongoing corpus luteal function rather than the temporary progesterone level in the blood at the time of vein puncture. However, the proportion of progesterone that is converted to and excreted in the urine as pregnanediol is quite variable. Progesterone metabolite secretion in urine can vary from 15% to 75% of progesterone synthesis, and only half of this is pregnanediol.[16] Thus urinary pregnanediol levels are not clinically useful. Single and multiple serum progesterone levels have been proposed to diagnose LPD. In

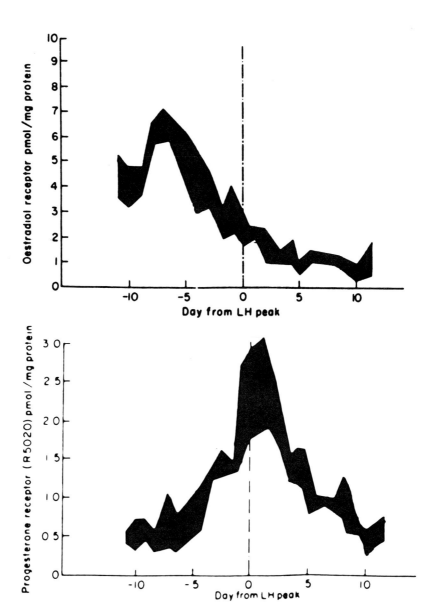

Figure 11–3. Levels of inactivated (cytoplasmic) estradiol and progesterone receptors in the endometrium during the menstrual cycle. Note that peak level of progesterone receptors occurs at ovulation. (Reproduced with permission from Edman.[27])

Table 11–1. Concentration of Cytoplasmic and Nuclear Receptors During Various Phases of the Menstrual Cycle[a]

Day of Cycle	Estradiol Receptor fmol/mg DNA			Progesterone Receptor fmol/DNA		
	Total	Cyto-plasm	Nucleus	Total	Cyto-plasm	Nucleus
Proliferative						
−8 to −5	1540	1130	410	1520	1220	300
−4 to 0	1930	1030	900	3010	2450	560
Secretory						
+1 to +6	1210	400	810	1890	860	1030
+7 to +12	640	260	380	880	660	220

[a] While the concept of cytoplasmic and nuclear receptors is under revision, the basic concept of induction of receptors remains valid. In the endometrium, estradiol and progesterone receptors increase throughout the proliferative phase. Activated (nuclear) estradiol receptors peak in the late proliferative and early secretory phase, then decrease as receptor levels fall in the secretory phase with the activation of the progesterone-progesterone receptor complex. Progesterone receptors peak at ovulation. Receptor activation (nuclear receptors) then occurs in the secretory phase. Estradiol and progesterone receptors decrease markedly under the influence of progesterone. It is clear from these data that the ideal time to analyze adequacy of progesterone receptor induction is at ovulation. (Reproduced with permission from Edman.[27])

single assay techniques the level of progesterone suggested to represent normal ovulation has increased from 3 ng/ml[17] and 5 ng/ml[18] to 10 mg/ml.[19] Abraham suggested that a more accurate approach would be multiple (3) drawings in the mid-luteal phase with a total above 15ng/ml considered normal.[20] This latter approach is, however, clinically cumbersome and relatively expensive, leading most proponents of progesterone levels to utilize the single draw approach.

Healy, using the rhesus monkey[21], and Crowley, in human beings,[22] have both presented evidence that calls into question the underlying tenet of this approach, i.e., that a single assay is a true reflection of functional progesterone synthesis and therefore corpus luteal function. The pulsatile nature of GnRH while slowed in the luteal phase is still present.[9] This results in a pulsatile release of FSH and LH and, in turn, pulsatile stimulation of corpus luteal cells. Progesterone release could be pulsatile at 2- to 3-hour intervals. Since the half-life of progesterone is much shorter than this, 15 to 20 minutes, serum levels of progesterone might demonstrate considerable variation. This is precisely what Healy and Crowley found. Progesterone varied 2- to 10-fold and in a pulsatile manner (Figure 11–4). Progesterone levels were both above and below the 10ng/ml level most commonly used to diagnose luteal phase defect. It is difficult to reconcile these data on pulsatile progesterone serum levels with the use of a single progesterone assay to diagnose luteal phase defect.

Endometrial biopsy is the "gold standard" for diagnosing dysfunctional ovulation. As noted earlier, the maturation of the endometrium is dependent on both follicular and luteal steroidogenesis. Therefore the endometrial biopsy is, for all practical purposes, a bioassay for cyclic ovarian function. To maximize the usefulness of this test it should be performed on the 12th day of temperature increase, i.e., the 26th day of the ideal 28-day menstrual cycle. Moreover, to make the diagnosis of dysfunctional ovulation (LPD) by endometrial biopsy, the biopsy must be accurately dated histologically. The guidelines for reading endometrial biopsies have changed little since Noyes' lead article in the first issue of Fertility and Sterility in 1950.[23]

The assessment of maturation of the endometrial glands relates primarily to dating of biopsies performed in the first week of the luteal phase and is inadequate for the diagnosis of LPD. The glands initially show a pattern of subnuclear vacuolization, which is actually a collection of secretory granules, on the basal side of the nucleus on days 16 and 17. These secretory elements subsequently move to the luminal side of the nucleus by days 18 and 19. By days 20 and 21 the cells appear "exhausted" but are actually still quite active, with the secretory granules being rapidly released. The glands then show accumulation of secretions in the lumens and irregular infolding. This is the appearance that should be present in an adequately timed biopsy in the second week of the luteal phase.

In vitro studies of estradiol-primed proliferative-phase endometrium have revealed that some of these changes, particularly subnuclear vacuolization, can occur with the withdrawal of estradiol stimulation and in the absence of progesterone (Figure 11–5).[24] This effect of estradiol withdrawal, resulting in early secretory changes in glandular cells, may explain the histologic reading of "early secretory endometrium" in endometrial biopsy or curettage specimens in women who are anovulatory by all other criteria.

An adequately timed endometrial biopsy for the diagnosis of dysfunctional ovulation (LPD) is performed late in the second week of the luteal phase. It is the endometrial stroma that is used to date the adequacy of endometrial maturation. Traditionally, four factors are examined to determine dating based on Noyes' criteria: edema, decidualization, mitosis and infiltration of neutrophils and mononuclear cells. The changes in the degree of mitosis in the stroma are relatively subtle, difficult to assess, and are generally not used in dating. It is not known whether they correlate with impending menses or stromal maturation. The degree of leukocytic and especially neu-

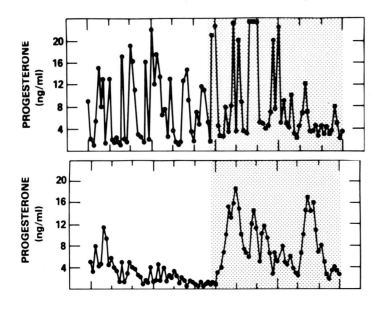

Figure 11–4. Serum levels of progesterone have been found to vary markedly during the day, the variation being consistent with episodic GnRH pulses as 2-3 hour intervals. This variation is pulsatile and probably due to episodic LH release from the pituitary. The variation in progesterone is up to 10-fold and averages 3-5-fold. It is difficult to envision how a single serum progesterone can be used to summarize the luteal phase given this pattern of progesterone levels. (Reproduced from Healy[21] with permission.)

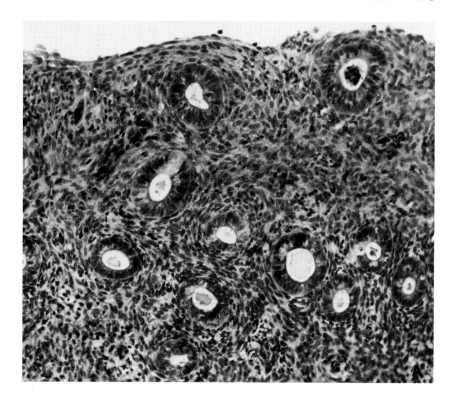

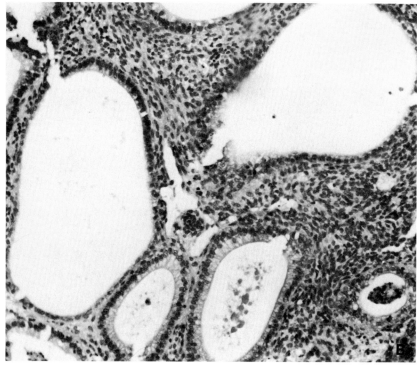

Figure 11–5. A. *In vitro* culture of estrogen-primed late proliferative endometrium in estradiol-containing medium reveals persistence of small glands without secretory activity. B. The culture of the same endometrium in estradiol- and progesterone-free medium reveals glandular secretory activity, although the stromal changes normally associated with secretory endometrium do not occur.

trophilic infiltration should not be used to date endometrial biopsies intended to diagnose LPD since such findings have been demonstrated to correlate more strongly with the occurrence of subsequent menses than with the assessment of endometrial maturation based on the degree of edema and decidualization.[25] Therefore, the dating of biopsies performed in the second week of the luteal phase is based on changes in edema and in the extent of decidualization (Figure 11–6).

Stromal edema changes overlap with the final changes in glandular morphology. Edema increases through days 19 to 20, peaks by days 21 to 22, and gradually resolves through day 25. The term *edema* implies that some osmotic gradient is established that results in an influx of water or that some change occurs in the vasculature of the endometrium leading to an increased loss of fluid into the interstitial space. Both of these possibilities seem unlikely based on the changes observed in *in vitro* deci-

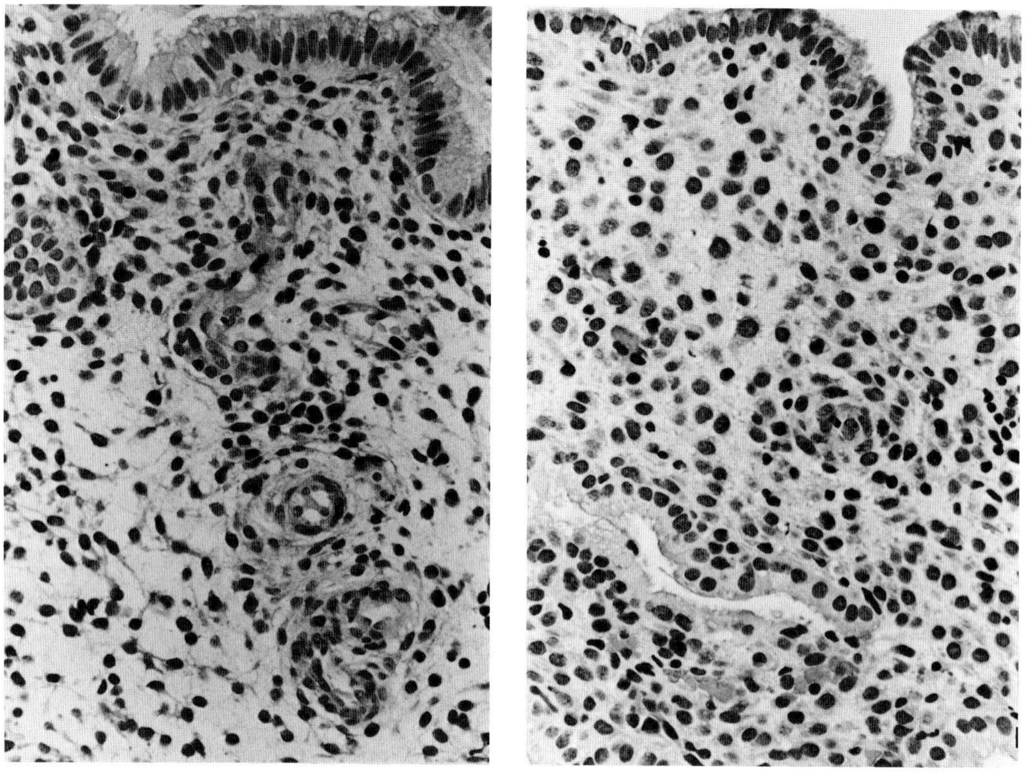

Figure 11–6. A. The changes in the second week of the luteal phase that are important in dating relate to the gradual decidualization of the stroma. This begins around the spiral arteries of the upper endometrium on day 23 and increases to 2 to 4 layers on day 24. At this stage the endometrial stroma is still edematous. B. By day 25 the subepithelial stromal cells are decidualizing and the edema is less apparent as the decidualization around the vessels increases. By days 26 and 27 these areas of decidualization become confluent, the vessels less apparent and the edema less marked (See Figure 11-8B).

dualized explants of proliferative endometrium.[24] These explants, lacking both an intact vasculature and an intact epithelial capsule that could allow for the development of an osmotic gradient, nonetheless undergo an edema stage prior to decidualization (Figure 11–7). It would therefore appear that the edema stage is actually caused by the endometrial stroma cells physically dispersing themselves by their thin cytoplasmic appendages. When viewed as a mechanical event, the edema phase can be seen to merge with the decidualization phase in that the area initially occupied by extracellular fluid during the edema phase is gradually replaced by expanding cytoplasm of the decidualizing stromal cells (i.e. the stromal cells may be making room for their own increase in volume).

It is the development of decidualization that is the final criterion for assessing endometrial maturation. Day 22 is associated with the ability to clearly delineate the terminal spiral arteries in the portion of the endometrium near the surface. The more basal endometrium will demonstrate vascular changes and decidual cuffing when more superficial regions do not. If relied upon for dating, the basal endometrium can give inaccurate impressions and should be avoided. By day 23 a cuff of decidualizing cells with expanding cytoplasm will be present, and by day 24 this cuff will have extended to 2 to 4 cells in thickness. On

day 25 decidual cells begin to appear below the surface epithelium and by days 26 and 27 the regions of decidualization are becoming confluent. The changes of early menstruation begin to disrupt the architecture of the endometrium making assessment of the degree of decidualization difficult or impossible. Therefore, biopsies on the first day of menses should be avoided. Biopsies of the lower uterine segment endometrium, identified by elongated nuclei in the glandular cells and more densely packed spindle-shaped stromal cells, should not be used in making a histologic diagnosis (Figure 11–8) since they do not correlate with the timing of the changes occurring in the fundal endometrium, where pregnancy normally occurs.

Returning to the physiologic model of endometrial maturation, the probable reason for this pattern of decidualization is apparent. Since the estradiol that generates progesterone receptors in the follicular phase and the progesterone that stimulates them in the luteal phase are both delivered via the spiral arteries, it is logical that the stromal cells around the arteries would receive the greatest steroid exposure in both phases. It has been shown that estradiol receptors are more prevalent in gland cells than in stroma cells in general, and this correlates with the more rapid response of these cells to hormonal stimulation.[26] It would also seem logical that, depending on

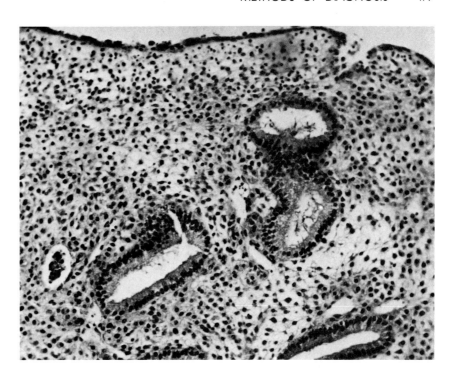

Figure 11–7. Proliferative endometrium decidualized *in vitro* with progesterone reveals the typical patterns of edema and decidualization. The development of edema in this culture, in the absence of either an intact epithelium or vasculature, would suggest that it is probably a result of active mechanical separation of the stromal cells rather than passive separation caused by true edema.

the degree of estradiol and progesterone stimulation in each phase of the cycle, that progression of decidualization might cease or be slowed at any point in the process. Following this rationale, biopsies should be performed only on days 12 ± 1 of the luteal phase if all patients whose decidualization process is inadequate are to be detected. A biopsy performed on day 9 of the luteal phase, for example, would potentially miss a luteal phase defect in a patient whose decidualization proceeded normally to day 9 of the luteal phase (day 23 of the ideal cycle) but then ceased due to inadequate stimulation of the stromal cells distant from the spiral arteries and capillaries.

Prolactin and Decidual Proteins

While the histologic pattern of decidualization is useful for dating endometrium, the relevance of this to implantation and successful pregnancy can still be debated. Evidence for the physiologic importance of decidualization is actually quite sparse and indirect. The most thoroughly studied of the decidual proteins is prolactin and the reason for its presence remains an enigma. However, the pattern of prolactin induction in decidualization does represent a reasonable model for speculation on the importance of decidualization. Other endometrial proteins, including the enzyme hydroxysteroid dehydrogenase, various proteases and lysosomal enzymes, have been studied in normal cycles but not in relation to LPD.[27] Likewise information on the relative activity of prostaglandins in LPD is not available.[28]

Prolactin was first clearly identified in human beings and a radioimmunassay developed in 1971.[29] This was followed shortly after by the demonstration of high prolactin levels in the amniotic fluid of pregnancies and the subsequent demonstration of decidual prolactin synthesis by a number of independent laboratories.[30,31] Riddick demonstrated that prolactin from the decidua was capable of being preferentially transported across the chorioamniotic membrane and was therefore the probable source of amniotic fluid prolactin.[32] Maslar extended the observations on decidual prolactin with evidence of prolactin synthesis during decidualization of the late luteal phase endometrium.[14] This work was extended to reveal that the induction of prolactin synthesis was correlated with decidualization. In biopsies performed in luteal phase deficient cycles, there was, based on histologic appearance, inadequate prolactin synthesis for the ideal menstrual day compared to biopsies from normal cycles (Figure 11–9).[33] This has been confirmed in immunohistochemical analyses which failed to demonstrate the presence of prolactin in LPD specimens. Prolactin was only demonstrated where decidualization had occurred.[34] It is not unreasonable to suspect that other proteins synthesized by decidua would follow a similar pattern and thereby result in an inadequate environment for implantation. Joshi[35] has isolated and studied a glandular protein, PEP, produced in the early secretory endometrium, which is released into the circulation and becomes detectable in the mid-luteal phase. In two patients suspected of having LPD, PEP was not detectable. Joshi suggests that LPD endometrial glandular function may also be suboptimal, at least as reflected in PEP synthesis and release.[35] This assumes that decidual proteins are necessary for implantation as modifiers or stimulants of trophoblastic invasion, or as modifiers of the body's immunologic response to the syncytiotrophoblast. Evidence for this in the human is not available.

Since prolactin synthesis in the endometrium parallels decidualization, the evaluation of prolactin synthesis is a useful model for monitoring endometrial decidualization

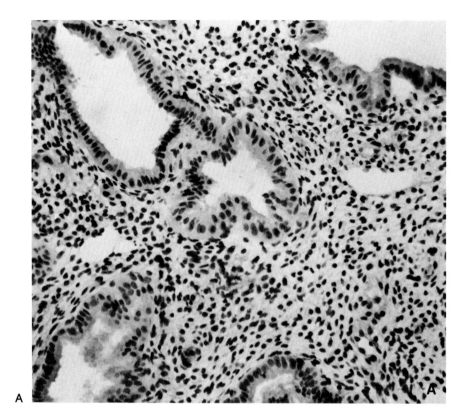

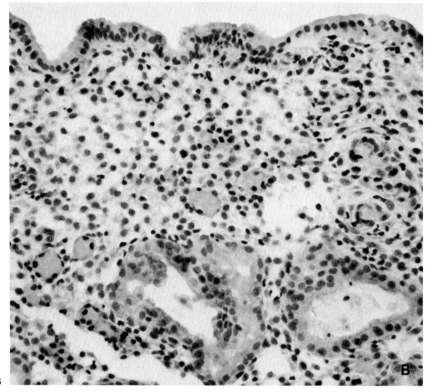

Figure 11–8. A. The lower uterine segment does not go through the same changes as fundal endometrium. The stroma is more densely packed with cells and its edema phase is minimal. The glands, while secretory, have elongated nuclei and narrow cells. B. The fundal endometrium from the same biopsy reveals a normal day 26 pattern of decidualization.

both *in vitro* and *in vivo*. During *in vitro* decidualization of estradiol-primed proliferative endometrium, it has been shown that estradiol slows the decidualization process both physiologically and histologically (Figure 11–10).[24] Preliminary evidence indicates that this effect of estradiol is dose-dependent. The rate of decidualization is positively correlated with progesterone concentration in preliminary dose response studies. In a combination of *in vitro* and *in vivo* studies it has also been shown that when endometrial tissue from patients with LPD was cul-

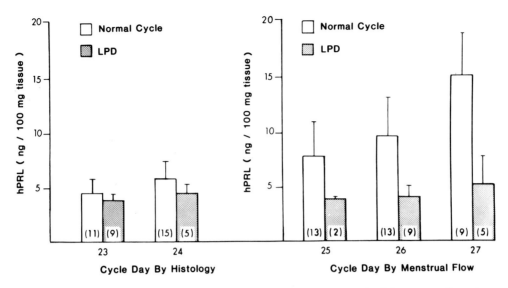

Figure 11–9. Synthesis of human prolactin from endometrial biopsies gradually increases with endometrial maturation. Luteal phase defect endometrium synthesizes normal amounts of prolactin for the histologic day of the cycle but, when compared to the menstrual day, the synthesis is suppressed below normal levels. This would indicate that the physiologic activity of luteal phase defect endometrium is abnormal for the menstrual day. (Reproduced from Daly et al.,[33] with permission.)

tured with progesterone only some of the samples responded with accelerating prolactin synthesis (Figure 11–11).[36] Further, when endometrial samples from patients undergoing treatment for luteal phase defect and whose biopsy specimens were corrected *in vivo* were subjected to *in vitro* studies, the prolactin synthesis from these samples was normal.[37] The first observation indicates that not all endometrium is functionally capable of responding to progesterone with complete decidualiza-

tion, presumably because of a lack of functional progesterone receptors. This observation would predict that some patients will require treatment with medications to improve the follicular phase. Attempts to measure progesterone receptors in the late luteal phase are complicated by the low levels of receptors that exist even in normal endometrium by the late luteal phase, and results for these studies are in conflict.[38,39,40] To truly assess whether progesterone receptor induction has been adequate, the assessment of receptor concentration should be done at ovulation. However, in an infertility population, biopsies at mid-cycle are not indicated for diagnostic or therapeutic reasons at the present time and this information is not now available. The second observation strongly links histologic correction of LPD with physiologic correction of endometrial function.

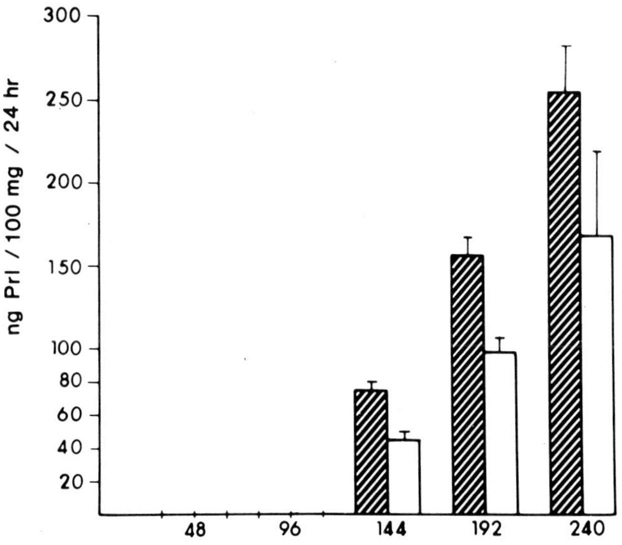

Figure 11–10. Proliferative endometrium decidualizes *in vitro* when progesterone (20 ng/ml) alone is added to the culture (hatched bars). When progesterone (20 ng/ml) and estradiol (200 pg/ml) are added, the rate of decidualization is slowed and prolactin synthesis is comparatively suppressed (open bars). (Reproduced from Daly et al.,[24] with permission.)

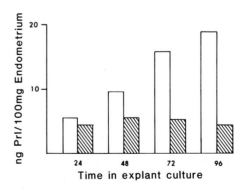

Figure 11–11. The *in vitro* culturing of day 12 post-ovulation endometrial biopsies demonstrating luteal phase defect changes reveals that some specimens complete decidualization and increase prolactin synthesis (open bars) while other specimens do not complete decidualization, and prolactin synthesis is static (hatched bars). (Reproduced from Daly et al.,[36] with permission.)

TREATMENT

Diagnosis of luteal phase defect requires demonstration of the abnormality in at least 2 cycles, preferably based on endometrial biopsy criteria. Treatment has traditionally been with either progesterone suppositories, 25mg BID, or with clomiphene citrate. There has been a tendency

for clinicians who utilize endometrial biopsy evaluation to treat with progesterone suppositories, while those clinicians utilizing serum progesterone levels for diagnosis tend to treat with clomiphene. The results of these therapies reported in the literature reveal an amazingly consistent pregnancy rate of about 50%.[19,41–45] This success rate has changed little over time. To help define why half the

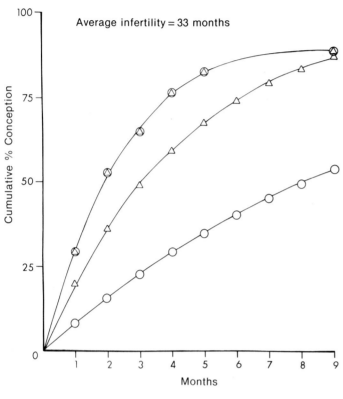

A

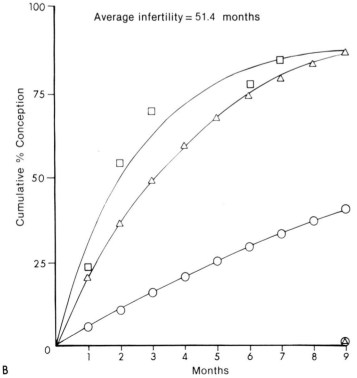

B

Figure 11–12. Our standard treatment for LPD has been progesterone suppositories. A. Progesterone responders. In patients who correct their biopsies on progesterone (△-△), the conception rate is comparable to a theoretical normal population (Δ-Δ) and significantly better than would be anticipated in a group of patients with 33 months of infertility (O-O). B. Progesterone nonresponders. Those who did not correct did not conceive until treated with a variety of ovulation induction techniques and correction accomplished (□-□). The conception rate was then comparable to the normal population. (Reproduced with permission from Daly *et al.*[46])

patients failed to conceive and to try to improve overall conception rates, a sequential treatment protocol was formulated and all patients diagnosed as having LPD, based on adequately timed biopsies, entered into the protocol.[46]

Protocol

1. Diagnosis based on 2 abnormal biopsy cycles
2. Serum prolactin, thyroid function, and DHEA-S
3. Patients with abnormal prolactin were treated with bromocriptine (16%). Patients with abnormal thyroid were treated with Synthroid (2%).
4. The remainder of patients were treated by a sequential protocol with a biopsy performed at each treatment and therapy continued for 6 months, regardless of the outcome of the biopsy. (Two patients did conceive prior to the biopsy.)
   A. Progesterone suppositories 25mg BID
   B. Clomiphene 50mg days 5-9
   C. Addition of dexamethasone or progesterone to clomiphene if biopsy or serum DHEA-S indicated
   D. Low-dose pergonal 1 amp IM days 6-11
   E. Full-dose pergonal by standard protocols

With this protocol it was found that no single therapy was effective for all patients. Sixteen percent of the patients were found to have elevated prolactin. These patients showed improvement in their biopsies and eventually conceived when treated with bromocriptine. This agrees with other studies showing elevated prolactin as a cause of LPD.[47] Approximately half of the patients failed to respond to progesterone supplementation with correction of their biopsy findings and none of these patients had viable pregnancies. However, in the patients with correction of their biopsy specimens, the conception rate based on life table analysis was nearly identical to a theoretical normal population (Figure 11–12). This pat-

tern of endometrial biopsy correction and conception was seen in each treatment group through low-dose pergonal. When the patients as a whole were analyzed by life table statistics based on the conception rate after correction of the biopsy, regardless of the therapy, the results revealed a fecundability similar to a normal population and a projected pregnancy rate of 80% at 6 months of treatment. Since few dropouts occurred in the study, over 75% of couples conceived within 6 months of correction of the LPD based on biopsy results, a rate significantly higher than in any of the single therapy protocols.

The failure of half the patients to respond to treatment with progesterone suppositories would be anticipated by the theoretical model previously constructed. This model predicted that in a proportion of patients, the quality of follicular development would be inadequate for the induction of decidualization in the endometrium when it was exposed to progesterone in the luteal phase, or the quality of follicular development would be inadequate for actual physical ovulation to occur—the LUFS syndrome (luteinized unruptured follicle syndrome). The former concept is supported by the failure of the endometrium of some patients to respond to progesterone both *in vivo* and *in vitro*.[36,37] To assess the latter possibility subsequent patients with a diagnosis of LPD underwent serial ultrasound tests to determine the growth pattern of the follicle and whether rupture of the follicle occurs (Figure 11–13). The incidence of LUFS in an apparently normally ovulating population has been reported as 4.9%.[48] In patients with unexplained infertility the incidence was 9%, with half of the cases being nonrecurrent.[49] Another 9% of these patients had follicular growth patterns that varied significantly from the normal (Figure 11–14). Prospective ultrasound data in patients with diagnosed LPD indicate that 10% to 30% of LPD patients also demonstrate a LUFS pattern and another 20% to 40% have an abnormal growth pattern.[50,51] Certainly the patients with LUFS cannot respond to proges-

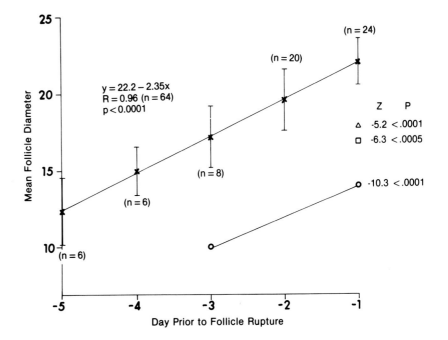

Figure 11–13. For a specified population and ultrasound machine, a follicular growth curve can be generated and an expected follicular size at ovulation estimated. Some follicles rupture at smaller size. This occurs more commonly in luteal phase defects. It appears that a minimal follicle size of 16 mm to 18 mm (depending on the machine) is required for an ovulation to result in a viable conception. (Reproduced with permission from Daly et al.[49])

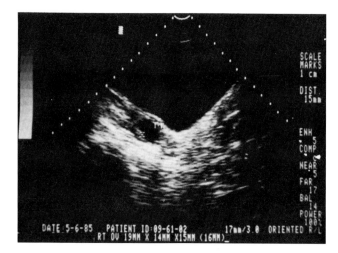

Figure 11–14. This follicle measures 19 × 14 × 15, mean diameter 16 mm. The following day the BBT was elevated and the follicle had ruptured at an abnormally small size. The patient had been diagnosed as having LPD and did not respond to progesterone suppositories.

terone suppositories with conception. Since nearly all the patients who showed improvement in their biopsies with progesterone conceived, it seems likely that many of the progesterone non-responders have follicular development that is so inadequate that not only is the endometrium inadequately prepared to respond to progesterone but ovulation is absent as well. The other progesterone non-responders may consist of patients whose follicular growth was less than adequate, but in whom follicular rupture did occur. Whether normal ovum maturation occurs in such patients is unknown. It seems probable that these patients would be more likely to conceive on clomiphene or other ovulation induction medications.

TYPES OF LUTEAL PHASE DEFECT

It is now possible to hypothesize several varieties of dysfunctional ovulation based on two determinants: 1. Has adequate estradiol stimulation of the endometrium occurred in the follicular phase to allow correction of LPD with the addition of progesterone? 2. Has the development of the dominant follicle demonstrated a normal growth pattern and has physical ovulation occurred? With these two determinants in mind, an effective protocol for the diagnosis and treatment of dysfunctional ovulation can be devised.

After an ovulatory pattern has been demonstrated by BBT, after a major male factor has been eliminated by semen analysis, and after a post-coital test is normal:

1. An endometrial biopsy is performed on the 12th day ± 1 of temperature elevation based on BBT. If the biopsy is normal then dysfunctional ovulation has been ruled out.

2. If abnormal, then the patient is scheduled for serial ultrasound tests during the ovulatory period to deter-

mine the growth pattern of the follicle and the presence or absence of physical ovulation (LUFS). (Serial ultrasound testing may also be done at the time of the post-coital test and, if already performed and normal, would not be repeated.)

If a LUFS is demonstrated than this second cycle would be considered abnormal and a second biopsy deemed unnecessary. Since physical ovulation is not occurring, the treatment of choice would be the same as if the patient were anovulatory. Serum prolactin, thyroid function, and DHEA-S are assessed and the patient is started on whatever medication is indicated by this screen.

3. If LUFS is excluded, an endometrial biopsy would be performed in this second cycle. If abnormal, then the diagnosis of LPD without LUFS would be made and, again, after excluding an abnormality of prolactin, thyroid, or adrenal androgen function, the patient would be started on therapy, although this time progesterone suppositories would be the treatment of choice. (Under ideal circumstances this second biopsy could also be sent for *in vitro* culture to determine whether it responds to progesterone stimulation.)

By this protocol two groups of patients are defined: 1. LPD without physical ovulation or with abnormal follicle development, which is treated like anovulation, and 2. LPD with normal follicle development and physical ovulation, which is initially treated with progesterone suppositories. However, regardless of the initial therapy, it is necessary to confirm by endometrial biopsy that correction of the luteal phase defect has occurred on therapy. This protocol should allow for maximum efficiency of diagnosis and treatment of dysfunctional ovulation within our current knowledge limitations.

References

1. Jones GES: Some newer aspects of management of infertility. JAMA 141:1123, 1949.
2. Speroff L, Glass RH, Kase NG: Investigation of the infertile couple. *In* Clinical Gynecologic Endocrinology and Infertility, 3rd Ed. Baltimore Williams and Wilkins, 1983.
3. Green JD, Harris GW: The neurovascular link between the neurohypophysis and adenohypophysis. J Endocrinology 5:136–146, 1947.
4. Knobil E, Plant TM, Wildt L, et al.: Control of the rhesus monkey menstrual cycle: permissive role of hypothalamic gonadotropic releasing hormone (GnRH). Science 207:1371–1373, 1980.
5. Wildt L, Hausler A, Marshall G, et al.: Frequency and amplitude of gonadotropin-releasing hormone stimulation and gonadotropic secretion in the rhesus monkey. Endocrinology 109:376, 1981.
6. Norman RL, Gliessman P, Lindstrom SA, et al.: Reinitiation of ovulatory cycles in pituitary-stable-sectional rhesus macaques, evidence for a specific hypothalamic message for the preovulatory release of luteinizing hormone. Endocrinology 111:1874, 1982.
7. Klibanski A, Beitins IZ, Merriam GR, et al.: Gonadatropin and prolactin pulsations in hyperprolactinemic women be-

fore and during bromcriptase therapy. J Clin Endocrinol Metab 58:1141–1147, 1984.

8. Reame NE, Sauder SE, Case GD, et al.: Reduced GnRH pulse frequency in hypothalamic amenorrhea: a cause for absent cyclicity. Program of the 65th Annual Meeting of the Endocrine Society. San Antonio, Texas, p. 110 (Abstr 117) 1983.

9. Reame N, Sauder SE, Kelch RP et al.: Pulsatile gonadotropin secretion during the human menstrual cycle: evidence for altered frequency of gonadotropin releasing hormone secretion. J Clin Endocrinol Metab 59:328–337, 1984.

10. Crowley WF, McArthur JW: Stimulation of the normal menstrual cycle in Kallmann's syndrome by pulsatile administration of luteinizing hormone releasing hormone (LHRH). J Clin Endocrinol Metab 51:173, 1980.

11. Chang RJ, Mandel FP, Lu JK, et al.: Enhanced disparity of gonadotropin secretion by estrone in women with polycystic ovarian disease. J Clin Endocrinol Metab 54:490, 1982.

12. Lasley BL, Wang CF, Yen SSC.: The effects of estrogen and progesterone on the functional capacity of the gonadotropin. J Clin Endocrinol Metab 41:820–826, 1975.

13. Stouffer RL, Hodgen GD: Inductional luteal phase defects in rhesus monkeys by follicular fluid administration at the onset of the menstrual cycle. J Clin Endocrinol Metab 51:669, 1980.

14. Maslar IA, Riddick DH: Prolactin production by human endometrium during the normal menstrual cycle. Am J Obstet Gynecol 135:751, 1979.

15. Bayard F, Damilano S, Robel P, et al.: Cytoplasmic and nuclear estradiol and progesterone receptors in human endometrium. J Clin Endocrinol Metab 46:635, 1978.

16. Gallagher TF, Bradlaw HL, Fukusheina DK: Studies of the metabolites of isotopic steroid hormones in man. Recent Prog Horm Res 9:411, 1954.

17. Israel R, Mishell DR, Stone SC, et al.: Single luteal phase serum progesterone assay as an indicator of ovulation. Am J Obstet Gynecol 112:1043, 1972.

18. Ross GT, Cargille CM, Lipsett MD, et al.: Pituitary and gonadal hormones in women during spontaneous and induced ovulatory cycles. Recent Prog Horm Res 26:1, 1970.

19. Radwanska E, Swyer GI: Plasma progesterone estimation in infertile women and in women under treatment with clomiphene and chorionic gonadotropin. J Obstet Gynaecol Br Common 81:107, 1974.

20. Abraham GE, Maroulis GB, Marshall JR: Evaluation of ovulation and corpus luteal function, using measurement of plasma progesterone. Obstet Gynecol 44:522, 1974.

21. Healy DL, Schenken RS, Lynch A, et al.: Pulsatile progesterone secretion: its relevance to clinical evaluational of corpus luteum function. Fertil Steril 41:114, 1984.

22. Filicosi M, Butler JP, Crowley WF: Neuroendocrine regulation of the corpus luteum in the human. Evidence for pulsatile progesterone secretion. J Clin Invest 73:1638, 1984.

23. Noyes RW, Hertig A, Rock J: Dating the endometrial biopsy. Fertil Steril 1:3, 1950.

24. Daly DC, Maslar IA, Riddick DH: Prolactin production during in vitro decidualization of proliferative endometrium. Am J Obstet Gynecol 145:672–678, 1983.

25. Daly DC, Tohan N, Doney TJ, et al.: The significance of lymphocytic-leukocytic infiltrates in interpreting late luteal phase endometrial biopsies. Fertil Steril 37:786, 1982.

26. Press MF, Nousek-Goebl N, King WJ, et al.: Immunohistochemical assessment of estrogen receptor distribution in the human endometrium throughout the menstrual cycle. Lab Invest 51:495, 1984.

27. Edman CD.: The effects of steroids on the endometrium. Semin Reprod Endocrinol 1:179–188, 1983.

28. Schwarz BE.: The production and biologic effects of uterine prostaglandins. Semin Reprod Endocrinol 1:189–195, 1983.

29. Hwang P, Guyda H, Friesen H: A radio-immunoassay for human prolactin. Proc Natl Acad Sci USA 68:1902–1906, 1971.

30. Riddick DH, Luciano AA, Kusmik WF, et al.: De novo synthesis of prolactin by human decidua. Life Sci 23:1913, 1978.

31. Healy DL, Kimpton WG, Muller HK, et al.: The synthesis of immunoreactive prolactin by decidua-chorion. Br J Obstet Gynaecol 86:307, 1979.

32. Riddick DH, Maslar IA: The transport of prolactin by human fetal membranes. J Clin Endocrinol Metab 52:220, 1981.

33. Daly DC, Maslar IA, Rosenberg SM, et al.: Prolactin production by luteal phase defect endometrium. Am J Obstet Gynecol 140:587, 1981.

34. Kauma SW, Shapiro SS: Immunoperoxidase localization of prolactin in human endometrium during normal menstrual cycles and luteal phase defect cycles. 41st Annual Meeting of the American Fertil Society. Chicago, (Abstr 73) 1985.

35. Joshi, SG. Progestin-regulated proteins of the human endometrium. Semin Reprod Endocrinol. 1:221–236, 1983.

36. Daly DC: The endometrium and the luteal phase defect. Semin Reprod Endocrinol 1:237–43, 1983.

37. Ying YK, Walters CA, Kuslis S, et al.: Prolactin production by explants of normal, luteal phase defective, and corrected luteal phase defective late secretory endometrium. Am J Obstet Gynecol 151:801–804, 1985.

38. Levy C, Robel P, Gautray JP, et al.: Estradiol and progesterone receptors in human endometrium: normal and abnormal menstrual cycles and early pregnancy. Am J Obstet Gynecol 136:646, 1980.

39. Gravanis A, Zorn JR, Tanguy G, et al.: The "dysharmonic luteal phase" syndrome: endometrial progesterone receptor and estradiol dehydrogenase. Fertil Steril 42:730–735, 1984.

40. Chong A, Daly DC, Riddick D, et al.: Cytoplasmic estradiol and progesterone receptors in human endometrium: their possible clinical use in luteal phase deficiency. Society for Gynecologic Investigation. Phoenix AZ, (Abstr 261T) 1985.

41. Rosenberg SM, Luciano AA, Riddick DH: The luteal phase defect—the relative frequency of an encouraging response to treatment with vaginal progesterone. Fertil Steril 34:17, 1980.

42. Wentz AC, Herbert CM, Maxson WS, et al.: Outcome of progesterone therapy of luteal phase inadequacy. Fertil Steril 41:856, 1984.

43. Hammond MG, Talbert LM: Clomiphene citrate therapy of infertile women with low luteal phase progesterone levels. Obstet Gynecol 59:275, 1982.

44. Downs KA, Gibson M: Clomiphene citrate therapy for luteal phase defects. Fertil Steril 39:34, 1983.

45. Soules MR, Wiebe RH, Aksel S, et al.: The diagnosis and therapy of luteal phase deficiency. Fertil Steril 28:1033, 1977.

46. Daly DC, Walters CA, Soto-Albors CE, et al.: Endometrial biopsy during treatment of luteal phase defects is predictive of therapeutic outcome. Fertil Steril 40:305–10, 1983.

47. Del Pozo E, Wyss H, Tollis G, et al.: Prolactin and deficient luteal function. Obstet Gynecol 53:282, 1979.

48. Kerin JF, Kirby C, Morris D, *et al.*: Incidence of the luteinized unruptured follicle phenomenon in cycling women. Fertil Steril 40:620, 1983.

49. Daly DC, Soto-Albors C, Walters C, *et al.*: Ultrasonographic assessment of luteinized unruptured follicle syndrome in unexplained infertility. Fertil Steril 43:62–65, 1985.

50. Ying YK, Randolf JF, Daly DC, *et al.*: Ultrasonic monitoring of folliculogenesis for luteal phase defect. American Fertility Society. Chicago, IL, (Abstr. 46) 1985.

51. Check JH, Goldberg BB, Kurtz A, *et al.*: Pelvic sonography to help determine the appropriate therapy for luteal phase defects. Int J Fertil 29:156–158, 1984.

12. Hypothalamic–Pituitary Abnormalities in Ovulatory Disorders

K. Kovacs and E. Horvath

Ovulation plays a fundamental role in keeping the human species alive. Superficially, it appears to represent a single event which is easy to perceive. However, in fact it is a complicated process which requires the complex interaction of several hormones and nonhormonal mechanisms. The study of ovulation has attracted the energy and imagination of the best scientists; although they invested unlimited time, effort and talent to shed light on the various aspects of the ovulatory process, it happened only in the last two decades that a deeper insight has been achieved on the regulatory machinery leading to ovulation and the various abnormalities affecting the normal sequence of events. The introduction of several sensitive and sophisticated methods resulted in unprecedented progress in this area of research and allowed for a better understanding of fertility and infertility, the menstrual cycle and ovulation—a prerequisite of human reproduction.

This chapter focuses on the disorders of ovulation, especially disturbances of hypothalamic-pituitary function which interfere with the physiologic regulation. Before discussing the pathology, the current knowledge on the physiology of the menstrual cycle and ovulation will be summarized briefly. One should keep in mind that there are several abnormalities which affect ovulation independent of or only secondarily involving the activity of the hypothalamus and pituitary.

PHYSIOLOGY

In describing the physiology of menstruation and ovulation, the excellent textbook of Wilson *et al.*[1] is used as a guideline. The menstrual cycle, pivotal event in the life of women in the reproductive age, can be divided into two phases: 1. follicular or proliferative phase, 2. luteal or secretory phase. The actual menstruation is the cyclic discharge of blood and portions of disintegrating endometrium from the uterus to the vagina. The follicular phase begins with commencement of menstrual bleeding and ends with ovulation. The luteal phase begins following ovulation and lasts until the onset of menstruation.

The normal menstrual cycle depends primarily on the synchronized interaction of the hypothalamus, anterior pituitary, and ovaries. These three endocrine tissues form the hypothalamic-hypophysial-ovarian axis. The hypothalamic-hypophysial regulation of gonadal function and the causes of ovulatory disorders were dealt with in detail in several recent publications.[2–12]

Certain specialized neurons of the hypothalamus synthesize gonadotrophin-releasing hormone (GnRH, LRH or LHRH). This decapeptide is discharged from the nerve cells, is transported along the nerve fibers to the capillary plexus of the median eminence, enters the portal vessels, is carried via the hypophysial stalk to the anterior pituitary, and stimulates pituitary gonadotrophs, evoking FSH and LH release. According to current knowledge, only one gonadotrophin-releasing hormone is produced in the hypothalamus: GnRH which releases both FSH and LH. Immunocytologic, biochemical, electron microscopic, and tissue culture studies conclusively prove that the two gonadotroph hormones are synthesized and stored in one single cell type: the gonadotroph or FSH/LH-producing cell. The gonadotrophs are medium-sized, oval, or irregular basophilic cells, with PAS positive cytoplasmic secretory granules. They are located throughout the entire anterior lobe, often in close proximity to prolactin cells. Electron microscopy demonstrates that gonadotroph cells have all the organelles required for hormone secretion; they possess well-developed rough endoplasmic reticulum membranes, conspicuous Golgi complexes, and membrane-bound, spherical secretory granules varying slightly in electron density and measuring 100-350 nm in their largest diameter. Although the majority of gonadotroph cells produce two hormones, some contain only FSH or LH. Whether this means that these cells are in a different secretory phase, or that specific subclones of gonadotrophs exist which are capable of synthesizing only FSH or LH remains to be elucidated.

The two gonadotroph hormones stimulate the ovary. FSH induces growth and maturation of follicles whereas LH causes ovulation and luteinization. FSH and LH are not released steadily from the pituitary but in a cyclic and pulsatile fashion.[13]

This work was supported in part by Grant MT-6349 awarded by the Medical Research Council of Canada. The authors wish to thank Mrs. G. Ilse, Mrs. N. Losinski, and Mrs. N. Ryan for their contribution in the morphologic studies, and Mrs. W. Wlodarski for secretarial work.

Estrogen secreted by the ovary has a multiple function in the entire ovulatory process. Estradiol, the principal estrogen, exerts a negative feedback effect on the hypothalamus and anterior pituitary. The low estrogen concentrations, during the first few days of the menstrual period, elicit the secretion of GnRH and subsequently FSH-LH which stimulate follicular growth and estrogen synthesis. In addition to their effect on the hypothalamus and anterior pituitary, estrogens play a role in follicular maturation by increasing FSH binding to receptors within the granulosa cell, as well as the sensitivity of the follicle to FSH. Estrogen concentrations gradually rise during the follicular phase, reaching the maximum before ovulation. The elevated estrogen levels inhibit FSH secretion by blocking the discharge of GnRH from the hypothalamus and evoke the mid-cycle surge of LH to induce ovulation. Following ovulation, the secretion of LH and estrogens continues at a lower level, whereas secretion of progesterone increases markedly, concurrent with a slight rise in estrogen production. High blood levels of these hormones are maintained until about days 23-24 of the menstrual cycle. At that point, the corpus luteum begins to regress if the ovum remains unfertilized. The loss of hormone support to the endometrium is followed by its disintegration and menstrual bleeding. The low concentrations of ovarian hormones stimulate the hypothalamus and the anterior pituitary and a new menstrual cycle begins.

Estrogens are synthesized in the cells of the maturing follicle and theca interna, and progesterone in the granulosa cells.[14] The theca cells use progesterone as a precursor for estrogen synthesis during the first half of the menstrual cycle. During the second half, the corpus luteum cells mainly produce progesterone and, to a lesser extent, estrogens. Blood progesterone levels peak approximately 7 days after ovulation. The main effects of progesterone are the induction of secretory activity in the endometrial glands, decidualization of the endometrial stromal cells, the preparation of a suitable site for nidation of the fertilized ovum and the inhibition of LH secretion. The discussion of other effects of progesterone is beyond the scope of this review.

The so-called third gonadotroph hormone, prolactin or lactotroph hormone or mammotroph hormone acts mainly on the mammary gland. It has been claimed that prolactin is involved in the preservation of the corpus luteum.[15] This suggestion, however, has not been proved conclusively, and it appears that prolactin has no major role in the regulation of human ovarian function. Prolactin secretion is inhibited by the hypothalamus. Dopamine, synthesized in the hypothalamus and transported to the anterior pituitary by the portal circulation, is the main prolactin-inhibiting factor. TRH and estrogens, on the other hand, stimulate prolactin release. Whereas FSH and LH are produced in basophilic, PAS-positive gonadotrophs, prolactin is synthesized in a different adenohypophysial cell type, the prolactin cells or lactotrophs or mammotrophs. These cells, depending on the size and number of cytoplasmic secretory granules, are slightly or strongly acidophilic and PAS negative. They are usually small, angular, or irregular cells, distributed throughout the anterior lobe; they show positive staining with Herlant's erythrosin as well as Brookes' carmoisin; the most conclusive procedure which identifies them is the immunoperoxidase method. By immunocytologic techniques, applying antiprolactin as specific antiserum, prolactin can be localized convincingly in the cytoplasm of prolactin cells.

Ovulation is the rupture of the mature follicle and the release of the ovum. Due to the effect of FSH, a group of follicles begins to enlarge in the ovary. These growing follicles secrete some estrogen which is needed to produce a mature follicle in every cycle. At the preovulatory phase, estrogen binding to granulosa cells and FSH sensitivity are increased. The remaining follicles regress and become atretic. In the gradually maturing follicle, the granulosa cell lining becomes cuboidal and multilayered, and a central cavity is formed which is filled with the liquor folliculi. The ovum is in the central cavity. When the follicle is matured, the LH surge causes its rupture, with the discharge of the ovum from the central cavity and opening up capillary lumina leading to bleeding. The spilled follicular fluid is replaced by blood and a hemorrhagic follicle is formed. Due to continuous LH action, the granulosa cells soon undergo luteinization, resulting in the formation of the corpus luteum. The corpus luteum continues to grow and produce hormones until about day 23-24 of the menstrual cycle, when it starts to regress. If the discharged ovum becomes fertilized, no regression of corpus luteum occurs. During the preovulatory phase, the theca cells of the growing follicles secrete increasing quantities of estrogen. After ovulation, the cells lining the hemorrhagic follicle and the corpus luteum continue to produce estrogen and increasing amounts of progesterone. When the corpus luteum regresses, estrogen and progesterone secretion is sharply reduced, leading to menstruation, and the commencement of a new cycle. The suggested mechanisms responsible for menstrual bleeding and the uterine changes will not be dealt with here.

PATHOLOGY

Anovulation, the absence of ovulation, can be associated with bleeding or amenorrhea.[16-18] Anovulatory bleeding refers to the occurrence of cyclic uterine hemorrhage which is not preceded by ovulation and formation of corpus luteum. The bleeding occurs in response to a reduction or relative decrease in circulating estrogen; it may be regular or irregular, short or long, slight or excessive. If estrogen concentrations are steady, amenorrhea results.

The underlying causes for anovulation are numerous. Besides pregnancy and lactation, anovulation is most frequently due to an imbalance in the functional activity of the hypothalamic-pituitary-ovarian axis. The circulating estrogen levels are regarded as important factors. If estrogen concentrations do not drop sufficiently in the postmenstrual period, their negative feedback effect on the hypothalamus and pituitary will suppress FSH secretion.

An estrogen peak at midcycle provides the positive feedback effect for the LH surge necessary to induce ovulation.

Anovulation often occurs around the beginning and end of reproductive life. The adolescent girl may have regular menstrual periods without ovulation. Similarly, anovulatory cycles may be common in women approaching the menopause. A frequent cause of anovulation is extragonadal estrogen production. Obesity may cause a rise in estrogen concentrations; the accumulating fatty tissue can convert androstenedion to estron. Stressful situations may increase the secretion of adrenocortical estrogen and estrogen precursors. Liver damage may interfere with intrahepatic metabolism of estrogen and lead to an increase in blood estrogen levels. Primary diseases of the ovary may affect the growth, maturation, or rupture of the follicle and cause anovulation. Since this chapter focuses on the abnormalities of the hypothalamus and pituitary, only those disease will be dealt with which primarily affect the functional activity of the hypothalamic-pituitary axis.

A common cause of anovulation is a disturbance in the secretion of pituitary FSH and LH. The finding of low serum FSH-LH values associated with primary or secondary amenorrhea strongly suggests that the primary site of the disease lies either in the hypothalamus or the anterior pituitary, or both. Major advances in diagnostic techniques recently have made it possible to distinguish between primary hypothalamic and primary pituitary abnormalities. Sophisticated imaging techniques may also be helpful in localizing the primary site of the lesion.

There are two types of hypothalamic-hypophysial involvements—functional and organic.

In functional hypothalamic-hypophysial disorders, morphologic techniques fail to reveal any conclusive lesion. Various situations, such as stressful conditions, psychosis, anorexia nervosa, malnutrition, obesity, strenuous exercise, severe illness, systemic disease, etc., may lead to abnormal function of the hypothalamus-pituitary axis.[19-25] Among long-distance runners, ballet dancers, anovulation and amenorrhea are not uncommon. The mechanism responsible for disturbed hypothalamic-pituitary function in these women is still not completely understood and more work is required to shed light on the causes which account for the development of ovulatory disorders. Administration of several drugs can result in anovulation and amenorrhea. These drugs will not be listed and their mechanism of action will not be discussed. Non-endocrine diseases, perhaps by interfering with intermediary estrogen metabolism or the synthesis of GnRH, may lead secondarily to dysfunction of the hypothalamus-pituitary axis and, subsequently, anovulation and amenorrhea.

Several organic diseases, affecting the hypothalamus-pituitary stalk or adenohypophysis can be associated with menstrual and ovulatory disorders.[26-29] It should be emphasized that, unrelated to the morphologic findings, every disease which destroys a large area of the hypothalamic production site of GnRH or interferes with its release and its transport to the pituitary can cause anovulation and amenorrhea. Clinically, similar endocrine changes may become manifest in patients with primary damage of the adenohypophysis. In these cases, the loss of FSH-LH-producing pituitary gonadotrophs makes FSH-LH secretion impossible. Disorders involving primarily the hypothalamus can be distinguished from those of the pituitary, since in women with diseases located in the hypothalamus, a normal number of gonadotrophs is present in the pituitary, and administration of GnRH can cause a rise in blood FSH-LH.[30,31] However, in abnormalities of hypophysial origin, the gonadotrophs capable of releasing FSH-LH are lost and GnRH cannot cause an elevation in blood FSH-LH levels. The low blood FSH-LH concentrations in patients with hypothalamic or pituitary hypogonadism is in sharp contrast to those seen in patients with primary hypogonadism, the cause of which resides in the ovary. In patients with primary hypogonadism, because of lack of negative feedback effect of ovarian steroids, blood FSH-LH levels are abnormally high.

The hypothalamus can be affected by several diseases which may impair the production site of GnRH, cause loss of GnRH secretion and, subsequently, anovulation or amenorrhea.[32] Various inflammatory processes, granulomas, tuberculosis, sarcoidosis, histiocytosis X several primary and secondary neoplasms may lead to GnRH deficiency.[33-35] In cases of Kallmann's syndrome, which may develop not only in men but also in women, amenorrhea, hypogonadism, and anosmia are the leading alterations.[36-39] The cause of this rare disease is the defective development of those areas of the hypothalamus which regulate FSH-LH secretion and account for the sense of smell.

Compression, destruction, and interruption of the pituitary stalk blocks the delivery of GnRH from the hypothalamus or median eminence to the anterior pituitary. The loss of stimulation of pituitary gonadotrophs results in a decrease of FSH and LH release and subsequent anovulation and amenorrhea. Several organic diseases, such as inflammation, granulomas, tumors, and surgical intervention can interrupt the hypophysial stalk and the transport of GnRH to the anterior pituitary, bringing about hypogonadotrophinism.

The anterior lobe can be the target of several diseases which damage FSH-LH-producing cells. It is obvious that the loss of a large portion of the anterior lobe causes a reduction in the secretion of FSH-LH. The reserve capacity of the anterior pituitary is remarkable. If 50% of the anterior lobe is lost, no conspicuous endocrine symptoms develop. At least 90–95% of the adenohypophysis must be impaired before symptoms of severe hypopituitarism become clinically manifest.

Circulatory disturbances can result in the development of large adenohypophysial infarcts which can cause hypopituitarism including various degrees of hypogonadotrophinism.[40] In Sheehan's syndrome, about the time of delivery, circulation is arrested in the vessels supplying the pituitary with blood. Depending on the extent and duration of ischemia, portions of the anterior lobe undergo infarction.[41,42] The pathogenesis of ischemia is not clear; embolism, thrombosis, intravascular coagulation, platelet aggregation, vascular compression, and vasospasm have been suggested to account for the arrest of blood flow to the pituitary.[43] During pregnancy, the pituitary gradually enlarges and the adenohypophysial cells may be more sensitive to hypoxia, or the vessels supplying the anterior pituitary with blood may become more susceptible to develop spasm. In severe cases large areas of the anterior lobe undergo ischemic necrosis. Since adenohypophysial cells are not capable of sufficient regeneration, the cells lost during the ischemic period will not be substituted. The necrotic area is gradually replaced by connective tissue which shrinks and becomes a fibrous scar. In patients with Sheehan's syndrome, if the initial vascular catastrophe is sufficiently extensive, various degrees of hypopituitarism ensue.

Inflammatory processes, abscesses, and granulomas can damage large areas of the pituitary gland.[44-50] Tuberculosis, syphilis, various fungal, bacterial, and parasitic diseases, giant cell granulomas, sarcoidosis, and histiocytosis X can be located in the pituitary.[49,51] In these diseases the hypothalamus is often involved and the reduction of FSH-LH production is due rather to decreased secretion of GnRH than to mechanical injury and unresponsiveness of the anterior lobe.

Lymphocytic hypophysitis is an uncommon disease which has created considerable interest recently.[52-59] The lesion is morphologically similar to that seen in autoimmune diseases of other endocrine glands, such as the thyroid, adrenal cortex, or testis. In the anterior lobe, a massive cellular infiltrate can be detected which is composed mainly of lymphocytes, plasma cells, and macrophages. The adenohypophysial cells are gradually destroyed and replaced by inflammatory exudate and subsequently by fibrous scar. Lymphocytic hypophysitis can lead to various degrees of hypopituitarism, including anovulation and amenorrhea. It is noteworthy that most of the cases which have been described so far occurred in young women, often associated with pregnancy.

In amyloidosis, amyloid fibers are deposited between the pituitary cells and blood vessels.[60] Accumulation of amyloid material may directly damage hypophysial cells or may interfere with their blood supply; alternatively, amyloid deposition may suppress the delivery of GnRH to gonadotrophs or the transport of FSH-LH to the circulation. Pituitary amyloidosis is always secondary and represents a very infrequent cause of hypogonadism.

In hemochromatosis or hemosiderosis, iron pigment is deposited in several tissues including the pituitary gland.[61] The anterior lobe can be extensively involved in this uncommon disease. The gonadotrophs appear to be more prone to storing iron pigment than other adenohypophysial cell types. Thus, it is not surprising that the gonadotroph function is probably the most vulnerable in cases of iron overload, and decreased FSH-LH secretion may be the first sign indicating the involvement of anterior pituitary.[62]

Several benign and malignant neoplasms are important causes of hypopituitarism leading to anovulation, amenorrhea, infertility, and hypogonadism. If the tumors are large enough to destroy substantial areas of the adenohypophysial parenchyma including pituitary gonadotrophs, FSH-LH secretion may decrease to such a low level that hypogonadism will develop. Another mechanism responsible for adenohypophysial injury is the in-

terference with pituitary blood supply by expanding or invading tumors. If the portal circulation is arrested and blood flow to the anterior lobe is blocked, the adenohypophysial parenchyma undergoes ischemic necrosis. Since the dying gonadotrophs will not be replaced, it is obvious that, in cases of large infarcts, the secretion of FSH and LH will diminish. Alternatively, the growing tumor may compress or damage the median eminence or the hypothalamus. In these cases, hypopituitarism develops but the endocrine abnormality is of hypothalamic origin and GnRH administration elicits a rise in serum FSH and LH levels.

Any tumor located in the region of the sella turcica can lead to decreased secretion of FSH-LH either by a direct effect on the pituitary or indirectly by interfering with the synthesis, release, or adenohypophysial transport of GnRH.[63] It should be mentioned, however, that secondary tumor deposits rarely cause hypopituitarism.[64] Although metastatic tumors in the pituitary are noted not infrequently during autopsy in patients with disseminated carcinoma, they are usually found in the late phase of the disease and do not occupy large areas of the anterior lobe.[65] In the substantial majority of cases, the patients succumb before clinical symptoms become obvious.[66] The most frequent primary site of tumors giving rise to metastasis to the pituitary is the breast.[67] However, carcinomas of other locations, such as cancer of the bronchus, gastrointestinal tract, pancreas, prostate, etc., can cause metastasis to the anterior lobe. Some carcinomas arising in the neighborhood of the sella turcica can invade the pituitary directly, or can interfere with its blood supply.[68] The most frequent endocrine abnormality developing in patients with metastatic carcinoma is diabetes insipidus.[64,69,70] In these patients, polyuria and polydipsia are the dominant clinical symptoms and tumor metastases are located either in the posterior lobe, in the pituitary stalk, or in supraoptic and paraventricular nuclei, the so-called magnocellular nuclei of the hypothalamus, the production sites of vasopressin and oxytocin.

Rarely, tumors other than metastatic carcinomas, such as Hodgkin's disease, other lymphomas, and various sarcomas, can involve the pituitary. However, massive tumor deposits are uncommon and endocrine symptoms, except for diabetes insipidus, rarely develop. A description of the morphologic appearance of numerous tumor types occurring in the sella region is beyond the scope of this review.

Besides pituitary adenomas, benign tumors in the sella region are rarely located in the pituitary. These tumors infrequently impair sufficient numbers of adenohypophysial cells to cause endocrine abnormalities. They can compress the hypothalamus, damage the hypothalamic nerve cells which synthesize GnRH, impinge upon the pituitary stalk, thus blocking the transport of GnRH from the hypothalamus to the anterior pituitary.

In patients with tumors in the sella region, the two most frequent endocrine abnormalities are diabetes insipidus and hyperprolactinemia.

Diabetes insipidus is due to the deficiency of vasopressin, secondary to damage of the vasopressin-producing nerve cells of the hypothalamus, or to injury of nerve fibers transporting vasopressin to the median eminence or to impairment of the pituitary stalk causing an interruption of vasopressin transport to the posterior lobe, or to destruction of the posterior lobe where the hormone is stored and subsequently released to the circulation.

Hyperprolactinemia can be associated with various diseases in the sella region.[71-75] The mechanism responsible for increased pituitary prolactin secretion is complex. The hypothalamus regulates prolactin secretion primarily via dopamine, which, synthesized in the hypothalamus and carried through the portal vessels to the adenohypophysis, inhibits the secretory activity of prolactin cells. If the hypothalamic centers are damaged or compressed by a growing tumor or the portal circulation in the stalk is interrupted, dopamine does not reach the anterior pituitary; hence prolactin cells escape from dopaminergic inhibition, resulting in increased prolactin secretion and hyperprolactinemia.[76,77] Craniopharyngiomas, germinomas, meningiomas, metastatic carcinomas, or several non-neoplastic lesions occurring in the sella region can lead to hyperprolactinemia by the above-described mechanism.

Pituitary adenomas can be associated with a great variety of endocrine symptoms; they can cause hypogonadism, anovulation, amenorrhea, and infertility.

The occurrence of pituitary adenomas is not uncommon. They represent 10%-15% of surgically-removed intracranial tumors and can be found in approximately 10%-20% of unselected adult autopsies.[78-81] In the substantial majority of cases, they are slow-growing, histologically and biologically benign tumors. A few exceptions, however, are known to occur. Some pituitary adenomas exhibit a more rapid growth rate, show histologic signs of pleomorphism, and invade neighboring tissues spreading outside the sella turcica. Endocrinologically, pituitary adenomas can produce various hormones or are non-functioning, unassociated with clinical or biochemical evidence of hormone excess.

Earlier, on the basis of tinctorial characteristics of the cell cytoplasm, pituitary adenomas were classified into three entities: acidophilic, basophilic, and chromophobic types. It was claimed that acidophilic adenomas produce growth hormone and are associated with acromegaly or gigantism. Basophilic adenomas were assumed to secrete ACTH and to be accompanied by Cushing's disease. Chromophobic adenomas were thought to be endocrinologically inactive tumors. Classification on the grounds of staining affinities of the cell cytoplasm has not much value because it provides no information on the hormonal function of the tumor and does not permit one to correlate histologic features with endocrine activity. Electron microscopic studies show that pituitary adenomas invariably contain cytoplasmic secretory granules and, if fixation and tissue processing is adequate, secretory granules can be detected in every pituitary adenoma even by conventional histologic or histochemical techniques. Thus, chromophobic cells, in fact do not exist and, using the old terminology, misleading conclusions can be drawn.

The introduction of sophisticated morphologic techniques has demonstrated that acidophilic adenomas may not necessarily be associated with growth hormone secretion; these tumors can produce prolactin or can be functionally inactive. Basophilic adenomas most often secrete ACTH, but they can produce TSH, FSH, LH, or α-subunit as well. Moreover, some highly active prolactin-producing adenoma cells may have a basophilic tint in their cytoplasm due to the basophilic staining of the RNA-rich rough-surfaced endoplasmic reticulum network, as shown in electron micrographs. Chromophobic adenomas can be endocrinologically inactive tumors, but they are often hormonally active, capable of producing all the known adenohypophysial hormones, GH, PRL, ACTH, TSH, FSH, LH, or α-subunit. Although it is clear that classification of pituitary adenomas, on the grounds of their staining characteristics, has only limited value, this terminology should not be discarded for it is simple and it may be useful, especially in those hospitals where immunocytology and electron microscopy are not available.

The application of immunocytology and electron microscopy led to a new pituitary adenoma classification which separates pituitary adenomas into distinct morphologic entities based on their hormone content, ultrastructural features, cellular composition, and cytogenesis.[82-84] This new classification, which is widely used in many medical centers, has not only theoretical but also practical value, since it allows for the correlation of morphologic features with endocrine function and secretory activity. The various pituitary adenoma types and their prevalence, based on our surgical material, is shown in Table 12-1. It can be seen from the table that, morphologically, several well-defined adenoma types can be distinguished, and that all five cell types known to occur in the adenohypophysis can give rise to and constitute the adenoma. It can also be established that prolactin-producing adenomas represent the most frequent adenoma type in the human pituitary.

The detailed morphology of the various adenoma

Table 12-1. Classification and Frequency of Pituitary Adenoma Types

Type		Frequency in Percentage
Growth hormone cell		16.1
Densely granulated	7.0	
Sparsely granulated	9.1	
Prolactin cell adenoma		26.9
Densely granulated	0.2	
Sparsely granulated	26.7	
Corticotroph cell adenoma		14.6
Endocrinologically active	8.7	
Endocrinologically silent	5.9	
Thyrotroph cell adenoma		0.7
Gonadotroph cell adenoma		4.5
Null cell adenoma		24.7
Nononcocytic	17.8	
Oncocytic	6.9	
Plurihormonal adenoma		12.5
Mixed growth hormone cell-prolactin cell adenoma	4.7	
Acidophil stem cell adenoma	3.1	
Mammosomatotroph cell adenoma	1.5	
Other	3.2	
Total		100.0

types will not be described here; their pertinent features will be shown on a few selected representative electron micrographs (Figures 12–1 to 12–8). Many articles have been published from which the interested reader can obtain more information relevant to the morphologic diagnosis of pituitary adenomas.[82,83,85–88]

Certain pituitary adenomas can be associated with anovulation, amenorrhea, infertility, and hypogonadism. There are several possible mechanisms by which pituitary tumors can interfere with and affect the function of gonads. Pituitary adenomas, if large, may compress and damage the nontumorous adenohypophysis, reducing the number of gonadotrophs to such an extent that FSH—LH secretion will greatly diminish. The growing adenomas can interfere with the blood supply of the nontumorous adenohypophysis. Compression of blood vessels blocks circulation and the subsequent ischemia causes infarction and permanent loss of gonadotroph cells. The compression of the hypothalamus and pituitary stalk can suppress the synthesis, release, and adenohypophysial transport of GnRH. In these cases, hypothalamic hypogonadism develops which can be distinguished from hypogonadism of hypophysial origin. The differential diagnosis between these two conditions has been discussed before.

All pituitary adenoma types can interfere with FSH-LH secretion and can lead to hypogonadism. The mechanism accounting for decreased FSH-LH secretion may be the tumor's large size which damages the pituitary or interferes with its blood supply or with the synthesis, release, or adenohypophysial transport of GnRH. In some patients with acromegaly, Cushing's disease, or so-called nonfunctioning tumors, even a small pituitary adenoma can cause hypogonadism which cannot be explained on the basis of loss of adenohypophysial parenchyma or lack of stimulation. In these patients, the mechanism of decreased FSH-LH secretion is obscure.

There are two pituitary adenoma types which are frequently associated with hypogonadism: the prolactin-producing adenoma and the FSH-LH-producing adenoma.

In prolactin-producing pituitary adenomas, the mechanism of functional abnormality of the hypothalamic-pituitary-ovarian axis is complex.[89] These patients frequently have anovulation, amenorrhea, galactorrhea, and infertility. It appears that prolactin excess can suppress FSH-LH secretion either by a direct effect exerted on the pituitary or by blocking the synthesis and/or release of hypothalamic GnRH.[90] Bromocriptine, a dopaminergic agonist, decreases serum prolactin levels, restores menstruation and fertility, stops lactation and normalizes serum FSH-LH concentrations.[91–94] Similarly, after successful surgical removal of prolactin-producing adenomas, amenorrhea, galactorrhea, and infertility disappear and gonadal function becomes normal.[95] In cases of recurrence, serum prolactin levels begin to rise again and gonadal function deteriorates with anovulation, amenorrhea, galactorrhea, and infertility.

Prolactin excess may interfere with the endocrine activity of the adrenal cortices and ovaries. These effects, however, are not clearly understood, and more work is required to reveal the mechanism whereby prolactin excess influences adrenocortical and ovarian function.

Gonadotroph cell adenomas of the pituitary have been only recently recognized. During the past few years, several cases have been published which show convincingly that gonadotroph adenomas represent a distinct morphologic entity.[96–102] By immunocytology, these tumors contain FSH or LH or both. The most frequent type contains only FSH, suggesting that the tumors arose from a special subclone of gonadotrophs capable of secreting only FSH. Alternatively, it is possible that the tumors originate in FSH-LH-producing cells which, as a result of neoplastic transformation or subsequent proliferation, have lost the capacity to produce both gonadotroph hormones. By electron microscopy, gonadotroph adenomas are seen to consist of gonadotroph cells which show various degrees of differentiation. It is noteworthy that a sexual dichotomy exists between gonadotroph adenomas of male and female patients.[102] Gonadotroph adenomas of men are composed of less differentiated cells which are often easier to immunostain for FSH-LH. In contrast, gonadotroph adenomas of women are composed of more differentiated cells containing prominent, honeycomb-like Golgi complexes and more developed cytoplasm. These tumors are more difficult to immunostain for FSH-LH than their male counterparts.

Gonadotroph adenomas produce FSH or LH or both, and occur primarily in older men and women. Their clinical diagnosis is difficult, since high serum FSH-LH levels are known to occur in older subjects without the development of pituitary tumor. After menopause, the secretion of ovarian steroids is greatly diminished and the lack of negative feedback inhibition brings about increased FSH-LH secretion. Thus, it may be impossible to establish with certainty whether FSH-LH are released in excess from the tumor or from hyperactive nontumorous gonadotrophs.

Very little information is available on the results of functional endocrine tests in patients harboring pituitary gonadotroph adenomas.[99,103–106] In some patients, the sensitivity of adenomatous gonadotrophs may be increased in response to endocrine stimuli, such as GnRH. However, in other patients with gonadotroph adenomas, serum FSH-LH levels remain unchanged following administration of GnRH or estrogen. Some gonadotroph adenomas may secrete abnormal gonadotroph hormones or only fragments of the molecules which may lack biological and/or immunological activity.[107] Recently, several cases of α-subunit-secreting pituitary adenomas have been described.[108–110]

Clinically, several patients with gonadotroph adenoma show signs indicating various degrees of hypogonadism. The reasons for decreased gonadal function are not clear. It may be that, in some patients, abnormal gonadotroph hormones are produced which have no biologic activity and, occupying the receptor sites in the ovary, block the effect of FSH-LH discharged from the nontumorous portion of the adenohypophysis. This problem is not easy to resolve as the majority of patients with gonadotroph adenoma are old and are hypogonadal, exhibiting amenorrhea and anovulation. Ovarian hypofunction in these patients cannot be restored even if large amounts of FSH-LH are constantly secreted by the adenoma cells.

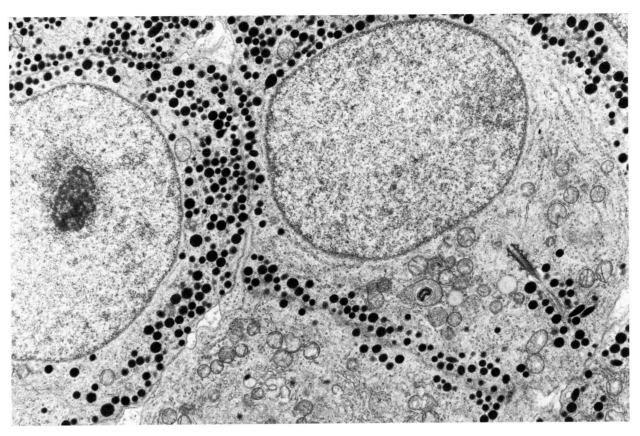

Figure 12–1. Densely granulated growth hormone cell adenoma. The well differentiated cytoplasm contains numerous large secretory granules. (×9,650)

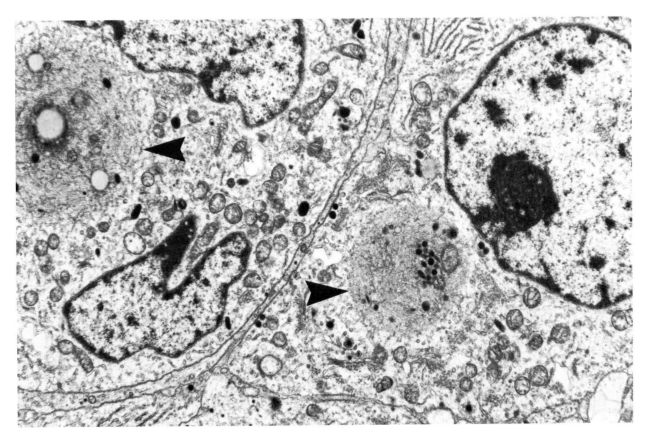

Figure 12–2. Sparsely granulated growth hormone cell adenoma with irregular nuclei, dispersed RER, sparse, small secretory granules and fibrous bodies (arrowheads). (×9,300)

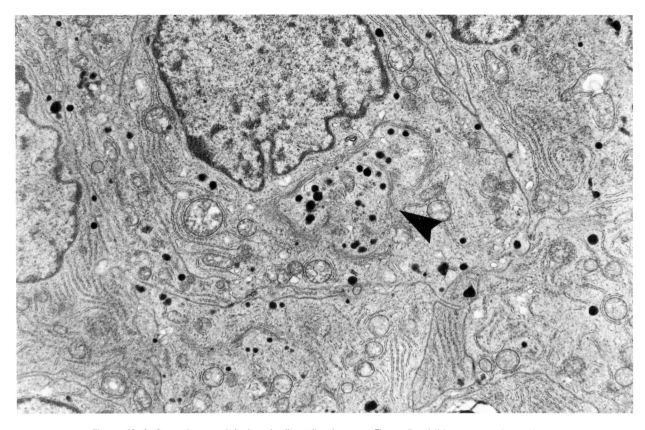

Figure 12–3. Sparsely granulated prolactin cell adenoma. The cells of this common tumor type possess abundant RER and prominent Golgi complex (arrowhead), often harboring pleomorphic forming granules. (×9,650)

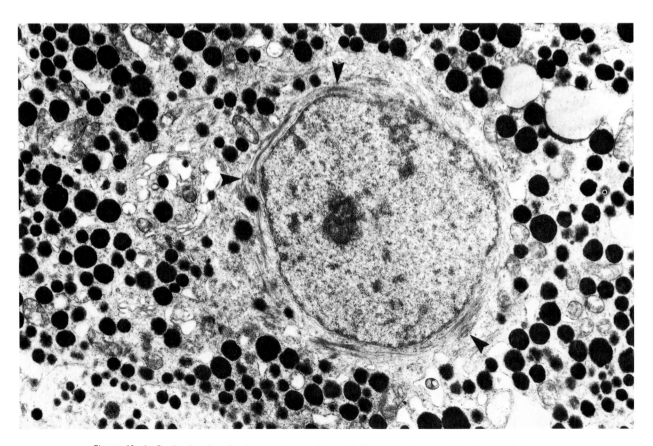

Figure 12–4. Corticotroph cell adenoma in a patient with Cushing's disease. Note the slightly irregular secretory granules and bundles of type I microfilaments (arrowheads), characteristic features of human corticotrophs. (×13,150)

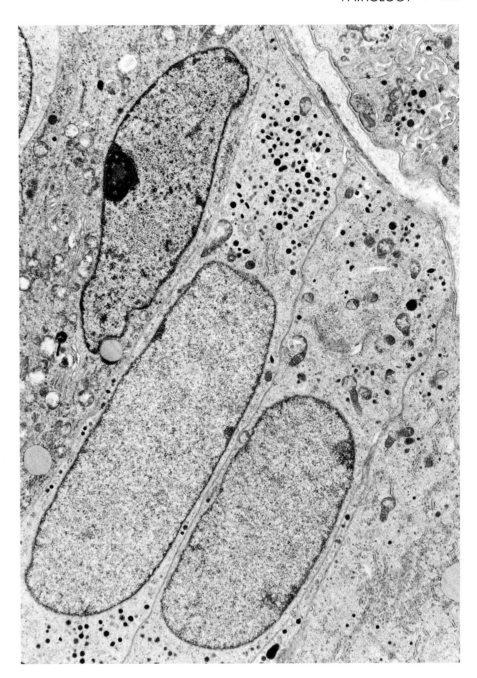

Figure 12–5. Gonadotroph cell adenoma, male type. The elongated cells contain a varying number of small secretory granules. The Golgi complex shows no unusual features. (×8,400)

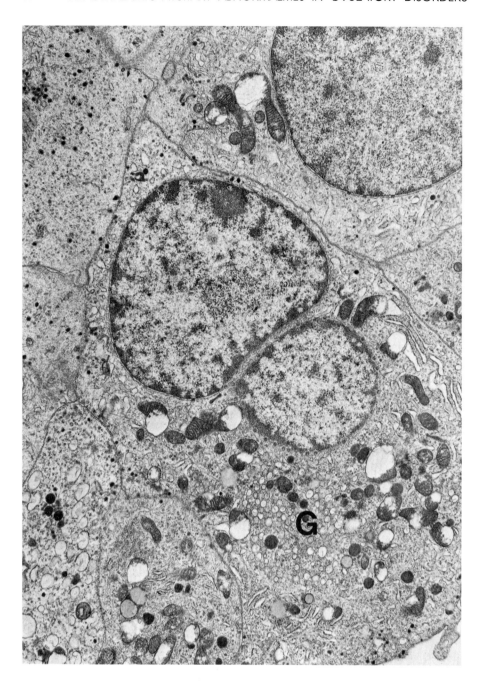

Figure 12–6. Gonadotroph cell adenoma, female type with abundant RER, small, very sparse secretory granules and the characteristic "honeycomb Golgi complex" (G). (×10,300)

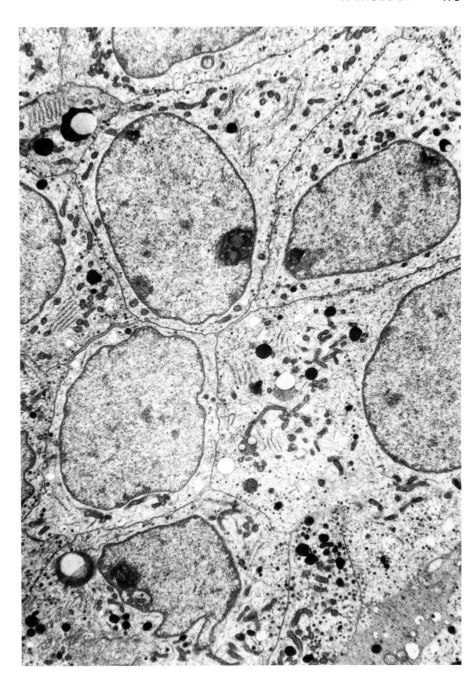

Figure 12–7. Null cell adenoma composed of small, polyhedral cells with poorly developed cytoplasm and a few, small secretory granules. (×7,100)

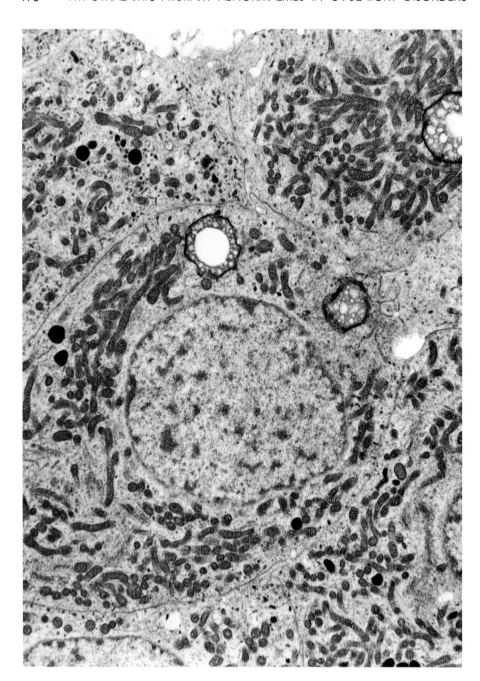

Figure 12–8. Pituitary oncocytoma exhibiting mitochondrial abundance, the morphologic marker of this tumor type. (×9,300)

References

1. Wilson JR, Carrington ER, Ledger WJ: Obstetrics and Gynecology. St. Louis, Mosby, 1983.
2. Knobil E: The neuroendocrine control of the menstrual cycle. Recent Prog Horm Res 36:53–88, 1980.
3. Savoy-Moore RT, Schwartz NB: Differential control of FSH and LH secretion. Int Rev Physiol 22:203–248, 1980.
4. Turgeon JL: Neural Control of ovulation. Physiologist 23:56–62, 1980.
5. Burger, H. G.: Neuroendocrine control of human ovulation. Int J Fertil 26:153–160, 1981.
6. Clayton RN, Calt KJ: Gonadotropin-releasing hormone receptors: characterization, physiological regulation, and relationship to reproductive function. Endocr Rev 2:186–209, 1981.
7. Belchetz PE: Gonadotrophin regulation and clinical applications of GnRH. Clin Endocrinol Metab 12:619–640, 1983.
8. Chappel SC, Ulloa-Aguirre A, Coutifaris C: Biosynthesis and secretion of follicle-stimulating hormone. Endocr Rev 4:179–211, 1983.
9. Van Rees GP, Schuiling GA, de Koning J: Effects of LH-RH on the secretion of LH. Neuroendocrinol Perspect 2:173–198, 1983.
10. Barnes ER, Naftolin F, Tolis G, et al.: Hypothalamic amenorrhea syndromes. In JR Givens, AE Kitabchi, JT Robertson (eds) The Hypothalamus. Chicago, Year Book Med Publ Inc, pp 147–170, 1984.
11. Besser GM: Sex hormones and the hypothalamus. In JR Givens, AE Kitabchi, JT Robertson (eds) The Hypothalamus. Chicago, Year Book Med Publ Inc, pp 129–146, 1984.
12. Schinfeld JS: Sex steroid metabolism in the hypothalamus. In JR Givens, AE Kitabchi, JT Robertson (eds) The Hypothalamus. Chicago, Year Book Med Publ Inc, pp 189–203, 1984.
13. Backstrom CT, McNeilly AS, Leask RM, et al.: Pulsatile secretion of LH, FSH, prolactin, oestradiol, and progesterone in the human menstrual cycle. Clin Endocrinol 17:29–42, 1982.
14. Marut EL, Huang SC, Hodgen GD: Distinguishing the steroidogenic roles of granulosa and theca cells of the dominant ovarian follicle and corpus luteum. J Clin Endocrinol Metab 57:925–930, 1983.
15. Richardson DW, Goldsmith LT, Pohl CR, et al.: The role of prolactin in the regulation of the primate corpus luteum. J Clin Endocrinol Metab 60:501–504, 1985.
16. Hull MGR: Ovulation failure and induction. Clin Obstet Gynaecol 8:753–785, 1981.
17. Reindollar RH, McDonough PG: Adolescent menstrual disorders. Clin Obstet Gynecol 26:690–701, 1983.
18. Kim MH, Cheng FE: Chronic anovulation. Clin Obstet Gynaecol 27:941–952, 1984.
19. Warren MP, Siris E, Petrovich C: The influence of severe illness on gonadotropin secretion in the postmenopausal female. J Clin Endocrinol Metab 45:99–104, 1977.
20. Molitch ME, Hou SH: Neuroendocrine alterations in systemic disease. Clin Endocrinol Metab 12:825–851, 1983.
21. Warren MP: Effects of undernutrition of reproductive function in the human. Endocr Rev 4:363–377, 1983.
22. Bates GW, Whitworth NS: Effects of body weight on female reproductive function. In JR Givens, AE Kitabchi, JT Robertson (eds) The Hypothalamus. Chicago, Year Book Med Publ Inc, pp 97–114, 1984.
23. Rebar RW: Effects of exercise on reproductive function in females. In JR Givens, AE Kitabchi, JT Robertson (eds) The Hypothalamus. Chicago, Year Book Med Publ Inc, pp. 245–262, 1984.
24. Ronkainen H, Pakarinen A, Kirkinen P: Physical exercise-induced changes and season-associated differences in the pituitary-ovarian function of runners and joggers. J Clin Endocrinol Metab 60:416–422, 1985.
25. Woolf PD, Hamill RW, McDonald JV, et al.: Transient hypogonadotropic hypogonadism caused by critical illness. J Clin Endocrinol Metab 60:444–450, 1985.
26. Korsgaard O, Lindholm J, Rasmussen P: Endocrine function in patients with suprasellar and hypothalamic tumours. Acta Endocrinol (Copenh) 83:1–8, 1976.
27. Goodrich I, Lee KJ: The differential diagnosis of sellar and parasellar diseases. Clinical and radiographic features. Otolaryngol Clin North Am 14:355–378, 1981.
28. Sheehan HL, Kovacs K: Neurohypophysis and hypothalamus. In JMB, Jr Bloodworth (ed) Endocrine Pathology, General and Surgical (2nd ed). Baltimore, Williams and Wilkins, pp 45–99, 1982.
29. Lamberton RP, Jackson IMD: Investigation of hypothalamic-pituitary disease. Clin Endocrinol Metab 12:509–534, 1983.
30. Miller DS, Reid RR, Cetel NS, Pulsatile administration of low-dose gonadotropin-releasing hormone. Ovulation and pregnancy in women with hypothalamic amenorrhea. JAMA 250–2937–2941, 1983.
31. Leyendecker G, Wildt L: Pulsatile administration of GnRH in hypothalamic amenorrhea. Ups J Med Sci 89:19–32, 1984.
32. Kovacs K, Bilbao JM, Asa SL: The pathology of parasellar and hypothalamic lesions. In JR Givens, AE Kitabchi, JT Robertson (eds) The Hypothalamus. Chicago, Year Book Med Publ Inc, pp 17–38, 1984.
33. Brust JCM, Rhee RS, Plank CR, et al.: Sarcoidosis, galactorrhea, and amenorrhea: 2 autopsy cases, 1 with Chiari-Frommel syndrome. Ann Neurol 2:130–137, 1977.
34. Vesely DL, Meldonodo A, Levey GS: Partial hypopituitarism and possible hypothalamic involvement in sarcoidosis. Report of a case and review of the literature. Am J Med 62:425–431, 1977.
35. Stewart CA, Neelan FA, Lebovitz HE: Hypothalamic insufficiency: the cause of hypopituitarism in sarcoidosis. Ann Inter Med 88:589–594, 1978.
36. Soules MR, Hammond CB: Female Kallmann's syndrome: evidence for a hypothalamic luteinizing hormone-releasing hormone deficiency. Fertil Steril 33:82–85, 1980.
37. Kovacs K, Sheehan HL: Pituitary changes in Kallmann's syndrome: a histologic, immunocytologic, ultrastructural, and immunoelectron microscopic study. Fertil Steril 37:83–89, 1982.
38. Lieblich JM, Rogol AD, White BJ, et al.: Syndrome of anosmia with hypogonadotropic hypogonadism (Kallmann's syndrome). Clinical and laboratory studies in 23 cases. Am J Med 73:506–519, 1982.
39. Crowley WF Jr, McArthur JW: Simulation of the normal menstrual cycle in Kallmann's syndrome by pulsatile administration of luteinizing hormone-releasing hormone (LHRH). J Clin Endocrinol Metab 51:173–175, 1980.

40. Kovacs K: Necrosis of anterior pituitary in humans. Neuroendocrinology 4:170–199, 201–241, 1969.

41. Sheehan, HL: Postpartum necrosis of the anterior pituitary. J Path Bact 45:189–214, 1937.

42. Sheehan HL, Davis JC: Postpartum hypopituitarism. Thomas Publ. Springfield, 1982.

43. Sheehan HL, Stanfield JP: The pathogenesis of postpartum necrosis of the anterior lobe of the pituitary gland. Acta Endocrinol (Copenh) 37:479–510, 1961.

44. Domingue JN, Wilson CB: Pituitary abscesses. Report of seven cases and review of the literature. J Neurosurg 46:601–608, 1977.

45. Blackett PR, Bailey, JD, Hoffman HJ: A pituitary abscess simulating an intrasellar tumor. Surg Neurol 14:129–131, 1980.

46. Del Pozo JM, Roda JE, Montoya JG, et al.: Intrasellar granuloma. Case report. J Neurosurg 53:717:719, 1980.

47. Scanarini M, Cervellini P, Rigobello L, et al.: Pituitary abscesses: report of two cases and review of the literature. Acta Neurochir (Wien) 51:209–217, 1980.

48. Taylon C, Duff TA: Giant cell granuloma involving the pituitary gland. Case report. J Neurosurg 52:584–587, 1980.

49. Asa SL, Kovacs K: Histologic classification of pituitary disease. Clin Endocrinol Metab 12:567–596, 1983.

50. Bjerre P, Riishede J, Lindholm J: Pituitary abscess. Acta Neurochir (Wien) 68:187–193, 1983.

51. Ezrin C, Chaikoff R, Hoffman H: Panhypopituitarism caused by Hand-Schüller-Christian disease. Can Med Assoc J 89:1290–1293, 1963.

52. Goudie RB, Pinkerton PH: Anterior hypophysitis and Hashimoto's disease in a young woman. J Path Bact 83:584–585, 1962.

53. Lack EE: Lymphoid "hypophysitis" with end organ insufficiency. Arch Pathol 99:215–219, 1975.

54. Gleason TH, Stebbins PL, Shanahan MF: Lymphoid hypophysitis in a patient with hypoglycemic episodes. Arch Pathol Lab Med 102:46–48, 1978.

55. Mayfield RK, Levine JH, Gordon L, et al.: Lymphoid adenohypophysitis presenting as a pituitary tumor. Am J Med 69:619–623, 1980.

56. Asa SL, Bilbao JM, Kovacs K, et al.: Lymphocytic hypophysitis of pregnancy resulting in hypopituitarism: a distinct clinicopathologic entity. Ann Intern Med 95:166–171, 1981.

57. Portocarrero CJ, Robinson AG, Taylor AL, et al.: Lymphoid hypophysitis. An unusual cause of hyperprolactinemia and enlarged sella turcica. JAMA 246:1811–1812, 1981.

58. Baskin DS, Townsend JJ, Wilson CB: Lymphocytic adenohypophysitis of pregnancy simulating a pituitary adenoma: a distinct pathological entity. Report of two cases. J Neurosurg 56:148–153, 1982.

59. Sobrinho-Simoes M, Brandao A, Paiva ME, et al.: Lymphoid hypophysitis in a patient with lymphoid thyroiditis, lymphoid adrenalitis, and idiopathic retroperitoneal fibrosis. Arch Pathol Lab Med 109:230–233, 1985.

60. Las MS, Surks MI: Hypopituitarism associated with systemic amyloidosis. NY State J Med 83:1183–1185, 1983.

61. Bergeron C, Kovacs K: Pituitary siderosis: a histological, immunocytologic, and ultrastructural study. Am J Pathol 93:295–309, 1978.

62. Livados DP, Sofroniadou K, Souvatzoglou A, et al.: Pituitary and thyroid insufficiency in thalassemic hemosiderosis. Clin Endocrinol 20:435–443, 1984.

63. Bunich EM, Hirsh LF, Rose LI: Panhypopituitarism resulting from Hodgkin's disease of the nasopharynx. Cancer 41:1134–1136, 1978.

64. Teears RJ, Silverman EM: Clinicopathologic review of 88 cases of carcinoma metastatic to the pituitary gland. Cancer 36:216–220, 1975.

65. Kovacs K: Metastatic cancer of the pituitary gland. Oncology 27:533–542, 1973.

66. Duchen LW: Metastatic carcinoma in the pituitary gland and hypothalamus. J Path Bact 91:347–355, 1966.

67. Roessmann U, Kaufman B, Friede RL: Metastatic lesions in the sella turcica and pituitary gland. Cancer 25:478–480, 1970.

68. Wolfowitz BL, Fernandes C: Panhypopituitarism in a case of nasopharyngeal carcinoma. S Afr Med J 45:601–602, 1971.

69. Max MB, Deck MDF, Rottenberg DA: Pituitary metastasis: incidence in cancer patients and clinical differentiation from pituitary adenoma. Neurology 31:998–1002, 1981.

70. Kimmel DW, O'Neill BP: Systemic cancer presenting as diabetes insipidus. Clinical and radiographic features of 11 patients with a review of metastatic-induced diabetes insipidus. Cancer 51:2355–2358, 1983.

71. Ezrin C, Kovacs K, Horvath E: Hyperprolactinemia. Morphologic and clinical considerations. Med Clin North Am 62:393–408, 1978.

72. McCarty KS. Jr, Dobson CE II: Pituitary pathology associated with abnormalities of prolactin secretion. Clin Obstet Gynecol 23:367–384, 1980.

73. Nakasu Y, Nakasu S, Handa J, et al.: Amenorrhea-galactorrhea syndrome with craniopharyngioma. Surg Neurol 13:154–156, 1980.

74. Shah RP, Leavens ME, Samaan NA: Galactorrhea, amenorrhea, and hyperprolactinemia as manifestations of parasellar meningioma. Arch Int Med 140:1608–1612, 1980.

75. Franz S, Jacobs HS: Hyperprolactinaemia. Clin Endocrinol Metab 12:641–668, 1983.

76. Turkington RW, Underwood LE, Van Wyk JJ: Elevated serum prolactin levels after pituitary-stalk section in man. N Engl J Med 285:707–710, 1971.

77. Lundberg PO, Osterman PO, Wide L: Serum prolactin in patients with hypothalamus and pituitary disorders. J Neurosurg 55:194–199, 1981.

78. Burrow GN, Wortzman G, Rewcastle NB, et al.: Microadenomas of the pituitary and abnormal sellar tomograms in an unselected autopsy series. N Engl J Med 304:156–158, 1981.

79. Parent AD, Bebin J, Smith RR: Incidental pituitary adenomas. J Neurosurg 54:228–231, 1981.

80. Parent AD, Brown B, Smith EE: Incidental pituitary adenomas: a retrospective study. Surgery 92:880–883, 1982.

81. McComb DJ, Ryan N, Norvath E, et al.: Subclinical adenomas of the human pituitary. New light on old problems. Arch Pathol Lab Med 107:448–491, 1983.

82. Horvath E, Kovacs K: Pathology of the pituitary gland. In C Ezrin, E Horvath, B Kaufman, et al. (eds) Pituitary Diseases. Boca Raton, CRC Press, pp 1–83, 1980.

83. Esiri MM, Adams CBT, Burke C, et al.: Pituitary adenomas: immunohistology and ultrastructural analysis of 118 tumors. Acta Neuropathol (Berl) 62:1–14, 1983.

84. Kovacs K, McComb DJ, Horvath E: Subcellular investigation of experimental and human pituitary adenomas. Neuroendocrinol Perspect 2:251–291, 1983.

85. McCarty KS. Jr, Bredesen DE, Vogel FS: Neoplasms of the anterior pituitary. Neurosurgery 3:96–104, 1978.

86. Martinez AJ, Lee A, Moossey J, et al. Pituitary adenomas: clinicopathological and immunohistochemical study. Ann Neurol 7:24–36, 1980.

87. Kovacs K, Horvath E: Pathology of pituitary adenomas. In JR Givens (ed) Hormone Secreting Pituitary Tumors. Chicago, Year Book Med Publ Inc, pp 97–119, 1982.

88. Kovacs K, Horvath E: Morphology of adenohypophyseal cells and pituitary adenomas. In H Imura (ed): The Pituitary Gland. New York, Raven Press, pp 25–55, 1985.

89. Kovacs K, Horvath E, Corenblum B, et al.: Pituitary chromophobe adenomas consisting of prolactin cells. A histologic, immunocytological, and electron microscopic study. Virchows Arch [A] 366:113–123, 1975.

90. McNeilly AS, Glasier A, Jonassen J, et al.: Evidence for direct inhibition of ovarian function by prolactin. J Reprod Fertil 65:559–569, 1982.

91. Tindall GT, Kovacs K, Horvath E, et al.: Human prolactin-producing adenomas and bromocriptine: a histological, immunocytochemical, ultrastructural, and morphometric study. J Clin Endocrinol Metab 55:1178–1183, 1982.

92. Klibanski A, Beitins IZ, Zervas NT, et al.: α-subunit and gonadotropin responses to luteinizing hormone-releasing hormone in hyperprolactinemic women before and after bromocriptine. J Clin Endocrinol Metab 56:774–780, 1983.

93. Bassetti M, Spada A, Pezzo G, et al.: Bromocriptine treatment reduces the cell size in human macroprolactinomas: a morphometric study. J Clin Endocrinol Metab 58:268–273, 1984.

94. Klibanski A, Beitins IZ, Merriam GR, et al.: Gonadotropin and prolactin pulsations in hyperprolactinemic women before and during bromocriptine therapy. J Clin Endocrinol Metab 58:1141–1147, 1984.

95. Koizuni K, Aono T, Koike K, et al.: Restoration of LH pulsatility in patients with prolactinomas after transsphenoidal surgery. Acta Endocrinol (Copenh) 107:433–438, 1984.

96. Kovacs K, Horvath E, Van Loon GR, et al.: Pituitary adenomas associated with elevated blood follicle-stimulating hormone levels: a histologic, immunocytologic, and electron microscopic study of two cases. Fertil Steril 29:622–628, 1978.

97. Kovacs K, Horvath E, Rewcastle NB, et al.: Gonadotroph cell adenoma of the pituitary in a woman with long-standing hypogonadism. Arch Gynecol 229:57–65, 1980.

98. Trouillas J, Girod C, Sassolas G, et al.: Human pituitary gonadotropic adenoma: histological, immunocytochemical, and ultrastructural and hormonal studies in eight cases. J Pathol 135:315–336, 1981.

99. Nicolis GL, Modhi G, Gabrilove JL: Gonadotropin-producing pituitary adenomas. A case report and review of the literature. Mt Sinai J Med (NY) 49:297–304, 1982.

100. Harris RI, Schatz NJ, Gennarelli T, et al.: Follicle-stimulating hormone-secreting pituitary adenomas: correlation of reduction of adenoma size with reduction of hormonal hypersecretion after transsphenoidal surgery. J Clin Endocrinol Metab 56:1288–1293, 1983.

101. Borges JLC, Ridgway EC, Kovacs K, et al.: Follicle-stimulating hormone-secreting pituitary tumor with concomitant elevation of serum α-subunit levels. J Clin Endocrinol Metab 58:937–941, 1984.

102. Horvath E, Kovacs K: Gonadotroph adenomas of the human pituitary: sex-related fine structural dichotomy. A histologic, immunocytochemical, and electron microscopic study of 30 tumors. Am J Pathol 117:429–440, 1984.

103. Friend JN, Judge DM, Sherman BM, et al.: FSH-secreting pituitary adenomas: stimulation and suppression studies in two patients. J Clin Endocrinol Metab 43:650–657, 1976.

104. Snyder PJ, Sterling FH: Hypersecretion of LH and FSH by a pituitary adenoma. J Clin Endocrinol Metab 42:544–550, 1976.

105. Demura A, Kubo O, Demura H, et al.: FSH and LH secreting pituitary adenoma. J. Clin. Endocrinol. Metab. 45:653–657, 1977.

106. Miura M, Matsukado Y, Kadama T, et al.: Clinical and histopathological characteristics of gonadotropin-producing pituitary adenomas. J Neurosurg 62:376–382, 1985.

107. Wide L, Lundberg PO: Hypersecretion of an abnormal form of follicle-stimulating hormone associated with suppressed luteinizing hormone secretion in a woman with a pituitary adenoma. J Clin Endocrinol Metab 53:923–930, 1981.

108. Ridgway EC, Klibanski A, Ladenson PW, et al.: Pure alpha-secreting pituitary adenomas. N Engl J Med 304:478–480, 1970.

109. Kourides, IA, Weintraub BD, Rosen SW, et al.: Secretion of alpha subunit of glycoprotein hormones by pituitary adenomas. J Clin Endocrinol Metab 43:97–106, 1976.

110. MacFarlane IA, Beardwell CG, Shalet SM, et al.: Glycoprotein hormone α-subunit secretion by pituitary adenomas: influence of external irradiation. Clin Endocrinol Metab 13:215–222, 1980.

13. Genetic and Infectious Causes of Habitual Abortion

Donald B. Maier

Recurrent early pregnancy loss, commonly referred to as habitual abortion, is a frustrating problem for patient and physician alike. For the patient there is the repeated tragedy of spontaneous abortion and the fear of future pregnancy losses. For the physician there is the uncertainty about the natural history of habitual abortion, the inability to find a clear-cut etiology in many cases, and the controversy over the importance of many of the proposed causes.

The concept of habitual abortion has been greatly influenced by a 1937 paper by Malpas.[1] He used clinical data and a mathematical model to predict the risk of subsequent pregnancy losses in women with a history of prior losses (Table 13–1). While later clinical studies[2,3] proved these predictions to be unduly pessimistic, the statistics were used for many years in evaluating therapy for habitual abortion instead of using control groups. The work still influences the way many investigators define habitual abortion. It proposed that there are two groups of women: those with nonrepeating pregnancy losses from "random" factors, and those with repetitive losses from "recurrent" factors. Because these "recurrent" factors would be operative in all of an affected woman's pregnancies, these "habitual aborters" would have an unbroken succession of pregnancy losses. From this model, Malpas predicted that the chance of a subsequent pregnancy loss was 38% after two losses, 73% after three losses, and 94% after four losses. These statistics had a bimodal distribution with a sharp increase in the chance of repeated losses after two losses; therefore, women with a history of one or two losses were more likely to be sporadic aborters with a favorable outcome in subsequent pregnancies, while women with three or more losses were more likely to be habitual aborters and have subsequent losses.

The classic definition of habitual abortion therefore became the consecutive loss of three or more pregnancies, usually before 20 weeks of gestation.[4] All three parts of this definition are arbitrary. Contrary to Malpas' assumption, not all causes of recurrent abortion will result in loss of every pregnancy, and thus the abortions may not be consecutive. Clinical data show that, while the chance of subsequent pregnancy loss increases with the number of previous losses, there is no clear bimodal distribution (see Table 13–1). Therefore, women with

three or more losses are not a distinct group. Finally, some causes of repeated loss may result in either early or late pregnancy loss, and the exclusion of women with later losses is also artificial. It is preferable to avoid a strict, arbitrary definition of habitual abortion. In this chapter, habitual abortion will be broadly defined as the loss of two or more pregnancies before fetal viability.

It must be noted that many or most pregnancy losses are undetected because they occur very early in gestation. One study indicates that 57% of pregnancies abort before they are clinically apparent.[5] This high rate is disputed by some,[6] but, regardless of the exact incidence of unrecognized losses, it must be kept in mind that all studies of habitual abortion are limited to clinically recognized cases. The extent to which unrecognized losses occur on a repetitive basis can only be speculated.

The natural history of habitual abortion is unknown; there are no prospective studies of untreated women with repeated pregnancy losses. There is continued debate on the etiologies and therapy of repeated pregnancy loss. To resolve the confusion surrounding this issue it is necessary to consider the question of habitual abortion in a critical manner. Data on supposed causation must be reviewed to exclude mere association. Results of therapy must be compared with outcomes in a well-matched, untreated control group. This chapter will consider potential genetic and infectious causes of habitual abortion in just such a critical fashion. Other potential causes are considered elsewhere in this book. These include uterine malformations (Chapter 3) and luteal phase defects (Chapter 11). The reader is referred elsewhere for discussions of possible autoimmune[7] and immune[8] causes of habitual abortion.

GENETIC CAUSES OF HABITUAL ABORTION

Genetic causes of habitual abortion may be either single-gene defects or chromosomal abnormalities. The vast majority of the literature deals with the latter; the role of single-gene defects remains almost entirely speculative. It is reasonable to assume that, just as there are recessive genes causing late fetal or newborn demise, there may be

Table 13–1. Percentage of Subsequent Pregnancies Aborted After (N) Abortions

	(N = 1)	(N = 2)	(N = 3)	(N = 4)
Malpas[1a]	22	38	73	94
Warburton[2b]	24	26	32	26
Poland[3c]	19	35	47	—

[a] Statistical calculations.

[b] All women in this study also had at least one liveborn.

[c] Clinical study.

similar genes that cause repeated early pregnancy loss. Simpson[9] feels that these as-yet-undiscovered genes account for much of the loss of chromosomally normal pregnancies. Potential support for their existence is found in FitzSimmons and colleagues' study[10] which showed high incidence of a family history of repeated pregnancy loss in chromosomally normal habitual aborters. Whether these defects will ever be specifically identified is uncertain as the ability to study early abortuses and their biochemistry is severely limited.

So this section on genetic factors will deal with chromosomal abnormalities associated with repeated pregnancy loss. It is necessary first to review the role of these abnormalities in all spontaneous pregnancy losses. The first chromosomally abnormal abortus was documented in 1961,[11] and since then a large body of data on the chromosomal status of spontaneous abortuses has accumulated. Five large studies have been summarized by Sankaranarayanan[12] (Table 13–2). These series show that 50% of spontaneous abortions are chromosomally abnormal. Of these abnormalities, most are numerical: 53% are trisomies, 19% are monosomy 45,X, 16% are triploidies, 6% are tetraploidies, and 2% are mosaics and others. The minority are structural abnormalities, primarily translocations. They represent only 4% of all abnormalities but are quite important in habitual abortion. The earlier the abortion, the higher the chance of chromosomal abnormality. In the Boués' study,[13] 66% of abortions at 2 to 7 weeks were abnormal, while the percentage fell to 23% for abortions at 8 to 12 weeks.

Chromosomal abnormalities also play a role in later pregnancy wastage. Abnormalities are found in 12% of macerated stillbirths, 4% of nonmacerated stillbirths, and 5% of early neonatal deaths.[12] By comparison, the rate of chromosomal abnormalities in all newborns is 0.63%.[12]

Table 13–2. Relative Frequencies of Types of Chromosomal Abnormalities in Spontaneous Abortions[a]

Examined		3375
Abnormal		1698 (50.3%)
Numerical:	Trisomies	905 (53.3% of abnormals)
	Monosomy 45,X	319 (18.8% of abnormals)
	Triploidy	279 (16.4% of abnormals)
	Tetraploidy	95 (5.6% of abnormals)
	Mosaics	26 (1.5% of abnormals)
Structural		69 (4.1% of abnormals)

[a] Data from studies collected by Sankaranarayanan.[12]

Structural abnormalities either arise *de novo* or are inherited. Numerical abnormalities result from errors during chromosomal segregation at meiosis (nondisjunction or anaphase lag) or during fertilization (dispermy). These errors are usually random events, but there may be factors which increase their likelihood. A couple would be predisposed to repeated pregnancy loss by the presence of either parental structural abnormalities or any factors affecting the randomness of numerical abnormalities. Most studies have been directed toward evaluating parental structural abnormalities. These studies will be reviewed first, followed by reviews of studies of parental chromosomal mosaicism and studies of fetal chromosomes.

Translocations

Translocations are the most common chromosomal abnormalities in habitual aborters. Reciprocal translocations arise when a crossover between nonhomologous chromosomes occurs during meiosis (Figure 13–1). If both translocated chromosomes segregate together, no genetic material is lost from the gamete. The resulting phenotypically normal individual is a balanced translocation carrier. This individual will produce abortuses or abnormal offspring if one, but not both, of the translocated chromosomes is transmitted in his or her gametes (Figure 13–2). This would result in an unbalanced conceptus with partial monosomy and partial trisomy.

The specific chromosomes transmitted in the gametes are determined during meiosis. At meiosis I, a quadrivalent is formed involving the normal and translocated chromosomes (Figure 13–2). The alignment that gives the greatest amount of homologous pairing occurs. The chromosomes may then undergo either disjunction, with two chromosomes migrating to each daughter cell, or 3 : 1 nondisjunction, with three chromosomes migrating to one cell and only one to the other cell. There are two types of disjunction: alternate, which is most common, results in a normal segregant and a balanced segregant; and adjacent, which results in two unbalanced segregants. The type of disjunction which will occur will be influenced by certain physical characteristics of each translocation and may be predicted by the relative lengths of the different branches of the quadrivalent cross.[15] For example, adjacent disjunction is favored by factors such as equal-sized chromosomes, metacentric chromosomes, translocations of approximately equal

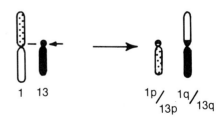

Figure 13–1. Diagrammatic representation of reciprocal translocation formation of chromosomes 1 and 13. Crossing-over occurs at arrows. 1p is stippled for easier visualization.

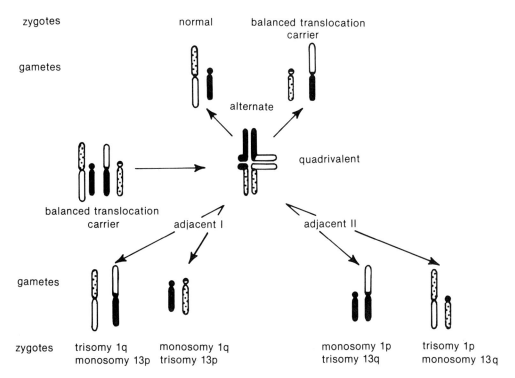

zygotes normal balanced translocation carrier

gametes

alternate

quadrivalent

balanced translocation carrier adjacent I adjacent II

gametes

zygotes trisomy 1q monosomy 1q monosomy 1p trisomy 1p
monosomy 13p trisomy 13p trisomy 13q monosomy 13q

Figure 13–2. Possible outcomes of meiosis in a balanced translocation carrier. The translocation involves chromosomes 1 and 13, as shown in Figure 13–1; 1p is stippled for easier visualization. At meiosis, a quadrivalent is formed which maximizes pairing between the 2 normal and 2 translocation chromosomes. If the alternate (opposite) chromosomes of the quadrivalent segregate together, the gametes will each receive a normal genetic complement and the zygotes will either be normal or balanced translocation carriers. Alternate segregation is favored in most translocations. If adjacent chromosomes of the quadrivalent segregate together, 2 different groupings are possible (adjacent I and II). All the gametes will have genetic excesses and deficiencies, and the zygotes will be partial monosomies and partial trisomies.

length, and chiasmata involving terminal but interstitial segments.[6] The less common 3 : 1 nondisjunction is favored by disparities in length between the translocated chromosomes, short interstitial segments, and acrocentric chromosomes.[6]

A Robertsonian translocation results from a crossover in the area of the centromere between two acrocentric chromosomes of the D or G groups (Figure 13–3). The long arms of these two chromosomes unite to form one metacentric chromosome; the short arms form a small fragment which is subsequently lost. The loss of this genetic material apparently has no phenotypic effect on the carrier, but the total chromosome number is reduced from 46 to 45. If the "two-in-one" translocation chromosome segregates with one of the normal chromosomes at meiosis, a trisomy or monosomy will result, leading to probable abortion in either case (Figure 13–4).

To date there have been over fifty studies of karyotypic analyses of couples with repeated pregnancy losses. The introduction of banding techniques in the early 1970's gave much greater precision in detecting structural abnormalities than could be achieved previously. Many small abnormalities were undoubtedly not detected in earlier studies; these have been reviewed by Khudr.[16] This discussion will deal only with studies in which banding was used.

The incidence of translocations found in these studies ranges from 0%[17,18] to 50%.[19] The studies vary widely in criteria for patient selection and methodology, and much has been made of these variations in explaining the wide range of results. While most studies include patients with two or more losses (not necessarily consecutive), others include couples with only one loss, or exclude couples with less than three. Some studies exclude patients with other apparent causes of habitual abortion, but most do not. Certain studies expressly include or exclude couples with later pregnancy losses or malformed offspring. Despite all these variations, probably the most crucial variable is sample size. This ranges from 4[19] to 1,068 cou-

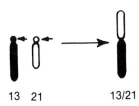

13 21 13/21

Figure 13–3. Diagrammatic representation of Robertsonian translocation of chromosomes 13 and 21. Crossing-over occurs at arrows. The short arms are lost and the total chromosome number is reduced to 45.

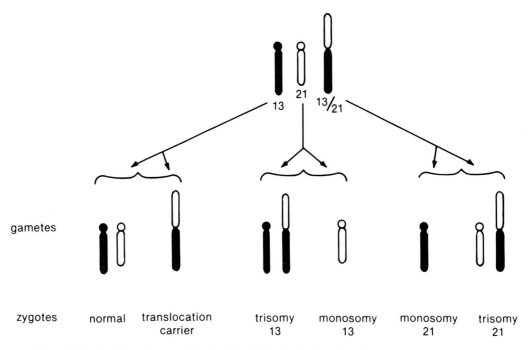

Figure 13–4. Possible outcomes of meiosis in a Robertsonian translocation carrier. The translocation involves chromosomes 13 and 21, as shown in Figure 13–3. The 2 normal and 1 translocation chromosomes may segregate in 3 possible ways, leading to 6 possible gametes. If the translocation chromosome segregates alone, the zygotes produced after fertilization will be phenotypically normal. If the translocation chromosome segregates with 1 of the other chromosomes, the zygotes will be either monosomic or trisomic.

ples,[20] and Lippman-Hand[21] has presented statistical evidence showing that this variation alone could account for all the variations seen in results. In addition, if one considers only several large recent studies of over 200 couples each,[20-30] one finds very consistent results. Therefore, it seems appropriate to combine the results from the published series in order to ascertain the overall incidence of translocations in couples with habitual abortion. Table 13–3 presents the available data. The number of individuals examined is now quite large, and the data indicate that the chance of finding a balanced translocation in an individual in a couple with habitual abortion is 2% to 3%. Some prefer to express the incidence per couple: this would be 4% to 6%.

Certain factors might be expected to influence a couple's likelihood of having a balanced translocation. One of these is the number of abortions. Turleau,[29] whose study included couples with only one abortion, found that the incidence of translocation rose from 1.5% of individuals in that group to 3.2% in the group with two abortions; the incidence did not increase further with additional pregnancy losses. Schwartz[34] and Husslein[37] showed a progressive increase in the incidence of translocations as the number of losses increased; however, neither of these studies was large. Lippman-Hand,[21] in reviewing data through 1983, found no effect of an increased number of losses above two. Fryns[20] and Sachs,[26] in their recent large studies involving over 3,000 individuals, also found no effect.

Similarly, a couple's chance of having a translocation does not seem to be markedly influenced by their having had a normal, live offspring. While some investigators have found a slightly higher rate of translocations in such couples,[22,34] others have found either no effect[29] or a

Table 13–3. Structural Chromosomal Abnormalities in Habitual Aborters[a]

Subjects	Structural Abnormalities			
	Reciprocal Translocations	Robertsonian Translocation	Inversions[b]	Total
13,302	208	85	20	317
(6754 females, 6548 males)	(1.56%)	(0.64%)	(0.15%)	(2.38%)

[a] From data summarized in reference 31 and from references 20, 21, 23–26, 33–36.

[b] Does not include inv(9).

lower incidence.[33] This is not unexpected, for, as will be seen, a phenotypically normal liveborn is the usual outcome of pregnancy in most couples with a translocation.

One factor which does influence the chance of finding a translocation in habitual aborters is the history of a stillborn or malformed infant. While Lippman-Hand's review[21] and Fryn's study[20] found no increase in translocations in couples who had such an infant, other reviews consistently show a 2.5- to 3-times increased rate.[38,39] Simpson noted that this increase was greater for females than for males; 16.4% of women with abortions and stillbirths or abnormal liveborns had balanced translocations, as opposed to 4.2% of males with such a history.[39]

Within habitually aborting couples in general, translocations are detected twice as frequently in females as in males. This was found in Lippman-Hand's review,[21] analyzing over 3,000 couples. Data which have accumulated since then, again on over 3,000 couples, give the same results.[20,22–26,33–37,40] In Fryn's large study there was no sex difference in the rate of reciprocal translocations but a threefold female predominance in Robertsonian translocations.[20] No other study has shown a difference between the types of translocations. Two somewhat opposing theories have been put forward to explain the sex difference in the incidence of translocations. The first is that males with translocations may have a high rate of infertility, and, as the chance of such a male fathering a pregnancy decreases, the percentage of females with translocations in habitual aborting couples is relatively increased. Alternatively, it has been postulated that a translocation is a less severe defect in a male than in a female because sperm with unbalanced translocations may have a defect in motility or fertilizing capacity. This would decrease the chance of such a male fathering an unbalanced conceptus and decrease the chance of his causing recurrent pregnancy loss. Support for this latter theory is found in the data on D/G translocations which predispose to trisomy 21. A male carrier is one-quarter as likely to produce a child with this anomaly as a female carrier of the same translocation.[41] Some form of gamete selection is presumed to be the explanation for this finding.

Despite the lower yield, karyotyping of the male should still be performed. If a translocation is found, the couple may be offered the option of artificial insemination with donor sperm.

Once a balanced translocation has been detected, the couple should receive genetic counseling, and other family members should be karyotyped for the same translocation. Identification of carriers among relatives is important because they should also receive counseling and because this will provide a larger population for studying the reproductive consequences of a specific translocation.

The data available for counseling show that the risks of subsequent abortions and malformed infants vary with the type of translocation and the sex of the carrier. Robertsonian translocations are a more homogeneous group, and so the information on them is the most consistent. Neri and co-workers[42] found that carriers of these translocations had a 20% to 25% risk of spontaneous abortion; this was in agreement with other studies that

they reviewed. D/D carriers may have a worse prognosis than D/G carriers.[42] The only exceptions are translocations involving homologous chromosomes. If, for example, both copies of chromosome 22 fuse, the carrier should produce only trisomy 22 or monosomy 22 conceptuses, all of which would abort. Carriers of this type of translocation should therefore have a 100% rate of pregnancy loss, but two unexplained normal offsprings from such carriers have been reported.[43,44]

There is a small risk for a subsequent malformed infant in couples with a Robertsonian translocation who have a history of previous abortions. It is very important to distinguish this from the much higher risk in carriers ascertained because of a previous malformed infant. Boué and Gallano reported on 1,356 amniocenteses in pregnancies of translocation carriers.[45] These included 106 Robertsonian translocation carriers ascertained because of spontaneous abortions, and 209 carriers ascertained because of an infant with an unbalanced translocation. The distribution of the specific chromosomes in the translocations was striking: only 11% of the translocations ascertained through abortion involved chromosome 21, as opposed to 83% of the translocations ascertained through an anomalous infant. The importance of this difference is made clear by the fact that 27 of the 28 unbalanced translocations found at amniocentesis involved chromosome 21. Therefore, Robertsonian translocations of this chromosome are likely to result in repetitive anomalous infants, while translocations not involving it are associated with recurrent early losses. Translocation carriers are a heterogeneous group and must be categorized by their previous reproductive history. Boué and Gallano also noted that unbalanced translocations were only detected in cases where the mother was the carrier.

Studies of subsequent abortions in carriers of reciprocal translocations give rates which vary from 20% to 47%.[42] This variation results from small sample sizes and the heterogeneous nature of these translocations. The lack of adequate data on any specific translocation limits the accuracy of counseling for the individual couple. However, the couple can be reassured that the risk of a malformed infant is low. Boué and Gallano[45] showed a 3.4% rate of unbalanced karyotypes when the reciprocal translocation had been ascertained because of habitual abortion. This contrasted sharply with the 20.8% rate found when the translocation had been ascertained because of a previous malformed infant. In contrast to the data on Robertsonian translocations, the sex of the carrier had no effect.

It is apparent that only large studies in which data are categorized by the method of ascertainment should be used to counsel habitual aborters. Pooling data on the reproductive histories of all individuals with translocations will give a falsely pessimistic prognosis. Because of the increased risk of an abnormal liveborn, amniocentesis should be offered in all cases.

The recent availability of chorionic villus sampling for first trimester chromosome analysis will provide more information on the frequency of unbalanced translocations in conceptuses of translocation carriers.[46] Data from Mikkelsen quoted by Simpson[6] show the rate to be approximately three times that detected by Boué and Gallano's study[45] of midtrimester amniocenteses. This higher rate might be expected, as many of these abnormal conceptuses would abort spontaneously between the first and second trimesters. If the rate of pregnancy loss following sampling proves to be acceptable, this technique will provide much useful data about translocation carriers.

Despite the large body of data on parental translocations, there is very little information correlating the specific parents' karyotypes with those of their abortuses. To prove that a parental balanced translocation causes habitual abortion, repetitive unbalanced fetal karyotypes should be demonstrated. Kajii and Ferrier[47] karyotyped 425 female and 358 male members of habitually aborting couples and 310 of their abortuses. Out of this large group, they found only five couples in whom one member had a balanced translocation and the karyotype of their abortus was known. Four abortuses showed an unbalanced translocation inherited from the parent (Figure 13–5) and one had a balanced translocation with a trisomy. Five additional unbalanced abortuses were found with normal parental karyotypes. Reviewing the literature, Jacobs found that of 76 cases of unbalanced translocations in abortuses, half were inherited while the remainder arose *de novo*.[48] Thus it cannot be assumed that translocations detected in abortuses indicate the presence of parental translocations. Conversely, abortuses of couples with a balanced translocation cannot be assumed to have an unbalanced translocation. Indeed, it has been suggested that translocations may cause abortion other than by transmission in an unbalanced state. Translocations may have interchromosomal effects which interfere with the segregation of other chromosomes. If this is so, it would result in an increased incidence of trisomic conceptuses in couples with translocations. While such phenomena have been reported in studies, such as that of Kajii and Ferrier,[47] it is uncertain whether this is an increase over the normal incidence of trisomies in abortuses. This question has been reviewed by Stoll[49] and can only be resolved by karyotypic study of a large number of abortuses from couples with a balanced translocation. Accumulating such information will be difficult.

Inversions

Inversions represent another structural parental chromosomal anomaly which may result in habitual abortion. Inversions arise when two break points in the same chromosome result in a temporary free segment. This segment is then reinserted in reversed order (Figure 13–6). Heterozygote carriers will be normal as long as no genes are altered or lost and the placement of genes next to new neighbors does not alter their expression ("position effect").[50] If the break points are on different sides of the centromere, the inversion is termed pericentric; if they are on the same side, the inversion is paracentric. Pericentric inversions may alter the relative lengths of the chromosome arms and change the position of the centro-

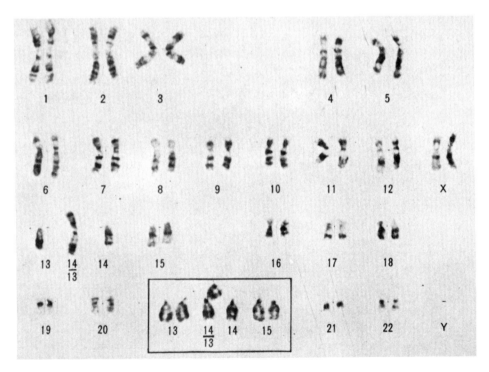

Figure 13–5. Karyotype of translocation carrier and partial karyotype of abortus (insert), showing the transmitted unbalanced translocation. Cases such as this, in which the karyotypes of both parent and abortus are known, are uncommon but provide the only direct evidence that a parental translocation has caused a particular abortion. (Reprinted from Kajii T, Ferrier A: Cytogenetics of aborters and abortuses. Am J Obstet Gynecol 131:33, 1978, with permission from CV Mosby Co.)

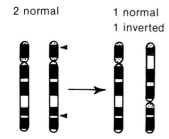

2 normal   1 normal
            1 inverted

Figure 13–6. Formation of a pericentric chromosomal inversion. One of the pair of normal chromosomes undergoes breakage at 2 points (small arrows). The intervening segment is inverted. Areas of the short arm are stippled for easier visualization. Note that the change in the position of the centromere is the most obvious result.

mere. They may thus be more easily detectable than paracentric inversions, which will only alter the banding pattern. Regardless of type, inversions may be hard to detect even with excellent technique, and this difficulty may partially account for their apparent low incidence in couples with habitual abortion (Table 13–3).

Unlike balanced translocations, in which chromosomally abnormal conceptuses result from the pattern of chromosomal segregation at meiosis, inversions probably cause abortions through the formation of abnormal chromosomes during meiotic crossing over. At that time, an inversion chromosome will form a loop at the inverted segment to allow it to pair with the normal homologous chromosome (Figure 13–7). If a single crossover occurs, the result is an abnormal recombinant chromosome with duplications and deficiencies of the material outside the inverted segment. The larger the inversion, the larger the resultant loop, and the greater the chance

for crossing over in the loop. However, the smaller the inversion, the larger the amount of unbalanced material in recombinants and the greater the potential phenotypic effect.[6]

With pericentric inversions the recombinants each have one centromere. With paracentrics—because the exchanged material outside the inversion includes the centromere—the recombinants will have either two centromeres (dicentric) or none (acentric). The latter are lost in future cell divisions because they cannot undergo disjunction.

By far the most commonly reported inversion in couples with habitual abortion is the small pericentric inversion of chromosome 9, inv(9) (p12q13). There is considerable controversy about this inversion, as many researchers consider it to be a normal variant.[24,25,47] This view is not held by all, however. Tibiletti *et al.*[51] found this inversion in 4.1% (11 of 264) of members of couples with habitual abortion, a significant increase over the 1.4% incidence in a newborn control population. Six of these eleven individuals were males. Lyberatou-Moraitou and coworkers[52] found 8 cases of inv(9) in 150 couples; 6 were males. They felt this overall incidence of 3% was significant but did not have a control group. On the other hand, Ward[17] found no increase in inv(9) in his controlled study of 100 couples with two consecutive abortions. De la Chapelle and colleagues,[53] in a review of their experience with this inversion, concluded that there was no attributable increased risk of pregnancy loss.

Inversions other than inv(9) have been reported much less frequently (See Table 13–3). Only one paracentric inversion has been reported in a habitual aborter.[54]

Counseling habitual aborters with inversions is difficult because of the controversy about the importance of

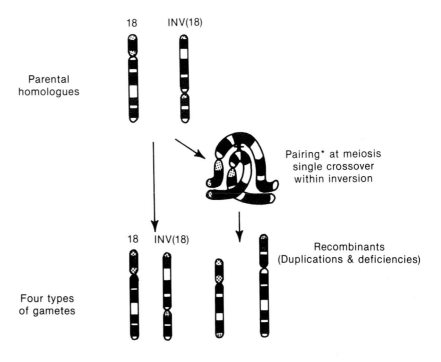

Parental homologues

18   INV(18)

Pairing* at meiosis single crossover within inversion

18   INV(18)   Recombinants (Duplications & deficiencies)

Four types of gametes

Figure 13–7. Potential gametes from an individual with an inversion. Pairing at meiosis requires the formation of a loop; if a single crossover occurs within the loop, abnormal recombinants with duplications and deficiencies will result. Areas of the short arm are stippled for easier visualization. (Reprinted, with slight modifications, from Martin AO, Simpson JL, Deddish RB, *et al.*: Clinical Implications of chromosomal Inversions. Am J Perinatol 1:1, 1983.)

*Only 2 of the 4 strands are shown

inv(9) and the paucity of data on other inversions. Overall, parental inversions carry a 4% to 8% risk for abnormal liveborns.[45] Since this is based on pooled data it is uncertain if inversions ascertained specifically through investigation of habitual abortion confer such as increased risk. Simpson[39] states that abnormal liveborns are likely to occur if the inversion involves 50% or more of the chromosome, but the precise relationship of inversion length to the likelihood of abortion is unknown. Since the combination of abortions and abnormal liveborns has occurred with some inversions, prenatal diagnosis should be offered.

Heterochromatin

Variations in the amount of heterochromatin have also been evaluated as a possible parental chromosomal cause of habitual abortion. Heterochromatin is the darkly staining area of chromosomes which remains condensed during interphase. Such areas consist of repeated base pair sequences which do not code for protein synthesis. As has been noted, the introduction of banding techniques highlighting the heterochromatin has allowed for more detailed chromosomal analysis and enhanced the detection of structural abnormalities such as translocations. These techniques also provoked interest in the heterochromatin itself. At present, the literature on the importance of variations in heterochromatin is contradictory. The amount of heterochromatin varies widely among different populations, and there is no standardized objective measurement technique.

Heterochromatin variation on the Y chromosome has received the most attention. Heterochromatin is present on the terminal portion of the Y; an increase results in a "big Y" (Yq+). Interest was initially generated by the studies of Nielsen[55] and Patil and Lubs.[56] They addressed the question indirectly by screening newborn males for Yq+. Evaluation of the previous reproductive performance of the mothers of Yq+ boys showed that they had an abortion rate twice that of the mothers of boys with normal Y's. Both of these studies concluded that paternal Yq+ caused an increased rate of pregnancy loss. Genest,[57] in an uncontrolled study, looked for Yq+ in couples with two or more abortions and found it in 10 of 51 men (19.6%). However, several larger and controlled studies have not confirmed this finding,[33,58,59] and at present there is no good evidence for a detrimental effect of Yq+.

Variations in heterochromatin on other chromosomes have also been evaluated. Nordenson[60] claimed that 25% of individuals had increased chromosome 1 heterochromatin in a very small but controlled study of twenty couples with fetal wastage. The criteria for judging the amount of heterochromatin to be increased were not mentioned. It was postulated that the larger heterochromatic areas increased the rate of nondisjunction. However, using C-banding and more careful techniques in a larger controlled study of 50 couples with three or more abortions, Hemming and Burns[61] found no increase in heterochromatic polymorphism for either chromosome 1 or 9.

Ward[17] and Blumberg et al.[33] confirmed these findings in their controlled studies.

Erdtmann,[62] in reviewing the whole topic of heterochromatin, concluded that the available data are often subjective and need to be better controlled. He felt that while there are not yet any definitive data, the majority of the available evidence shows a very minor or nonexistent role for heterochromatin in reproductive fitness. Still, the phenomenon noted by Nielsen[55] and by Patil and Lubs[56] remains unexplained.

Mosaicism

To this point only structural abnormalities have been discussed. An unexpected numerical abnormality has been found in some studies. This is an apparent increased incidence of mosaicism, especially involving the X chromosome.

Mosaicism, the existence of two or more different cell lines, arises after zygote formation either by anaphase lag or by nondisjunction. In anaphase lag, one chromosome fails to segregate into either of the two daughter cells and is lost in future cell generations. If the X is involved, a 45,X/46,XX mosaic results. In nondisjunction, both X chromosomes migrate to the same cell. This results in 45,X and 47,XXX lines which, in association with a normal line, give a 45,X/46,XX/47,XXX mosaic. Subsequent loss of the 45,X line in this case would explain the occurrence of 46,XX/47,XXX mosaics. Multiple nondisjunctional events would result in cells with 48 or more chromosomes. The relative percentage of each cell line depends on both the embryological timing of the lines' formation and their relative viability.

Mosaicism can only be detected if an adequate number of cells is studied. Since the emphasis in most studies of parental karyotypes has been on structural abnormalities, the number of each individual's cells examined is often low, as few as six.[24] Such a small number would be insufficient to evaluate possible mosaicism, especially if one line were present in a low percentage of cells. To establish a 25% level of mosaicism with 95% confidence, examination of as few as 23 cells may suffice;[63] to establish a 3% mosaicism with similar confidence may require examination of as many as 100 to 150 cells.[64] Routine evaluation of such a high number of cells is rarely done. Because of this methodologic problem in detecting mosaicism, this review will be confined to those studies of habitual aborters in which mosaicism is specifically investigated and in which an adequate number of cells is studied.

Initial studies of mosaicism and habitual abortion were all case reports. Singh et al.[63] reviewed this literature and added data from their study of 23 couples with 2 or more losses. By studying an average of 55 cells in each individual, they found 5 women who had 47,XXX in 15% to 95% of their cells. This study was followed by 2 controlled studies[65,66] which showed habitual aborters to have an increased incidence of hyperploid cells (cells with one or more extra chromosomes). Holzgreve and co-workers[67] studied 30 or more cells in both members of 144 habitually aborting couples and found 1 man and 11 women (4.1% of the individuals studied) who had X mosaicism in a small percentage (2% to 5%) of their cells. Hecht[68] found similar mosaicism in 3% of the males and 10% of the females in 183 individuals from habitually aborting couples. This was 3 times the rate of structural abnormalities in the same group. In their large study of 500 couples, Sachs and colleagues[26] found 16 women and 2 men with sex chromosomal mosaicism and 3 women and 2 men with autosomal mosaicism; the total rate was 5%, similar to the rate of structural abnormalities in that population. As with all the other studies except Singh's,[63] the percentage of aneuploid cells was low, 4% to 10%.

One controlled study[69] did not find an increase in X chromosomal mosaicism in habitual aborters. In addition, it is possible that the observed mosaicism may only be an artifact of increased patient age. Habitual aborters with sex chromosome mosaicism tend to be older than similar patients with normal chromosomes, and several studies[70-72] have noted a general age-related increase in the occurrence of X chromosome aneuploidy. However, this increase is not significant until after age 40 and is much stronger for the occurrence of 45,X than for 47,XXX lines. Therefore, while some mosaicism may simply be a phenomenon of increased age, this does not seem to account for all cases, nor for patients with hyperploidy.

While there is a reasonable body of evidence favoring a connection between sex chromosome mosaicism and habitual abortion, the potential mechanism involved is speculative. Three main possibilities have been proposed. The first is that lymphocytic mosaicism reflects germ cell mosaicism.[73] Fertilization of an oocyte lacking an X chromosome would result in either a 45,X or a 45,Y conceptus. The former would abort in 98% of the cases and the latter in 100%. However, as chromosomal analysis of individual germ cells would be technically very difficult, there are no pertinent data at this time.

Alternatively, lymphocytic mosaicism may indicate the existence of genes favoring a tendency toward anaphase lag or nondisjunction. Such genes might cause abnormal spindle assembly or increased chromosomal association.[66] Abnormal segregation of autosomes would result in the loss of conceptuses with autosomal monosomies or trisomies.

A final potential mechanism is that women with sex chromosomal mosaicism may have an increased tendency toward ovarian dysfunction,[74] specifically luteal phase defects, which would result in abortion because of insufficient progesterone support of the pregnancy. This possibility is based on the fact that women with sex chromosomal mosaicism, especially involving 45,X, have an increased incidence of premature ovarian failure;[75] in general, ovarian failure may be preceded by luteal phase defects.[76] It remains to be shown that women with aneuploidy ascertained through premature ovarian failure represent the same group as those ascertained through habitual abortion. If they do, one would expect an increase in the loss of chromosomally normal conceptuses.

Counseling couples with mosaicism is difficult, since the empirical evidence is quite limited. As with translocations, the chance of having abnormal liveborns is strongly dependent on the method of ascertainment. In his review of reproductive outcomes in women with 45,X and 47,XXX mosaicism, Dewhurst points out that women in whom mosaicism is detected because of repeated losses or an abnormal child have a much worse subsequent pregnancy outcome than women in whom mosaicism is discovered because of other indications.[77] This study implies that there may be different subsets of mosaicism which have different effects on reproduction. Pooled data from different sources are therefore not valid in counseling habitual aborters. In addition, some studies of mosaicism[67,68] specifically exclude couples with an abnormal offspring. Hence the frequency with which mosaicism may cause recurrent losses and anomalous liveborns in the same family is unknown. The only prospective data available are those of Hecht,[68] who has followed 12 pregnancies in habitual aborters with mosaicism. Of these, 3 resulted in chromosomally abnormal abortions (1 45,X, 1 trisomy and 1 triploidy) and 1 in a liveborn with trisomy 21. While such findings hint at an increase in chromosomally abnormal conceptuses in these patients, the numbers are obviously too small to draw any conclusions. The infant with trisomy 21 does raise the possibility of an increased incidence of abnormal liveborns in these patients.

It is apparent that several areas of research will shed more light on this topic. These areas include karyotypic investigation of other cell lines, investigation for luteal phase defects, follow-up for possible premature ovarian failure, and karyotyping of the abortuses. Through such studies the true role of mosaicism in pregnancy loss will be clarified and information may be gained on basic mechanisms involved in chromosome segregation.

Abortus Karyotypes

Besides studies of parental karyotypes, the other approach to evaluating chromosomal causes of habitual abortion is the karyotypic examination of the aborted conceptuses themselves. The relative frequency of chromosomal anomalies in all spontaneous abortions has been presented in Table 13–2. It should be noted that the vast majority of this information has been obtained from sporadic losses; little specific information is available on the karyotypes of abortuses of habitual aborters. Such data would help answer two important questions: First, are the percentages of normal and abnormal karyotypes in habitual abortuses the same as those in spontaneous abortuses in general? Second, are there any specific chromosomal abnormalities which tend to repeat in recurrent pregnancy loss?

These questions can be answered by the published data on the karyotypes of successive abortuses of 156 couples[78-80] (Table 13–4). These data show that the distribution of normal and abnormal karyotypes is similar to that seen in all spontaneous abortions: 56% are normal; and, of the abnormal karyotypes, 61% are trisomic, 11% are monosomic, 16% are polyploid, and 9% are translocations. In comparison with the data in Table 13–2, these

Table 13–4. Karyotypes of Two Consecutive Abortions[a]

First Abortion	Second Abortion					
	Normal	Monosomy	Trisomy	Polyploidy	Translocation	All
Normal	74	2	6	5	0	87
Monosomy	7	1	4	1	0	13
Trisomy	14	1	29	4	0	48
Polyploidy	6	1	4	2	0	13
Translocation	1	0	0	0	6	7
Total	102	5	43	12	6	168

[a] From references 78, 79 and from studies compiled in reference 80.

data do show a slight increase in normals, trisomics, and translocations, and conversely, they show a slight decrease in monosomics and polyploids. However the same general patterns hold true. What is noteworthy is the pattern of recurrence. If the first abortus was normal, the second was also normal in 85% (74 of 87) of the cases, significantly greater than the 50% rate that would have been predicted by random chance. Likewise, abnormal karyotypes were followed by a second abnormality in 65% (53 of 81) of the cases. Most striking is the nonrandom distribution of trisomics: when the first abortus was trisomic, 60% of the subsequent abortuses were also trisomic. This is three times the expected incidence if the distribution of karyotypic abnormalities were random. These trisomies are not limited to any specific chromosomes, nor is the extra chromosome in the second trisomic necessarily the same as that in the first.[79] Some feel that this pattern is related to the increase in trisomics that occurs with increased maternal age. Hassold states that this age-related effect does play a role, but that age-independent factors also exist.[79]

There are several important findings from these data. The first is that couples who have repeated pregnancy losses tend to fall into two groups; those who repeatedly abort normal fetuses, and those who repeatedly abort abnormal ones. This has obvious implications for the etiology of the recurrent abortions in these two groups and suggests that the focus of the couple's evaluation might be influenced by the abortus karyotype.

The second implication is that women who have a pattern of conceiving and aborting trisomic fetuses may have an increased risk of having a liveborn trisomic. As mentioned above, this phenomenon is not limited to any one chromosome, so that a nonviable trisomy 16 may be followed by a viable trisomy 21. This possibility is supported by Alberman's data showing that the incidence of Down's syndrome in siblings of trisomic abortuses was 2%, eight times the incidence in siblings of normal abortuses in her study.[81] It should be noted that these groups were not age-matched. A similar phenomenon is shown in the study by Hecht indicating an increased incidence of Down's syndrome in siblings of liveborn trisomic 18 infants.[82] Using a variety of statistics, Lippman-Hand predicted that the chance of a liveborn trisomic following an aborted trisomic was 1%, equivalent to the risk following the birth of a liveborn trisomic.[83] She felt that this neces-

sitated amniocentesis in the subsequent pregnancies of any woman who had been shown to have a trisomic abortus. Because the karyotype of most abortuses is unknown, Elias and Simpson have recommended amniocentesis for all women with a history of three or more previous abortions.[84]

It has been mentioned that parental X chromosome mosaicism may be a marker for a tendency toward nondisjunction, resulting in repeated monosomic or trisomic conceptuses. Certainly, the apparent repetitive nature of trisomic abortuses strengthens this possibility, but it is too early to make a definite connection. More data are needed to confirm the incidence of parental mosaicism and of repeated trisomic abortuses. Most importantly, parental karyotypes must be matched with those of abortuses to show that these are not merely two isolated phenomena. Such data are not yet available and will take a considerable amount of time and effort to accumulate.

Pathology of Chromosomally Abnormal Abortuses

In keeping with this volume's emphasis on pathology, it is appropriate to consider the potential value of examining abortuses for pathologic changes, in addition to studying them karyotypically. Chromosomal abnormalities in liveborns may cause characteristic phenotypic changes; this is most clearly seen in syndromes such as Down's, Edward's, Patou's, and Turner's. If chromosomally abnormal abortuses also have characteristic pathologic changes, such changes might prove valuable in the study of recurrent abortuses by providing clues as to the karyotype.

The mechanism by which chromosomal abnormalities result in abortion is still unclear. Available data indicate that a prolonged cell cycle is characteristic of aneuploid cells in culture.[85] If this phenomenon also occurs *in vivo,* then placenta and organ hypoplasia or alterations in the timing of induction of organ development would be the most likely causes of embryonic demise. Alternatively, metabolic abnormalities may cause both the altered cycle length and death of the conceptus. In either case, growth disorganization and retardation would be expected in chromosomally abnormal abortuses; such abnormalities are indeed seen. Two large studies have correlated chromosomal abnormalities with developmental abnormalities in abortuses.[85,86]

In triploidy, the conceptus usually develops to a stage consistent with approximately 5 weeks' gestation; however, a wide range is seen.[86] The gestational sac is disproportionately large, and the small embryo may be incomplete or have neural tube defects.[86] The placental tissue contains very characteristic macroscopic and microscopic cystic changes which become more conspicuous as gestation progresses.[87] The villi are generally avascular, and there are frequent intrachorial thromboses.[86] Tetraploid conceptuses are arrested at an even earlier stage, usually between two and three weeks of gestation.[86] Embryonic tissue is either absent or severely disorganized. Cystic placental changes with hypovascular villi are seen.[87]

Monosomy X abortuses present a different picture. Mean pregnancy duration is usually longer, approximately 6 weeks.[86] In early abortuses, the sac is usually empty or contains only a cord stump.[86] Later abortuses may show findings similar to those in liveborn Turner's syndrome, such as horseshoe kidneys and generalized edema.[86] Cystic hygromas are a very characteristic finding. Many of the embryos may appear normal, and Boué has suggested that embryonic death in these cases is secondary to a placental defect. The placenta, while frequently grossly normal and the least immature of chromosomally abnormally conceptuses, may have small hypovascular villi.[87] Subchorial thromboses are frequent. It is unclear why the 45,X karyotype can result in such a spectrum of outcomes ranging from anembryonic conceptuses to liveborn individuals with a relatively normal lifespan.

Trisomic abortuses show a wide range of pathologic changes, with the findings being to some extent dependent on the particular extra chromosome.[86] Anembryonic empty sacs or small, severely disorganized embryos are most frequently seen in trisomies A, E, and F, and, to a lesser extent, in trisomies B and C. Advanced development is seen in some trisomies C and D; the latter may also have a characteristic median facial cleft.[88] In general, the most severe growth disorganization is seen in the abortuses with the shortest gestational age. Placental changes are less variable. Grossly, placentas may appear normal or may show a range of cystic changes; microscopically, however, the villi are characteristically hypovascular, the trophoblast is underdeveloped, and large isolated cytotrophoblastic cells are frequently seen.[86,87] While Boué and colleagues feel that specific placental changes may be correlated with certain chromosomes,[86] Honoré and coworkers could not make that distinction.[87]

Because of their infrequent occurrence, sufficient data are not available on the pathologic changes in abortuses with translocations. As with trisomies, a wide range of changes would be expected.

Examination of the fetus and placenta will give some clues as to the presence of a chromosomal abnormality and its particular type. However, the specificity of pathologic findings may be inadequate. Poland and Miller categorized a total of 123 karyotypically normal and abnormal abortuses into 4 groups based on the amount of growth disorganization.[89] They found "no clearly defined association of phenotype with karyotype," and, in addition, found that many chromosomally normal abortuses were phenotypically similar to chromosomally abnormal ones. They postulated that single gene mutations could produce growth disorganization similar to that produced by chromosomal abnormalities.

It should be noted that neither Poland and Miller's classification, nor the more recent system of Rushton,[90] was devised to distinguish abortuses by karyotype. Perhaps a system specifically designed with that goal in mind would give a better correlation between karyotypic and pathologic findings. At present, examination of an abortus has limited value in determining the karyotype, and standard chromosomal studies should still be done when possible.

There is only one report of examination of successive abortuses from couples with recurrent losses. Poland and Yuen found that successive losses were usually at the same stage of development.[78] Normal abortuses were usually followed by another normal abortus, while the same repetitive pattern held true for phenotypically abnormal losses. These data tend to support the karyotypic findings found in Table 13–3.

Summary of Genetic Causes of Habitual Abortion

In conclusion, translocations are the most important genetic cause of habitual abortion; they are found in 4 to 6% of couples with repeated pregnancy loss and cause fetal wastage by being transmitted in the unbalanced state. Possible interchromosomal effects may also occur, but the evidence for this is meager. Mosaicism may be found as frequently as translocations, but it is still debatable whether or not it causes habitual abortion and, if it does, what mechanisms are involved. More careful studies of this topic will undoubtedly be forthcoming. Inversions other than inv(9) are a very infrequent finding in habitual aborters. The roles of heterochromatin abnormalities and of inv(9) remain unclear; most likely, these represent normal variants.

More study of abortus karyotypes and the more widespread use of chorionic villus biopsy will help define the importance of recurrent fetal trisomies. Because this may be a more common occurrence than unbalanced translocations, further work in this area is obviously needed.

INFECTIOUS CAUSES OF HABITUAL ABORTION

Infections have long been associated with spontaneous pregnancy losses. Infection may cause pregnancy loss by one of several mechanisms. The first involves direct embryonic or fetal effects such as sepsis, interference with organogenesis, or chromosomal damage. The second involves placental effects such as infarction or endometrial effects, such as endometritis or impaired implantation. The third includes maternal effects, such as toxin release or hyperthermia, which would secondarily affect the pregnancy. While any of these mechanisms may explain sporadic pregnancy losses caused by infection, certain requirements must be met for an infectious agent to cause recurrent pregnancy losses. If the infection is acute, then coincidental reinfection or recurrence must occur during each pregnancy. If the infection is chronic, then it would need to cause minimal, or no, clinical signs in the mother in order to escape recognition and treatment. Certain organisms thought to be commensals or normal flora may therefore be pathogenic during pregnancy.

Certain methodologic problems exist in attempting to prove an infectious cause of habitual abortion. One potential approach, isolation of organisms from the abortus, has two major difficulties. The first is avoiding contamination by maternal organisms during the process of abortion. While this may be avoided to some extent by culturing only internal organs, this approach is practically impossible because of the macerated state of most abortuses. The second major problem, even if the fetus is shown to be infected and not contaminated, is the difficulty of establishing a cause-and-effect relationship. A fetus dying from any cause may be more susceptible to infection. This problem is also quite difficult to deal with, and therefore isolation of infectious agents from the mother is potentially a more useful approach.

Studying the mother has its own problems. The first is the question of which site to study. Cervical or vaginal sampling is simple. However, since the cervix usually acts as a barrier to ascending infection, the relevance of lower genital tract flora to intrauterine fetal death is questionable. In addition, there is still much controversy about what organisms are normal vaginal and cervical flora, and also about the potential interactions between different organisms. The multitude of the organisms found, the difficulty in adequately culturing all of them, and the microbial changes which may occur cyclically and with pregnancy make an adequate study of lower tract flora a formidable task. Study of the upper tract has its own drawbacks, the most apparent being the difficulty in avoiding contamination from the lower tract when sampling the uterus transcervically. All of these points must be kept in mind, as studies of this topic will only be useful if they can avoid these potential pitfalls.

Numerous organisms have been considered as possible causes of habitual abortion.[4] The evidence for most is scanty, and only those that have been well studied will be considered (see Table 13–5).

Listeria Monocytogenes

The first bacterium to be associated with habitual abortion was *Listeria monocytogenes*. In this case, the initial

Table 13–5. Possible Infectious Causes of Habitual Abortion

Bacteria—*Listeria monocytogenes*
Protozoa—*Toxoplasma gondii*
Virus—*Herpes simplex*
Mollicute—*Ureaplasma urealyticum*

positive report has not been confirmed by several later studies. Rappaport et al.,[91] in a study from Israel, claimed to have isolated the organism from the cervices of 25 of 34 women with a history of "repeated abortion" in whom other potential causes of pregnancy loss had apparently not been ruled out. No positive cultures were found in a control group of 87 women. Ruffolo et al.,[92] in a more general study, were unable to isolate Listeria from the cervices of 80 women, including an unspecified number with repeated abortions. Stronger evidence is found in the further studies summarized by Bottone.[93] In these studies the organism was not found in any of a total of 708 patients with a history of repeated abortions or perinatal wastage. Bottone noted that these studies did find some microorganisms superficially resembling *L. monocytogenes* which were shown to be another species. Therefore, the results of Rappaport's study may be at least partly attributable to inaccurate microbiological examination. At present the majority of the evidence shows no role for *Listeria monocytogenes* in causing habitual abortion.

Toxoplasma

The protozoon *Toxoplasma gondii* has also been proposed as a cause of habitual abortion. This organism can cause congenital fetal infection by hematogenous spread during the primary maternal infection. It has been postulated that chronic maternal infection, which is not associated with congenital fetal infection, may cause repeated early pregnancy loss. *T. gondii* forms cysts in several tissues, including muscle. These cysts may rupture, releasing the organisms contained therein. If these cysts were present in the uterine musculature, they might be caused to rupture by placental ingrowth or uterine distention during or after implantation. The local release of the parasites might then cause acute pregnancy loss.[94] To date, there is no good histopathological evidence for this proposed mechanism.

Several recent studies have examined serologic evidence of toxoplasmosis in women with repeated pregnancy losses. In general, the results have shown no apparent association. As part of a prospective study, Kimball et al.[95] evaluated 73 pregnant women with a history of three or more previous losses. The percentage of positive Sabin-Feldman dye tests was not significantly different in the group that later had a subsequent successful pregnancy from the group that later had a subsequent pregnancy loss. Southern[96] found the same percentage of positive tests in women with a history of two or more losses and in a group of fertile controls without a history of abortion. Stray-Pedersen[97] used the dye test and an IgG indirect fluorescent antibody test to study 11,736 pregnant women in Norway. The two tests showed a good correlation, and the 14.5% rate of positives in 83 women with three or more pregnancy losses was no different from the 13.7% rate in the other women in the study. Giorgino and Mega[94] studied 41 women in whom other causes of habitual abortion had been ruled out and also found no difference from controls.

The issue cannot be considered to be completely settled however. Megafu,[98] using an indirect hemagglutination test, found a 25% positive rate in Nigerian habitual aborters compared with a 6% rate in controls. The population studied was one with a generally high positive rate due to poor sanitation, and these data may therefore not be applicable to more developed countries.

Thus, while there is some very minimal theoretical and clinical evidence that toxoplasmosis may cause habitual abortion, the weight of evidence favors an infrequent or nonexistent role. Demonstration of such a role in individual cases would probably require documentation of *T. gondii* cysts in uterine tissue.

Herpes Simplex

There is little information on the possible role of viral infections in habitual abortion. *Herpes simplex* is a good candidate for an infectious cause of recurrent pregnancy loss because it is a chronic, recurrent pelvic infection. The virus may remain dormant in nerve roots and become activated by a variety of events. To date, most interest has centered on herpes in the third trimester because of the severity of neonatal infection. Consequently, it is usual to culture for herpes only in the third trimester, and its effects in early pregnancy are not well studied. In one relevant study by Nahmias and colleagues,[99] spontaneous abortion occurred in 34% of cases in which herpes was detected before 20 weeks of gestation. Unfortunately, the study was not controlled, and the organism was detected by Pap smear and not by culture. Because the rate of abortion in cases of primary infection was twice that in cases of recurrent infection, this study does not provide strong support for the role of herpes in recurrent abortion. Because of the recent increased incidence in this infection, more studies are clearly needed.

Mycoplasmas

The mycoplasmas, especially *Ureaplasma urealyticum,* are now the leading candidates for an infectious cause of habitual abortion. There is a large literature, much of it conflicting, on the potential roles of these organisms in gynecologic and obstetrical disorders. Because infertility and early abortion might both be caused by the same infectious agent, the literature on ureaplasma and infertility will be briefly reviewed before examining the studies concerning habitual abortion.

Some peculiarities of the microbiology of these organisms should be noted.[100] Mycoplasmas are the smallest, self-replicating, free-living organisms. They are neither bacteria, as they do not produce a cell wall, nor are they viruses, as they are free-living. *Mycoplasma* and *Ureaplasma* are the two genera of the family Mycoplasmataceae. Ureaplasmas, of which *U. urealyticum* is the only species, are capable of hydrolyzing urea. None of the seven species of mycoplasmas possesses this capability. Before this biochemical difference was known, *U. urealyticum* was referred to as T-strain mycoplasma. There are at least 14 different serotypes of *U. urealyticum.*[101]

Tetracycline and its derivatives are the drugs of choice for treatment of mycoplasma infections. Doxycycline is most frequently used, at a dosage of 100 mg BID for 10 to 14 days. Therapy is usually started in the early follicular phase of the menstrual cycle to avoid possible exposure of the conceptus. Tetracycline resistance occurs in approximately 10% of strains.[103,104] Erythromycin is used in resistant cases or when therapy is given during pregnancy.

Techniques for isolation, culture, and identification of these organisms have been standardized. These techniques, and the special precautions needed in sample collection, are described elsewhere.[102] Methodologic differences in sampling may account for varying rates of isolation in different studies, as isolation rates vary by site.[105]

Certain epidemiologic factors are crucial in determining the isolation rates of these organisms from different populations. For both *M. hominis* and *U. urealyticum,* isolation rates are highest during early adulthood, in women, in blacks, in individuals in lower socioeconomic groups, and, most importantly, in individuals with multiple sexual partners.[100] The failure to control for any of these important variables is one of the major drawbacks of all studies of the Mollicutes and casts considerable doubt on the reliability of their conclusions.

Studies investigating the potential connection between *U. urealyticum* and infertility may be divided into three groups: studies of cervical isolation, studies of endometrial isolation, and treatment trials. These three groups should be considered separately, as each approach has its own limitations. The initial study, by Gnarpe and Friberg in 1972,[105] found cervical ureaplasma in 91% of a group of women with unexplained infertility and in 23% of a group of pregnant women. This study, which sparked interest in this field, showed a greater difference in isolation rates between infertile patients and controls than has been found in any subsequent study. Styler and Shapiro[100] have reviewed the more recent studies involving infertile couples with complete or incomplete infertility investigations. These studies generally failed to show a difference in the incidence of ureaplasma from that in either pregnant or nonpregnant controls. When differences were found, they were not as great as those found by Gnarpe and Friberg and were usually not statistically significant. As mentioned previously, none of these studies was adequately controlled for important epidemiologic variables.

Because one- to two-thirds of women with successful pregnancies are colonized, the mere existence of cervical ureaplasma is obviously not detrimental in all cases. A positive culture may be significant either as a marker for the same organism elsewhere in the genital tract or as a marker for some other pathogenic organism. Alternatively, it may be that only certain specific serotypes of ureaplasma are pathogenic. In line with the first of these possibilities, some have studied the endometrium for the presence of ureaplasma. The first study, by Horne *et al.,*[107] described a "characteristic focal accumulation of subacute inflammatory cells . . . below the surface epithelium, around a spiral arteriole, or beside a gland" which they correlated with the presence of cervical ureaplasma. They felt that the histologic finding was evidence of subclinical endometritis. This inflammatory pattern has not been confirmed by other investigators.[108,109] Koren and Spigland[110] used an endometrial jet washing technique and isolated ureaplasma from 25% of women with unexplained infertility and 6% of controls. Stray-Pedersen et al.[111] studied cervical mucus and endometrium in 379 women with infertility from a variety of causes. Fifty-seven percent of these women and 48% of controls had positive cervical cultures; in the infertile women, the isolation rate was the same regardless of the cause of infertility or the finding of unexplained infertility. Endometrial cultures were positive in 26% of infertile women and 8% of controls; again, the type of infertility had no effect. Ninety percent of the women with positive endometrial cultures also had positive cervical cultures. They concluded that there was a significant difference in endometrial, but not cervical, colonization in infertile women compared with controls. However, the fact that this was true of patients with tubal abnormalities, male infertility, other known causes, and unexplained infertility makes it difficult to understand the potential role of endometrial ureaplasma in promoting infertility; indeed, it raises the possibility that infertility of any cause somehow results in endometrial ureaplasma colonization.

The most recent study of this type, by Cassell et al.,[112] found endometrial ureaplasma in 0.05% of an infertility population. There is no apparent reason for the difference in their results and those of Stray-Pedersen other than differences in collection technique. Cassell's group, in an effort to avoid cervical contamination, enclosed the endometrial curette in a sealed polyethylene sheath which was withdrawn after the curette was passed through the endocervix. Such techniques were not used in Stray-Pedersen's study, and indeed there were bacteria in 14% of the ureaplasma positive cultures in his study. However, this does not explain entirely the different results in these studies. At this time the possibility that endometrial ureaplasma plays a role in infertility cannot be dismissed, but there is a definite need for a more careful study in order to clarify the differences between previous investigations.

The third way of examining the potential relationship between ureaplasma and infertility is by evaluating the result of treatment. In Gnarpe and Friberg's[113] population, a 29% pregnancy rate resulted after treatment of the ureaplasma positive group. This study was not controlled, but the pregnancy rate was felt to be higher than would be expected in such a group of patients with a history of unexplained infertility of five or more years. However, all subsequent studies have failed to show a positive effect of treatment.[100] This includes studies in which there was or was not a significantly higher rate of cervical ureaplasma among infertile women compared with controls. These studies used several different types of methodology, including randomization, placebo, and randomized double-blind cross-over. These treatment trials are subject to criticism, however, because any positive effect may be related to eradication of organisms other than ureaplasmas. Furthermore, if ureaplasma does truly cause infertil

ity in a small percentage of colonized women, then a beneficial effect of antibiotics on that small subgroup would be obscured by the lack of effect in the majority. Finally, the failure in most of the studies to obtain posttreatment cultures to document successful therapy further clouds the issue.

In summary, the data relating infertility with ureaplasma are inconclusive. A variety of types of methodologic failures makes the results unreliable, and the high rate of cervical colonization in fertile women necessitates that future studies be made more specific, either in terms of the site of culture or the serotype of the organism. Unfortunately, studies associating ureaplasma with habitual abortion are subject to the same uncertainties. In addition, the high spontaneous "cure" rate for habitual abortion mandates the use of an appropriate control group. Driscoll's[114] initial study reported the isolation of ureaplasma from four of five women with recurrent pregnancy loss. All women were treated with declomycin. Subsequent pregnancies in four of these five women progressed beyond 34 weeks, while only one pregnancy ended as a recurrent loss. A study such as this, in which the evaluation for other potential causes of pregnancy loss is not detailed and in which there is no control group, cannot be counted as showing an effect of either ureaplasma or treatment.

Stray-Pedersen,[115] in a study similar to his work on infertile women, evaluated uterine ureaplasma colonization in 46 women with habitual abortion of unknown etiology. Cervical cultures were positive in 61% compared to 49% in controls, and endometrial cultures were positive in 28% compared to 7% in controls. However, the strong possibility of cervical contamination or the effect of other bacteria is raised by the fact that a variety of bacterial isolates from the endometrium were found in 41% of the habitual aborters as opposed to 13% of the controls, with a strong correlation between the growth of ureaplasma and bacteria. Subsequent pregnancy outcome was much better in culture-positive patients who were treated than in culture-negative patients who received no treatment. However, this again cannot be taken to show either a causative role for the infection or a positive effect of treatment.

In a later study by Foulon,[116] a higher rate of cervical colonization (67%) was found in women with two or more spontaneous abortions than in women with an induced abortion (49%) or normal pregnant women (40%). In addition, the habitual aborters had a 71% isolation rate from trophoblast compared with a 22% rate in the group with induced abortion. Again, the latter statistic may simply reflect acquisition of the organism after fetal death rather than abortion caused by the organisms.

Harger et al.[35] isolated cervical ureaplasma in 48% of 155 women with two or more consecutive pregnancy losses. One-quarter of these women also had either a genetic or uterine abnormality which may have contributed to their reproductive failure. More than half of them were treated with doxycycline and 70% had negative follow-up cultures. It is interesting that the rate of subsequent spontaneous abortion was lowest in the treated group with positive follow-up cultures, next lowest in the untreated group, and worst in the group with negative follow-up cultures. But the numbers are small and the groups are not subdivided by the presence or absence of other factors influencing pregnancy loss.

Two studies by Quinn and associates[117,118] add some information about the possible association of ureaplasma and habitual abortion. They studied 71 couples with previous pregnancy wastage; of these 22 had lost only one previous pregnancy. *U. urealyticum* was isolated from 79% of the women and 62% of the men in these couples, compared with rates of 22% and 18%, respectively, in 51 fertile controls without a history of abortion. Isolation rates were the same, irrespective of the number of previous losses. They studied the effect of doxycycline treatment before conception, erythromycin treatment from the second or third week of pregnancy until delivery, and both. Comparison was made with an ill-defined retrospective control group of mycoplasma-positive women. Pregnancy loss was broadly defined as spontaneous abortion, stillbirth, premature infants who died, and term infants who died from congenital pneumonia felt to be caused by *U. urealyticum*. The loss rate was 96% in the untreated pregnancies, 49% when only doxycycline was given before conception, 15% when only erythromycin was given during pregnancy, and 17% when both therapies were used. They also studied maternal and infant serologic response to *U. urealyticum* at delivery in 14 successful pregnancies in women with a history of previous pregnancy losses. Forty-three percent of these women had positive titers. Elevated maternal and infant titers to the relatively uncommon serotypes 4 and 8 were found, while there were no differences from controls in positive titers to the more common serotypes.

Quinn's studies, unfortunately, have many defects. Cultures were taken from the cervix, vagina, and urine; all positives were grouped together. Women with other factors linked to habitual abortion were included randomly. Subjects were not randomized, and the control group was retrospective and poorly defined. Data on ureaplasma and other mycoplasmas were combined, and various types of pregnancy losses were grouped together. Thus, while these studies do hint at possible roles for specific serotypes in recurrent pregnancy losses, the findings need to be confirmed.

As mentioned earlier, infectious agents might cause pregnancy loss by several mechanisms. For *U. urealyticum* specifically, three possibilities have been proposed. The first is interference with placentation because of endometrial colonization. The second is direct fetal infection; this is suggested by the isolation of *U. urealyticum* from internal organs of mid-trimester abortuses.[119] The third is induction of chromosomal abnormalities; this is suggested by cytogenetic effects of other mycoplasmas on cells in culture.[120] The major task at hand, however, is to determine whether, and not how, these relatively ubiquitous organisms cause pregnancy losses in a few women. As suggested in this discussion, this will necessitate well-controlled studies involving sampling from different sites, serotyping of organisms, correlation with the presence of other infectious agents, and double-blind randomized treatment studies. Until these studies are available, finding the organism should not deter the physician from looking for other, better documented causes of habitual abortion, but such a finding should not be ignored. The most prudent approach is to culture habitual aborters for vaginal, cervical, and endometrial ureaplasmas, treat both partners when cultures are positive, obtain post-treatment cultures to document eradication of the organisms, and to complete the remainder of the evaluation for habitual abortion.

Summary of Infectious Causes of Habitual Abortion

There is no well-documented infectious cause of habitual abortions. All studies to date which show positive results have some methodologic flaw which casts doubt on the conclusions obtained, and better-designed studies are needed. It is appealing to think that there may be an infectious agent which causes recurrent pregnancy wastage since such an agent may be eradicated with appropriate therapy. The combination of the microbiological complexity of the female genital tract and the clinical complexity of recurrent pregnancy loss will continue to challenge researchers.

References

1. Malpas P: A study of abortion sequences. J Obstet Gynaecol Brit Emp 45:932–949, 1938.
2. Warburton D, Fraser FC: Spontaneous abortion risks in man: data from reproductive histories collected in a medical genetics unit. Hum Genet 16:1–25, 1964.
3. Poland BJ, Miller JR, Jones DC, et al.: Reproductive counseling in patients who have had a spontaneous abortion. Am J Obstet Gynecol 127:685–691, 1977.
4. Rock JA, Zacur HA: The clinical management of repeated early pregnancy wastage. Fertil Steril 39:123–140, 1983.
5. Miller JF, Williamson EM, Glu J: Fetal loss after implantation. Lancet 1:554–556, 1981.
6. Simpson JL, Bombard A: Chromosomal abnormalities in spontaneous abortion: frequency, pathology, and genetic counseling. In DK Edmonds, MJ Bennett (eds) Spontaneous Abortion. London: William Heineman, in press.
7. Lubbe WF, Liggins GC: Lupus anticoagulant and pregnancy. Am J Obstet Gynecol 153:322–327, 1985.
8. Gall SA: Immunologic factors influencing pregnancy. In RM Wynn (ed) Obstetrics and Gynecology Annual, Vol 14. Norwalk CT, Appleton-Century-Crofts, 1985.
9. Simpson JL: Genes, chromosomes, and reproductive failure. Fertil Steril 33:107–116, 1980.
10. FitzSimmons, J, Tunis S, Jackson D, et al.: Factors related to subsequent reproductive outcome in couples with repeated pregnancy loss. Am J Med Genet 18:407–411, 1984.
11. Penrose LS, Delhanty JDA: Triploid cell cultures from a macerated foetus. Lancet 1:1261–1262, 1961.
12. Sankaranarayanan K: Genetic Effects of Ionizing Radiation in Multicellular Eukaryotes and the Assessment of Genetic Radiation Hazards in Man. Amsterdam, Elsevier Biomedical Press, 1982.
13. Boué A, Boué J: Chromosome abnormalities and abortion. In EM Coutinho, F Fuchs (eds) Physiology and Genetics of Reproduction. Part B. New York, Plenum Press, 1975.

14. Lucas M, Wallace I, Hirschhorn K: Recurrent abortions and chromosome abnormalities. J Obstet Gynaecol Brit Common 79:1119–1127, 1972.

15. Jalbert P, Sele B, Jalbert H: Reciprocal translocations: a way to predict the mode of imbalanced segregation by pachytene-diagram drawing. Human Genet 55:209–222, 1979.

16. Khudr G: Cytogenetics of habitual abortion. Obstet Gynecol Surv 29:299–310, 1974.

17. Ward BE, Henry GP, Robinson A: Cytogenetic studies in 100 couples with recurrent spontaneous abortions. Am J Hum Genet 32:549–554, 1980.

18. Kardon NB, Davis JG, Berger AL, et al.: Incidence of chromosomal rearrangements in couples with reproductive loss. Hum Genet 53:161–164, 1980.

19. Sulewski JM, Dang TP, Ferguson KA, et al.: Chromosomal abnormalities associated with infertility. Obstet Gynecol 55:469–475, 1980.

20. Fryns JP, Kleczkowska A, Kublen E, et al.: Cytogenetic survey in couples with recurrent fetal wastage. Human Genet 65:336–354, 1984.

21. Lippman-Hand A, Vekemans M: Balanced translocation among couples with two or more spontaneous abortions: are males and females equally likely to be carriers? Hum Genet 63:252–257, 1983.

22. Fitzsimmons J, Wapner RJ, Jackson LG: Repeated pregnancy loss. Am J Med Genet 16:7–13, 1983.

23. Michels VV, Medrano C, Venne VL, et al.: Chromosome translocations in couples with multiple spontaneous abortions. Am J Hum Genet 34:507–513, 1982.

24. Osztovics MK, Toth SP, Wessely JA: Cytogenetic investigations in 418 couples with recurrent fetal wastage. Ann Genet 25:232–236, 1982.

25. Pantzar JT, Allanson JE, Kalousek DK, et al.: Cytogenetic findings in 318 couples with repeated spontaneous abortion: a review of experience in British Columbia. Am J Med Genet 17:615–620, 1984.

26. Sachs ES, Jahoda MGJ, Van Hemel JO, et al.: Chromosome studies of 500 couples with two or more abortions. Obstet Gynecol 65:375–378, 1985.

27. Stoll C, Flori E, Rumpler Y, et al.: Cytogenetic findings in 217 couples with recurrent fetal wastage. Clin Genet 17:88, 1980.

28. Tsenghi C, Metaxotou C, Kalpini-Mavrov A, et al.: Parental chromosome translocations and fetal loss. Obstet Gynecol 58:456–458, 1981.

29. Turleau C, Chavin-Colin F, deGrouchy J: Cytogenetic investigation in 413 couples with spontaneous abortions. Eur J Obstet Gynecol Reprod Biol 9:65–74, 1979.

30. Vulkova G: Chromosomal aberrations and chromosomal polymorphism in families with reproductive failure. Folia Med 25:11–18, 1983.

31. Kleinhout J, Madan K: Repeated abortions and chromosome analysis. In ESE Hafez (ed) Spontaneous Abortion. Lancaster, MTP Press Limited, 1984.

32. Schempp W, Wolff G: Cytogenetic studies in couples with multiple spontaneous abortions. Acta Anthropogenetica 7:113–118, 1983.

33. Blumberg BD, Shulkin JD, Rotter JI, et al.: Minor chromosomal variants and major chromosomal anomalies in couples with recurrent abortion. Am J Hum Genet 34:948–960, 1982.

34. Schwartz S, Palmer CG: Chromosomal findings in 164 couples with repeated spontaneous abortions with special consideration to prior reproductive history. Hum Genet 63:28–34, 1983.

35. Harger JH, Archer DF, Marchese SG, et al.: Etiology of recurrent pregnancy losses and outcome of subsequent pregnancies. Obstet Gynecol 62:574–581, 1983.

36. Stray-Pedersen B, Stray-Pedersen S: Etiologic factors and subsequent reproductive performance in 195 couples with a prior history of habitual abortion. Am J Obstet Gynecol 148:140–146, 1984.

37. Husslein P, Huber J, Wagenbichler P, et al.: Chromosome abnormalities in 150 couples with multiple spontaneous abortions. Fertil Steril 37:379–383, 1982.

38. Toth A, Gaal M, Bosze P, et al.: Chromosome abnormalities in 118 couples with recurrent spontaneous abortion. Gynecol Obstet Invest 18:72–77, 1984.

39. Simpson JL, Elias S, Martin AO: Parental chromosomal rearrangements associated with repetitive spontaneous abortions. Fertil Steril 36:584–590, 1981.

40. Davis JR, Weinstein L, Veomett IC, et al.: Balanced translocation karyotypes in patients with repetitive abortion. Am J Obstet Gynecol 144:229–233, 1982.

41. Opitz JM, Shapiro SS, Uehling DT: Genetic causes and work-up of male and female infertility. 2. Abnormalities presenting between birth and adult life. Postgrad Med 65(6):157–166, 1979.

42. Neri G, Serra A, Campana M, et al.: Reproductive risks for translocation carriers: cytogenetic study and analysis of pregnancy outcome in 58 families. Am J Med Genet 16:535–561, 1981.

43. Kirkels VGHJ, Hustinx TWJ, Scheres JMJC: Habitual abortion and translocation (22q; 22q): unexpected transmission from a mother to her phenotypically normal daughter. Clin Genet 18:456–461, 1980.

44. Palmer CG, Schwartz S, Hodes ME: Transmission of a balanced homologous t(22q; 22q) translocation from mother to normal daughter. Clin Genet 17:418–422, 1980.

45. Boué A, Gallano P: A collaborative study of the segregation of inherited chromosomal structural rearrangements in 1356 prenatal diagnoses. Prenat Diag 4:45–67, 1984.

46. MacKenzie IZ, Lindenbaum RH, Patel C, et al.: Prenatal diagnosis of an unbalanced chromosome translocation identified by direct karyotyping of chorionic biopsy. Lancet 2:1426–1427, 1983.

47. Kajii T, Ferrier A: Cytogenetics of aborters and abortuses. Am J Obstet Gynecol 131:33–38, 1978.

48. Jacobs PA, Hassold TJ: The origin of chromosome abnormalities in spontaneous abortion. In IH Porter, EB Hook (eds) Human Embryonic and Fetal Death. New York, Academic Press, 1980.

49. Stoll CG, Flori E, Beshara D: Interchromosomal effect in balanced translocations. Birth Defects 14(6C): 393–398, 1978.

50. Martin AD, Simpson JL, Deddish RB, et al.: Clinical implication of chromosomal inversions. Am J Perinatol 1:81–86, 1983.

51. Tibiletti MG, Simoni G, Terzoli GL, et al.: Pericentric inversion of chromosome 9 in couples with repeated spontaneous abortion. Acta Eur Fertil 12:245–248, 1981.

52. Lyberatou-Moraitou E, Grigori-Kostaraki P, Retzepopoulou Z, et al.: Cytogenetics of recurrent abortions. Clin Genet 23:294–297, 1983.

53. de la Chapelle A, Schroder J, Stenstrand K, et al.: Pericen-

tric inversions of human chromosomes 9 and 10. Am J Hum Genet 26:746–766, 1974.

54. Stetten G, Rock JA: A pericentric chromosomal inversion associated with repeated early pregnancy wastage. Fertil Steril 40:124–126, 1983.

55. Neilsen J: Large Y chromosome (Yq+) and increased risk of abortion. Clin Genet 13:415–416, 1978.

56. Patil SR, Lubs HA: A possible association of long Y chromosomes and fetal loss. Human Genet 35:233–235, 1977.

57. Genest P: Chromosome variants and abnormalities detected in 51 married couples with repeated spontaneous abortions. Clin Genet 16:387–389, 1979.

58. Robertson RD, Leddet I, Funderburk SI, et al.: Chromosomal variants and abnormalities in couples with repeated spontaneous pregnancy loss. Clin Res 29:116A, 1981.

59. Verma RS, Shah JV, Dosik H: Size of Y chromosome not associated with abortion risk. Obstet Gynecol 61:633–634, 1983.

60. Nordenson I: Increased frequencies of chromosomal abnormalities in families with a history of fetal wastage. Clin Genet 19:168–173, 1981.

61. Hemming L, Burns C: Heterochromatic polymorphism in spontaneous abortion. J Med Genet 16:358–362, 1979.

62. Erdtmann B: Aspects of evaluation, significance, and evolution of human C-band heteromorphism. Hum Genet 61:281–294, 1982.

63. Singh DN, Hara S, Foster HW, et al.: Reproductive performance in women with sex chromosome mosaicism. Obstet Gynecol 55:608–611, 1980.

64. McCorquodale MM, Bowdle FC: Two pregnancies and the loss of the 46,XX cell line in a 45,X/46,XX Turner mosaic patient. Fertil Steril 43:229–233, 1985.

65. Stallard R, Haney N, Frank P, et al.: Detecting inherent parental tendency to nondisjunction. Am J Hum Genet 33:123A, 1981.

66. Staessen C, Maes AM, Kirsch-Volders M, et al.: Is there a predisposition for meiotic nondisjunction that may be detected by mitotic hyperploidy? Clin Genet 24:184–190, 1983.

67. Holzgreve W, Schonberg SA, Douglas RG, et al.: X-chromosome hyperploidy in couples with multiple spontaneous abortions. Obstet Gynecol 63:237–240, 1984.

68. Hecht F, Hecht BK, Berger C: Aneuploidy in recurrent spontaneous aborters: the tendency to parental nondisjunction. Clin Genet 26:43–45, 1984.

69. Reinisch LC, Silvey KL, Dumars KW: Sex chromosome mosaicism in couples with repeated fetal loss. Am J Hum Genet 33:117A, 1981.

70. Jacobs PA, Brunton M, Court-Brown WM, et al.: Change of human chromosome count distributions with age: evidence for a sex difference. Nature 197:1080–1081, 1963.

71. Fitzgerald PH: A mechanism of X chromosome aneuploidy in lymphocytes of aging women. Humangenetik 28:153–158, 1975.

72. Galloway SM, Buckton KE: Aneuploidy and ageing: chromosome studies on a random sample of the population using G-banding. Cytogenet Cell Genet 20:78–95, 1978.

73. Hus LYF, Garcia FEP, Grossman D, et al.: Fetal wastage and maternal mosaicism. Obstet Gynecol 40:98–103, 1972.

74. Diedrich U, Hansmann I, Janke D, et al.: Chromosome anomalies in 136 couples with a history of recurrent abortions. Hum Genet 65:48–52, 1983.

75. Coulam CB: Premature gonadal failure. Fertil Steril 38:645–655, 1982.

76. Upton GV: The perimenopause. J Reprod Med 27:1–27, 1982.

77. Dewhurst J: Fertility in 47,XXX and 45,X patients. J Med Genet 15:132–135, 1978.

78. Poland BJ, Yuen BH: Embryonic development in consecutive specimens from recurrent spontaneous abortions. Am J Obstet Gynecol 130:512–515, 1978.

79. Hassold TJ: A cytogenic study of repeated spontaneous abortions. Am J Hum Genet 32:723–730, 1980.

80. Warburton D, Stein Z, Kline J, et al.: Chromosome abnormalities in spontaneous abortion: data from the New York City study. In IH Porter, EB Hook (eds) Human Embryonic and Fetal Death. New York, Academic Press, 1980.

81. Alberman E, Elliott M, Creasy M, et al.: Previous reproductive history in mothers presenting with spontaneous abortions. Br J Obstet Gynaecol 82:366–373, 1975.

82. Hecht F, Bryant JS, Gruber D, et al.: The nonrandomness of chromosomal abnormalities. N Engl J Med 271:1081–1086, 1964.

83. Lippman-Hand A: Genetic counseling and human reproductive loss. In IH Porter, EB Hook (eds) Human Embryonic and Fetal Death. New York, Academic Press, 1980.

84. Elias S, Simpson JL: Evaluation and clinical management of patients at apparent increased risk for spontaneous abortions. In IH Porter, EB Hook (eds) Human Embryonic and Fetal Death. New York, Academic Press, 1980.

85. Cure S, Boué A, Boué J: Consequence of chromosomal anomalies on cell multiplication. In A Boué, C Thibault (eds) Les Accidents Chromosomiques de la Réproduction. Paris, INSERM, 1973.

86. Boué J, Philippe E, Giroud A, et al.: Phenotypic expression of lethal chromosomal anomalies in human abortuses. Teratol 14:3–20, 1976.

87. Honoré LH, Dill FJ, Pocano BJ: Placental morphology in spontaneous human abortuses with normal and abnormal karyotypes. Teratol 14:151–166, 1977.

88. Roux C: Étude morphologique des embryons humains atteints d'abérrations chromosomiques. Presse Med 78:647–652, 1970.

89. Poland BJ, Miller JR: Effect of karyotype on zygotic development. In A. Boué, C Thibault (eds) Les Accidents Chromosomiques de La Reproduction. Paris, INSERM, 1973.

90. Rushton DI: Examination of products of conception from previable human pregnancies. J Clin Pathol 34:819–835, 1981.

91. Rappaport F, Rabinovitz M, Toaff R, et al.: Genital listeriosis as a cause of repeated abortion. Lancet 1:1273–1275, 1960.

92. Ruffolo EH, Wilson RB, Weed LA: Listeria monocytogenes as a cause of pregnancy wastage. Obstet Gynecol 19:533–536, 1962.

93. Bottone EJ, Sierra MF: Listeria monocytogenes: another look at the "Cinderella among pathogenic bacteria," Mt Sinai J Med 44:42–59, 1977.

94. Giorgino FL, Mega M: Toxoplasmosis and habitual abortion. Clin Exp Obstet Gynecol 8:132–134, 1981.

95. Kimball AC, Kean BH, Fuchs F: The role of toxoplasmosis in abortion. Am J Obstet Gynecol 111:219–226, 1971.

96. Southern PM: Habitual abortion and toxoplasmosis. Obstet Gynecol 39:45–47, 1972.

97. Stray-Pedersen B, Lorentzen-Styr A-M: The prevalence of toxoplasma antibodies among 11736 pregnant women in Norway. Scand J Infect Dis 11:159–165, 1979.

98. Megafu U, Ugwuegbulam I: Incidence of positive toxoplasmosis hemagglutination test in Nigerian (Ibo) women with recurrent abortions. Int J Fertil 26:132–134, 1981.

99. Nahmias AJ, Josey WE, Naib ZM, et al.: Perinatal risk associated with maternal genital herpes simplex virus infection. Am J Obstet Gynecol 110:825–834, 1971.

100. Styler M, Shapiro SS: Mollicutes (mycoplasma) in infertility. Fertil Steril 44:1–12, 1985.

101. Robertson JA, Stemke GW: Expanded serotyping scheme for Ureaplasma urealyticum strains isolated from humans. J Clin Microbiol 15:873–878, 1982.

102. Taylor-Robinson D, McCormack WM: Mycoplasmas in human genitourinary infections. In JG Tully, RF Whitcomb (eds) The Mycoplasmas. New York, Academic Press, 1979.

103. Evans RT, Taylor-Robinson D: The incidence of tetracycline-resistant strain of Ureaplasma urealyticum. J Antimicrobial Chemotherapy 4:57–63, 1978.

104. Spaepen MS, Knudsin RB, Horne HW: Tetracycline-resistant T-Mycoplasmas (Ureaplasma urealyticum) from patients with a history of reproductive failure. Antimicrobiol Agent and Chemotherapy, 9:1012–1018, 1976.

105. McCormack WM, Rankin JS, Lee Y-H: Localization of genital mycoplasmas in women. Am J Obstet Gynecol 112:920–923, 1972.

106. Gnarpe H, Friberg J: Mycoplasma and human reproductive failure. I. The occurrence of different mycoplasmas in couples with reproductive failure. Am J Obstet Gynecol 114:727–731, 1972.

107. Horne HW, Hertig AT, Kundsin RB, et al.: Sub-clinical endometrial inflammation and T-mycoplasma. Int J Fertil 18:226–231, 1973.

108. Bercovici B, Haas H, Sacks T, et al.: Isolation of mycoplasmas from the genital tract of women with reproductive failure, sterility, or vaginitis. Isr J Med Sci 14:347–352, 1978.

109. Gump DW, Gibson M, Ashikaga T: Lack of association between genital mycoplasmas and infertility. N Engl J Med 310:937–941, 1984.

110. Koren Z, Spigland I: Irrigation technique for detection of mycoplasma intrauterine infection in infertile patients. Obstet Gynecol 52:588–590, 1978.

111. Stray-Pedersen B, Bruu A-L, Molne K: Infertility and uterine colonization with Ureaplasma urealyticum. Acta Obstet Gynecol Scand 61:21–24, 1982.

112. Cassell GH, Younger JB, Brown MB, et al.: Microbiologic study of infertile women at the time of diagnostic laparoscopy. N Eng J Med 308:502–504, 1983.

113. Gnarpe H, Friberg J: Mycoplasma and human reproductive failure. III. Pregnancies in "infertile" couples treated with doxycycline for T-mycoplasmas. Am J Obstet Gynecol 116:23–26, 1973.

114. Driscoll SG, Kundsin RB, Horne HW, et al.: Infections and first trimester losses: possible role of mycoplasmas. Fertil Steril 20:1017–1019, 1969.

115. Stray-Pedersen B, Eng J, Reikvam TM: Uterine T-mycoplasma colonization in reproductive failure. Am J Obstet Gynecol 130:307–311, 1978.

116. Foulon W, Naessens A: Role of Ureaplasma urealyticum and mycoplasma hominis in spontaneous abortion. In ESE Hafez (ed) Spontaneous Abortion. Lancaster, MTP Press Limited, 1984.

117. Quinn PA, Shewshuk AB, Shuber J, et al.: Efficacy of antibiotic therapy in preventing spontaneous pregnancy loss among couples colonized with genital mycoplasmas. Am J Obstet Gynecol 145:239–244, 1983.

118. Quinn PA, Shewchuk AB, Shuber J, et al.: Serologic evidence of Ureaplasma urealyticum infection in women with spontaneous pregnancy loss. Am J Obstet Gynecol 145:245–250, 1983.

119. Dische MR, Quinn PA, Czegledy-Nagy E, et al.: Genital mycoplasma infection. 1. Intrauterine infection: pathologic study of the fetus and placenta. Am J Clin Pathol 72:167–174, 1979.

120. McGarrity GJ, Vanaman V, Sarama J: Cytogenetic effects of mycoplasmal infection of cell cultures: a review. In vitro 20:1–18, 1984.

14. Development of the Testis and Associated Disorders

Bernard Gondos

The developing testis plays a key role in the establishment of male reproductive function. Male and female gonads originate in a similar manner and undergo parallel patterns of differentiation, but there are two striking differences related to the major functions of gamete production and sex hormone secretion. While oogenesis is initiated soon after gonadal differentiation, development of testicular germ cells is characterized by a delay in maturation, with spermatogenesis beginning only at the time of puberty. In regard to hormone production, the fetal testis is extremely active, in contrast to the relatively inactive fetal ovary, and secretes high levels of hormones essential for the formation of the male reproductive system. These differences bear directly on the understanding of abnormalities of gonadal development.

Endocrine activity in the fetal testis regulates the differentiation of male internal and external genital structures. These effects are of critical importance for the later development of sexual maturation and reproductive capacity. The fetal testis is also the source of the definitive germ cells. Although spermatogenesis does not begin until puberty, the pool of spermatogenic stem cells present in the postnatal testis is derived entirely from fetal precursors.

This chapter will review the development of the fetal and postnatal testis and consider pathologic changes which occur during the early differentiation period.

TESTICULAR DEVELOPMENT

The adult testis contains two main compartments: seminiferous tubules and interstitial tissue. The tubules are involved in the formation of spermatozoa, while the interstitial tissue is the source of testosterone production. Cellular changes within these two compartments begin early in development, involving the principal cellular elements: germ cells, Sertoli cells, Leydig cells, and peritubular cells. The main changes occurring at different stages of development are indicated in Table 14–1. Establishment of external influences involving the hypothalamic-pituitary-testicular axis also occurs at an early stage. Both intrinsic and extrinsic interactions evolve in a complex manner during fetal and postnatal development.

Fetal Testis

Testicular differentiation begins at 6 to 7 weeks gestation with the formation of groups of germ cells and differentiating Sertoli cells surrounded by a basal lamina, and development of a tunica albuginea in the outer cortical region.[1] As discussed in Chapter 8, primitive germ cells migrate to the genital ridge from the yolk sac region and undergo proliferation within the developing gonad. Differentiation of testicular structures depends on the presence of a Y chromosome (46,XY).

Initially the groups of germ cells and Sertoli cells are arranged in plate-like structures.[2] The germ cells, referred to as gonocytes, are randomly distributed among the more numerous Sertoli cells. Subsequently the plates are transformed into cell cords, the seminiferous cords, and the gonocytes begin to move to a peripheral location (Figure 14–1). These cells become situated along the basal lamina in the position of spermatogonia, but still retain the general appearance of precursor cells, and are therefore designated as prespermatogonia (Figure 14–2). There is only limited mitotic activity at this time and the cords are compact, lacking the lumen characteristic of seminiferous tubules in the adult. Large numbers of germ cells degenerate during the early differentiation period. The surviving fetal gonocytes and prespermatogonia are the source of the definitive population of germ cells involved in spermatogenesis in the adult testis.[3]

Sertoli cells are the first cells to exhibit evidence of differentiation shortly after testis formation. Particularly noteworthy is the presence of cytoplasmic organelles associated with protein production (Figure 14–3). This correlates with the appearance of antimüllerian hormone, a large protein which is responsible for regression of the müllerian ducts.[4,5] AMH has been found to originate from Sertoli cells.[5,6] Inhibitory activity can be demonstrated as early as 7 to 8 weeks.[7] Müllerian duct regression is observed at 8 weeks in male fetuses,[8] indicating a close temporal association with the development of inhibitory activity (Table 14–2).

Leydig cells with characteristic ultrastructural features of steroid-secreting cells begin to appear in the interstitial regions at 8 weeks,[9] correlating with the onset of

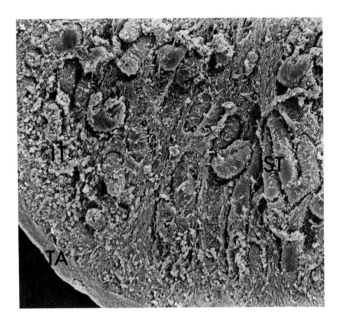

Figure 14–1. Human fetal testis, early differentiation. Scanning electron micrograph shows tunica albuginea (TA), seminiferous cords (ST) and interstitial tissue (IT). (×50)

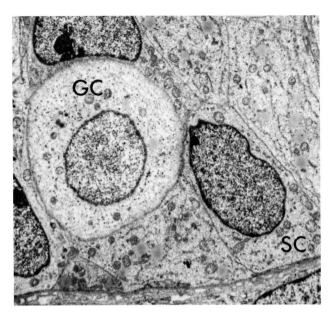

Figure 14–3. Fetal Sertoli cells (SC) with numerous polyribosomes and abundant rough endoplasmic reticulum. GC, gonocyte. (×6,000)

testosterone production.[10] This is followed by growth of the wolffian ducts, lengthening of the urogenital distance, fusion of the labioscrotal swelling and closure of the urethral groove. Differentiation of the wolffian ducts into the epididymis, vas deferens, and seminal vesicles occurs under the direct influence of testosterone.[11] The reduced form of testosterone, dihydrotestosterone, regulates the differentiation of the external genitalia.[11]

Testosterone synthesis by the testis and serum levels reach a peak during the early second trimester (Figure 14–4).[12] At this time, large sheets of Leydig cells fill the interstitial regions. The fetal Leydig cells have an appearance identical to that in the adult except for absence of Reinke crystals (Figure 14–5). At midgestation, the Leydig cells undergo regression[13] and there is a corresponding fall in testosterone production.[10]

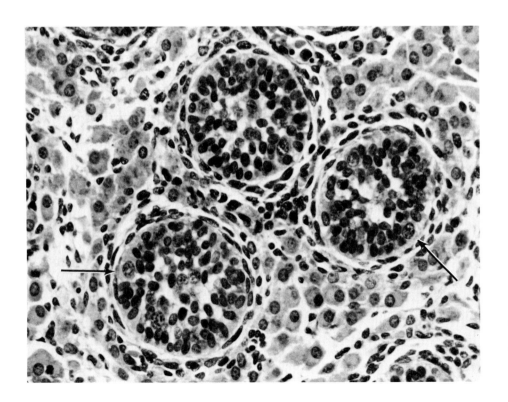

Figure 14–2. Light micrograph of fetal testis, 12 weeks gestation. Note abundant Leydig cells in interstitium. Arrows indicate prespermatogonia at periphery of seminiferous cords. (×250)

Table 14–1. Appearance of Testis at Different Stages of Development

Age	Tubules	Interstitium
Fetus		
6–8 wk	Seminiferous cords (primitive tubules) contain randomly distributed germ cells (gonocytes) among more numerous Sertoli cells	Undifferentiated mesenchyme
8–24 wk	Sertoli cells, immature type, predominate; germ cells present as individual central gonocytes and paired peripheral prespermatogonia	Groups of fully differentiated, Leydig cells
24 wk–term	As above	Undifferentiated mesenchyme and partially differentiated Leydig cells
Childhood	Gradually increasing diameter, germ cells move to periphery; Sertoli cells continue to predominate, undergo differentiation and elongation	As above
Puberty	Spermatogenesis begins, germ cells predominate; Sertoli cells cease dividing, form occlusive junctions resulting in basal and adluminal compartments	Groups of fully differentiated Leydig cells with Reinke crystals; prominent peritubular tissue including myoid cells

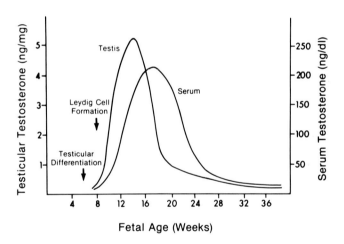

Figure 14–4. Testosterone levels in testis and serum during fetal development. (Data from Refs.[11,13])

Gonadotropin regulation of fetal testosterone production is indicated by several observations. The fetal testis has receptors for LH and hCG, to which it responds *in vitro* with increased synthesis of testosterone.[14] Maternal serum hCG levels, resulting from placental production, peak at 8 to 10 weeks, corresponding to the time of onset of testosterone production. Gonadotropins can be detected in fetal pituitary extracts as early as 10 weeks[15] when gonadotrophs first appear.[16] Concentrations of LH reach peak levels in the pituitary at about 20 weeks and in the serum at 12 to 16 weeks.[15,17] These observations suggest dual placental and pituitary regulation of fetal testosterone production.

Hypothalamic regulation of gonadotropin secretion by the fetal pituitary is suggested by a close temporal relationship in the anatomical and functional development of the fetal hypothalamus and pituitary. A large increment in hypothalamic gonadotropin-releasing hormone content

Table 14–2. Fetal Testicular Hormones[a]

Type	Source	Peak Activity	Effect
Antimüllerian hormone (AMH)	Sertoli cells	7–10 wk	Regression of müllerian ducts
Testosterone	Leydig cells	8–16 wk	Growth of wolffian ducts, differentiation of epididymis, vas deferens, and seminal vesicles[b]

[a] See text for references.

[b] Additional effects dependent on dihydrotestosterone.

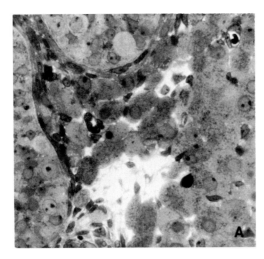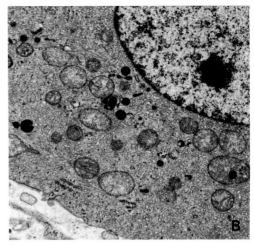

Figure 14–5. Fetal Leydig cells with abundant cytoplasm, well-developed smooth endoplasmic reticulum, and prominent tubulovesicular mitochondria. A. Light micrograph. Toluidine blue (×250). B. Electron micrograph. (×9,000)

occurs between 8 and 18 weeks.[18] This correlates with the time of maximal *in vitro* and *in vivo* effects of LHRH on gonadotropin release[19] and with the peak of FSH and LH content in the pituitary during the second trimester.[20] The subsequent decline in gonadotropins and testosterone later in gestation reflects a complex interrelationship of testicular, pituitary, and hypothalamic function during fetal development.

In the latter part of gestation, the testis completes its descent into the scrotum. At approximately the seventh month, the processus vaginalis grows rapidly and the inguinal canal increases in diameter. Descent occurs as a result of degeneration of the portion of the gubernaculum in contact with the epididymis and testis, allowing both to move through the dilated inguinal canal into the scrotum. Numerous studies on experimental cryptorchidism as well as clinical observations have been evaluated in an attempt to define the precise function of androgens and gonadotropins in testicular descent. A clear picture is yet to emerge and, consequently, there is still considerable controversy on this subject.

Postnatal Testis

The structure of the testis during the late fetal and postnatal period shows relatively little change and reflects a general lack of functional activity. There is a slight increase in size as the seminiferous cords gradually increase in diameter, but the cellular arrangement remains essentially unchanged. The number of germ cells is relatively stable, indicating limited mitotic activity, although there is a slight increment in germ cell number between 5 and 10 years of age.[21]

Sertoli cells continue to proliferate during this time and also show evidence of cellular differentiation, including increased cytoplasmic complexity, nucleolar enlargement, and cellular elongation (Figure 14–6). Nonocclusive attachments can be found between Sertoli cells at this time, but occlusive tight junctions of the type seen in the adult are not present.[22]

Interstitial regions are characterized by the presence of undifferentiated mesenchymal cells and only small numbers of partially differentiated Leydig cells, the result of regressive changes in the latter part of gestation in association with falling gonadotropin levels. Testosterone production is similarly at a low level. There is a transient, but significant, rise in the neonatal period which lasts until approximately 6 months.[23] Subsequently, testosterone levels remain low until the immediate prepubertal period. Mature Leydig cells are not present in childhood, but the mesenchymal precursor cells are capable of undergoing Leydig cell differentiation with secretion of high levels of testosterone in response to gonadotropin stimulation.[24]

Germ cells in the postnatal testis are of prespermatogenic type. Although spermatogenic maturation can be seen in early childhood in cases of precocious puberty[25] or following gonadotropin treatment,[26] under normal conditions germ cells in the testes of young boys are principally prespermatogonia. The distinction between prespermatogonia and spermatogonia (see below) is rather difficult at the light microscopic level, and consequently many reports on the developing human testis refer to the presence of spermatogonia. While a few such cells may be present prior to the onset of spermatogenesis, the majority of germ cells encountered would be precursor forms.

The peritubular, or boundary, tissue of the seminiferous tubules is an important component of the adult testis involved in metabolic transport and tubular contractility. This tissue is of relatively simple structure in the developing testis. In the childhood period, a thin basal lamina is the principal component, surrounded by scattered fibroblasts and bundles of collagen.

Pubertal Development

The changes that occur in the prepubertal and pubertal testis are complex, affecting all of the major cell types. The principal effects are the onset of spermatogenesis

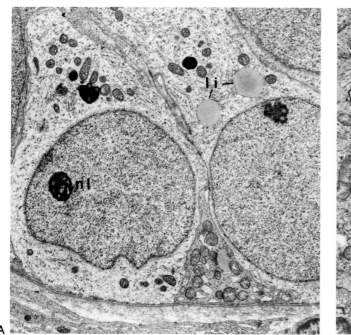
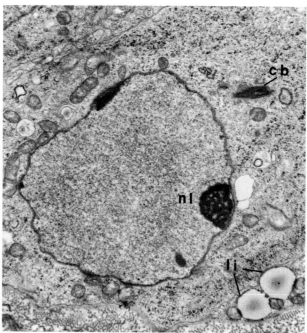

Figure 14–6. Appearance of Sertoli cells during postnatal development. A. Late childhood period. B. At puberty. nl, nucleolus, li, lipid. cb, Charcot-Böttcher crystal. (×7,500)

and establishment of the adult pattern of testosterone production.

The onset of spermatogenesis indicates the capacity of the germ cells to progress through the stages of maturation leading to sperm formation. The progression within the seminiferous tubules consists of a series of mitotic divisions (spermatogonia), two successive meiotic divisions (spermatocytes), morphologic transformation from round to elongated forms (spermatids), and release into the tubular lumen (spermatozoa) (Table 14–3). This sequence of events generally develops at 10 to 12 years of age. Onset of active mitotic division and accumulation of large numbers of cells undergoing spermatogenesis correlates with a sharp increase in testicular size at this time.[27,28] During the progression through puberty, there is a doubling of mean testis length[27] and a six-fold increase in testicular volume.[29] Spermaturia and the first conscious ejaculation occur between 12 and 14 years.[30]

The key morphologic change signaling initiation of spermatogenesis is the differentiation and proliferation of spermatogonia, followed by entry into meiosis. Spermatogonia differ from prespermatogonia in that their basal margin is flattened and directly aligned along the basal lamina (Figure 14–7). Nuclear chromatin is relatively dense, nucleoli are compact and eccentrically located, and cytoplasmic organelles are dispersed. In contrast, prespermatogonia show only partial association with the basal lamina, irregular cell shapes, loosely distributed chromatin, large central nucleoli, and clustering of cytoplasmic organelles. The distinction, which is best visualized by electron microscopy, may be important in conditions requiring determination of the precise level of germ cell maturation.

Once spermatogenesis begins, there is a continued cyclic pattern associated with waves of maturation throughout the seminiferous tubules. The initial cycle may be

Table 14–3. Types of Germ Cells Present Before and During Spermatogenesis

Type	Stage	Activity	Shape	Location
Prespermatogenesis	Fetus/child			
Gonocytes		Mitosis[a]	Round	Central
Prespermatogonia		Mitosis[a]	Round	Peripheral
Spermatogenesis	Puberty/adult			
Spermatogonia		Mitosis	Round	Basal
Spermatocytes		Meiosis	Round	Adluminal
Spermatids		Maturation	Round to elongated	Adluminal
Spermatozoa		Transport	Elongated	Luminal

[a] Limited mitotic activity.

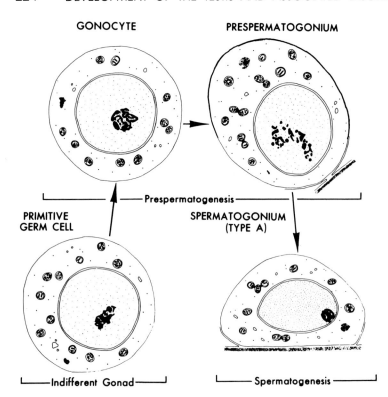

GONOCYTE

PRESPERMATOGONIUM

PRIMITIVE GERM CELL

SPERMATOGONIUM (TYPE A)

Prespermatogenesis

Indifferent Gonad

Spermatogenesis

Figure 14–7. Diagram illustrating developmental stages of testicular germ cells based on electron microscopic observations. Note differences between prespermatogonium and spermatogonium. (Reproduced from Gondos,[3] with permission.)

slightly shorter than later cycles, but the basic pattern of cellular growth and differentiation is established from the start. The resulting cyclic pattern enables production of spermatozoa from spermatogonia without interruption. An important feature of spermatogenesis is spermatogonial renewal, whereby continued maturation of spermatogonia takes place without exhausting the supply of stem cells. Maintenance of a pool of stem cells allows recovery of the testis from pathologic effects associated with germ cell damage.

Sertoli cells are considered to play a key role in supporting the maturation and function of germ cells throughout their development. At the time of puberty, a number of changes in Sertoli cells can be recognized.[33] These include increased nucleolar complexity, extensive cytoplasmic differentiation resulting in marked cellular elongation and the appearance of distinctive cytoplasmic inclusions, Charcot-Böttcher crystals (Figure 14–6). A particularly interesting feature is the development of occlusive tight junctions between adjacent Sertoli cells. The formation of such junctions, which occurs at the time of the initial spermatogenic cycle, results in the establishment of basal and adluminal compartments within the seminiferous tubule. Tubular lumen opening also occurs at this time. The junctions are considered to be the morphologic basis for the blood-testis barrier, which restricts passage of materials into the interior of the seminiferous tubules.[31] Once Sertoli cells have completed their differentiation, they cease dividing. As a result, a stable population is established at the time of puberty.

Differentiation of the adult generation of Leydig cells takes place during the prepubertal period (Figure 14–8). This is a redifferentiation process resembling the earlier phase in the fetus but developing more gradually over a longer time period. Mesenchymal and partially differentiated cells in the interstitial regions respond to rising gonadotropin levels by increasing in size and cytoplasmic complexity and developing the capacity for steroid hormone production. The fully differentiated Leydig cells are characterized by round, eccentric nuclei, abundant smooth endoplasmic reticulum and tubulovesicular mitochondria, and the presence of prominent Golgi areas, collections of glycogen and Reinke crystals in the cytoplasm (Figure 14–9). Initially small groups of Leydig cells are seen at 10 to 11 years, with larger aggregates beginning to appear at 12 to 13 years.

Testosterone levels show a similar pattern (Figure 14–10). After the transient neonatal elevation, they remain low throughout childhood. A gradual rise begins at 10 years of age, followed by a sharp 20-fold increase between ages 11 and 17.[27,32] When analyzed in terms of pubertal development, there is similarly a modest rise in plasma testosterone from P1 to P2 and then a sharp rise in later stages.[29] In addition to the rise in testosterone production, there are important changes in androgen biosynthetic pathways accompanying sexual maturation.[33]

Leydig cell differentiation at puberty, as in the fetus, appears to be under gonadotropin control. However, there are differences in the duration of the differentiation process and in the pattern of responsiveness of the Leydig cells in the two generations. The process is more prolonged in the pubertal testis and desensitization, whereby down regulation occurs in response to hCG administration, is seen in the adult generation of Leydig cells which develops at puberty but not in the fetus.[34] These differences are most likely related to changes in hypothalamic-pituitary-testicular interaction which take

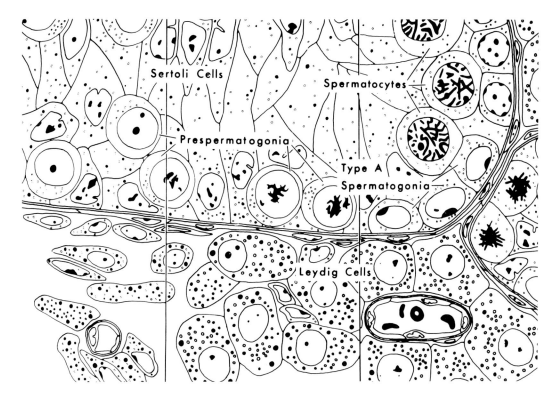

Figure 14-8. Diagram showing testicular maturation from prepubertal appearance at left, to onset of spermatogenesis at right. Interstitial cells undergo changes in shape, size, and arrangement in the process of Leydig cell differentiation. (Reproduced from Gondos,[3] with permission.)

place during prepubertal and pubertal development. In addition, there is evidence that intratesticular mechanisms, such as Sertoli cell regulation, may modulate changes in Leydig cell function.[35]

A marked increase in responsiveness of Leydig cells to gonadotropins occurs at the time of puberty. Although administration of hCG can induce Leydig cell differentiation and functional activity in prepubertal boys, the response is slower and weaker than in pubertal subjects.[36] Available data indicate that the shift in responsiveness

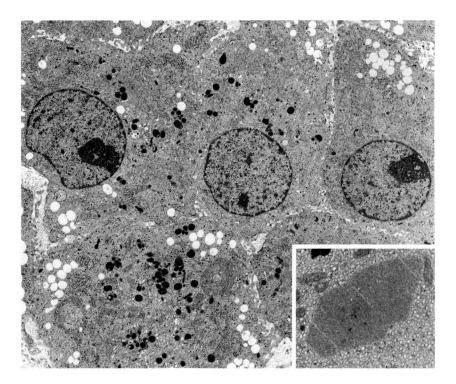

Figure 14-9. Electron micrograph of fully differentiated Leydig cells at early puberty, showing extensive development of cytoplasmic organelles. (×3,400). Inset, Reinke crystal. (×9,500)

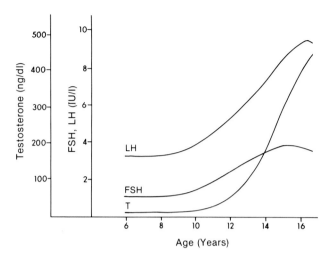

Figure 14–10. Testosterone, FSH and LH levels in boys during childhood and pubertal development. (Data from Refs.[27,98])

occurs at the time of entry into puberty (stage P2). Significant changes in hCG-induced responses occur in parallel with rises in androstenedione, 17α-hydroxyprogesterone and estradiol production.[37] The early pubertal testis already exhibits the refractoriness to hCG administration characteristic of adult Leydig cells. This has led to the suggestion that a single hCG-injection test could serve as a marker of normal sexual maturation.[38]

The sharp rise in testosterone secretion at puberty, associated with increased testicular sensitivity to gonadotropins, correlates with increasing gonadotropin production. Gonadotropin levels are low at birth, rise transiently during the first few months of life, and then remain low from 6 months to approximately 10 years of age.[27,32] A gradual rise in FSH and LH occurs during puberty, mediated by changes at the hypothalamic and pituitary level. There is an increase in pituitary sensitivity to GnRH, which appears to result from increasing GnRH secretion and changes in the physiologic status of the gonadotrophs.[39,40] These effects may in turn be related to extra-hypothalamic central nervous system changes which result in pulsatile LH release. Early in puberty, these pulses occur only during sleep, but as puberty progresses they increase in magnitude and occur throughout the day and night.[41] Another key element in the process is the decreased sensitivity of the hypothalamic-pituitary unit to inhibition by gonadal steroids at puberty.[39,40]

The peritubular tissue at puberty becomes a complex structure consisting of several layers of basal lamina, fibroblasts, and collagen fibers. The fibroblastic cells develop elaborate cytoplasmic extensions containing bundles of filaments, and numerous pinocytotic vesicles are present at the cell margins. These are features characteristic of smooth muscle and the name, myoid cells, has been used for the peritubular cells which do indeed exhibit contractile activity. The development of the peritubular tissue is evidently under hormonal control. In hypogonadotropic hypogonadism, the peritubular tissue is poorly organized, but after treatment with FSH and LH it attains the adult appearance.[42] The effect could be the result of stimulation of testosterone production by the interstitial tissue.[43]

CHROMOSOMAL AND GENETIC DISORDERS

Chromosome abnormalities and gene defects associated with male infertility need to be understood in terms of cytogenetic considerations which are discussed in detail in the following chapter. In some of the conditions, the diagnosis is not established until the time of adulthood in relation to impaired fertility. Other chromosomal and genetic disorders may be associated with pathologic effects at birth, during childhood, or at the time of puberty. In all of these conditions, the underlying cause and pathogenesis are based on early events affecting testicular differentiation or androgen action.

Morphologic changes occurring in the developing testis and associated functional abnormalities are considered here in relation to early pathologic effects. In those conditions producing intersex disorders and ambiguous genitalia, distinction between developmental abnormalities of the ovary and testis is not always possible or meaningful. From a clinical standpoint, distinction on a phenotypic or karyotypic basis may be most useful, and the terms, male pseudohermaphroditism and female pseudohermaphroditism, have provided some aid in this regard. However, from the standpoint of pathogenesis, it is important to try to distinguish the specific structural and functional changes responsible for the different disorders. While this is not always possible, advances in understanding have provided considerable information on mechanisms of pathogenesis and pathologic effects.

Gonadal Dysgenesis

Conditions in which gonadal dysgenesis is associated with a female phenotype have been discussed in the chapter on ovarian developmental disorders. Male phenotypic changes occurring with gonadal dysgenesis may appear in individuals with mosaicism including a 45,X cell line and at least one line containing a Y chromosome. In such cases, dysgenetic testes are usually present, either unilaterally or bilaterally.[44] There can be a spectrum of phenotypes ranging from almost normal males with cryptorchidism or hypospadias to females with the findings characteristic of Turner's syndrome.[45] Patients with ambiguous external genitalia having one streak gonad and a contralateral dysgenetic testis are referred to as having mixed gonadal dysgenesis.

A point discussed previously that needs to be amplified here relates to individuals with a male phenotype and testicular tissue in whom gonadal preservation is a consideration (see Chapter 8). The risk for neoplasia in gonadal dysgenesis has been considered to relate to the presence of a Y chromosome.[46] The gonads in individuals with mixed dysgenesis are at high risk for undergoing neoplastic transformation. It has been suggested that a possible exception is the group with a male phenotype and palpable scrotal testes.[47] This would imply that lack of descent is the key risk factor. Others have suggested that the presence of immature or dysgenetic testicular tissue represents the main basis for neoplastic changes.[48] Clearly, more information is needed on whether the risk for neoplasia relates to genetic or chromosomal factors, testicular abnormalities, or location of the gonad. Such information, which is not currently available, would be required to assess reliably the potential risk for neoplasia in patients in whom gonadal preservation for future fertility is being considered.

Klinefelter Syndrome

The pathogenetic mechanisms and pathologic changes in the testes of individuals with Klinefelter syndrome are described in Chapters 15 and 16. The diagnosis is generally not made until adulthood when the basis for unex-

plained infertility is sought. Since the etiology is on a chromosomal basis, changes in the testis might be expected to be present early in development. However, testicular biopsies in prepubertal boys with Klinefelter syndrome show only decreased tubular diameter and not the marked germ cell depletion, peritubular thickening, and Leydig cell abnormalities seen later.[49] Characteristic clinical and endocrine findings, similarly, are generally absent prior to puberty.[50]

We have had the opportunity to perform electron microscopic studies on the testes of a fetus with a 47,XXY karyotype aborted at 18 weeks gestation. There were no specific abnormalities in germ cells or Sertoli cells. Leydig cells showed some regressive changes, but others were well developed, findings consistent with the age of the fetus (Figure 14–11).

Since extensive damage to germ cells can occur in the adult, it appears that the effects only become manifest after puberty. Increased degeneration of germ cells and

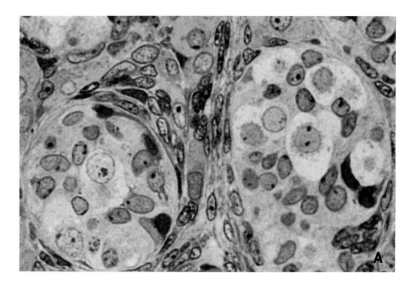
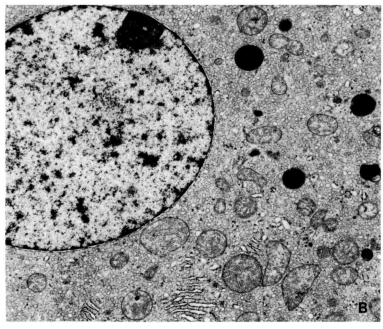

Figure 14–11. Testicular tissue from 47,XXY fetus, 18 weeks gestation. A. Light micrograph indicating normally-formed germ cells and Sertoli cells. Toluidine blue (×500). B. Leydig cell with ultrastructural features of fully differentiated cell. (×9,000)

depletion of spermatogenic elements in the postpubertal testis correlates with advancing age. Thus, one might draw an analogy with Turner's syndrome (see Chapter 8) since the chromosomal anomaly does not affect formation, migration, or early differentiation of the germ cells, but has its principal effect during meiosis, when extensive germ cell loss occurs. Furthermore, there is variation in the extent of damage in different individuals, and some patients with Klinefelter syndrome, particularly those with mosaicism, have demonstrated normal spermatogenesis and apparent fertility.[51]

Androgen Biosynthesis Defects

Developmental disorders related to defective androgen biosynthesis are of two main types: enzyme deficiencies in testosterone synthesis and a deficiency in the enzyme required for the reduction of testosterone to dihydrotestosterone. The first type includes a series of enzymes present in the testis that are involved in conversion of cholesterol to testosterone. The second type involves a single enzyme, 5α-reductase, present in target tissues which are under the influence of dihydrotestosterone.

Enzyme Deficiencies in Testosterone Synthesis

Enzyme deficiencies leading to decreased secretion of testosterone can result in incomplete virilization during fetal development. Five enzymatic defects in testosterone biosynthesis have been described, one at each of the enzymatic steps required for the conversion of cholesterol to testosterone. Three of the reactions (cholesterol desmolase complex, 3β-hydroxysteroid dehydrogenase and 17α-hydroxylase) are also involved in glucocorticoid synthesis and, consequently, a deficiency will produce both adrenal and gonadal effects (see Chapter 10). The remaining two (17,20-desmolase and 17-ketosteroid reductase) are unique to the androgen pathway and only affect genital tract development.

The disorders are inherited in an autosomal recessive or X-linked recessive fashion.[52] Some individuals are severely affected, with little or no virilization. Others have minimal abnormalities and older children with less severe defects are increasingly being recognized.

Diagnosis is suspected in individuals with hypospadias or ambiguous genitalia which, depending on the particular defect, may be associated with adrenal insufficiency. Determination of a 46,XY karyotype with low plasma testosterone and elevated gonadotropin levels provides supporting evidence. Further steroid analysis can lead to identification of the specific defect.

Pathogenesis relates to the failure in normal virilization of the wolffian ducts, urogenital sinus, and urogenital tubercle. The degree of abnormality depends on the level of testosterone, which varies in different individuals most likely relating to the severity of the enzymatic defect involved. The absence of müllerian duct derivatives indicates that production of antimüllerian hormone by Sertoli cells is not affected.

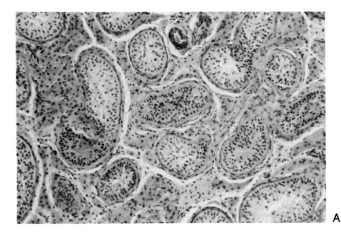

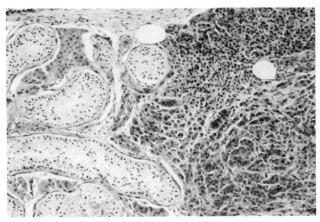

Figure 14–12. Appearance of Leydig cells in developmental disorders. A. 17-ketosteroid reductase deficiency. B. Complete androgen insensitivity syndrome. See the Color Plate after page 84.

Pathologic changes in the testis are secondary. The testes may be abdominal, inguinal, or in the labioscrotal folds.[45] There is typically an abundance of Leydig cells (Figure 14–12A), which may seem paradoxical in view of the deficiency in testosterone production. However, this finding results from the elevated gonadotropin levels which are related to the low testosterone and associated decreased negative feedback effect on LH production. The abundance of Leydig cells reflects a hyperplastic response to persistent gonadotropin stimulation. The Leydig cells have typical features of fully differentiated steroidogenic cells.[53] However, Reinke crystals are not seen, indicating that the cells are of fetal type. Germ cells are markedly reduced in number and most areas show only Sertoli cells within the seminiferous cords (Figure 14–13).

5α-Reductase Deficiency

This disorder is characterized by ambiguous genitalia at birth, but subsequent normal male development and virilization at puberty.[54] Also called pseudovaginal perineoscrotal hypospadias, the condition results from deficiency of the enzyme required for conversion of

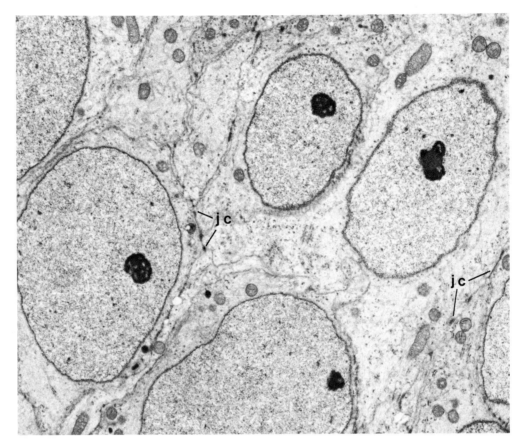

Figure 14–13. Electron microscopic appearance characteristic of androgen biosynthesis defects. Sertoli cells predominate in seminiferous cords and show normal cellular differentiation. jc, junctional complexes. (×6,000)

testosterone to dihydrotestosterone.[55] Testes are normal in size and testosterone production is normal. The defect in reduction of testosterone affects functions of the important androgen, dihydrotestosterone. Since the latter is responsible for the virilization of the external genitalia, the effects of a deficiency are evident at birth. The defect is transmitted in an autosomal recessive fashion.[52]

Testicular changes are variable. Leydig cells may be present in normal or increased numbers. A diminution in germ cells and effects on maturation at the time of spermatogenesis can be seen. Normal maturation has also been found. Since the basic defect is not within the testis but in target tissues, testicular effects, as in the steroidogenic defects, are of a secondary nature.

The pathogenesis of this condition may be more closely related to the androgen receptor disorders (see below) than to the testicular enzyme deficiencies. Recent clinical studies suggest some overlap in the manifestations of 5α-reductase deficiency and androgen receptor disorders, with combined defects in the same family and even the same individual having been described.[56] The question of fertility in those individuals with complete spermatogenesis remains unanswered. Most patients have significant seminiferous tubule damage, probably related to the cryptorchidism often present, at least until puberty.[57]

Androgen Receptor Disorders

Androgen receptor disorders include several different syndromes in which there is abnormal development of phenotypic sex in 46,XY individuals with bilateral testes. Testosterone synthesis and müllerian regression are normal. The abnormality resides in some aspect of androgen action in target tissues. The result is androgen insensitivity, either complete or incomplete, associated with varying degrees of defective virilization. Despite differences in clinical presentation and molecular aspects, the disorders share basic genetic, endocrine, and pathophysiologic features.[58] Four distinct forms have been recognized.

Complete Androgen Insensitivity

The complete androgen insensitivity form, also known as complete testicular feminization, is an X-linked recessive disorder characterized by a female phenotype. External genitalia, breast development, and distribution of body fat are unambiguously female. There is decreased or absent axillary and pubic hair, and the vagina is short and blind-ending. Patients come to medical attention because of an inguinal hernia or primary amenorrhea. There is often a history of similarly affected family members, but about a third of patients have negative family histories.

The testes may be located in the abdomen, inguinal canal, or labia majora. Seminiferous tubules are poorly developed and resemble the cord-like structures of the fetal testis.[59] Germ cells, which are few in number, are of prespermatogenic type. Sertoli cells have an immature appearance and peritubular tissue is minimally developed.[60] Absence of Reinke crystals in the Leydig cells is consistent with the fetal generation.[59] Numerous lipid inclusions may be present. In some cases, there is a hyperplastic response of the Leydig cells (Figure 14–12B).

Incomplete Androgen Insensitivity

This form is much less common than the complete form, and resembles it, except for some ambiguity of the external genitalia, normal pubic hair, and some virilization as well as feminization at the time of puberty. There is usually partial fusion of the labial folds and some clitoromegaly. In contrast to the complete form, wolffian duct derivatives are usually present although not completely normal. Family history in most cases is not informative, but in several instances an X-linked pattern of inheritance has been identified.

The testes in this form may exhibit spermatogenic maturation but not spermatozoa.[61] Sertoli cells are generally of mature type. Diffuse proliferation of Leydig cells is characteristically seen.

Reifenstein Syndrome

Several different forms of androgen insensitivity associated with a predominantly male phenotype have now been grouped in this category.[58] There is a spectrum of defective virilization, ranging from gynecomastia and azoospermia to more severe defects such as hypospadias and the presence of a pseudovagina. Axillary and pubic hair is normal, but chest and facial hair is minimal.

Cryptorchidism is common and the testes are often smaller than normal. Spermatogenesis is incomplete in most cases. However, some patients are able to produce spermatozoa.[61] The appearance of Leydig cells is similar to that in the other forms.

Infertile Male Syndrome

This syndrome includes individuals with normal external genitalia, apparently normal wolffian duct structures, and infertility resulting from azoospermia in whom a receptor abnormality has been demonstrated.[62] Limited information is available on the endocrine and pathologic changes in this form.

The hormonal pattern appears to be similar in the different forms of androgen receptor disorders. Plasma testosterone levels and rates of production by the testes are normal or elevated. The elevated testosterone production is secondary to increased LH levels resulting from defective regulation caused by resistance to androgen action at the hypothalamic-pituitary level. Elevations

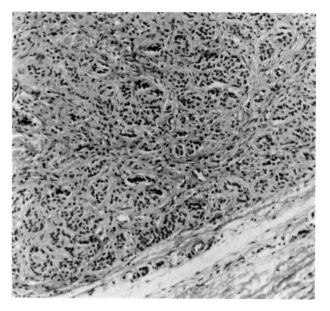

Figure 14–14. Testis from 46,XY phenotypic female with complete androgen insensitivity includes nodule containing cords filled with Sertoli cells and intervening fibrous tissue. (×150)

in LH are believed to be responsible for increased estrogen secretion by the testes. Thus, variable degrees of androgen resistance coupled with enhanced production of estradiol result in varying degrees of defective virilization and feminization in the different androgen receptor disorders.

The testes of patients with testicular feminization are at risk for neoplastic transformation.[47] The incidence of tumor development increases with advancing age.[45] Removal of the testes after puberty has been recommended,[45,46] although there are instances when prepubertal gonadectomy is indicated.[46,63]

An appearance resembling Sertoli cell tumor is occasionally seen in testicular feminization, consisting of circumscribed nodular formations which may be single or multiple.[59] The nodules are composed of seminiferous cords filled with Sertoli cells (Figure 14–14). The terms tubular adenoma and microadenoma have been used for these nodules which are probably developmental malformations rather than truly neoplastic.[61,64] Similar nodules occur in the cryptorchid testis where it is felt they are a result of maldevelopment and therefore the designation of adenoma is unjustified.[65]

LEYDIG CELL HYPOPLASIA

Deficiency in testosterone production may be a result of Leydig cell hypoplasia or agenesis.[66,67] In this condition, there are female-type external genitalia and undescended testes. No müllerian structures are present. There is development of normal wolffian structures, including epididymis and vas deferens.

Diagnosis should be suspected in a phenotypic female with primary amenorrhea and delayed sexual develop-

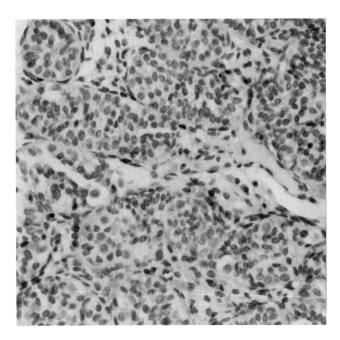

Figure 14–15. Testis in Leydig cell hypoplasia. Interstitial areas include undifferentiated mesenchymal cells. H & E (×250). (Provided by Dr. C. Eil).

ment who demonstrates a 46,XY karyotype. Gonads may be palpable in the inguinal region. Plasma LH is elevated, while FSH is normal. Testosterone levels are low and unresponsive to hCG stimulation.

Pathogenesis may be related to defective Leydig cell differentiation or unresponsiveness to gonadotropins during fetal development. The lack of responsiveness is evident in clinical studies of affected individuals, suggesting, but not necessarily proving, that a similar defect could be present in the fetus. Complete agenesis is unlikely in most cases, since normal wolffian duct differentiation is present.[68] This would mean that fetal Leydig cells are functional during early development. Secondary hypoplasia would better explain the findings.

Pathologic findings in the testes consist of a paucity of Leydig cells (Figure 14–15). This is in direct contrast to the prominence of Leydig cells seen in conditions in which defective virilization is a result of errors in testosterone synthesis or action. In other respects there is a similar immature appearance of the seminiferous tubules which contain numerous Sertoli cells and scattered prespermatogenic germ cells. Tubular boundary tissue is thin and unremarkable.

PERSISTENT MÜLLERIAN DUCT SYNDROME

This disorder is characterized by male external genitalia, bilateral testes, presence of wolffian duct derivatives, and a uterus and fallopian tubes.[69] The latter are usually discovered during repair of an inguinal hernia. The condition, also known as uteri herniae inguinale, was recog-

nized before the identification of antimüllerian hormone. It is now clear that defective AMH production or responsiveness explains the findings.[12] There are no defects in Leydig cell function either during early development or at puberty. Familial cases have been described.

Diagnosis is made in individuals with unilateral or bilateral cryptorchidism associated with the presence of uterine and tubal structures. The vas deferens is often attached to or embedded in the uterus. Testosterone and gonadotropin levels are normal. Karyotype is 46,XY.

Pathogenesis is related to failure of regression of müllerian duct structures. This results from either deficient antimüllerian hormone production by fetal Sertoli cells or refractory response of the müllerian ducts. Deficient production could be a result of defective Sertoli cell differentiation or function. The mechanism appears to be related to locally induced effects on the müllerian ducts. For example, in cases of dysgenesis associated with a testis on one side and a streak on the other, a single uterine horn and tube can be demonstrated on the side contralateral to the testis and therefore lacking in Sertoli cells.[70]

Pathologic changes in the testes include reduction in tubular diameter and defective spermatogenesis, changes associated with cryptorchidism. Leydig cells are abundant and often hyperplastic. An increased incidence of germ cell tumors has been described in patients with müllerian duct persistence.[71] This could be related to the cryptorchid location,[72] although limited information is available because of the relative rarity of this syndrome. Development of embryonal carcinoma has been described in a patient in whom neonatal orchiopexy was performed.[73]

TESTICULAR REGRESSION SYNDROME

The testicular regression syndrome refers to a clinical range of conditions in 46,XY individuals with female, ambiguous, or male phenotype, microphallus, and rudimentary internal genital structures.[74,75] Gonads are absent or small testes may be present. Various terms have been used for cases exhibiting these findings, including gonadal agenesis, anorchia, agonadism, rudimentary testis syndrome, embryonic testicular dysgenesis, vanishing testis syndrome, and Swyer's syndrome. The designation of testicular regression syndrome for the spectrum of disorders encountered seems most appropriate in indicating the probable pathogenesis.[74]

Diagnosis is made in patients with ambiguous or rudimentary external genitalia, micropenis, and elevated gonadotropin levels. Karyotype of 46,XY can be demonstrated in various tissues including gonadal and internal genital structures. If present, testes are very small.

Pathogenesis relates to developmental defects during early testicular differentiation. No genetic or chromosomal abnormalities have been identified. The range in disorders probably relates to the timing of the insult, as has been shown by analyzing the varying effects on mül-

Table 14–4. Major Types of Disorders of Testicular Development

Type	Etiology	Phenotype	Karyotype	Testicular Changes
Gonadal dysgenesis	Chromosome abnormality	Variable (male, female, or ambiguous)	Variable	Streak gonad/immature testis/may be associated w. gonadoblastoma, GC tumors
Klinefelter syndrome	Chromosome abnormality	Male	Variable; 47,XXY most frequent	Peritubular fibrosis, GC depletion, and LC hyperplasia develop at puberty
Testosterone synthesis defects	Gene-related enzyme defects	Variable	46,XY	LC hyperplasia, GC depletion
5α-Reductase deficiency	Gene-related enzyme defect	Ambiguous at birth; male at puberty	46,XY	Usually minimal or no effects on testis
Androgen insensitivity syndrome (TF, Reifenstein syndrome, infertile male syndrome)	Gene-related androgen receptor disorders	Female or male, depending on type	46,XY	LC proliferation/hyperplasia, GC depletion, often w. nodular malformations
Leydig cell hypoplasia	Unknown	Female	46,XY	Absent or sparse LC, lack of tubular development
Persistent müllerian duct syndrome	AMH defect; underlying cause unknown	Male	46,XY	Reduction in tubular diameter, abundant LC
Testicular regression syndrome	Unknown	Variable	46,XY	Streak gonads/rudimentary testes/absent gonadal tissue
Germ cell aplasia	Unknown	Male	46,XY	Tubules lined by SC, normal appearance of LC
Cryptorchidism	Unknown	Male	46,XY	Variable, depending on age; progressive GC depletion and interstitial fibrosis w. advancing age

Abbreviations: GC, germ cell; SC, Sertoli cell; LC, Leydig cell; TF, testicular feminization; AMH, antimüllerian hormone.

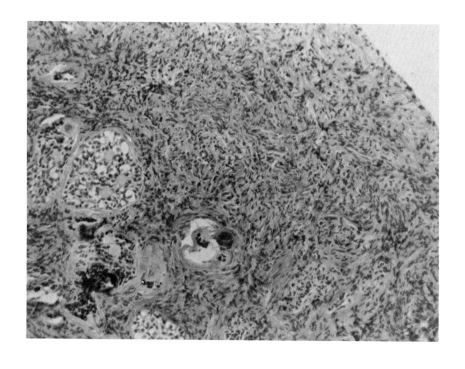

Figure 14–16. Five-year-old 46,XY phenotypic female had fibrous band on left and apparent gonad on right with associated fallopian tube. Gonadal tissue consists principally of fibrous elements, but a few cord-like structures are evident. The findings are consistent with the testicular regression syndrome. (×150)

lerian and wolffian duct development in different cases.[76] It is doubtful that true gonadal agenesis accounts for a significant proportion of the cases, since some degree of fetal testicular function is usually evident.

Pathologic changes are variable. In some cases, thorough search fails to reveal any gonadal tissue, while in other streak gonads can be identified. In still others, rudimentary testes may be present (Figure 14–16). When this is the case, only sparse testicular structures are recognizable, but occasional germ cells, Sertoli cells, and Leydig cells have been described.

GERM CELL APLASIA

The condition referred to as Sertoli-cell-only syndrome or del Castillo syndrome is better designated on the basis of pathogenesis as germ cell aplasia or hypoplasia. Although less commonly used, the latter term is probably more accurate because some germ cells are generally present. For this reason, it is likely that the condition is usually acquired rather than congenital as originally thought by those who first observed the disorder and assumed that no germ cells were present during early differentiation.

As with the testicular regression syndrome, multiple etiologies are possible since there are various mechanisms for eliminating germ cells. Drug effects, radiation, and infection are among the possible causes, but these conditions, which are usually recognized on the basis of history and other findings, represent a small proportion of the cases in which the syndrome is diagnosed. Karyotype studies typically demonstrate a 46,XY pattern and there are generally no associated abnormalities to suggest a genetic or chromosomal basis. It has been suggested that an inherited defect could be present in some

cases, based on studies of genetically determined infertility in animals.[51]

Testicular biopsy establishes the nature of the defect by revealing the lack of germ cells within the tubules but almost always fails to provide evidence of specific etiology. Leydig cells have a normal morphologic appearance and Sertoli cells are of adult type, although some ultrastructural and functional abnormalities have been described.[77] Seminiferous tubules are well formed with wide open lumina for the most part (Figure 14–17). These observations suggest that the pathophysiologic effects are produced late in development and probably are not present prior to puberty.

CRYPTORCHIDISM

Pathologic changes in the testis associated with cryptorchidism are discussed in detail in Chapter 16. Lesions affecting all of the major cellular components of the testis have been reported in children with cryptorchid testes.[78,79] From infancy, the seminiferous cords may be reduced in diameter with decreased numbers of germ cells compared to the normal testis. Progressive fibrosis in the testicular interstitium has been described. It is unclear whether or not there are specific alterations affecting surviving cells. Leydig cells which develop at puberty generally appear normal and testosterone levels reflect adequate Leydig cell function. Germ cells present in the childhood period are comparable in appearance in normal and cryptorchid testes, as is the pattern of seminiferous cord development (Figure 14–18). Consequently, morphologic assessment of the cryptorchid testis in young boys may show no significant deviation from normal.

On the basis of careful anatomic studies, it has been

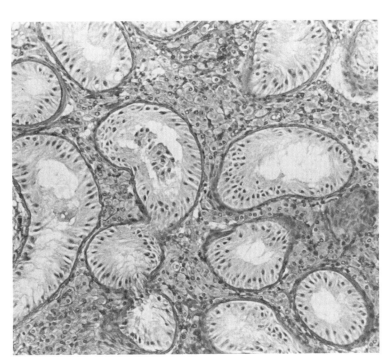

Figure 14–17. Germ cell aplasia, testicular biopsy. Although absence of germ cells suggests immature appearance, Sertoli cells are of mature type and tubular lumen opening is well developed. (×250)

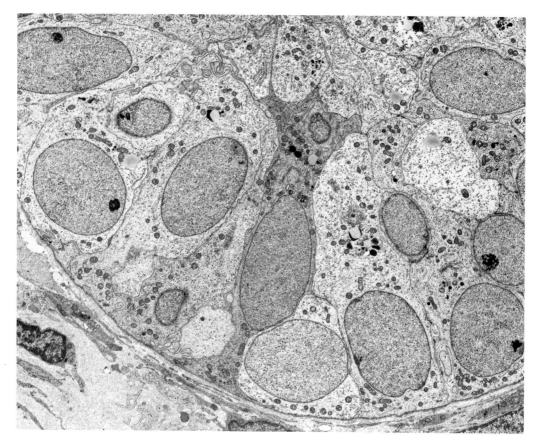

Figure 14–18. Cryptorchid testis, in 12-year-old, with fully differentiated Sertoli cells. (×3,000)

suggested that the epididymis plays a key role in normal testicular descent.[78] Hormonal factors most likely play a role as well, based on clinical and experimental observations. Association of epididymal abnormalities and cryptorchidism with maternal diethylstilbestrol exposure has been described,[80,81] but the precise relationship of these changes is not clear. A particular need exists for information to indicate whether there are intrinsic defects present in the testes of cryptorchid children. Such information is critical for assessment and management related to establishment of subsequent testicular function.

Association of cryptorchidism and germ cell neoplasia is a well established phenomenon, suggesting intrinsic germ cell abnormalities in the cryptorchid testis from an early stage of development. However, the tumors most frequently encountered, such as seminoma and embryonal carcinoma, generally appear in adults and follow a similar pattern in descended and undescended testes. Germ cell tumors in general represent a much lower proportion of testicular neoplasms in children then in adults, and the type most frequently seen in the childhood testis is the yolk sac carcinoma,[82] which is relatively rare in adults. The recently described entity of intratubular germ cell neoplasia (carcinoma *in situ* of the testis), a precursor lesion of the common germ cell neoplasms, has been reported in young boys (Figure 14–19), but

these cases have been associated with gonadal abnormalities other than cryptorchidism.[63,83,84]

Still unresolved is the question of whether the cryptorchid testis which is brought down into the scrotum during childhood remains at risk for neoplasia or should be expected to differentiate and function in a normal manner. Studies on subsequent fertility and incidence of neoplasia following orchiopexy are needed. In a recent retrospective survey, fertility rates of 80% in unilateral cryptorchidism and 35% in bilateral cryptorchidism as compared with age-matched controls were reported after 12 years of follow-up.[85] The authors concluded that the findings challenge the concept that there is an inherent testicular defect in patients with cyrptorchidism. Further studies on the pathophysiologic mechanisms involved in cryptorchidism are required to shed additional light on this controversial subject.

RADIATION EFFECTS

The adult testis is known to be extremely sensitive to the effects of external radiation (See Chapter 16). Although less information is available on damage to the developing testis, several studies have been described on effects in response to treatment of childhood leukemia and other forms of cancer.[86,87]

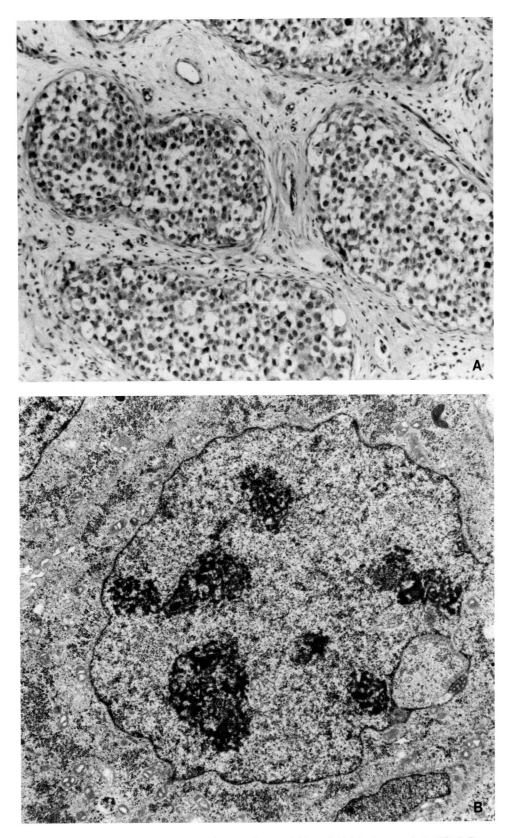

Figure 14–19. Intratubular germ cell neoplasia, 9-year-old boy. A. Light micrograph. (×150). B. Electron micrograph of abnormal germ cell shows multiple nucleoli and abundant glycogen (×6,500)

The reports indicate that radiation may be responsible for severe damage to germ cells and Leydig cells. In one study, 8 of 10 men treated for Wilms tumor during early childhood had either oligospermia or azoospermia.[86] FSH levels were normal prior to puberty and became abnormal only at puberty, indicating that damage can be present in spite of initially normal studies. Effects on Leydig cell function were noted in boys who required testicular irradiation for leukemic infiltration of the testes.[88,89] After treatment there was no testosterone response to hCG stimulation, while there had been a normal response prior to treatment. The effect on Leydig cell function was found to be dose-dependent.

In individuals with delayed pubertal maturation following testicular irradiation, the results of Leydig cell damage could be corrected by androgen replacement therapy.[88] However, when there was damage to germ cells, this was apparently permanent.

DRUG EFFECTS

Effects of cytotoxic drugs in the treatment of childhood cancer and nephrotic syndrome have indicated that severe testicular damage can result.[88,90] Alkylating agents, such as cyclophosphamide and chlorambucil, have been implicated in single-agent therapy. Several studies have described the effects of combination therapy in boys with leukemia and Hodgkin's disease.

The most frequent gonadal alterations described include fibrosis and thickening of the peritubular tissue, partial or total loss of germ cells, and, after puberty, de-

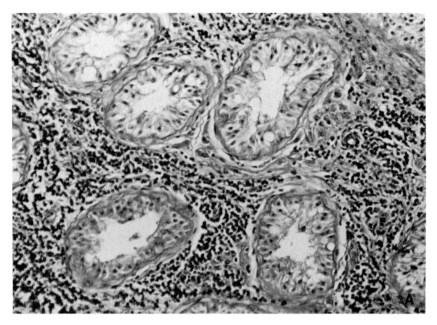

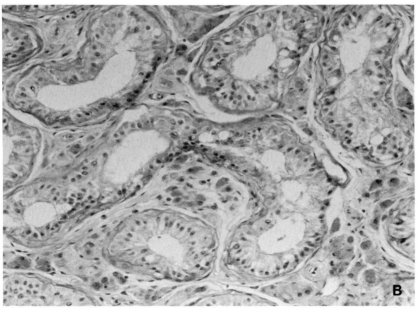

Figure 14–20. Testicular tissue, in 19-year-old, following treatment for acute lymphoblastic leukemia. A. Germ cell depletion associated with leukemic infiltration. B. Contralateral uninvolved testis showing similar changes. (×250)

creased or arrested spermatogenesis (Figure 14–20). Sherins *et al.* found germ cell depletion and markedly elevated FSH levels in pubertal boys receiving a combination of mustine, vincristine, procarbazone, and prednisolone.[91] Effects on Leydig cell function were also evident, as indicated by elevated serum LH and low normal testosterone levels. In another study of men who had been treated with a similar regimen during childhood, semen analysis revealed azoospermia.[92] Some of these individuals had demonstrated normal basal gonadotropin levels and response to GnRH stimulation while still prepubertal. These findings indicate that gonadotropin function and normal progression through puberty may occur in the presence of severe testicular damage from chemotherapy. A number of patients initially assumed to be unaffected subsequently developed evidence of testicular damage.[93]

Since the most sensitive germ cells are the proliferating spermatogonia,[94] the extent of damage should be greatest when treatment is given after the initiation of spermatogenesis. Prior to the onset of spermatogenesis, prespermatogonia are in a slowly cycling state. Such cells are generally assumed to have limited sensitivity to cytotoxic agents. However, prespermatogenic germ cells may be critical targets for long-term effects in view of the profound testicular damage seen after treatment in the prepubertal period.[95] Clinical data currently available suggest that effects of chemotherapeutic agents on potential fertility depend on dose, age, and pubertal status, but further long-term studies are needed.

PREMATURE DEVELOPMENT

Precocious development of testicular function is associated with appearance of testosterone-dependent secondary sex characteristics and initiation of spermatogenesis prior to the normal time of puberty. Onset of significant androgen production and development of pubertal changes before 9 years of age indicates premature testicular function.[96]

True or central precocious puberty arises from disturbed neural function resulting in a pubertal level of hypothalamic-pituitary-testicular activity. The effect on the testis is LH-induced Leydig cell function resulting in gonadotropin-dependent sexual precocity. The pathologic effects include Leydig cell hyperplasia and premature initiation of spermatogenesis. The hyperplastic process is usually bilateral and diffuse, the cells filling the interstitial regions without destroying or disrupting the seminiferous cords (Figure 14–21). Preservation of the seminiferous structures is helpful in distinguishing hyperplasia from tumor.[65] Stimulation of spermatogenic maturation is secondary to the high levels of testosterone produced by the Leydig cells. The extent of spermatogenesis is variable, but complete maturation with spermatogonia, spermatocytes, spermatids, and spermatozoa is frequently observed. Differential diagnosis is directed toward determining the cause of the premature stimulation of Leydig cell activity.

Leydig cell tumors may arise during childhood and produce pubertal changes resulting from premature testosterone secretion. Since this is on a local rather than central basis and not dependent on activation of the hypothalamic-pituitary axis, the changes are referred to as precocious pseudopuberty. Leydig cell tumors constitute approximately 10% of testicular tumors in young boys. They have a peak incidence in mid-childhood, most cases being diagnosed between 3 and 7 years of age.[82] Nocturnal emission and precocious sexual behavior are frequent findings. Gynecomastia may also be present. Diagnosis is established by clinical and endocrine findings of

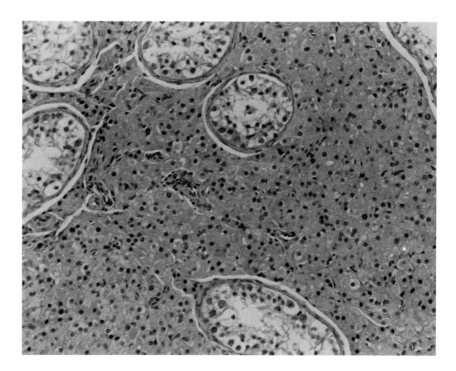

Figure 14–21. Leydig cell hyperplasia, 3-year-old boy. Note preservation of seminiferous cords. (×350)

premature testicular function associated with the presence of unilateral scrotal enlargement. Occasionally, bilateral tumors may be present. In some instances, the tumors are small and nonpalpable, in which case appropriate endocrine studies are needed to rule out adrenal source of the androgens. Gross examination typically reveals a discrete yellow to brown nodule. The microscopic appearance consists of sheets of uniform polyhedral

Leydig cells replacing the testicular parenchyma but not infiltrating surrounding tissue. Reinke crystals are generally absent in the childhood tumors. Leydig cell tumors are almost always benign and successfully treated by orchiectomy. However, androgenic effects on accelerated bone growth may not be entirely reversible.

A familial form of gonadotropin-independent male sexual precocity has recently been described.[96] Desig-

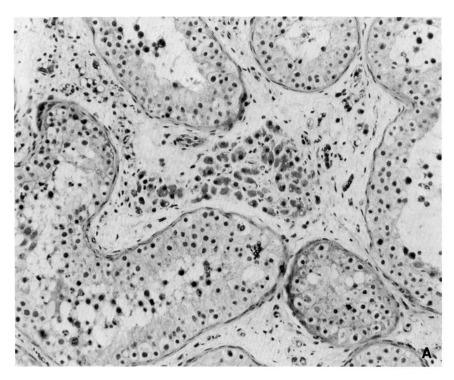

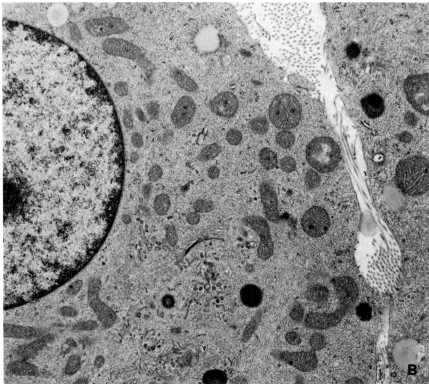

Figure 14–22. Testicular changes in familial gonadotropin-independent sexual precocity. A. Light micrograph showing fully differentiated Leydig cells and seminiferous tubules with lumen formation and spermatogenesis. Toluidine blue (×150). B. Electron micrograph of Leydig cells. (×6,000)

nated as familial testotoxicosis, the condition is characterized by premature Leydig cell development and spermatogenesis in the absence of pituitary gonadotropin stimulation (Figure 14–22). The findings are consistent with an inherited autosomal dominant intratesticular defect. A majority of cases of familial male sexual precocity seem to be examples of this disorder rather than central precocious puberty. The testicular findings in boys with this condition include effects of various kinds.[97] There is a diffuse, patchy proliferation of Leydig cells which lack Reinke crystals. Germ cells at all stages of spermatogenesis are present, but with evident disorganization of maturation. Sertoli cells also show evidence of premature differentiation, including the presence of tight junctional attachments. In adults, there is marked oligospermia and Leydig cells contain numerous cytoplasmic inclusions. Since gonadotropin stimulation is not involved, the pathogenesis appears to be of intratesticular origin, possibly related to defects in local cellular interactions.

DELAYED MATURATION

Delayed onset of Leydig cell function and spermatogenesis can be associated with absent or delayed development of secondary sex characteristics and failure of normal sperm production. Intrinsic testicular disorders may be involved, including the conditions already discussed and those considered in Chapter 16. Since pathologic changes of various types can be associated with delayed testicular development, identification of the specific type of abnormality is essential to proper management and determination of the potential for fertility. In those conditions in which the disorder is of extrinsic origin, the changes in the testes will depend on the type and severity of the disorder. Hypogonadotropic hypogonadism, a major cause of delayed maturation, is discussed in detail in Chapter 17. Various other extratesticular abnormalities may also be responsible for problems in development of testicular function. Differential diagnosis should be directed to identifying the specific source and cause of the abnormality.

References

1. van Wagenen G, Simpson ME: Embryology of the Ovary and Testis: *Homo sapiens* and *Macaca mulatta.* New Haven, Yale University Press, 1965.
2. Elias W: Frühentwicklung des Samenkanälchen beim Menschen. Verh Anat Ges 68:123–131, 1974.
3. Gondos B: Testicular development. *In* AD Johnson, WR Gomes (eds) The Testis (Vol. 4). New York, Academic Press, 1977.
4. Josso N, Picard JY, Tran D: The anti-müllerian hormone. Recent Prog Horm Res 33:117–167, 1977.
5. Donahoe PK, Budzik GP, Trelstad R, *et al.:* Müllerian inhibiting substance: an update. Recent Prog Horm Res 38:279–330, 1982.
6. Tran D, Josso N: Localization of anti-müllerian hormone in the rough endoplasmic reticulum of the developing bovine Sertoli cell, using immunocytochemistry with a monoclonal antibody. Endocrinology 111:1562–1567, 1982.
7. Taguchi O, Cunha GR, Lawrence WD, *et al.:* Timing and irreversibility of müllerian duct inhibition in the embryonic reproductive tract of the human male. Dev Biol 106:394–398, 1984.
8. Jirasek JE: Morphogenesis of the genital system in the human. *In* RJ Blandau, D Bergsma (eds) Morphogenesis and Malformation of the Genital System. New York, Alan R Liss, 1977.
9. Pelliniemi LJ, Niemi M: Fine structure of the human foetal testis. I. The interstitial tissue. Z Zellforsch 99:507–522, 1969.
10. Siiteri PK, Wilson JD: Testosterone formation and metabolism during male sexual differentiation in the human embryo. J Clin Endocrinol Metab 38:113–135, 1974.
11. Wilson JD: Sexual differentiation. Annu Rev Physiol 40:279–306, 1978.
12. Reyes FI, Winter JSD, Faiman C: Studies on human sexual development. I. Fetal gonadal and adrenal sex steroids. J Clin Endocrinol Metab 37:74–78, 1973.
13. Faiman C, Winter JSD, Reyes FI: Endocrinology of the fetal testis. *In* H Burger, D de Kretser (eds) The Testis. New York, Raven Press, 1981.
14. Huhtaniemi IT, Korenbrot CC, Jaffe RB: hCG binding and stimulation of testosterone biosynthesis in the human fetal testis. J Clin Endocrinol Metab 44:963–967, 1977.
15. Kaplan SL, Grumbach, MM, Aubert ML: The ontogenesis of pituitary hormones and hypothalamic factors in the human fetus: maturation of central nervous system regulation of anterior pituitary function. Recent Prog Horm Res 32:161–243, 1976.
16. Baker BL, Jaffe RB: The genesis of cell types in the adenohypophysis of the human fetus as observed with immunocytochemistry. Am J Anat 143:137–162, 1975.
17. Hagen C, McNeilly AS: Identification of human luteinizing hormone, follicle-stimulating hormone, luteinizing hormone β-subunit and gonadotropin α-subunit in fetal and adult pituitary glands. J Endocrinol 67:49–57, 1975.
18. Clements JA, Reyes FI, Winter JSD, *et al.:* Ontogenesis of gonadotropin releasing hormone in the human fetal hypothalamus. Proc Soc Exp Biol Med 163:437–444, 1980.
19. Goodyer CG, St George Hall C, Guyda H, *et al.:* Human fetal pituitary in culture: hormone secretion and response to somatostatin, luteinizing hormone releasing factor, thyrotropin releasing factor, and dibutyryl cyclic AMP. J Clin Endocrinol Metab 45:73–85, 1977.
20. Takagi S, Yoshida T, Tsubata K, *et al.:* Sex differences in fetal gonadotropins and androgens. J Steroid Biochem 8:609–620, 1977.
21. Hadziselimovic F: Cryptorchidism: Ultrastructure of Normal and Cryptorchid Testis Development. Berlin, Springer-Verlag, 1977.
22. Nagano T, Suzuki F: Cell junctions in the seminiferous tubule and the excurrent duct of the testis: freeze-fracture studies. Int Rev Cytol 81:163–190, 1983.
23. Forest MG, Sizonenko PC, Cathiard AM, *et al.:* Hypophysogonadal function in humans during the first year of life. I. Evidence for testicular activity in early infancy. J Clin Invest 53:819–828, 1974.
24. Chemes HE, Gottlieb SE, Pasqualini T, *et al.:* Response to acute hCG stimulation and steroidogenic potential of

Leydig cell fibroblastic precursors in humans. J Androl 6:102–112, 1985.

25. Steinberger E, Root A, Ficher M, et al.: The role of androgens in the initiation of spermatogenesis in man. J Clin Endocrinol Metab 37:746–751, 1973.

26. Bergada C, Mancini RE: Effect of gonadotropins in the induction of spermatogenesis in human prepubertal testis. J Clin Endocrinol Metab 37:935–943, 1973.

27. Winter JSD, Faiman C: Pituitary-gonadal relations in male children and adolescents. Pediat Res 6:126–135, 1972.

28. Sizonenko PC, Schindler A, Cuendet A: Clinical evaluation and management of testicular disorders before puberty. In H Burger, D de Kretser (eds) The Testis. New York, Raven Press, 1981.

29. August GP, Grumbach MM, Kaplan SL: Hormonal changes in puberty: III. Correlation of plasma testosterone, LH, FSH, testicular size, and bone age with male pubertal development. J Clin Endocrinol Metab 34:319–326, 1972.

30. Laron Z, Dickerman Z, Arad J, et al.: Age at first conscious ejaculation. In E Cacciari, A Prader (eds) Pathophysiology of Puberty. New York, Academic Press, 1980.

31. Gilula NB, Fawcett DW, Aoki A: The Sertoli cell occluding junctions and gap junctions in mature and developing mammalian testis. Dev Biol 50:142–168, 1976.

32. Swerdloff RS: Physiological control of puberty. Med Clin North Am 62:351–366, 1978.

33. Forti G, Facchinetti F, Sardelli S, Spermatic and peripheral venous plasma concentrations of progesterone, 17α-hydroxyprogesterone, and 20α-dihydroprogesterone in prepubertal boys. J Clin Endocrinol Metab 56:831–834, 1983.

34. Leinonen PJ, Jaffe RB: Leydig cell desensitization by human chorionic gonadotropin does not occur in the human fetus. J Clin Endocrinol Metab 61:234–238, 1985.

35. de Kretser DM: Sertoli cell-Leydig cell interaction in the regulation of testicular function. Int J Androl Suppl 5:11–17, 1982.

36. Scholler R, Roger M, Leymarie P, et al.: Evaluation of Leydig cell function in normal prepubertal and pubertal boys. J Steroid Biochem 6:95–99, 1975.

37. Forest MG, Lecoq A, Saez JM: Kinetics of human chorionic gonadotropin-induced steroidogenic response of the human testis. II. Plasma 17α-hydroxyprogesterone, Δ^4-androstenedione, estrone, and 17β-estradiol: Evidence for the action of human chorionic gonadotropin on intermediate enzymes implicated in steroid biosynthesis. J Clin Endocrinol Metab 49:284–291, 1979.

38. Forest MG: Maturation of the human testicular response to hCG. Ann NY Acad Sci 438:304–328, 1984.

39. Roth JC, Grumbach MM, Kaplan SL: Effect of synthetic luteinizing hormone-releasing factor on serum testosterone and gonadotropins in prepubertal, pubertal, and adult males. J Clin Endocrinol Metab 37:680–686, 1973.

40. Swerdloff RS, Heber D: Endocrine control of testicular function from birth to puberty. In H Burger, D de Kretser (eds) The Testis. New York, Raven Press, 1981.

41. Boyar R, Perlow M, Hellman L, et al.: Twenty-four-hour pattern of luteinizing hormone secretion in normal men with sleep stage recording. J Clin Endocrinol Metab 35:73–81, 1972.

42. de Kretser DM, Burger H: Ultrastructural studies of the human Sertoli cell in normal men and males with hypogonadotrophic hypogonadism before and after gonado-

trophic trestment. In BB Saxena, CG Beling, HM Gandy (eds) Gonadotrophins. New York, Wiley, 1972.

43. de Kretser DM, Kerr JB, Paulsen CA: The peritubular tissue in the normal and pathological human testis: an ultrastructural study. Biol Reprod 12:317–324, 1975.

44. Robboy SJ, Miller T, Donahoe PK, et al.: Dysgenesis of testicular and streak gonads in the syndrome of mixed gonadal dysgenesis. Hum Pathol 13:700–716, 1982.

45. Grumbach MM, Conte FA: Disorders of sex differentiation. In RH Williams (ed) Textbook of Endocrinology (6th ed). Philadelphia, WB Saunders, 1981.

46. Manuel M, Katayama KP, Jones HW, Jr: The age of occurrence of gonadal tumors in intersex patients with a Y chromosome. Am J Obstet Gynecol 124:293–300, 1976.

47. Simpsom JL: Genetic disorders of gonadal development in humans. In PG Crosignani, BL Rubin, M Fraccaro (eds) Genetic Control of Gamete Production and Function. London, Academic Press, 1982.

48. Ishida T, Tagatz GE, Okagaki T: Gonadoblastoma: ultrastructural evidence for testicular origin. Cancer 37:1770–1781, 1976.

49. Rubin P, Mattei A, Cesarini JP, et al.: Étude en microscopie électronique de la cellule de Leydig dans la maladie de Klinefelter en périodes pré- per- et postpubertaires. An Endocrinol 32:671–687, 1971.

50. Salbenblatt JA, Bender BG, Puck MH, et al.: Pituitary-gonadal function in Klinefelter syndrome before and during puberty. Pediatr Res 19:82–86, 1985.

51. Bardin CW, Paulsen CA: The testes. In RH Williams (ed) Textbook of Endocrinology (6th ed). Philadelphia, WB Saunders, 1981.

52. Wilson JD, Goldstein JL: Classification of hereditary disorders of sexual development. Birth Defects 11(4):1–16, 1975.

53. Longo FJ, Coleman SA, Givens JR: Ultrastructural analysis of the testes in male pseudohermaphrodism due to deficiency of 17-ketosteroid reductase. Am J Clin Path 64:145–154, 1975.

54. Peterson RE, Imperato-McGinley J, Gautier T, et al.: Male pseudohermaphroditism due to steroid 5α-reductase deficiency. Am J Med 62:170–191, 1977.

55. Wilson JD: Dihydrotestosterone formation in cultured human fibroblasts. Comparison of cells from normal subjects and patients with familial incomplete male pseudohermaphroditism, type 2. J Biol Chem 250:3498–3504, 1975.

56. Jukier L, Kaufman M, Pinsky L, et al.: Partial androgen resistance associated with secondary 5α-reductase deficiency: identification of a novel qualitative androgen receptor defect and clinical implications. J Clin Endocrinol Metab 59:679–688, 1984.

57. Imperato-McGinley J, Peterson RE, Gautier T: Primary and secondary 5α-reductase deficiency. In M Serio, M Motta, M Zanisi, et al. (eds) Sexual Differentiation: Basic and Clinical Aspects. New York, Raven Press, 1984.

58. Griffin JE, Wilson JD: Disorders of androgen receptor function. Ann NY Acad Sci 438:61–71, 1984.

59. Ferenczy A, Richart RM: The fine structure of the gonads in the complete form of testicular feminization syndrome. Am J Obstet Gynecol 113:399–409, 1972.

60. Damjanov I, Drobnjak P: Ultrastructure of the gonad in the testicular feminization syndrome. Pathol Europ 9:249–257, 1974.

61. Nistal M, Paniagua R: Testicular and Epididymal Pathology. New York, Thieme-Stratton, 1984.

62. Aiman J, Griffin JE, Gazak JM, et al.: Androgen insensitivity as a cause of infertility in otherwise normal men. Engl J Med 300:223–227, 1979.

63. Müller J, Skakkebaek NE: Testicular carcinoma in situ in children with the androgen insensitivity (testicular feminisation) syndrome. Brit Med J 288:1419–1420, 1984.

64. Estima-Martins AM, Saleiro JV: Ultrastructural observations of a gonad in the testicular feminization syndrome. Pathol Europ 9:233–241, 1974.

65. Mostofi FK, Price EB: Tumors of the Male Genital System. Washington, Armed Forces Institute of Pathology, 1973.

66. Berthezéne F, Forest MG, Grimaud JA, et al.: Leydig-cell agenesis. A cause of male pseudohermaphroditism. N Engl J Med 295:969–972, 1976.

67. Brown DM, Markland C, Dehner LP: Leydig cell hypoplasia: a cause of male pseudohermaphroditism. J Clin Endocrinol Metab 46:1–7, 1978.

68. Eil C, Austin RM, Sesterhenn I, et al.: Leydig cell hypoplasia causing male pseudohermaphroditism: diagnosis 13 years after prepubertal castration. J Clin Endocrinol Metab 58:441–448, 1984.

69. Sloan WR, Walsh PC: Familial persistent müllerian duct syndrome. J Urol 115:459–461, 1976.

70. Bonaventura LM, Roth LM, Cleary RE: The Sertoli cell in mixed gonadal dysgenesis. Obstet Gynecol 53:324–329, 1979.

71. Simpson JL, Photopulos G: The relationship of neoplasia to disorders of abnormal sexual differentiation. Birth Defects 12(1):15–50, 1976.

72. Potashnik G, Sober I, Inbar I, et al.: Male müllerian hermaphroditism: a case report of a rare cause of male infertility. Fertil Steril 28:273–276, 1977.

73. Melman A, Leiter E, Perez JM, et al.: The influence of neonatal orchiopexy upon the testis in persistent müllerian duct syndrome. J Urol 125:856–858, 1981.

74. Edman CD, Winters AJ, Porter JC, et al.: Embryonic testicular regression: a clinical spectrum of XY agonadal individuals. Obstet Gynecol 49:208–217, 1977.

75. Josso N, Briard M: Embryonic testicular regression syndrome: variable phenotypic expression in siblings. J Pediat 97:200–204, 1980.

76. Coulam CB: Testicular regression syndrome. Obstet Gynecol 53:44–49, 1979.

77. Chemes HE, Dym M, Fawcett DW, et al.: Pathophysiologic observations of Sertoli cells in patients with germinal aplasia or severe germ cell depletion. Ultrastructural findings and hormone levels. Biol Reprod 17:108–123, 1977.

78. Hadziselimovic F: Cryptorchidism: Management and Implications. Berlin, Springer-Verlag, 1983.

79. Mininberg DT, Rodber JC, Bedford JM: Ultrastructural evidence of the onset of testicular pathological conditions in the cryptorchid human testis within the first year of life. J Urol 128:782–784, 1982.

80. McLachlan JA, Newbold RR, Bullock B: Reproductive tract lesions in male mice exposed prenatally to diethylstilbestrol. Science 190:991–992, 1975.

81. Gill WB, Schumacher GFB, Bibbo M: Pathological semen and anatomical abnormalities of the genital tract in human male subjects exposed to diethylstilbestrol in utero. J Urol 117:477–480, 1977.

82. Brosman SA, Gondos B: Testicular tumors in children. In WE Goodwin, JH Johnston (eds) Reviews in Paediatric Urology. Amsterdam, Excerpta Medica, 1974.

83. Wurzel R, Gondos B, Ratzan SK, et al.: Intratubular germ cell neoplasia associated with precocious puberty. J Androl 5:28P, 1984.

84. Müller J, Skakkebaek NE, Ritzen M, et al.: Carcinoma in situ of the testis in children with 45,X/46,XY gonadal dysgenesis. J Pediatr 106:431–436, 1985.

85. Gilhooly PE, Meyers F, Lattimer JK: Fertility prospects for children with cryptorchidism. Am J Dis Child 138:940–943, 1984.

86. Shalet SM, Beardwell CG, Jacobs HS, et al.: Testicular function following irradiation of the human prepubertal testis. Clin Endocrinol 9:483–490, 1978.

87. Leiper AD, Grant DB, Chessells JM: The effect of testicular irradiation on Leydig cell function in prepubertal boys with acute lymphoblastic leukemia. Arch Dis Child 58:906–910, 1983.

88. Shalet SM: The effects of cancer treatment on growth and sexual development. In A Aynsley-Green a (ed) Paediatric Endocrinology in Clinical Practice. Boston, MTP Press, 1984.

89. Brauner R, Czernichow P, Cramer P, et al.: Leydig-cell function in children after direct testicular irradiation for acute lymphoblastic leukemia. N Engl J Med 309:25–28, 1983.

90. Schilsky RL, Lewis BJ, Sherins RJ, et al.: Gonadal dysfunction in patients receiving chemotherapy for cancer. Ann Int Med 93:109–114, 1980.

91. Sherins RJ, Olweny CLM, Ziegler JL: Gynecomastia and gonadal dysfunction in adolescent boys treated with combination chemotherapy for Hodgkin's disease. N Engl J Med 229:12–16, 1978.

92. Whitehead E, Shalet SM, Morris Jones PH, et al.: Gonadal function after combination chemotherapy for Hodgkin's disease in childhood. Arch Dis Child 47:287–291, 1982.

93. Shalet SM: Effects of cancer chemotherapy on gonadal function of patients. Cancer Treat Rev 7:141–152, 1980.

94. Meistrich ML: Stage-specific sensitivity of spermatogonia to different chemotherapeutic drugs. Biomed Pharmacotherapy 38:137–142, 1984.

95. Matus-Ridley M, Nicosia SV, Meadows AT: Gonadal effects of cancer therapy in boys. Cancer 56:2353–2363, 1985.

96. Rosenthal SM, Grumbach MM, Kaplan SL: Gonadotropin-independent familial sexual precocity with premature Leydig and germinal cell maturation ("familial testotoxicosis"): Effects of a potent luteinizing hormone-releasing factor agonist and medroxyprogesterone acetate therapy in four cases. J Clin Endocrinol Metab 57:571–579, 1983.

97. Gondos B, Egli CA, Rosenthal SM, et al.: Testicular changes in gonadotropin-independent familial male sexual precocity: familial testotoxicosis. Arch Pathol Lab Med 109:990–995, 1985.

98. Apter D, Pakarinen A, Vikho R: Serum prolactin, FSH and LH during puberty in girls and boys. Acta Paediatr Scand 67:417–423, 1978.

15. Chromosome Anomalies and Male Infertility

Ting-Wa Wong, Keith A. Horvath, and Neil L. Kao

Infertility is a universal phenomenon observed in all species of the biological sphere, but only in man does the inability to have one's own progeny evoke so much turmoil and despair. In the United States, approximately 15% of the marriages are barren and produce no offspring; defects in the husband's reproductive system are responsible in about 50% of the cases.[1-3] In the majority of the instances of male infertility, impaired spermatogenesis is the immediate cause.[2,4] Spermatogenesis is a complex process which can be perturbed by a variety of intrinsic and extrinsic factors. Among the upsetting intrinsic influences are abnormalities in the chromosome constitution of the individual. The importance of chromosome aberrations as underlying causes of human male infertility has been increasingly recognized. Such aberrations are, for the most part, detectable by analysis of the chromosomes of somatic cells in mitosis. But in a fraction of the cases, the abnormalities can only be unveiled by studying the chromosomes of germ cells in meiosis, the mitotic chromosomes in somatic cells being normal. In Table 15–1, a brief outline of the more important mitotic and meiotic chromosome abnormalities associated with human male infertility is presented. This outline forms the basis of the following discussion.

PRINCIPLES AND METHODS OF CHROMOSOME ANALYSIS

Human chromosomes can be studied in three settings: 1. mitotic nuclei, 2. meiotic nuclei, and 3. nondividing, interphase nuclei.

Mitotic Chromosomes

In principle, mitotic chromosome analysis can be performed on any type of somatic cell which undergoes mitosis. But for ease of obtaining material for study, the lymphocytes from peripheral blood are most frequently employed.[5,6] Such chromosome analysis is usually carried out during metaphase of mitosis, because the chromosomes are darker and more discrete in metaphase than in any other stage of cell division and are consequently easier to separate and identify individually (Figure 15–1). The procedure may be summarized as follows. A sample of blood is drawn from the individual to be studied. Since blood normally contains no dividing lymphocytes, cell division must be stimulated artificially. This is usually accomplished by placing the blood in a culture medium containing phytohemagglutinin, which not only can agglutinate red blood cells and separate them from the white blood cells, but also has the ability

Table 15–1. Chromosome Aberrations Associated with Male Infertility

I. Aberrations detectable by mitotic chromosome analysis
  A. Sex chromosomes
    1. Numerical abnormalities
      a. Klinefelter's syndrome
        (1) Classical form (XXY)
        (2) Variant forms (examples: XXXY, XXYY, XXXXY, XXXYY)
        (3) Mosaicism (example: XY/XXY)
      b. XYY syndrome
    2. Structural abnormalities
      a. The Y chromosome
  B. Autosomes
    1. Autosomal reciprocal translocations
    2. Robertsonian translocations
  C. Both
    1. X-autosome reciprocal translocations
    2. Y-autosome reciprocal translocations
II. Aberrations detectable *only* by meiotic chromosome analysis
  A. Asynapsis
  B. Desynapsis
  C. Low chiasma counts
  D. Dissociation of the X and Y chromosomes

This study was supported by grant CA 28053 from the National Cancer Institute and by grant 84-35 from the American Cancer Society Illinois Division. The help of Cathy Hirsh and Charles Weber in the preparation of the illustrations is gratefully acknowledged.

to specifically stimulate lymphocytes to undergo mitosis. The lymphocytes are then allowed to grow and divide. After 48 to 72 hours of culture, colchicine is added to arrest mitotic nuclei in the metaphase stage, and the cells are recovered by centrifugation and treated with hypotonic saline. The resulting swelling not only causes the chromosomes to separate from one another, thereby avoiding overlap, but also makes their substructures easier to visualize. The cells are then fixed in a solution consisting of ethanol and acetic acid. Afterward, a drop of the cell suspension is placed on a glass slide and allowed to air-dry. The slide is next stained with either quinacrine mustard (a fluorescent dye) or Giemsa. By this staining procedure, a pattern of bands unique to each chromosome is revealed, enabling individual chromosomes and their component parts to be identified unequivocally.[7,8] The bands obtained with quinacrine staining are referred to as Q-bands, while those obtained with Giemsa staining are designated as G-bands. The fluorescent Q-bands tend to fade with time; in addition, they require ultraviolet illumination and a fluorescence microscope to visualize. In contrast, G-bands are permanent on storage and can be visualized with the ordinary light microscope. Therefore, most laboratories prefer G-banding for routine purposes. After staining, the chromosomes belonging to a single cell are photographed and greatly magnified in the printing process. The chromosome figures are then cut from the print and matched up in homologous pairs. Finally, the chromosome pairs are arranged in order of their size. This pictorial representation of an individual's chromosomes is called a karyotype (Figure 15–2). In humans, 22 of the 23 pairs of chromosomes occur in both sexes and are called autosomes. They are numbered 1 to 22 consecutively according to their size. The remaining pair of chromosomes are the sex chromosomes. These consist of two X chromosomes in females; but in males, the sex chromosomes are *un*like and consist of an X and a Y chromosome.

The autosomes are further characterized by two important variables: the length and the position of the centromere. By length, the 22 pairs of human autosomes are grouped into seven different classes from A to G (Figure 15–2). By position of the centromere, they are divided into the metacentric, submetacentric, and acrocentric varieties (Figure 15–3). If the centromere is located in the middle of the chromosome and divides it into two arms of equal length, the chromosome is termed metacentric. If the centromere is off-center, so that one arm of the chromosome is somewhat longer than the other, the chromosome is labeled submetacentric. Finally, if the centromere is situated near the end of the chromosome, so that one arm is considerably longer than the other, the chromosome is designated acrocentric. By these classifications, the chromosomes from Group A are metacentric, those from Groups B and C are submetacentric, while those from Groups D and G are acrocentric, and so forth (Figure 15–2). Such classifications are important, for the position of the centromere in a chromosome plays a role in determining its susceptibility to certain types of breakage and structural abnormalities. Many chromosome anomalies leading to male infertility are found to involve acrocentric chromosomes, as will be explained later.

Meiotic Chromosomes

Human chromosomes are less frequently studied during meiosis than during mitosis, because obtaining material for study usually presents a problem. To study meiosis in the human male, a testicular biopsy is required. The biopsy specimen is first treated briefly with a hypotonic solution before being fixed. The germ cells extruded

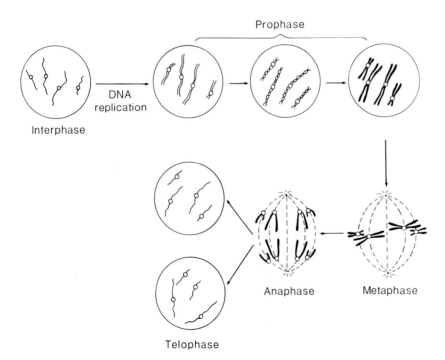

Figure 15–1. The stages of mitosis are illustrated using two pairs of homologous chromosomes. Only the nucleus is represented. Chromosomes are not normally visible as discrete structures during interphase, but for clarity of presentation they are so depicted. DNA synthesis leading to duplication of chromosomes takes place in interphase, immediately preceding the onset of prophase.

Interphase

DNA replication

Prophase

Metaphase

Anaphase

Telophase

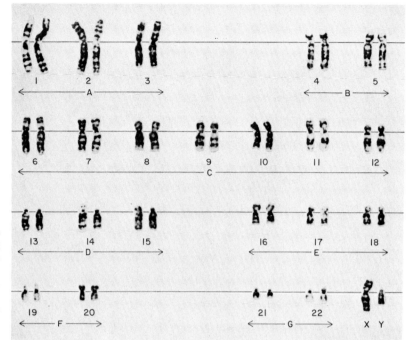

Figure 15–2. Karyotype from a normal male as revealed by mitotic chromosome analysis, using lymphocytes cultured from peripheral blood. The metaphase chromosomes have been stained with the Giemsa-banding method modified by pretreatment with trypsin. This procedure produces banding patterns specific for each chromosome, making it possible to identify all 46 chromosomes individually. (Contributed by K. Hirschhorn.)

from the seminiferous tubules are then processed with a DNA stain such as orcein or quinacrine mustard.[9,10] More recently, a silver stain for meiotic chromosomes has also become available.[11] In optimal material, all stages of meiosis can be examined in one specimen, particularly pachytene, diakinesis, and metaphase of the first meiotic division (Figure 15–4). In meiosis, the X-Y bivalent of normal males can be identified among the 22 autosome bivalents. In contrast to the autosomes, which pair side-by-side, the X and Y chromosomes are paired end-to-end in meiosis[12,13] (Figure 15–5a). The dissimilarity of the X and Y chromosomes and their end-to-end pairing during meiosis predispose the male to a variety of infertility problems not found in the female, as will be made clear later. Examination of meiotic chromosomes is essential to understanding how certain chromosome aberrations affect spermatogenesis and how the chromosome anom-

alies are passed on by the gametes to the next generation. In addition, certain infertile men who are karyotypically normal may harbor meiotic chromosome abnormalities that can only be detected by examining the germ cells in meiosis.

Interphase Chromosomes

The chromosomes of a nondividing, interphase nucleus are not usually visible as discrete structures. Some of the chromosomes lose their condensed appearance and become invisible to the light microscope, a form called euchromatin. Others appear as scattered, darkly staining areas throughout the nucleus, called heterochromatin. Euchromatin is invisible because it represents DNAs that have uncoiled into long thin threads, actively engaged in transcription concerned with the synthetic and metabolic functions of the cell during interphase. Heterochromatin, on the other hand, represents DNAs that are essentially inactive. Barr and Bertram were the first to report the presence of a mass of darkly staining heterochromatin at the periphery of the nucleus in resting ganglion cells of female cats but not of male cats.[14] This distinguishing feature of the female sex was subsequently found to hold true for all interphase somatic cells of eutherian mammals examined. For this reason, the mass of heterochromatin was named the sex chromatin body. The structure was also referred to as the Barr body, after the investigator who first reported it.[14] Later, it was shown by Ohno that the sex chromatin body in female somatic cells represents heterochromatin derived from a single X chromosome.[15] On the basis of these observations and the patterns of inheritance of X-linked traits, Lyon put forth the hypothesis that in female mammalian somatic cells,

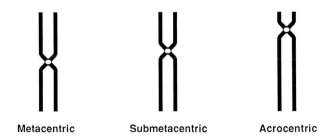

Metacentric **Submetacentric** **Acrocentric**

Figure 15–3. Classification of chromosomes. In a metacentric chromosome, the centromere is situated in the middle. In a submetacentric chromosome, the centromere is off-center. In an acrocentric chromosome, the centromere is located near the end. Each chromosome is shown in its duplicated state, with two sister chromatids joined by the centromere, as seen in karyotype analysis.

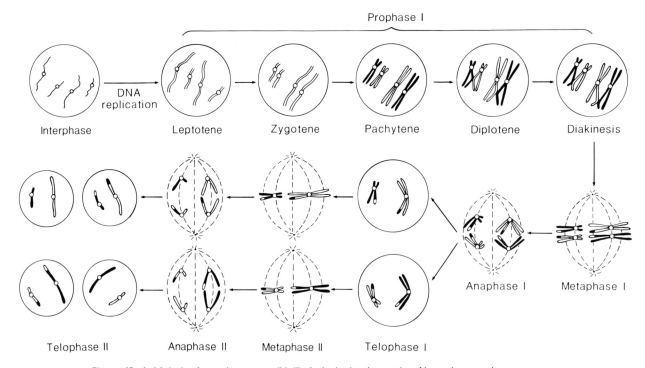

Figure 15–4. Meiosis of a male germ cell is illustrated using two pairs of homologous chromosomes. Only the nucleus is represented. To simplify the diagram, prophase II has been omitted. The original diploid cell gives rise to four haploid cells (spermatozoa).

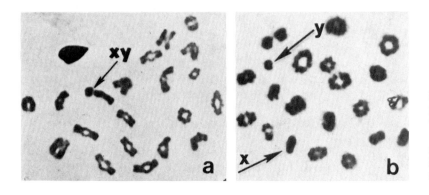

Figure 15–5. (a) Primary spermatocyte in metaphase I, from a normal male showing the usual end-to-end association of X and Y chromosomes (arrow). (From S Ohno, et al.[12]). (b) Primary spermatocyte in metaphase I, from a sterile male showing separate X and Y chromosomes (arrows). (From CV Beechey.[108])

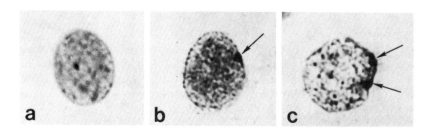

Figure 15–6. Interphase nuclei of cells from buccal smears showing sex chromatin bodies. The number of sex chromatin bodies in a given nucleus is one less than the number of X chromosomes it contains. Thus, a cell from a normal male (XY) will have no sex chromatin, as shown in (a). A cell from a normal female (XX), or a Klinefelter male with an XXY karyotype, will have one sex chromatin body, as demonstrated in (b). A cell from a Klinefelter male with the variant karyotype XXXY will have two sex chromatin bodies, as illustrated in (c). (Contributed by J de Grouchy.)

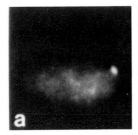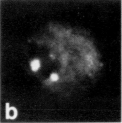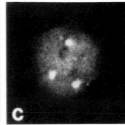

Figure 15–7. The number of fluorescent Y bodies in a given interphase nucleus is equal to the number of Y chromosomes it contains. In (a), one fluorescent Y body is seen in a fibroblast from a normal XY man. (Contributed by TR Chen.) In (b), two fluorescent Y bodies are seen in a primary spermatocyte prior to meiosis, from the testicular biopsy specimen of a man with an XYY somatic karyotype. (From A Baghdassarian, *et al.*[19]) In (c), three Y bodies are seen in a lymphocyte from an XYYY male. (From GS Schoepflin, WR Centerwall.[20])

only one X chromosome is genetically active; the second X chromosome is inactivated and converted to heterochromatin.[16,17] Normal males with XY cells, having only one X chromosome, will have no sex chromatin body, since the single X chromosome remains active and is in euchromatin form and hence is not visible. The consequence of inactivating one of two X chromosomes in female somatic cells is to equalize the amount of X-linked gene products in the female and the male. This phenomenon, by which one X chromosome in each female somatic cell is turned off to offset the sex differences in gene dosage, is known as dosage compensation. Further studies have established that regardless of how many X chromosomes a somatic cell possesses, only one X chromosome remains active; all X chromosomes in excess of one are inactivated and converted to sex chromatin bodies. As a result, in an abnormal male with an XXY karyotype, the somatic interphase nuclei will have one sex chromatin body; whereas in an abnormal male with an XXXY karyotype, the cells will have two sex chromatin bodies[18] (Figure 15–6). Thus an examination of the interphase nuclei of somatic cells, such as those obtained by gentle scraping of the buccal mucosa, can serve as a rough screening procedure for numerical abnormalities of the X chromosome. Cells containing one or more sex chromatin bodies are said to be sex chromatin-positive; those lacking sex chromatin bodies are labeled sex chromatin-negative.

In interphase nuclei stained with quinacrine mustard, the Y chromosome of the male can be identified as a bright fluorescent body, while the other chromosomes are usually too diffuse to be recognized (Figure 15–7a). The number of fluorescent Y bodies in an interphase nucleus is equal to the number of Y chromosomes it contains. An abnormal XYY cell will have two fluorescent Y bodies,[19] while an abnormal XYYY cell will have three[20] (Figures 15–7b,c). Therefore, quinacrine-stained interphase nuclei can provide hints of numerical abnormalities of the Y chromosome.

Once an individual has been found to have an abnormal number of sex chromatin bodies or fluorescent Y bodies in the interphase somatic nuclei, it is essential that a karyotype analysis be performed to ascertain the true nature of the sex chromosome anomaly.

MITOTIC CHROMOSOME ANOMALIES ASSOCIATED WITH MALE INFERTILITY

Of the chromosome anomalies associated with male infertility, most are diagnosable by mitotic chromosome analysis. Results from multiple large surveys indicate that among unselected men seen in infertility clinics, the overall incidence of mitotic chromosome aberrations ranges from 2% to 9%, with an average of about 5%.[21-25] The frequency of such aberrations increases as the sperm count of the patient decreases. Among azoospermic men, the incidence of mitotic chromosome anomalies has been reported to be as high as 15% to 20%.[21,23] These anomalies may involve the sex chromosomes, the autosomes, or both (Table 15–1). In the section to follow, the more important categories of these anomalies will be described.

Klinefelter's Syndrome

On the basis of chromosome constitution, three categories of Klinefelter's syndrome can be distinguished: 1. the classical form, 2. the variant forms, and 3. the mosaics. Of these, the classical form constitutes the majority.[26]

In the classical form of Klinefelter's syndrome, the patient exhibits a 47,XXY karyotype. Because of the presence of an extraneous X chromosome, the interphase nuclei of such patients possess a sex chromatin body (Figure 15–6b). The disorder appears to arise *de novo* rather than being inherited, since no increased incidence of the syndrome has been observed among the kindred of affected males. Studies using the dominantly inherited, X-linked blood group antigen Xg[a] have established that the extra X chromosome in 47,XXY males arises through unequal segregation (nondisjunction) of sex chromosomes during gametogenesis of one or the other parent, most frequently in the first meiotic division[27] (Figure 15–8). Pedigree studies of the inheritance of Xg[a] antigen indicate that approximately 60% of the nondisjunction is maternal in origin and about 40% paternal.[27]

Klinefelter's syndrome is a relatively common disor-

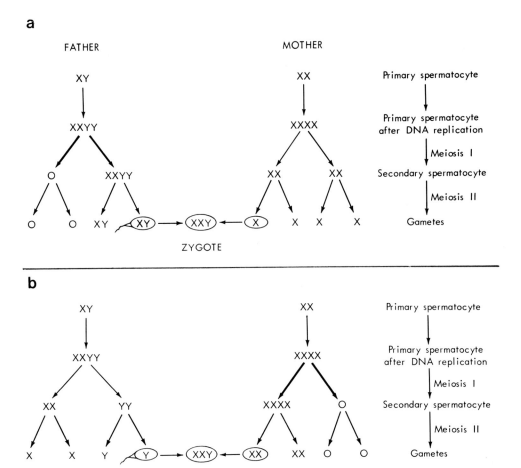

Figure 15–8. Classical Klinefelter's syndrome (XXY) most frequently arises through a single nondisjunctional event occurring in meiosis I of one or the other parent. In (a), the nondisjunction is depicted as occurring in meiosis I of the father. In (b), the nondisjunction is shown occurring in meiosis I of the mother. The heavy arrows indicate nondisjunction.

der. By mitotic chromosome analysis, the incidence of the XXY karyotype is found to be approximately 1 per 600 live-born males.[28] Among azoospermic men seen at infertility clinics, however, the frequency of this karyotype is considerably greater, and incidences as high as 10% to 13% have been reported,[23,29] making it the most common chromosomal anomaly associated with male infertility.[21–24]

The most consistent findings in patients with classical Klinefelter's syndrome are sclerosis of the testicular tubules and infertility, accompanied by varying degrees of Leydig cell dysfunction.[3,30] Although the gonadal abnormalities seldom attract attention prior to puberty, testicular biopsies performed on prepubertal boys with an XXY karyotype indicate that the inherent defects are present long before puberty.[31] Compared to normal controls of the same age obtained at necropsy, the seminiferous tubules of XXY boys are not only smaller but contain far fewer germ cells, with less than 5% of the tubules populated with the normal complement of spermatogonia. In contrast, over 90% of the tubules in most normal controls contain the full complement of spermatogonia.[31]

Despite these grave defects in the gonads, the full-blown clinical features of Klinefelter's syndrome are not usually apparent until puberty, when the intrinsically abnormal testes, unable to respond to pituitary gonadotropin stimulation, begin to undergo the typical pathological changes.[32] They fail to increase in size and instead become firmer and smaller because of progressive sclerosis of the seminiferous tubules.[33] Azoospermia and sterility soon ensue. The Leydig cells are usually increased in number.[33] But despite their hyperplastic appearance, these cells are functionally impaired, and androgen production is usually deficient.[34,35] Plasma testosterone is characteristically low to low-normal, and varying degrees of eunuchoidism and gynecomastia are often present. FSH is usually markedly elevated as a compensatory response to the loss of germ cells. LH is variably elevated, depending on the degree of androgen deficiency. Subnormal intelligence and personality disorders are found in about 25% of the cases.[36]

Variant forms of Klinefelter's syndrome with such karyotypes as 48,XXXY, 48,XXYY, 49,XXXXY, and 49,XXXYY are also known.[26,37] All of these are far less frequent than the 47,XXY karyotype associated with the classical form of Klinefelter's syndrome, undoubtedly because two nondisjunctional events, rather than one, are required for their occurrence (contrast Figure 15–9 with Figure 15–8). Patients with such variant karyotypes all show testicular sclerosis and sterility, often accompanied by cryptorchidism.[3,30] In addition, they appear to have more profound abnormalities of all types, including severe mental retardation.[36] In fact, most of these variant forms are detected through chromosome surveys of residents in mental institutions.

Various forms of mosaics involving the Klinefelter karyotype have also been reported.[3,26,30,37] As with any mosaic, the phenotype of the individual patient varies, depending on what fraction of the cells are aberrant and how the aberrant cells are distributed among the different tissues. The most frequently observed mosaic karyotype among Klinefelter patients is 46,XY/47,XXY. Not surprisingly, such mosaic males tend to exhibit a more normal phenotype and less severe testicular damage than 47,XXY males. The 46,XY germ cells in these mosaic individuals can undergo normal maturation, leading to the formation of spermatozoa. The ultimate sperm counts in such patients depend on the proportion of 46,XY germ cells in the gonads. A minority of them are reported to have normal-sized testes and to be fertile.[38] Studies of the inheritance of the X-linked blood group antigen Xg[a] in such patients indicate that the 46,XY/47,XXY mosaicism arises from mitotic loss of an X chromosome in some of the cell lines originating from an XXY zygote[27] (Figure 15–10).

XYY Syndrome

The incidence of the 47,XYY karyotype is approximately 1 per 1000 live-born males.[28] Quinacrine-stained interphase nuclei show two fluorescent Y bodies instead of

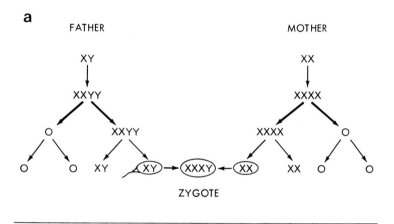

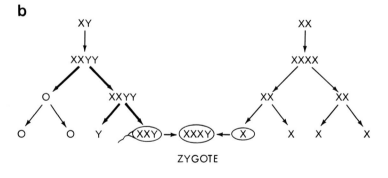

Figure 15–9. Ways by which a 48,XXXY zygote could be formed, all of which require two nondisjunctional events: (a) nondisjunction in the first meiotic division of both the father and the mother; (b) nondisjunction in the first and second meiotic divisions of the father; (c) nondisjunction in the first and second meiotic divisions of the mother. In each instance, nondisjunction is marked by heavy arrows.

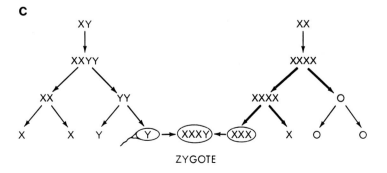

Chromosome loss as XXY cell divides

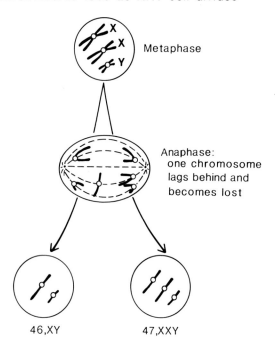

Figure 15–10. Mosaicism can arise through chromosome loss; that is, a chromosome may lag so far behind during the anaphase that it is not included in either daughter nucleus. If the original cell is XXY, then following the loss of an X chromosome, one daughter cell will be XY rather than XXY. As the two daughter cells continue to divide, they will give rise to two descendant cell lines, one XY and the other XXY. An individual who has a mixture of cells with different chromosome numbers is called a mosaic. In the above instance, the mosaicism which arises is 46,XY/47,XXY.

the usual one[19] (Figure 15–7b). The extra Y chromosome is believed to arise through nondisjunction in the second meiotic division of the father's germ cells (Figure 15–11).

The superfluous Y chromosome in the XYY karyotype appears to have a variable effect on fertility. The spermatogenic function of the affected individuals can be normal, minimally impaired, or severely deranged; on the whole, the gonadal dysfunction is much less severe than in Klinefelter's syndrome.[19,39] In cases of XYY males that are fertile, the offspring produced often have a normal number of sex chromosomes, either XX or XY, indicating

that a mechanism operates to eliminate the extra Y chromosome during gametogenesis.[3,23]

The XYY karyotype is often associated with excessively tall stature and a tendency to develop pustular acne. A number of such patients also tend to exhibit aggressive and criminal behavior.[3,37]

X-Autosome Reciprocal Translocations

In X-autosome reciprocal translocations, there is a breakpoint in the X chromosome and another in an autosome; the segments then rejoin in the wrong combinations.

In the mouse, most known X-autosome reciprocal translocations are radiation- or mutagen-induced and are "male-sterile," with spermatogenic arrest occurring at the pachytene stage of primary spermatocytes.[40,41] In man, X-autosome translocations are uncommon; those documented have been reported to be associated with spermatogenic arrest at the stage of primary spermatocytes,[24,42] similar to the findings in mice. There has been a large body of evidence indicating that inactivation of the X chromosome at a critical time is essential to the normal progression of spermatogenesis.[43] Such X-inactivation normally occurs during the early stage of prophase in meiosis I (Figure 15–4) of the male.[43–45] In X-autosome translocations, part of the X chromosome is translocated to an autosome and may be physically removed from the X-linked locus which normally controls X chromosome inactivation. The translocated X segment may therefore remain active longer than it should, leading to the synthesis of "nonpermissible" gene products which are lethal to the developing germ cells.[43] The consequence is spermatogenic arrest at the stage of primary spermatocytes. Since both X chromosomes normally remain active during oogenesis,[46–48] X-autosome translocations would not be expected to have the same adverse effect on germ cell maturation in females, and this is precisely what is observed.

Y-Autosome Reciprocal Translocations

Reciprocal translocations between the Y chromosome and an autosome are rare in most species. Those de-

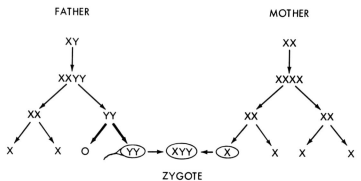

Figure 15–11. The XYY karyotype usually results from nondisjunction in meiosis II of the father, as shown here. Heavy arrows indicate nondisjunction.

scribed are associated with spermatogenic impairment in both mice[49,50] and men,[24,42,51-53] but the impairment is less severe than that observed with X-autosome translocations. Whereas the spermatogenic arrest associated with X-autosome translocations commonly occurs at the stage of primary spermatocytes, the arrest associated with Y-autosome translocations usually occurs later, at either the secondary spermatocyte or spermatid stage, and formation of spermatozoa in small numbers has been reported.[42]

Autosomal Reciprocal Translocations

In autosomal reciprocal translocations, two nonhomologous autosomes break and exchange segments, which need not be of the same size (Figure 15–12). If the chromosome segments involved in the exchange are intact, with no leftover pieces after the breakage and reunion, the translocation is said to be balanced. Since all of the genetic material is still present, though in a different arrangement, the phenotype of the individual is usually normal. Autosomal reciprocal translocations can occur in the heterozygous or homozygous state (Figure 15–12). In man, a proportion of the autosomal translocations detected by somatic karyotyping are associated with spermatogenic failure and sterility.[54-61]

Our knowledge of the way in which autosomal reciprocal translocations cause male infertility is gained largely through observations in the mouse, a species in which autosomal translocations can be induced with relative ease by x-rays or chemical mutagens.[49,50,62,63] More than 100 such experimentally induced autosomal reciprocal translocations have now been studied. Several features characterize these translocations: 1. The breakdown of gametogenesis affects only males; gametogenesis in females is not affected in the presence of the same chromosome rearrangement. 2. Sterility is observed only in males heterozygous for the translocation; homozygous males are fertile (Figures 15–13a,b). 3. Although all germ cells in a male heterozygote carry the same rearranged chromosomes, spermatogenic breakdown is not complete, and some spermatozoa may be formed. 4. If mating with a normal female results in pregnancy, the rate of spontaneous abortion is abnormally high. 5. If viable offspring are produced, about half of them will inherit the heterozygous state for the particular autosomal translocation. 6. The sterilizing effect of the translocations is not

linked to any particular autosome; in fact, in the experimentally induced translocations of the mouse, each autosome has been involved at least once. This observation suggests that the spermatogenic impairment is not due to the altered expression of a few specific genes at or near the breakpoint of a particular chromosome, but instead is caused by the grossly abnormal arrangement of the genome resulting from a translocation. In short, the deranged control mechanism brought on by an autosomal reciprocal translocation appears to be operating at the level of the chromosome rather than at the level of the gene.

These seemingly confusing observations were reconciled and made understandable by studies performed on the affected male germ cells in meiosis.[50,62,64-66] The meiotic behavior of germ cells bearing a heterozygous autosomal reciprocal translocation is complex and out of the ordinary. In the prophase of the first meiotic division, homologous chromosomes normally undergo side-by-side pairing in an extremely precise, gene-by-gene fashion. The translocated chromosomes, on the other hand, must form some unusual configuration in order to achieve pairing with their partners; in most autosomal reciprocal translocations, a distinctive cross-shaped quadrivalent, instead of the usual bivalent, is formed (Figure 15–14). Even with such peculiar configurations, however, there are pairing difficulties in certain portions of the translocation quadrivalent, which leave them free to interact and associate with the unpaired segments of the X chromosome in the X-Y bivalent.[64-66] This abnormal association can occur in the male because the X and Y chromosomes normally undergo end-to-end pairing (Figure 15–5a), rather than side-to-side pairing as in the case of the two X chromosomes of the female. As a result of the end-to-end pairing, large segments of the X chromosome in the X-Y bivalent remain unpaired. It has been postulated that abnormal association between the translocated autosomes and the unpaired portions of the X chromosome may interfere with X chromosome inactivation,[64-66] which normally occurs in early prophase of meiosis I. Delayed X inactivation can in turn lead to the persistence of gene products which are inappropriate and detrimental to a particular stage of germ cell maturation. Thus, spermatogenic arrest comes about by essentially the same mechanism as in X-autosome translocations.

There is good evidence in support of this hypothesis. First, abnormal contact of the translocation configuration with the X chromosome of the X-Y bivalent has been observed in all male-sterile autosomal translocations of the mouse examined thus far[64-66] (Figure 15–15). The severity of the spermatogenic arrest in each individual case is proportional to the percentage of pachytene spermatocytes showing such abnormal contact.[65,66] Those autosomal translocations which do not cause sterility are not accompanied by abnormal contact between the translocated autosomes and the X-Y bivalent.[65,66] Second, levels of X-linked (but not autosomal) enzymes are significantly higher in sterile males than in controls, particularly in late prophase, indicating an inappropriately high activity of X-linked genes at this stage.[67]

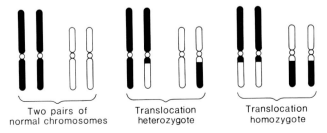

Two pairs of normal chromosomes   Translocation heterozygote   Translocation homozygote

Figure 15–12. Autosomal reciprocal translocation in the heterozygous and homozygous state.

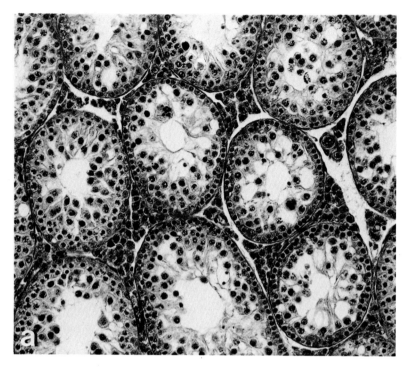

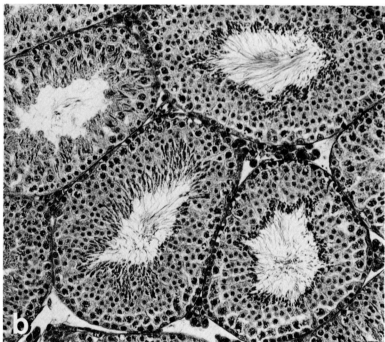

Figure 15–13. (a) Testis showing spermatogenic arrest at pachytene stage of primary spermatocytes, from a mouse heterozygous for the T(11;19)42H translocation. This reciprocal translocation between autosomes 11 and 19 was radiation-induced[63] and has since been maintained by breeding. H & E (X200). (b) Testis showing normal spermatogenesis, from a mouse homozygous for the T(11;19)42H translocation. H & E (X200). See text for explanation of sterility in heterozygous males and fertility in homozygous males.

If one accepts the hypothesis that in autosomal translocations, the spermatogenic arrest is due to interference of X inactivation through abnormal contact of the rearranged autosomes with the X-Y bivalent, then all of the characteristic features enumerated previously for autosomal translocations can be explained. 1. Germ cell maturation in females is not affected by such translocations, because both X chromosomes normally remain active in oogenesis.[46–48] Further, there are no unpaired segments between the two homologous X chromosomes in the female, in sharp contrast to the nonhomologous X and Y chromosomes in the male. 2. The sterility of the male heterozygote and the fertility of the male homozygote are also understandable. Since the homozygote has two identical translocated autosomes which can pair perfectly in meiosis, there will be no unpaired autosomal segments to engage in abnormal associations with the X-Y bivalent. 3. The incomplete spermatogenic arrest can be explained by the observation that, even though all germ cells in a male heterozygote carry the same auto-

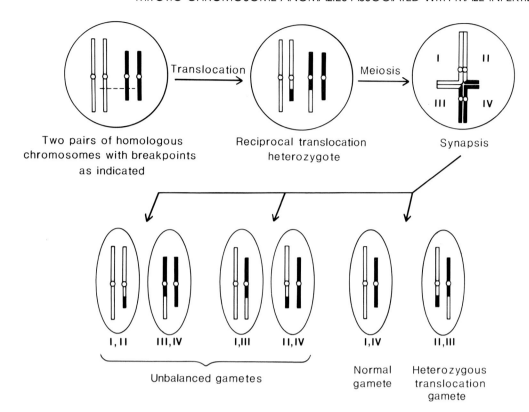

Two pairs of homologous chromosomes with breakpoints as indicated

Reciprocal translocation heterozygote

Synapsis

I, II   III, IV   I, III   II, IV   I, IV   II, III

Unbalanced gametes

Normal gamete

Heterozygous translocation gamete

Figure 15–14. Meiotic behavior of an autosomal reciprocal translocation heterozygote. The only way the two normal and two translocated chromosomes can pair gene-by-gene is for them to form a cross-shaped quadrivalent. From this configuration, the chromosomes can segregate in three possible ways at anaphase I: horizontally (I + II; III + IV), vertically (I + III; II + IV), or diagonally (I + IV; II + III), giving rise to six different combinations. Although the chromosomes are pictured as single rods for ease of presentation, in reality each of them is doubled (i.e., composed of two sister chromatids; see Figure 15–19). In meiosis II, the two sister chromatids separate longitudinally, one going to each haploid gamete. The overall result is as indicated in the bottom half of the diagram. Of the six possible types of gametes, four are unbalanced, with duplication of a segment of one chromosome and deficiency of a segment of the other chromosome. These gametes usually give rise to nonviable embryos and early abortions. Of the two balanced gametes, which carry a normal complement of genes, one has two normal chromosomes and the other two translocated chromosomes. The latter, if combined with a normal ovum, will again give rise to a translocation heterozygote.

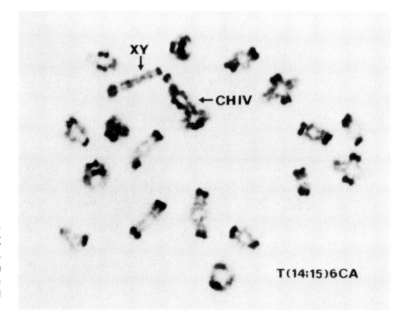

Figure 15–15. Abnormal association between the autosomal translocation quadrivalent (CHIV) and the X chromsome of the X-Y bivalent (XY) in metaphase I, from a male mouse heterozygous for the T(14;15)6Ca translocation. This heritable reciprocal translocation between autosomes 14 and 15 was radiation-induced originally.[63] (From J Forejt.[66])

somal translocation, not all primary spermatocytes exhibit the same abnormal association between the rearranged autosomes and the X-Y bivalent. In the various autosomal translocations, the frequency of such abnormal contact ranges from 30% to 90% of the pachytene spermatocytes examined.[65,66] Those translocations showing the highest percentage of abnormal contact are accompanied by the most profound disturbance in spermatogenesis. The spermatocytes in which such abnormal contact does not take place will be able to complete their differentiation into spermatozoa. 4. As a result of the formation of the cross-shaped quadrivalent in meiosis, of the spermatozoa that are formed, four out of every six will be genetically unbalanced, containing an excess of some genes and a deficiency in others (Figure 15–14). When such unbalanced spermatozoa combine with normal ova, the resulting zygotes will be destined for early embryo death and abortion. 5. Of the balanced spermatozoa produced by the translocation heterozygote, one-half will yield normal zygotes when combined with normal ova; the other half will give rise to the same type of translocation heterozygotes (Figure 15–14). Such a heterozygous state will again have an adverse effect on gametogenesis of the male but not that of the female. 6. If interference with X inactivation (and hence spermatogenic arrest) is due to abnormal association between the translocated autosomes and the X-Y bivalent during meiosis, it would explain why a large variety of seemingly unrelated autosomal translocations all have an adverse effect on spermatogenesis.

As a result of the studies performed on experimentally induced autosomal translocations, we now know that they affect fertility in two different ways: First, certain autosomal translocations cause infertility by arresting spermatogenesis, leading to reduced numbers or absence of spermatozoa. This adverse effect is restricted to the male, since it is a consequence of the abnormal contact between the X-Y bivalent and the translocated autosomes in meiosis. Oogenesis is not arrested. Second, autosomal translocations can cause reduced fertility postzygotically. In these instances, gametogenesis progresses to completion, but in the presence of the translocated autosomes, a fraction of the gametes produced are genetically unbalanced, giving rise to abnormal embryos that die *in utero*. As expected from the segregational events depicted in Figure 15–14, this postzygotic impairment in fertility affects males and females alike.

In man, the male-sterile autosomal reciprocal translocations reported thus far frequently involve acrocentric chromosomes (that is, those belonging to Groups D and G of the karyotype; see Figure 15–2).[68–70] As in the mouse, there is a tendency for the breakpoint on one chromosome to be close to the centromere and for the breakpoint on the second chromosome to be situated distally[50,68–70] (Figure 15–16). With such breakpoints, one translocated chromosome will be unduly long and the other unduly short; the quadrivalent formed during meiosis will very likely have one or two short arms (Figure 15–16), which can lead to imperfect pairing and failure of chiasma formation, predisposing them to abnormal contact with the X-Y bivalent.

Robertsonian Translocations

A Robertsonian translocation is a special type of reciprocal translocation between acrocentric chromosomes (Groups D and G, Figure 15–2). The two breakpoints in this type of translocation are usually situated very near or at the centromeres. The long arms of the two acrocentric chromosomes then fuse to yield a single large translocated chromosome (Figure 15–17). For this reason, such a translocation is also referred to as Robertsonian fusion.

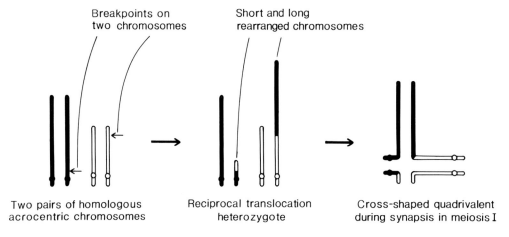

Breakpoints on two chromosomes

Short and long rearranged chromosomes

Two pairs of homologous acrocentric chromosomes

Reciprocal translocation heterozygote

Cross-shaped quadrivalent during synapsis in meiosis I

Figure 15–16. Male-sterile autosomal reciprocal translocations often involve acrocentric chromosomes, as shown above. One of the breakpoints is characteristically near the centromere of the first chromosome and the other breakpoint situated fairly distally on the second chromosome. The result is that one translocated chromosome will be unusually long and the other unusually short. At meiosis, pairing of chromosomes is achieved by the formation of a cross-shaped quadrivalent, which may have one or more short arms as a result of the positions of the breakpoints. Crossing over and chiasma formation often fail to take place in the short arms.

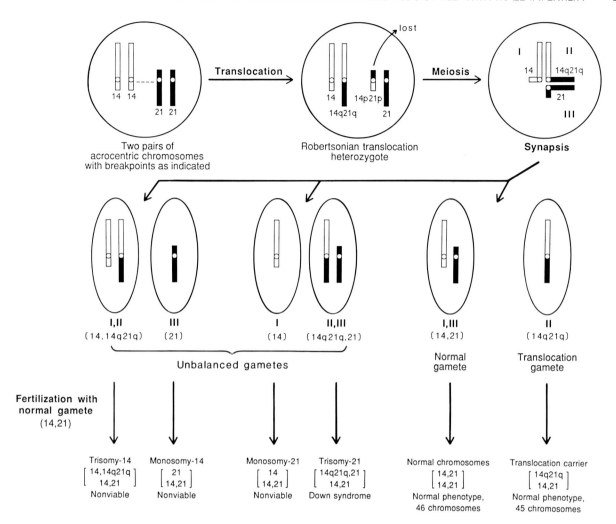

Figure 15–17. A Robertsonian translocation involving chromosomes 14 and 21, both of which are acrocentric. The two breakpoints are near the centromeres as indicated. By convention, the short arm of a chromosome is designated by the letter "p" (for petite) and the long arm by "q". Thus, in the diagram above, the chromosome formed by fusion of the long arms of chromosomes 14 and 21 is designated (14q,21q), while the chromosome formed by fusion of the short arms is designated (14p,21p). The latter, because of its small size, is usually lost. At meiosis, the normal chromosomes 14 and 21 and the large fused chromosome (14q21q) must form a trivalent to achieve synapsis. Subsequent segregation leads to the formation of six types of gametes, of which four are unbalanced and two balanced. Combination of the four unbalanced gametes with normal gametes leads to the formation of three nonviable embryos and one viable embryo afflicted with Down syndrome. Combination of the two balanced gametes with normal gametes leads to a normal individual and another phenotypically normal individual who is a heterozygote carrier for the same Robertsonian translocation as the parent.

The two very short arms may also join to form a chromosome which, due to its minute size, is ultimately lost. Because the two short arms seldom carry crucial genes, a heterozygous carrier of the large translocated chromosome is essentially genetically balanced and phenotypically normal, though he or she has only 45 chromosomes. Among Robertsonian translocations, that involving the long arms of chromosomes 13 and 14 is by far the most frequently encountered; next in frequency is that involving the long arms of chromosomes 14 and 21.[23–25,71–76] Robertsonian translocations between all other chromosomes are comparatively rare.[23–25,71]

A person carrying a Robertsonian translocation between chromosomes 14 and 21 is usually phenotypically normal. Three chromosomes in such a translocation heterozygote carry nearly all the genes present in the original four chromosomes. Even though the minute tips of chromosomes 14 and 21 have been lost, the fact that the translocation carrier is normal implies that no essential genes are missing. During meiosis, the large translocation chromosome and the normal chromosomes 14 and 21 must form a trivalent to achieve synapsis (Figure 15–17). In the male, such a trivalent usually engages in abnormal association with the X-Y bivalent, leading to interference with X chromosome inactivation and spermatogenic breakdown, as explained previously for autosomal reciprocal translocations.[76,77] Ultimately, there is a reduction in the number of spermatozoa formed; those formed are the results of three types of segregation as shown in Figure 15–17.[77] Of the six varieties of spermatozoa produced, four will be unbalanced and two balanced. Combination of the unbalanced spermatozoa with normal ova will lead to three types of nonviable zygotes; the remaining will be a zygote afflicted with Down syndrome (Figure 15–17). When the two balanced spermatozoa combine with normal ova, one zygote will have a normal karyotype with 46 normal chromosomes; the other zygote will be a heterozygous translocation carrier like the parent (Figure 15–17).

A Robertsonian translocation involving chromosomes 13 and 14, while behaving fundamentally like that involving chromosomes 14 and 21, tends to have a less severe and more variable effect on fertility.[24,42,54,74,75] Why certain heterozygous male carriers of a $^{13}/_{14}$ Robertsonian translocation are sterile while other males with the same translocation are fertile is not understood at present.[24,74,75]

In the female, because both X chromosomes remain active throughout oogenesis and are perfectly paired in meiosis, a Robertsonian translocation will not lead to arrest of germ cell maturation, although four-sixths of the ova formed will be unbalanced, which will ultimately lead to postzygotic embryo deaths and a high abortion rate, similar to the situation observed in male carriers of Robertsonian translocations.[77]

Structural Anomalies of the Y Chromosome

The Y chromosome plays a decisive role in male differentiation.[78] In its presence, the embryonic gonads develop into testes, and the organism becomes male.[79] In addition, the Y chromosome appears directly involved in the process of spermatogenesis.[79–81] Structural abnormalities of the Y chromosome can lead to abnormal testicular development or a disturbance in spermatogenesis. In both instances, the end result is infertility. Reviews on these subjects are available in the literature.[24,79–83]

Lyon's X Inactivation Hypothesis and Its Pertinence to Chromosome-Related Infertility

In the more than two decades since Lyon advanced her X inactivation hypothesis, it has become obvious that a striking feature of the X chromosome is its variable activity state.[79,84–90] Following is a summary of the cyclic variations of X chromosome activity in germ cells and somatic cells as we understand them today (Figure 15–18). At every stage, correct X chromosome dosage appears pivotal to normal differentiation and function of somatic cells and germ cells.

In male somatic cells, the lone X chromosome, which is maternally derived, is active from embryogenesis onward.

In the male germ cell line, the single X chromosome is active in spermatogonia and remains active as these stem cells undergo repeated mitoses to give rise to more spermatogonia during the fetal period.[91] From birth until puberty, the spermatogonia do not divide. Postpubertally, the spermatogonia resume their mitotic activities to replenish themselves and to give rise to primary spermatocytes; during this mitotic phase of proliferation, the single X chromosome remains active.[44,45,89] But as the primary spermatocytes enter the prophase of meiosis I, the X chromosome becomes inactivated; thereafter, the X chromosome remains inactive throughout spermatogenesis.[44,45,79,89]

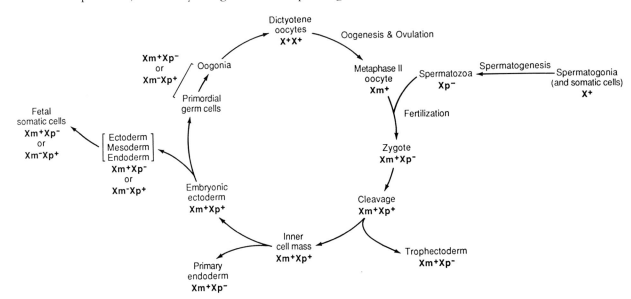

Figure 15–18. The cyclic variation of X chromosome activity in a female embryo. The active state is represented by **+**, and the inactive state by **−**. Maternal origin is denoted by **m**, and paternal origin by **p**. For detailed explanation, see text. (Modified from JL VandeBerg.[89])

In the female germ cell line, only one of the two X chromosomes is active in primordial germ cells and in oogonia; the other X chromosome is inactive.[91,92] This state persists as long as the oogonia are proliferating by mitotic divisions.[91,92] But as these cells differentiate into oocytes and enter meiosis, the inactive X chromosome becomes reactivated.[91,92] Thereafter, both X chromosomes remain active throughout oogenesis. Unlike meiosis in males, which begins at puberty, meiosis in female germ cells is initiated during the fetal period. By birth, the primary oocytes have progressed to late prophase of meiosis I and entered the quiescent, dictyotene stage, which is unique to oocytes.[89] They then remain suspended in the dictyotene stage until puberty. Postpubertally, with each monthly rise in pituitary gonadotropins, a particular oocyte is stimulated to complete meiosis I to become a secondary oocyte. Meiosis II then proceeds to the metaphase stage, at which time the secondary oocyte is released.[89] The secondary oocyte, plus the corona of cells which surround it, constitute the ovum. Completion of meiosis II takes place immediately after fertilization of the secondary oocyte by a spermatozoon.

At the time of fertilization and formation of a female zygote, the X chromosome contributed by the sperm is inactive, while the X chromosome contributed by the ovum is active. Shortly after fertilization, as the female embryo undergoes early cleavage divisions, there is a reactivation of the paternal X chromosome, so that by the 8-cell morula stage, both the paternal and the maternal X chromosomes are active in individual blastomeres.[86,87,89,90,93] The two X chromosomes remain active until the first sign of differentiation in the developing embryo, at which time one of the two X chromosomes in the embryonic cells again becomes inactivated. The X inactivation does not take place simultaneously in all cells of the female embryo but instead occurs in well-defined stages coincident with specific differentiative changes.[94] The first major differentiative event in embryogenesis is the formation of the trophectoderm; the second is the formation of the primary endoderm. In both of these tissues, which ultimately give rise to the extraembryonic placental membranes, the X inactivation is non-random, in that the paternally derived X is inactivated preferentially.[95,96] The third major differentiative event is the formation of the embryonic ectoderm, which will ultimately give rise to the definitive ectoderm, mesoderm, and endoderm (i.e., the somatic cells of the fetus), as well as the primordial germ cells.[87,89] With the differentiation of these tissues of the embryo proper, there is another wave of X inactivation. Unlike the situation in extraembryonic tissues, X inactivation in cells of the embryo proper is random.[87,89,94,97] Whether the paternal or maternal X chromosome is inactivated in any given somatic cell or primordial germ cell is a matter of chance. But once an X chromosome is inactivated in a particular cell, the same X chromosome will be inactivated in all its descendants by cell divisions. Clones of cells with one or the other X chromosome being inactivated are thereby produced, and every female is a mosaic with respect to X-linked genes in consequence.

Since the amount of gene products is proportional to the gene dosage, determinations of the activities of enzymes coded for by genes located on the X chromosome have been used extensively to study the variations in activity state of the X chromosome in somatic cells and germ cells in different developmental stages.

One of the most definitive proofs of X inactivation in female somatic cells came from studies of the inheritance of the enzyme glucose-6-phosphate dehydrogenase (G6PD),[98] the gene for which is located on the long arm of the X chromosome.[99] In the American black population, there are two variants of this enzyme distinguishable on electrophoresis: a fast-moving variant A and a slow-moving variant B.[98] Tissues from black males are found to exhibit either the fast-moving band A or the slow-moving band B, but never both, since males have only one X chromosome. Similarly, in black females homozygous for variant A or variant B, only one band is seen; quantitatively, the enzyme activity in each band is equivalent to that present in the same band of black males, indicating that one X is inactivated in each female somatic cell. Tissues from black female heterozygotes, on the other hand, are found to exhibit both bands. However, when single fibroblasts from heterozygous females are cloned by cell culture, each resulting clone shows either variant A or variant B, but not both. Together, these results indicate that in female heterozygotes, the gene for variant A, located on one X chromosome, is active in some cells; whereas the gene for variant B, located on the second X chromosome, is active in other cells. But once an X is inactivated in a particular somatic cell, the same X will be inactivated in all its descendants.

The same types of investigations were performed on germ cells. Studies involving human oocytes were aided by the fact that G6PD is a dimer molecule.[48] In the cells of a female heterozygote, the gene coding for variant A is located on one X chromosome, while the gene coding for variant B is located on the second X chromosome. If both X chromosomes are active in the same cell, a hybrid band AB, with an electrophoretic mobility between those of band A and band B, would be found. When oocytes of human adults and fetuses heterozygous for the variants A and B of G6PD were studied electrophoretically, a hybrid band AB was indeed observed, indicating that in human oocytes, both X chromosomes are active.[48,99]

In the mouse, oocytes of XX females have levels of activity of G6PD twice as high as those of oocytes of XO females, showing that in murine oocytes, both X chromosomes are active simultaneously as well.[46,47]

Further refinements of such biochemical studies involving various X-linked enzymes at different stages of embryogenesis and gametogenesis have led to the outline of X inactivation and reactivation described above,[91–97] as embodied in Figure 15–18.

Subsequent studies have indicated that X inactivation in somatic cells does not involve the entire X chromosome.[79,87,90,99] For if all X chromosomes in excess of one are completely inactivated in every somatic cell, patients with Turner's syndrome (XO) or classical Klinefelter's syndrome (XXY) would not be phenotypically abnormal. Similarly, patients with XXXY and XXXXY karyotypes would not be accompanied by progressively greater abnormality. From studies of genes located on different portions of the X chromosome, we now know that the inactivation process involves only the long arm of the chromosome; the short arm in the "inactivated" X remains active.[79,87,90] On the short arm are genes which must be present in duplicate if normal female somatic development is to take place. These observations explain why XO females are phenotypically different from normal XX females, because the former are deficient in genes on the short arm of X. Similarly, these findings explain why XXY males are somatically abnormal, since they possess an excess of genes on the short arm of X.

The importance of correct X chromosome dosage applies equally to germ cell maturation. In XO females, germ cells can be observed initially in the fetal ovaries, but all of them ultimately disappear prematurely, because in oogenesis involving XO germ cells, there can only be a maximum of one active X chromosome, instead of the usual two as in normal female XX germ cells.[85] The same detrimental effect of incorrect X chromosome dosage is seen in XXY male germ cells, in which both X chromosomes remain active early in spermatogenesis; the resulting excess of X-linked gene products causes the germ cells to degenerate.[85] Finally, in such chromosome anomalies as X-autosome translocations, autosomal reciprocal translocations, and Robertsonian translocations, X inactivation in primary spermatocytes is interfered with;[43,66,77] the consequence is spermatogenic arrest, apparently because of the persistence of gene products which are nonpermissible and lethal to the germ cells after a certain stage in spermatogenesis. Since in female germ cells, both X chromosomes normally remain active from meiotic prophase onward, processes which interfere with X inactivation and lead to male sterility would not have any adverse effect on the progression of oogenesis.

The mechanisms by which the X chromosome is inactivated and reactivated are not yet entirely elucidated. Nonetheless, it is obvious from the foregoing discussion that the presence of the proper dosage of X-linked genes at the proper stage, through timely inactivation and reactivation of the X chromosome, is critical for the normal development of somatic cells as well as germ cells. Any deviation from the normal dosage or schedule of X inactivation and reactivation will lead to developmental confusion, ending in permanent, irreversible damage.

MEIOTIC CHROMOSOME ANOMALIES ENCOUNTERED IN INFERTILE MEN WITH A NORMAL KARYOTYPE

In the preceding section, mitotic chromosome anomalies responsible for male infertility were described. These anomalies are all detectable by karyotype analysis, although to understand the manner in which they affect spermatogenesis, studies performed on germ cells in meiosis are often helpful. In connection with these studies, it became obvious that infertile men who have a

normal karyotype may nonetheless harbor abnormalities of the meiotic chromosomes that are detectable only by direct examination of the germ cells obtained by testicular biopsy.[22,23,100–102] Since histological examination of the biopsy usually takes precedence over cytogenetic studies, if a testicular biopsy is small, or if the seminiferous tubules are atrophic, there may not be sufficient germ cells to permit a satisfactory analysis of the meiotic chromosomes. Therefore, unlike somatic karyotyping, meiotic chromosome analysis is more frequently disappointing or yields inconclusive results. Despite these inherent difficulties, however, a number of anomalies are repeatedly observed in the meiotic chromosomes of oligospermic or azoospermic men with a normal karyotype, which strongly suggests that these anomalies are responsible for the impairment of spermatogenesis. The more common of these meiotic chromosome abnormalities are listed in Table 15–1. In one large series reported,[101] it was found that when only spermatocytes in metaphase I were examined, the incidence of meiotic chromosome anomalies in karyotypically normal, infertile men was a little over 1%. However, when all stages of meiosis, including pachytene, metaphase I, and metaphase II were analyzed, the incidence of meiotic chromosome anomalies in the same series of patients rose to 12%. This difference stresses the importance of including all stages of meiosis in the study, if the full spectrum of the chromosome anomalies is to be appreciated.[101] Considering the fact that a significant proportion of the testicular biopsies often show no meiotic cells because of extreme atrophy of the seminiferous tubules, the true incidence of such meiotic chromosome anomalies may well be higher than reported.[101]

Asynapsis, Desynapsis, and Reduced Chiasma Formation

The events which take place during the two meiotic divisions of germ cells are summarized briefly in Figure 15–19, using a pair of homologous chromosomes, one of which is derived from the father and the other from the mother originally. In the period preceding the first meiotic division, there is a duplication of each chromosome to form two chromatids. Each chromosome (consisting of two sister chromatids) then finds and pairs intimately with its homologue. This pairing process, or synapsis, is highly specific and occurs gene-by-gene along the chromosomal twosome. A structure called synaptonemal complex then forms between the paired chromosomes, physically linking them together in a zipperlike fashion[103] (Figure 15–20). After the formation of the synaptonemal complex, a process known as crossing over occurs, by which breakage and exchange of parts take place between nonsister chromatids, resulting in some shifting of genes from each chromosome to its homologue (Figure 15–19). The X-shaped connections formed between nonsister chromatids during crossing over are called chiasmata. Each of the above processes must progress normally before the succeeding one can take place. For example, failure of synapsis (asynapsis) will result in defective synaptonemal complex formation, which in

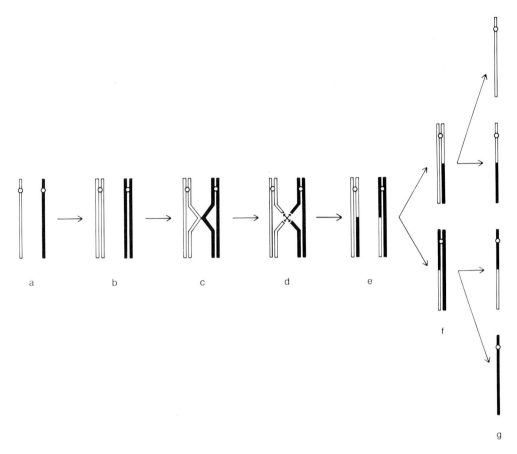

Figure 15–19. Events taking place in meiosis I and II, illustrated with a pair of homologous chromosomes, one of which is paternal and the other maternal in origin, as shown in (a). Prior to meiosis I, there is DNA duplication, leading to the formation of two sister chromatids for each chromosome (b); the homologous chromosome (each consisting of two sister chromatids) then pair side-by-side in an extremely precise, gene-by-gene fashion (b). Afterward, crossing over between two nonsister chromatids occurs, with chiasma formation at the point of crossing over (c). There is then breakage and reunion of the two nonsister chromatids at the point of crossing over, resulting in shifting of genes between homologous chromosomes (d and e). Meiosis I (f) and meiosis II (g) are then completed with results as shown.

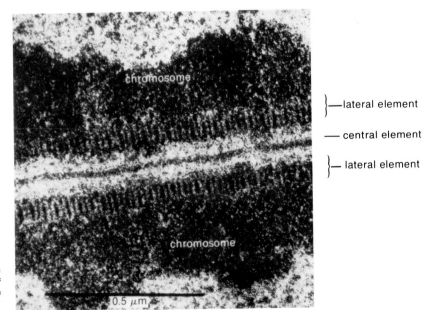

Figure 15–20. Electron micrograph of a portion of the synaptonemal complex, joining a pair of homologous chromosomes during prophase of meiosis I (X91,000). (From D von Wettstein.[103])

turn will interfere with crossing over and chiasma formation. In some instances, the initial synapsis and synaptonemal complex formation are normal, but there is premature separation of the paired homologous chromosomes (desynapsis); the consequence is that crossing over and chiasma formation fail to occur. Reduced numbers of chiasmata have been shown to be followed by spermatogenic arrest and sterility.[23,100–102]

In Drosophila and plants, asynapsis and desynapsis are both genetically determined, and mutants exhibiting each can be clearly identified.[104] In infertile men who have a normal somatic karyotype, asynaptic meiosis similar to that described in other organisms has been reported.[105,106] Electron microscopy reveals abnormal synaptonemal complex formation. Parental consanguinity and affected sibs in such cases suggest that a mutation is responsible for the meiotic abnormality. The trait is inherited as an autosomal recessive.[106] Degeneration of primary spermatocytes in these men is responsible for their oligo- or azoospermia and sterility. Genetically determined desynaptic meiosis has also been reported in infertile men; its mode of inheritance is not clear.[106,107]

Dissociation of X and Y Chromosomes

Proper association between the sex chromosomes at meiosis is a prerequisite to normal spermatogenesis.[108,109] As indicated earlier, in the male, the X and Y chromosomes of the germ cells are normally associated end-to-end at diakinesis and metaphase of the first meiotic division[12,13] (Figure 15–5a). In the mouse, germ cells with separate or dissociated X and Y chromosomes usually do not proceed beyond metaphase I, and no secondary spermatocytes, spermatids, or spermatozoa are formed.[108] If 100% of the germ cells show X-Y dissociation, complete maturation arrest at metaphase I and sterility are the result (Figure 15–5b). Evidence that this phenomenon also occurs in man was provided by meiotic studies performed on testicular biopsies of infertile men who had a normal somatic karyotype.[109] Such studies showed that individuals with a high proportion of unpaired sex chromosomes at metaphse I also had a low proportion of germ cells reaching metaphase II; histologically, the testicular biopsies of the same men showed maturation arrest at or soon after metaphase I. The cause of the X-Y dissociation is usually obscure. In one case report of an infertile man with complete X-Y dissociation, the Y chromosome was abnormal structurally in that it was ring-shaped, which made it impossible for the X and Y chromosomes to associate end-to-end.[110] In the two reported instances of sterile mice with complete X-Y dissociation, no such structural abnormalities of the sex chromosomes were apparent by light microscopy. However, the mice were offspring of fathers treated with x-rays[108] or mutagens;[111] hence there may have been structural abnormalities not visible at the light microscopic level. In both mouse and man, there is some evidence that the propensity for X-Y dissociation in germ cells is genetically determined and heritable.[109,112]

CONCLUSION

The adverse effect of chromosome aberrations on male infertility is by now well documented. Abnormalities of the karyotype detectable by mitotic chromosome analysis generally operate at the chromosomal level. They lead to impaired testicular development or defective spermatogenesis because of numerical abnormalities or gross structural aberrations and rearrangements of the chromosomes. In addition, those abnormalities involving chromosome rearrangements can cause postzygotic loss of fertility through the production of genetically unbalanced and nonviable embryos. By contrast, the abnormalities found in karyotypically normal men and detectable *only* by meiotic chromosome analysis tend to be point mutations and operate at the genic level. They disturb spermatogenesis by blocking a single step in the intricately interlocked and orderly events in meiosis. Because of their genic nature, their inheritance tends to obey Mendelian laws.

In recent years, the increasing use of mitotic and meiotic chromosome analysis in male infertility studies has helped to uncover a vast array of chromosome anomalies capable of causing male infertility. Experimental studies of analogous abnormalities in mice and other species have contributed greatly to our understanding of the abnormalities in man. In the early periods, both the clinical and experimental investigations were fundamentally cytogenetic and morphological in nature. While these studies have conclusively demonstrated certain chromosome aberrations as the basis of male infertility, they did not explain how these aberrations bring about defective spermatogenesis at the biochemical or molecular level. To a large extent, the inability to obtain pure populations of germ cells in different stages of maturation has consistently hampered such investigations. But as methods for separating the complex mixture of maturing germ cells become increasingly available, either by gradient centrifugation[113,114] or by cell-sorting,[115] the biochemical mechanisms responsible for normal and abnormal spermatogenesis are gradually amenable to stepwise dissection. Such biochemical studies, along with gene-mapping, may ultimately illuminate the many facets of human male infertility which today seem so very perplexing.

References

1. Simmons FA: Human infertility. N Engl J Med 255:1140–1146 and 1186–1192, 1956.
2. MacLeod J: Human male infertility. Obstet Gynecol Surv 26:335–351, 1971.
3. Paulsen CA: The testes. In RH Williams (ed) Textbook of Endocrinology, 5th ed. p323–367. Philadelphia, WB Saunders, 1974.
4. Wong TW, Jones TM: Evaluation of testicular biopsy in male infertility studies. In LI Lipshultz, SS Howards (eds) Infertility in the Male, p217–248. New York, Churchill Livingstone, 1983.
5. Yunis JJ (ed): Human Chromosome Methodology, 2nd ed. New York, Academic Press, 1974.

6. Priest JH: Medical Cytogenetics and Cell Culture, 2nd ed. Philadelphia, Lea and Febiger, 1977.

7. Caspersson T, Lomakka G, Zech L: The 24 fluorescent patterns of human metaphase chromosomes—distinguishing characters and variability. Heriditas 67:89–102, 1971.

8. Dutrillaux B, Lejeune J: New techniques in the study of human chromosomes: methods and applications. Adv Hum Genet 5:119–156, 1975.

9. Evans EP, Breckon G, Ford CE: An air-drying method for meiotic preparations from mammalian testes. Cytogenetics 3:289–294, 1964.

10. Hultén M, Lindsten J: Cytogenetic aspects of human male meiosis. Adv Hum Genet 4:327–387, 1973.

11. Fletcher JM: Light microscopic analysis of meiotic prophase chromosomes by silver staining. Chromosoma 72:241–248, 1979.

12. Ohno S, Kaplan WD, Kinosita R: On the end-to-end association of the X and Y chromosomes of Mus musculus. Exp Cell Res 18:282–290, 1959.

13. Egozcue J: The X chromosome in meiosis. In AA Sandberg (ed) Cytogenetics of the Mammalian X Chromosome, Part A: Basic Mechanisms of X Chromosome Behavior, p107–130. New York, Alan R Liss, 1983.

14. Barr ML, Bertram EG: A morphological distinction between neurons of the male and female, and the behavior of the nucleolar satellite during accelerated nucleoprotein synthesis. Nature 163:676–677, 1949.

15. Ohno S, Kaplan WD, Kinosita R: Formation of the sex chromatin by a single X chromosome in liver cells of Rattus norvegicus. Exp Cell Res 18:415–418, 1959.

16. Lyon MF: Gene action in the X-chromosome of the mouse (Mus musculus L.). Nature 190:372–373, 1961.

17. Lyon MF: Sex chromatin and gene action in the mammalian X-chromosome. Am J Hum Genet 14:135–148, 1962.

18. de Grouchy J, Turleau C: Clinical Atlas of Human Chromosomes, 2nd ed. New York, John Wiley, 1984.

19. Baghdassarian A, Bayard F, Borgaonkar DS, et al.: Testicular function in XYY men. Johns Hopkins Med J 136:15–24, 1975.

20. Schoepflin GS, Centerwall WR: 48,XYYY: a new syndrome? J Med Genet 9:356–380, 1972.

21. Kjessler B: Chromosomal constitution and male reproductive failure. In RE Mancini, L Martin (eds) Male Fertility and Sterility, p231–247, New York, Academic Press, 1974.

22. Koulischer L, Schoysman R: Chromosomes and human infertility. I. Mitotic and meiotic chromosome studies in 202 consecutive male patients. Clin Genet 5:116–126, 1974.

23. Chandley AC: The chromosomal basis of human infertility. Br Med Bull 35:181–186, 1979.

24. Zuffardi O, Tiepolo L: Frequencies and types of chromosome abnormalities associated with human male infertility. In PG Crosignani, BL Rubin, M Fraccaro (eds) Genetic Control of Gamete Production and Function, p261–273, New York, Grune and Stratton, 1982.

25. Mićić M, Mićić S, Diklić V: Chromosomal constitution of infertile men. Clin Genet 25:33–36, 1984.

26. Gorlin RJ: Classical chromosome disorders. In JJ Yunis (ed) New Chromosome Syndromes, p59–117. New York, Academic Press, 1977.

27. Race RR, Sanger R: Xg and sex-chromosome abnormalities. Br Med Bull 25:99–103, 1969.

28. Gerald PS: Current concepts in genetics. Sex chromosome disorders. N Engl J Med 294:706–708, 1976.

29. Williams DL, Runyan JW: Sex chromatin and chromosome analysis in the diagnosis of sex anomalies. Ann Intern Med 64:422–459, 1966.

30. Grumbach MM, Conte FA: Disorders of sex diferentiation. In RH Williams (ed) Textbook of Endocrinology, 6th ed, p423–514. Philadelphia, WB Saunders, 1981.

31. Ferguson-Smith MA: The prepubertal testicular lesion in chromatin-positive Klinefelter's syndrome (primary micro-orchidism) as seen in mentally handicapped children. Lancet 1:219–222, 1959.

32. Becker KL: Clinical and therapeutic experiences with Klinefelter's syndrome. Fertil Steril 23:568–578, 1972.

33. Wong TW, Straus FH, Warner NE: Testicular biopsy in the study of male infertility. I. Testicular causes of infertility. Arch Pathol 93:151–159, 1973.

34. Capell PT, Paulsen CA, Derleth D, et al.: The effect of short-term testosterone administration on serum FSH, LH and testosterone levels: evidence for selective abnormality in LH control in patients with Klinefelter's syndrome. J Clin Endocrinol Metab 37:752–759, 1973.

35. Humphery TJ, Rosen S, Casey JH: Klinefelter's syndrome. Experiences with 24 patients. Med J Austral 2:779–782, 1976.

36. Court-Brown WM: Sex chromosome aneuploidy in man and its frequency, with special reference to mental subnormality and criminal behavior. Int Rev Exp Path 7:31–97, 1969.

37. Schinzel A: Catalogue of Unbalanced Chromosome Aberrations in Man. New York, Walter de Gruyter, 1984.

38. Court-Brown WM, Mantle DJ, Buckton KE, et al.: Fertility in an XY/XXY male married to a translocation heterozygote. J Med Genet 1:35–38, 1964.

39. Skakkebaek NE, Hultén M, Jacobsen P, et al.: Quantification of human seminiferous epithelium. II. Histological studies in eight 47,XYY men. J Reprod Fertil 32:391–401, 1973.

40. Eicher EM: X-autosome translocations in the mouse: total inactivation versus partial inactivation of the X chromosome. Adv Genet 15:176–259, 1970.

41. Searle AG, Beechey CV, Evans EP, et al.: Two new X-autosome translocations in the mouse. Cytogenet Cell Genet 35:279–292, 1983.

42. Faed MJW, Lamont MA, Baxby K: Cytogenetic and histological studies of testicular biopsies from subfertile men with chromosome anomaly. J Med Genet 19:49–56, 1982.

43. Lifschytz E, Lindsley DL: The role of X-chromosome inactivation during spermatogenesis. Proc Natl Acad Sci USA 69:182–186, 1972.

44. Monesi V: Ribonucleic acid and protein synthesis during differentiation of male germ cells in the mouse. Arch Anat Microsc Morphol Exp 56(Suppl 3–4):61–74, 1967.

45. Monesi V, Geremia R, D'Agostino A, et al.: Biochemistry of male germ cell differentiation in mammals: RNA synthesis in meiotic and postmeiotic cells. Curr Top Dev Biol 12:11–36, 1978.

46. Epstein CJ: Mammalian oocytes: X chromosome activity. Science 163:1078–1079, 1969.

47. Epstein CJ: Expression of the mammalian X chromosome before and after fertilization. Science 175:1467–1468, 1972.

48. Gartler SM, Liskay RM, Campbell BK, et al.: Evidence for

two functional X-chromosomes in human oocytes. Cell Differ 1:215–218, 1972.

49. Cacheiro NLA, Russell LB, Swartout MS: Translocations, the predominant cause of total sterility in sons of mice treated with mutagens. Genetics 76:73–91, 1974.

50. Searle AG, Beechey CV, Evans EP: Meiotic effects in chromosomally derived male sterility of mice. Ann Biol Anim Biochim Biophys 18:391–398, 1978.

51. Smith A, Fraser IS, Elliott G: An infertile male with balanced Y;19 translocation. Review of Y; autosome translocations. Ann Genet 22:189–194, 1979.

52. Gonzales J, Lesourd S, Dutrillaux B: Mitotic and meiotic analysis of a reciprocal translocation t(Y;3) in an azoospermic male. Hum Genet 57:111–114, 1981.

53. Laurent C, Chandley AC, Dutrillaux B, et al.: The use of surface spreading in the pachytene analysis of a human t(Y;17) reciprocal translocation. Cytogenet Cell Genet 33:312–318, 1982.

54. Chandley AC, Christie S, Fletcher J, et al.: Translocation heterozygosity and associated subfertility in man. Cytogenetics 11:516–533, 1972.

55. Chandley AC, Seuánez H, Fletcher J: Meiotic behavior of five human reciprocal translocations. Cytogenet Cell Genet 17:98–111, 1976.

56. Laurent C, Biemont MC, Cognat M, et al.: Studies of the meiotic behavior of a translocation t(10;13)(q25;q11) in an oligospermic man. Hum Genet 39:123–126, 1977.

57. Léonard C, Bisson JP, David G: Male sterility associated with familial translocation heterozygosity t(8;15)(q22;p11). Arch Androl 2:269–275, 1979.

58. San Román C, Sordo MT, García-Sagredo JM: Meiosis in two human reciprocal translocations. J Med Genet 16:56–59, 1979.

59. Mićić MD, Mićić SR: Meiotic findings in human reciprocal 1;3 translocation. Hum Genet 57:442–443, 1981.

60. Egozcue J, Marina S, Templado C: Meiotic behaviour of two human reciprocal translocations. J Med Genet 18:362–365, 1981.

61. Mićić M, Mićić S: Meiotic studies in two infertile males with autosomal translocations. Hum Genet 65:308–310, 1984.

62. Lyon MF, Meredith R: Autosomal translocations causing male sterility and viable aneuploidy in the mouse. Cytogenetics 5:335–354, 1966.

63. Searle AG: Chromosomal variants. In MC Green (ed) Genetic Variants and Strains of the Laboratory Mouse, p324–359. Stuttgart, Gustav Fisher Verlag, 1981.

64. Forejt J, Gregorová S: Meiotic studies of translocations causing male sterility in the mouse. I. Autosomal reciprocal translocations. Cytogenet Cell Genet 19:159–179, 1977.

65. Forejt J, Gregorová S, Goetz P: XY pair associates with the synaptonemal complex of autosomal male-sterile translocations in pachytene spermatocytes of the mouse (Mus musculus). Chromosoma 82:41–53, 1981.

66. Forejt J: X-Y involvement in male sterility caused by autosome translocations—a hypothesis. In PG Crosignani, BL Rubin, M Fraccaro (eds) Genetic Control of Gamete Production and Function, p135–151. New York, Grune and Stratton, 1982.

67. Hotta Y, Chandley AC: Activities of X-linked enzymes in spermatocytes of mice rendered sterile by chromosomal alterations. Gamete Res 6:65–72, 1982.

68. Chandley AC: The origin of chromosomal aberrations in man and their potential for survival and reproduction in the adult human population. Ann Genet 24:5–11, 1981.

69. Chandley AC: Chromosomes and infertility. In GD Chisholm, DI Williams (eds) Scientific Foundations of Urology, 2nd ed, p564–572. London, AW Heinemann, 1982.

70. Chandley AC: Normal and abnormal meiosis in man and other mammals. In PG Crosignani, BL Rubin, M Fraccaro (eds) Genetic Control of Gamete Production and Function, p229–237. New York, Grune and Stratton, 1982.

71. Jacobs PA, Frackiewicz A, Law P, et al.: The effect of structural aberrations of the chromosomes on reproductive fitness in man. II. Results. Clin Genet 8:169–178, 1975.

72. Plymate SR, Bremner WJ, Paulsen CA: The association of D-group chromosomal translocations and defective spermatogenesis. Fertil Steril 27:139–144, 1976.

73. Mićić MD, Nikoliš JG, Mićić SR: 13/14 Translocation in a man with reproductive failure. Mitotic and meiotic studies. Hum Genet 55:137–139, 1980.

74. Templado C, Vidal F, Navarro J, et al.: Meiotic studies and synaptonemal complex analysis in two infertile males with a 13/14 balanced translocation. Hum Genet 67:162–165, 1984.

75. Luciani JM, Guichaoua MR, Mattei A, et al.: Pachytene analysis of a man with a 13q;14q translocation and infertility. Behavior of the trivalent and nonrandom association with the sex vesicle. Cytogenet Cell Genet 38:14–22, 1984.

76. Rosenmann A, Wahrman J, Richler C, et al.: Meiotic association between the XY chromosomes and unpaired autosomal elements as a cause of human male sterility. Cytogenet Cell Genet 39:19–29, 1985.

77. Gropp A, Winking H, Redi C: Consequences of Robertsonian heterozygosity: segregational impairment of fertility versus male-limited sterility. In PG Crosignani, BL Rubin, M Fraccaro (eds) Genetic Control of Gamete Production and Function, p115–134. New York, Grune and Stratton, 1982.

78. Welshons WJ, Russell LB: The Y-chromosome as the bearer of male-determining factors in the mouse. Proc Natl Acad Sci USA 45:560–566, 1959.

79. Gordon JW, Ruddle FH: Mammalian gonadal determination and gametogenesis. Science 211:1265–1271, 1981.

80. Tiepolo L, Zuffardi O: Localization of factors controlling spermatogenesis in the nonfluorescent portion of the human Y chromosome long arm. Hum Genet 34:119–124, 1976.

81. Yunis E, García-Conti FL, Torres de Caballero OM, et al.: Yq deletion, aspermia, and short stature. Hum Genet 39:117–122, 1977.

82. Ferguson-Smith MA: Karyotype-phenotype correlations in gonadal dysgenesis and their bearing on the pathogenesis of malformations. J Med Genet 2:142–156, 1965.

83. Jacobs PA: Structural abnormalities of the sex chromosomes. Br Med Bull 25:94–98, 1969.

84. Lyon MF: X-chromosome inactivation and developmental patterns in mammals. Biol Rev 47:1–35, 1972.

85. Lyon MF: Mechanisms and evolutionary origins of variable X-chromosome activity in mammals. Proc R Soc Lond [Biol] 187:243–268, 1974.

86. West JD: X chromosome expression during mouse embryogenesis. In PG Crosignani, BL Rubin, M Fraccaro (eds) Genetic Control of Gamete Production and Function, p49–91. New York, Grune and Stratton, 1982.

87. Martin GR: X-chromosome inactivation in mammals. Cell 29:721–724, 1982.

88. Lyon MF: The X chromosomes and their levels of activation. In AA Sandberg (ed) Cytogenetics of the Mammalian X Chromosome, Part A: Basic Mechanisms of X Chromosome Behavior, p187–204. New York, Alan R Liss, 1983.

89. VandeBerg JL: Developmental aspects of X chromosome inactivation in eutherian and metatherian mammals. J Exp Zool 228:271–286, 1983.

90. Gartler SM, Riggs AD: Mammalian X-chromosome inactivation. Annu Rev Genet 17:155–190, 1983.

91. Monk M, McLaren A: X-chromosome activity in foetal germ cells of the mouse. J Embryol Exp Morphol 63:75–84, 1981.

92. Kratzer PG, Chapman VM: X chromosome inactivation in oocytes of *Mus caroli.* Proc Natl Acad Sci USA 78:3093–3097, 1981.

93. Epstein CJ, Smith S, Travis B, et al.: Both X chromosomes function before visible X-chromosome inactivation in female mouse embryos. Nature 274:500–503, 1978.

94. Monk M, Harper MI: Sequential X chromosome inactivation coupled with cellular differentiation in early mouse embryos. Nature 281:311–313, 1979.

95. Takagi N, Sasaki M: Preferential inactivation of the paternally derived X chromosome in the extraembryonic membranes of the mouse. Nature 256:640–642, 1975.

96. West JD, Frels WI, Chapman VM, *et al.:* Preferential expression of the maternally derived X chromosome in the mouse yolk sac. Cell 12:873–882, 1977.

97. McMahon A, Fosten M, Monk M: Random X-chromosome inactivation in female primordial germ cells in the mouse. J Embryol Exp Morphol 64:251–258, 1981.

98. Davidson RG, Nitowsky HM, Childs B: Demonstration of two populations of cells in the human female heterozygous for glucose-6-phosphate dehydrogenase variants. Proc Natl Acad Sci USA 50:481–485, 1963.

99. Migeon BR: Glucose-6-phosphate dehydrogenase as a probe for the study of X-chromosome inactivation in human females. Isozymes: Curr Top Biol Med Res 9:189–200, 1983.

100. Luciani JM, Stahl A: Meiotic disturbances related to human male sterility. Ann Biol Anim Biochim Biophys 18:377–382, 1978.

101. Koulischer L, Schoysman R, Gillerot Y, *et al.:* Meiotic chromosome studies in human male infertility. *In* PG Crosignani, BL Rubin, M Fraccaro (eds) Genetic Control of Gamete Production and Function, p239–260. New York, Grune and Stratton, 1982.

102. Mićić M, Mićić S, Diklić V: Low chiasma frequency as an aetiological factor in male infertility. Clin Genet 22:266–269, 1982.

103. von Wettstein D: The synaptonemal complex and four-stranded crossing over. Proc Natl Acad Sci USA 68:851–855, 1971.

104. Baker BS, Carpenter ATC, Esposito MS, et al.: The genetic control of meiosis. Annu Rev Genet 10:53–134, 1976.

105. Hultén M, Solari AJ, Skakkebaek NE: Abnormal synaptonemal complex in an oligochiasmatic man with spermatogenic arrest. Heriditas 78:105–116, 1974.

106. Chaganti RSK, Jhanwar SC, Ehrenbard LT, et al.: Genetically determined asynapsis, spermatogenic degeneration, and infertility in men. Am J Hum Genet 32:833–848, 1980.

107. Chaganti RSK, German J: Human male infertility, probably genetically determined, due to defective meiosis and spermatogenic arrest. Am J Hum Genet 31:634–641, 1979.

108. Beechey CV: X-Y chromosome dissociation and sterility in the mouse. Cytogenet Cell Genet 12:60–67, 1973.

109. Chandley AC, MacLean N, Edmond P, et al.: Cytogenetics and infertility in man. II. Testicular histology and meiosis. Ann Hum Genet 40:165–176, 1976.

110. Chandley AC, Edmond P: Meiotic studies on a subfertile patient with a ring Y chromosome. Cytogenetics 10:295–304, 1971.

111. Cattanach BM, Pollard CE, Isaacson JH: Ethyl methanesulfonate-induced chromosome breakage in the mouse. Mutat Res 6:297–307, 1968.

112. Sotomayor RE, Cumming RB: XY dissociation in mice: a model that may account for sex aneuploidy in humans? Genetics 86:s60 (abstr), 1977.

113. Romrell LJ, Bellvé AR, Fawcett DW: Separation of mouse spermatogenic cells by sedimentation velocity. A morphological characterization. Dev Biol 49:119–131, 1976.

114. Chandley AC, Hotta Y, Stern H: Biochemical analysis of meiosis in the male mouse. I. Separation and DNA labelling of specific spermatogenic stages. Chromosoma 62:243–253, 1977.

115. Pfitzer P, Gilbert P, Rölz, G, et al.: Flow cytometry of human testicular tissue. Cytometry 3:116–122, 1982.

16. Pathological Changes of the Testis in Infertility

Ting-Wa Wong and Keith A. Horvath

Human reproductive failure, while not life-threatening, is a public health problem of major proportions. It has been estimated that 15% of the married couples in the United States are involuntarily childless and another 10% have fewer children than they desire.[1,2] Further, there are indications that the magnitude of the problem is increasing. In the male sex, a decline in fertility over the last two decades has been reported.[3-6] Changes in life style, rising incidence of venereal disease, increasing use of drugs, new occupational hazards, and multiplying environmental pollutants, including radiation, all appear to have contributed to such decline. Since some of the agents implicated are capable of causing chromosomal as well as genic damage, the potential harm they exert on male reproductive fitness is not confined to the present generation. Because so many etiological factors may be involved, modern diagnosis of male infertility often demands a multidisciplinary approach, in which the endocrinologist, urologist, cytogeneticist, microbiologist, immunologist, and pathologist all play a part. In this chapter, the pathological changes of the testis in infertility, as revealed by testicular biopsies, will be analyzed.

PROCESSING OF TESTICULAR BIOPSIES

Optimal interpretation of testicular biopsies depends on proper biopsy technique and on the care in handling and fixing the tissue obtained. Incisional biopsies performed under general or local anesthesia yield the most satisfactory tissue; needle biopsies are inadequate because of the attendant compression artifacts.[2,7,8] To avoid squeezing of the seminiferous tubules, the biopsy specimen should be obtained with a razor blade and dropped directly into the fixative without the use of forceps.[8] Although the two testes in the majority of men are similar histologically, differences are encountered sufficiently often to make

This study was supported in part by grants from the Cancer Research Foundation and the American Cancer Society Illinois Division. The help of Don Sitterly in the preparation of the photomicrographs is gratefully acknowledged.

biopsy of both sides prudent and preferable. This is especially true in cases where there is an appreciable difference in testicular size or in men with acquired obstructive azoospermia.

Prompt and proper fixation of the testicular biopsy specimen is of the utmost importance if histological preparations of good quality are to be obtained.[8] In our experience, Bouin's solution is the fixative of choice for as fragile a tissue as the testis. This fixative has the advantage of ensuring rapid and thorough fixation without causing shrinkage or distortion of testicular architecture; in addition, it achieves excellent preservation of nuclear details, thereby enabling germ cells in various stages of maturation to be recognized and analyzed histologically. It cannot be stressed too strongly that formalin fixation, while suitable for most other tissues, is virtually worthless for testicular biopsies; the shrinkage artifacts and disruptions produced make histological interpretation exasperating and futile.

CLASSIFICATION OF MALE INFERTILITY

Clinically, male infertility has been classified primarily on the basis of gonadotropin determinations. Depending on the levels of plasma gonadotropins, male infertility has been divided into three major categories: 1. hypogonadotropic, 2. hypergonadotropic, and 3. normal gonadotropic. This essentially biochemical classification has been pivotal in clarifying in a broad sense the nature of the abnormalities encountered in the various types of infertile men.

Our experience in examining testicular biopsies for infertility studies has led us to conclude that for the pathologist, a broad morphological-anatomical classification of male infertility paralleling the clinical-biochemical classification would be useful.[9-11] Such a classification is used in this chapter. It divides the fundamental causes of male infertility into three major categories: pretesticular, testicular, and posttesticular (Table 16–1).

An example of a pretesticular cause of infertility is pituitary failure, whether prepubertal or postpubertal in onset; as a result of impaired gonadotropin production by

Table 16–1. Classification of the Causes of Male Infertility

I. **Pretesticular causes**

  A. Hypogonadotropism

    1. Prepubertal onset

      a. Organic lesions in or near the pituitary (tumors, cysts, trauma, etc.)

      b. Genetic defects in gonadotropin secretion (hypo-gonadotropic eunuchoidism)

        1) Deficiency of FSH and LH

        2) Deficiency of LH

        3) Deficiency of FSH

    2. Postpubertal onset

      a. Organic lesions (pituitary tumors or trauma to pituitary fossa)

  B. Estrogen excess

    1. Endogenous

      a. Estrogen-producing tumors (of the adrenal cortex or the testis)

      b. Cirrhosis of the liver

    2. Exogenous

  C. Androgen excess

    1. Endogenous

      a. Adrenogenital syndrome

      b. Androgen-producing tumors (of the adrenal cortex or the testis)

    2. Exogenous

  D. Hyperprolactinemia

  E. Glucocorticoid excess

    1. Endogenous

      a. Cushing's syndrome

    2. Exogenous

      a. Treatment for ulcerative colitis

      b. Treatment for chronic asthma

  F. Hypothyroidism

  G. Hyperthyroidism

  H. Diabetes mellitus

II. **Testicular causes**

  A. Maturation arrest

  B. Hypospermatogenesis (proportional hypoplasia of all germ cells)

  C. Sertoli-cell-only syndrome (germ cell aplasia)

  D. Klinefelter's syndrome (XXY karyotype and its variants)

  E. XYY syndrome

  F. Other sex chromosomal or autosomal anomalies with gonadal involvement

  G. Male pseudohermaphroditism

    1. Defects in androgen production

    2. Defects in androgen action

    3. Defects in müllerian duct regression

  H. Cryptorchidism

  I. Radiation damage

  J. Chemotherapy damage

  K. Mumps orchitis

III. **Posttesticular causes**

  A. Block of ducts leading away from the testes

    1. Congenital

      a. Aplasia of the vas deferens

      b. Aplasia of the epididymis

    2. Acquired

      a. Infection

        1) Gonorrheal epididymitis

        2) Tuberculous epididymitis

        3) Others

      b. Surgical interruption of the vas deferens

        1) Voluntary

        2) Iatrogenic

  B. Impaired sperm motility (sperm counts adequate)

    1. Faulty maturation or improper storage of spermatozoa in the epididymis

    2. Biochemical abnormalities of the seminal plasma

    3. Defects of the sperm tail

      a. Genetic (the immotile-cilia syndrome)

      b. Acquired

the pituitary, the testes fail secondarily. An excess of circulating estrogen, whether associated with an estrogen-producing tumor of the adrenal cortex, with cirrhosis of the liver, or with exogenous estrogen therapy, by exerting a negative feedback effect on the hypothalamus and the pituitary, can also lead to suppressed gonadotropin production and secondary testicular failure. An excess of circulating androgen, whether endogenous or exogenous in nature, has similarly been shown to lead to secondary failure of the testes via its suppressive action on the hypothalamus and the pituitary. In short, any extra-gonadal endocrine disorder leading to defective spermatogenesis may be grouped under the pretesticular causes of infertility.

The testicular causes of infertility are conditions in which the primary defects reside in the testes.

The posttesticular causes of infertility consist mainly of obstructions of the ducts leading away from the testes. Cases in which the spermatozoa are normal in number but greatly impaired in motility, presumably due to faulty maturation or improper storage of the spermatozoa during their sojourn in the epididymides, or due to biochemical abnormalities of the seminal plasma (the nonspermatozoal portion of the semen), are also included in the posttesticular category.

In the remainder of this chapter, the above classification will be illustrated with testicular biopsies from patients with different causes of infertility, with emphasis on the light-microscopic findings. The cases were derived from an ongoing series of testicular biopsies performed at the University of Chicago for infertility studies or in association with orchiopexy for cryptorchidism. The first 25 years of the series have been reported in detail elsewhere.[9–13]

TESTICULAR CAUSES OF INFERTILITY

As shown in Table 16–2, the bulk of the male infertility patients in our series belongs to the testicular category, which constitutes 79.7% of the total cases. The conditions included in this category are listed in Table 16–1. The more important of them are described below.

For reference, a section of normal adult testis is demonstrated in Figure 16–1, showing the approximate size of the tubules and the thickness of the germinal epithelium. In the human male, fertility is continuous. Since it takes an average of 74 days for the progeny of a spermatogonium to mature into spermatozoa,[14] the continuous fertility implies that the development of any one generation of germ cells must go on concurrently with the development of earlier and later generations of germ cells at other portions of the seminiferous tubules. In consequence, a cross section of the human testis may show various stages of maturing germ cells bordering on the lumen of each seminiferous tubule. In one portion of the tubular lumen, spermatozoa may be seen, while in an adjacent area, spermatids or spermatocytes may predominate. On the whole, however, some spermatozoa can be found in the majority of the tubules at the level of section in any normal adult testis.

Maturation Arrest

One of the most prevalent conditions under the testicular causes of infertility in our series is maturation arrest[13] (Table 16–1), which is defined as a halt at some stage of spermatogenesis. As a general rule, arrest in early spermatogenesis carries a far worse prognosis than arrest in late spermatogenesis.

In a significant number of the cases, the maturation

Table 16–2. Distribution of Causes of Male Infertility as Revealed by Testicular Biopsy in a 25-Year Series at University of Chicago

Causes	Number of Cases	% of Total Cases
Pretesticular	15	8.0
Testicular	149	79.7
Posttesticular	23	12.3
Total	187	100.0

arrest occurs at the spermatid stage, and the arrest is incomplete. The consequence is a decrease in the number of spermatozoa formed in proportion to the population of spermatids present. Aside from the failure of spermatogenesis to reach its usual conclusion, however, there is usually no other defect in the testes of such patients, and no abnormalities are detectable in the Sertoli cells, the tunica propria of the seminferous tubules, or the Leydig cells on light microscopy.

Maturation arrest may also involve the primary spermatocytes. In these cases, the halt of spermatogenesis can occur at any one of multiple successive stages of the first meiotic division. If the arrest is extensive and involves nearly all of the germ cells, virtually no secondary spermatocytes, spermatids, or spermatozoa will be present, as illustrated in Figure 16–2. In recent years, it has been shown that when maturation arrest occurs at the early stage of primary spermatocytes, a gross chromosome anomaly such as an autosomal reciprocal translocation, X-autosome reciprocal translocation, or Robertsonian translocation may be present.[15,16] In other instances, the early maturation arrest may be caused by a genetic mutation affecting meiosis;[17,18] in these cases, abnormal synaptonemal complexes, defective chiasma formation, asynap-

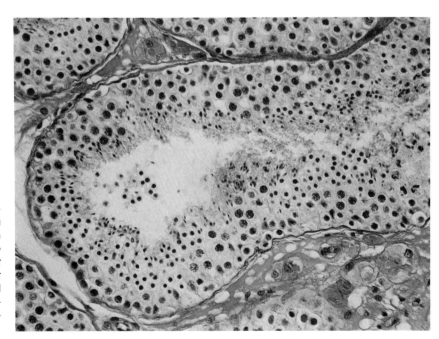

Figure 16–1. Normal testis showing spermatogenesis proceeding in different cycles along a tubule, with various cell types predominating in different portions of the circumference of the lumen. Thus, spermatozoa predominate at some stretches and spermatids at other stretches. Note the thickness of the germinal epithelium, the delicateness of the tunica propria, and the approximate diameter of the tubule. H & E (X250).

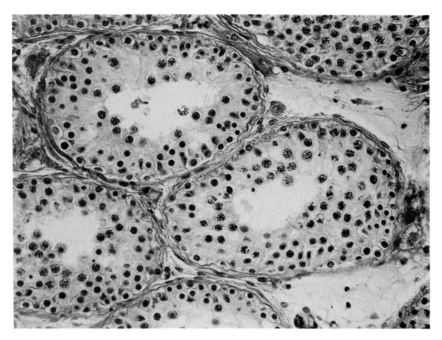

Figure 16–2. Biopsy specimen showing maturation arrest in spermatogenesis, from a 31-year-old man working in a petroleum cracking plant, with long-term exposure to gasoline, fuel oil, and other petroleum products as well as litharge. Despite the incriminating occupational exposures, mitotic and meiotic chromosome analyses, as well as electron microscopy of the germ cells in meiosis, should have been performed on this patient, since maturation arrest of this type can occur in individuals with chromosomal translocations or with genetic mutations affecting meiosis. Unfortunately, such analyses were not carried out. In this patient, maturation of the germ cells stops abruptly at the primary spermatocyte stage; no secondary spermatocytes, spermatids, or spermatozoa are formed. There is no thickening of the tunica propria. The diameter of the tubules is within normal limits. H & E (X250).

sis, or desynapsis may be seen involving the primary spermatocytes on electron microscopy,[18,19] and there is a tendency for the abnormalities to occur in families and to be inherited according to Mendelian laws.[18] For a more detailed discussion of these topics, see the chapter on chromosome anomalies and male infertility (Chapter 15).

Clinically, patients with maturation arrest in spermatogenesis are oligospermic or azoospermic, depending on the stage and extent of the arrest. Plasma FSH is often within normal limits if the arrest occurs late in spermatogenesis, but tends to be elevated if the arrest occurs early in spermatogenesis.[20,21] Plasma LH and testosterone are usually normal.

Hypospermatogenesis

Another prevalent condition under the testicular causes of infertility in our series is hypospermatogenesis[13] (Table 16–1). In this condition, all cell types, including spermatogonia, spermatocytes, spermatids, and spermatozoa, are present in approximately the usual proportion, but the number of each variety is decreased. The consequence of such a proportional hypoplasia is an overall thinning of the germinal epithelium, as shown in Figure 16–3. In contrast to maturation arrest, spermatogenesis does complete itself in the usual fashion in this condition. In most instances, some spermatozoa can be found. In

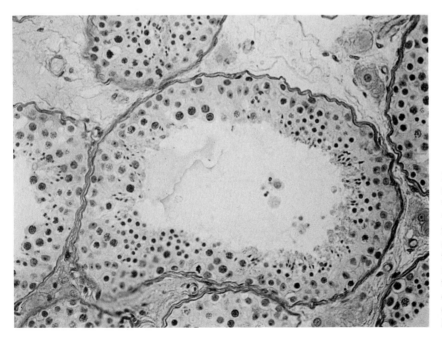

Figure 16–3. Biopsy specimen showing hypospermatogenesis, from a 27-year-old steel mill worker with daily exposure to high temperatures. Note overall thinning of the germinal epithelium due to proportional hypoplasia of all germ cells (compare with Figure 16–1). Despite the thinning of the germinal epithelium, spermatogenesis does complete itself in the usual fashion, and a small number of spermatozoa can be found. The tunica propria is not thickened. The diameter of the tubules and the Leydig cells are normal. H & E (X250).

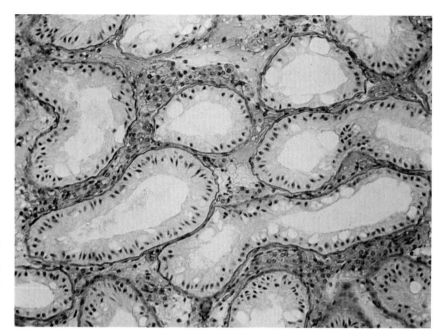

Figure 16–4. Biopsy specimen showing Sertoli-cell-only syndrome, from a 29-year-old man with azoospermia but normal secondary sex characteristics. The seminiferous tubules are lined by Sertoli cells exclusively. Many of the Sertoli cells have prominent cytoplasmic vacuoles. The tunica propria is usually thin and delicate. The tubular diameter is decreased. The Leydig cells appear normal. H & E (X150).

the majority of such testicular biopsies, the tunica propria of the tubules is not thickened, the Sertoli cells and Leydig cells appear normal, and the diameter of the tubules is within normal limits. In cases of severe hypospermatogenesis, however, some tubules may show thickening of the tunica, and occasional tubules may be completely sclerosed.

Clinically, patients with hypospermatogenesis are usually oligospermic. The majority of them have normal plasma FSH, LH, and testosterone.[21,22]

Sertoli-Cell-Only Syndrome (Germ Cell Aplasia)

In this disorder, the testicular tubules show a moderate decrease in diameter and are devoid of germ cells; they are lined by Sertoli cells exclusively (Figure 16–4). The cytoplasm of the Sertoli cells often contains a large number of clear vacuoles, which prove to be dilated endoplasmic reticulum ultrastructurally.[23] Such vacuoles are a commonly observed and nonspecific response of Sertoli

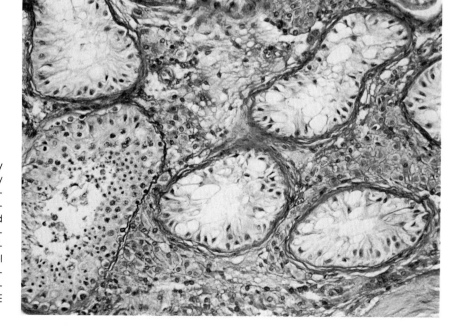

Figure 16–5. An occasional testicular biopsy specimen from patients with Sertoli-cell-only syndrome may have a rare tubule with preserved germ cells amidst a multitude of tubules lined only by Sertoli cells, as illustrated here. The Leydig cells appear somewhat increased in number in this instance. The specimen is from a 28-year-old man with normal secondary sex characteristics, chromatin-negative buccal smear, and severe oligospermia bordering on azoospermia. H & E (X170).

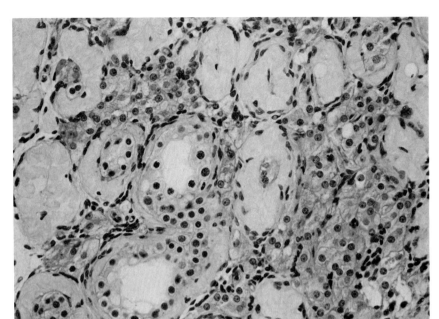

Figure 16–6. Testicular biopsy specimen from a 20-year-old man with Klinefelter's syndrome. A few tubules have sparse germ cells, atrophic Sertoli cells, and thickened tunica propria, while other tubules have lost all of their germ cells and Sertoli cells and are entirely obliterated by thickened, hyalinized, and contracted tunica propria. All tubules are markedly decreased in diameter. The Leydig cells are prominent and appear considerably increased in number focally. H & E (X250).

cells to a variety of noxious agents, and suggest that the testis may have been exposed to harmful influences. Generally, there is no thickening of the tunica propria of the tubules. The Leydig cells appear normal in most biopsies, but may be increased in number in some cases.

In a rare biopsy, one or several tubules may contain some residual germ cells in various stages of maturation, amidst a lawn of tubules lined only by Sertoli cells (Figure 16–5).

In a recent ultrastructural study,[24] the Sertoli cells in this disorder have been reported to be immature in appearance and to possess features seen in prepubertal Sertoli cells. These observations suggest that the Sertoli cells may be developmentally abnormal, but whether this inadequacy contributes to the loss of germ cells, or is merely a concomitant anomaly, is not known.

Clinically, most patients afflicted with Sertoli-cell-only syndrome have well-developed secondary sex characteristics. The testes are usually somewhat decreased in size. Azoospermia on repeated semen analyses is the rule, although an occasional patient may have a few spermatozoa in the semen, corresponding to the rare tubules with preserved germ cells seen in an occasional biopsy. The plasma FSH is almost always elevated as a response to the absence or near absence of spermatogenesis.[21,22,25] The plasma LH and testosterone are normal in most instances,

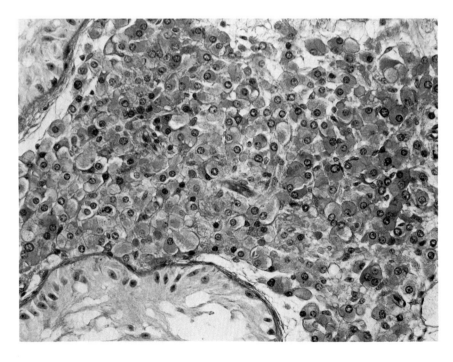

Figure 16–7. Tesicular biopsy specimen from a patient with Klinefelter's syndrome, showing a large mass of Leydig cells adjacent to a tubule which has lost all of its germ cells and is lined by Sertoli cells only. Such "adenomatous clumping" of Leydig cells is a common finding in Klinefelter's syndrome. This 30-year-old man had a chromatin-positive buccal smear, small firm testes, azoospermia, and signs of androgen deficiency. H & E (X250).

indicating adequate Leydig cell function. But in a minority of the cases, there is a small elevation in LH and either a normal or slightly decreased testosterone level, accompanied by a subnormal response of testosterone secretion to hCG stimulation and an exaggerated response of LH to GnRH infusion.[21,25] Taken together, these findings imply a state of compensated or mild Leydig cell failure, and tend to be associated with patients showing numerical increase in Leydig cells in their testicular biopsies.

Klinefelter's Syndrome

The testis in classical Klinefelter's syndrome shows a progressive failure of spermatogenesis, accompanied by tubular sclerosis and a marked increase in the number of Leydig cells (Figure 16–6). The earliest derangement is a reduction in spermatogenic activity, leading to gradual disappearance of the germ cells. In time, the loss of germ cells is followed by atrophy of the Sertoli cells and thickening of the tunica propria. Finally, both the germ cells and Sertoli cells disappear completely, and the lumens of the tubules are obliterated by thickened, hyalinized, and contracted tunica propria. By this series of events, the tubules are converted into shrunken collagenous cords. At first, these changes do not affect all tubules equally, and indeed, in the early stage of the syndrome, the testicular involvement is uneven and patchy, with tubules in the same biopsy showing markedly different degrees of change. But ultimately the entire testis is sclerosed. The Leydig cells are characteristically increased in number and often present a strikingly hyperplastic appearance.[9] At times, they form large aggregates described as "adenomatous clumping" (Figure 16–7).

Although the number of germ cells is significantly reduced and the size of the testes is smaller than normal in prepubertal boys with Klinefelter's syndrome,[26,27] the classical clinical signs usually do not appear until sometime after puberty, when the inherently abnormal testes fail to increase in size in response to pituitary gonadotropin stimulation, but instead become smaller and firmer because of unrelenting degeneration and sclerosis of the seminiferous tubules.[28–30] Leydig cell function is impaired to varying degrees despite the hyperplastic appearance of these cells seen on testicular biopsy.[28–30] If plasma testosterone is low, the patient exhibits incomplete development of the secondary sex characteristics, a eunuchoid appearance, and gynecomastia. If plasma testosterone is near normal, there is full development of the secondary sex characteristics. Semen analysis typically reveals azoospermia. Plasma FSH is characteristically high, reflecting the loss of germ cells. Plasma LH is variably elevated, depending on the degree of androgen deficiency.[28] Leydig cell reserve is diminished, as shown by a decreased response to the administration of hCG.[28] Subnormal intelligence and personality disorders are seen in a fraction of the cases.[29,30] In the classical form of Klinefelter's syndrome, the patient exhibits a 47,XXY chromosomal pattern. This karyotypic abnormality is one of the most commonly encountered among infertile men.[15,16]

XYY Syndrome

The majority of men with a 47,XYY karyotype show some defect in spermatogenesis, although the defect is on the whole much less severe than in Klinefelter's syndrome, and a minority of them are known to be fertile.[31] On testicular biopsy, the XYY syndrome has been reported to be associated with a spectrum of abnormalities in spermatogenesis ranging from mild maturation arrest and hypospermatogenesis to complete absence of germ cells.[31,32] Often, tubules exhibiting these diverse patterns of abnormalities coexist within the same biopsy.[32] Such heterogeneity of morphological changes appears to be a characteristic of patients with an XYY karyotype.[32]

Clinically, the patients show varying degrees of oligospermia. Most of them have normal plasma LH and testosterone levels. Plasma FSH can be normal or elevated, depending on the extent of germ cell damage.[29,31] The patients tend to be unusually tall and prone to develop pustular acne; some of them also exhibit aggressive behavior.[29]

Male Pseudohermaphroditism

Male pseudohermaphroditism is an anomaly of sex differentiation in which individuals with a 46,XY karyotype and male gonads exhibit abnormalities in the development of the male phenotype. Such inadequacy in virilization begins during embryogenesis and arises from one of three pathogenetic mechanisms, all of which appear to have a genetic basis, either autosomal or X-linked: 1. defects in androgen production, 2. defects in androgen action, and 3. defects in müllerian duct regression.[30,33,34] Of the three, defects in androgen action are by far the most common and account for three-fourths of the cases of male pseudohermaphroditism.[34]

Disorders in androgen production can be due to deficiencies in one of five sequential enzymes required for synthesis of testosterone from cholesterol,[30,33,34] or due to Leydig cell agenesis.[35,36] A deficiency of LH receptors in the Leydig cells, making it impossible for them to respond to pituitary LH, has also been reported to cause inadequacies in androgen production.[37]

Disorders in androgen action are either due to a lack of the enzyme 5α-reductase, involved in converting testosterone to 5α-dihydrotestosterone (a more potent androgen than testosterone),[33] or due to a quantitative or qualitative defect in androgen receptors in the target tissues, leading to androgen insensitivity.[34]

Defective müllerian duct regression (see Chapter 14) is the result of abnormalities in the synthesis or action of the müllerian inhibiting factor, normally provided by the Sertoli cells of the fetal testes.[30] The affected men have wolffian duct derivatives and male external genitalia but also possess a uterus and fallopian tubes.[30]

All of the above conditions are associated with impaired spermatogenesis. The testes are populated by immature seminiferous tubules showing varying degrees of germ cell loss and peritubular fibrosis and hyalinization.[30,34–36,38] In cases of Leydig cell agenesis, no Leydig cells are seen in the interstitium, even in the postpubertal period.[35,36] In instances of LH receptor deficiency, the Leydig cells are poorly differentiated and do not bind isotope-labeled LH.[37] In contrast, in patients with androgen insensitivity, the Leydig cells are hyperplastic.[34] In all these conditions, the testes are frequently decreased in size and may be maldescended.[30,34]

The syndromes due to androgen insensitivity are particularly varied in their manifestations. Depending on the nature and severity of the inherited defects, the phenotypic characteristics of the affected genetic males encompass a wide spectrum of abnormalities, ranging from individuals exhibiting only mild hypospadias to those who are phenotypically females and mistakenly reared as females.[30,34] The more severe cases, therefore, are unlikely to present themselves at male infertility clinics. But milder forms of such disorders are being detected with increasing frequencies. Patients with subtle androgen insensitivity due to partial deficiencies of androgen receptors, for example, may present as phenotypically normal males with oligospermia or azoospermia and infertility.[30,34,39–41] In studies performed on unselected men with the diagnosis of "idiopathic" oligospermia or azoospermia, the incidence of androgen receptor deficiency has been reported to be as high as 40%.[40] These finer shades of abnormalities are certain to assume increasing importance in future investigations of men with idiopathic infertility.[34,39,40]

Cryptorchidism

Cryptorchidism is etiologically complex. In some instances, a testis may fail to descend into the scrotum because of developmental malformations involving the spermatic cord or other structures along the path of descent. In other instances, the maldescent appears to be due to insufficient gonadotropin stimulation during early gonadal development, and in these cases, administration of gonadotropins may cause the testis to descend and to develop properly. In still other instances, cryptorchidism appears to be due to some inherent defect of the testis. Such an inherently defective testis often shows germ cell hypoplasia, even at an early age.[42–44] It is predominantly this last variety of cryptorchidism that is included in the testicular causes of infertility. All of the patients with cryptorchidism in our series had failed to respond to gonadotropin treatment before orchiopexy, and none of them was found to have anatomical abnormalities of the inguinal canal during the surgical procedure.

Histologically, a cryptorchid testis has small immature tubules with varying numbers of spermatogonia, depending in part on the severity of the intrinsic germ cell hypoplasia and in part on how long the testis has remained in the undescended position. By about 5 years of age, a lag of development of the undescended testis is histologically apparent.[44] Thereafter, the longer the testis remains undescended, the more pronounced is the retardation in maturation. After puberty, the germ cells in a cryptorchid testis rapidly disappear until the tubules are lined by Sertoli cells only (Figure 16–8). Later, the tubules become hyalinized and sclerotic. The Leydig cells, which are relatively resistant to elevated temperatures, develop properly as a result of gonadotropin stimulation and are often more prominent than usual. In some instances, the Leydig cells show marked cytoplasmic vacuolation.

Clinically, patients with bilateral cryptorchidism as children often show severely impaired spermatogenesis as adults, even when orchiopexy is performed prepubertally.[42,45] The plasma FSH is elevated, reflecting the loss of germ cells, but plasma LH and testosterone are usually normal, indicating adequate Leydig cell function. Patients

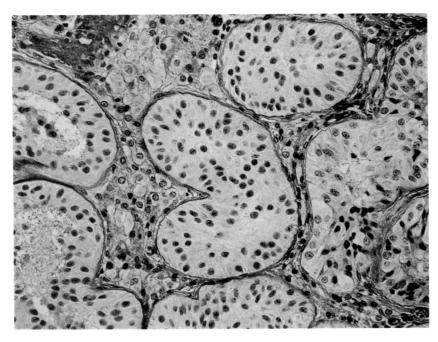

Figure 16–8. Biopsy specimen from a cryptorchid testis during orchiopexy, from a 15-year-old youth with bilateral cryptorchidism which had failed to respond to gonadotropin administration. Note virtual absence of germ cells. The tubules are lined by Sertoli cells only and are considerably smaller than usual in diameter. There is as yet no thickening of the tunica propria or tubular sclerosis. The Leydig cells are somewhat prominent. H & E (X250).

with unilateral cryptorchidism as children often also have lower than normal sperm counts and an exaggerated response of FSH to GnRH stimulation as adults.[44] These findings imply that the scrotal testis in the unilaterally cryptorchid patient is frequently also abnormal.

At times, maldescent of the testis is seen in Sertoli-cell-only syndrome, Klinefelter's syndrome, and various forms of familial male pseudohermaphroditism. The testicular maldescent associated with these disorders should not be confused with true cryptorchidism.

Damage by Radiation and Chemotherapy

Exposure to radiation leads to germ cell depletion that is dose-dependent. In contrast, the Leydig cells are relatively resistant. With single exposures below 600 rads, the germ cell damage appears reversible; above this level, permanent and complete depletion of germ cells is likely, as documented by serial testicular biopsies performed by Rowley and coworkers on normal volunteers exposed to graded doses of x-ray.[46] Of the different stages of maturing germ cells, spermatogonia are the most radiosensitive; of these, the premeiotic spermatogonia (type B) are more vulnerable than the stem cells (type A). By comparison, spermatocytes are considerably more resistant and spermatids even more so.[46]

Histologically, the germ cells undergo degeneration under the influence of radiation and are eventually lost. With more than 600 rads, the tubules are lined by Sertoli cells only (Figure 16–9). Their diameter becomes smaller and their tunica propria is progressively thickened (Figure 16–9). In time, there is total sclerosis of the tubules. The Leydig cells are usually better preserved and show no apparent dysfunction until the dosage of radiation is well over 800 rads.[29] It has been emphasized that

the return of spermatogenesis after exposure to radiation is a slow process; several years may elapse before the seminiferous tubules are repopulated by surviving stem cells. The recovery time, like the extent of the initial germ cell damage, is dose-dependent.[46]

In clinical situations, such as treatments for Hodgkin's disease and other lymphomas, the estimated dose of x-ray received by the testes, with gonadal shielding, is of the order of 200 rads. In radiotherapy for testicular tumors, the dose received by the contralateral testis, despite elaborate shielding, can be as high as 300 rads. Most such patients will be azoospermic for a period following irradiation. Only by long-term follow-up can the extent of recovery be assessed.[47,48]

A similar pattern of germ cell loss followed by slow recovery has been observed in patients who have undergone chemotherapy for various diseases.[48–50] Single-agent chemotherapy, as for example the administration of cyclophosphamide for nephrotic syndrome, is more likely to be followed by recovery of fertility,[51] whereas multiagent chemotherapy, such as the use of MOPP (mechlorethamine, vincristine, procarbazine, and prednisone) in the treatment of lymphomas and leukemias, or the use of VBP (vinblastine, bleomycin, and cis-platin) in the control of testicular malignancies, is often accompanied by complete germ cell loss as well as Leydig cell dysfunction, with a low incidence of recovery.[52–56]

A particularly grave situation is that of acute lymphocytic leukemia of childhood, which has a tendency to infiltrate the testes.[52,57] Since the testicular involvement may be detected during bone marrow remission and is often the first sign of a relapse of the disease, the clinical suspicion is that the leukemic cells in the testes are capable of re-seeding the bone marrow, leading to a systemic recrudescence of the disease with time.[57] For this reason, bilateral testicular biopsies are now routinely performed in most centers before systemic chemotherapy is

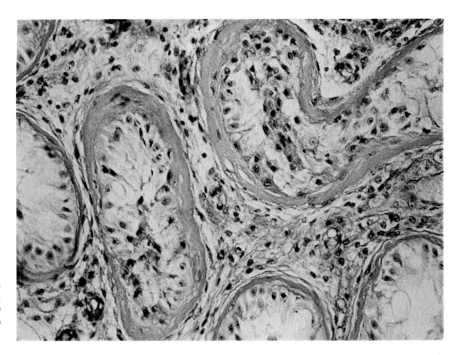

Figure 16–9. Testicular biopsy specimen from a 27-year-old engineer with several years of documented repeated exposures to x-ray. There is complete loss of germ cells, some thickening and hyalinization of the tunica propria, and diminution in size of the tubules. H & E (X250).

stopped; if testicular leukemic infiltrates are found, vigorous attempts are usually made to eradicate them. To achieve this goal, direct x-irradiation of the gonads with dosages as high as 2000 to 2500 rads is used, along with intensified multiagent chemotherapy. With such measures, not only the germ cells, but also the Leydig cells, are damaged beyond recovery, and androgen replacement therapy is often necessary to bring about pubertal development.[58-60] Clinically, the patients have elevated FSH and LH. The plasma testosterone is low and gives a less than normal response to hCG stimulation or not at all.[58-60] In patients who survive into the postpubertal period, azoospermia is common.

Since many young patients with lymphomas, leukemias, and testicular cancers are now enjoying long-term survival following high-dose radiation and combination chemotherapy, increasing attention is focused on the extent of damage to the gonads and the potential for future fertility following such modes of treatment. Because many of the agents used are not only toxic to the germ cells, but are also mutagenic and teratogenic, the problem is considerable.

Mumps Orchitis

Orchitis as a complication of mumps is relatively uncommon in children, and when it does occur before puberty, most patients will recover without dire consequences. During the pubertal and postpubertal periods, however, orchitis has been reported to occur in about 20% of the patients with mumps infection; among those affected by orchitis, the involvement is bilateral in about 15% to 30% of the cases,[61] and permanent damage to the seminiferous tubules often results.[29,62]

Biopsies performed at one time by Charny on patients suffering from acute mumps orchitis revealed that at this stage, there is interstitial edema, neutrophilic and mononuclear inflammatory infiltrate, and degeneration and sloughing of germ cells.[63]

After the acute inflammation has subsided, there are progressive chronic changes consisting of loss of germ cells and tubular hyalinization and sclerosis (Figure 16–10). Because of the slow evolution of the chronic changes, the full extent of the damage may not be apparent until 10 to 20 years after the acute infection.[29,62] Involvement is not uniform throughout the testis; some tubules are more affected than others. The Leydig cells seem, by comparison, far less susceptible than the germ cells to the action of the mumps virus and are usually preserved; often they are more prominent than usual, though seldom as striking as in Klinefelter's syndrome. A past history of acute mumps orchitis is necessary to confirm the histological diagnosis.

Clinically, the affected testis shows shrinking and softening. If involvement is unilateral, sperm density may be reduced but is generally compatible with fertility.[64] Bilateral testicular involvement is usually accompanied by severe oligospermia or azoospermia and sterility.[62,64] When the loss of germ cells is extensive, plasma FSH is elevated. Generally, plasma LH and testosterone are normal, but may be deranged if the orchitis leads to scarring of the interstitial areas with significant loss of Leydig cells, as indicated by a recent study.[65]

Comments on Testicular Causes of Infertility

The testicular causes of infertility are essentially primary defects of the testis. Among such causes, maturation

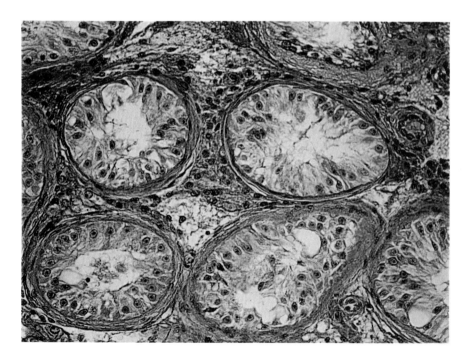

Figure 16–10. Testicular biopsy specimen from a 30-year-old man who had had bilateral acute mumps orchitis 3 years previously. Note loss of germ cells, thickening of the tunica propria, and decrease in size of the tubules. H & E (X250).

arrest and hypospermatogenesis represent the two most common conditions in our series; together they account for somewhat over 50% of the total cases.[13] The patients so afflicted generally have no manifestations of extragonadal endocrine disorders, and no evidence of anatomical block is found on vasography. The main abnormality appears to be subfertility or infertility, along with a defect of spermatogenesis demonstrable on testicular biopsy, in the form of maturation arrest or hypospermatogenesis. For this reason, we have placed these cases in the testicular category. Clinically, such cases are often grouped under the diagnosis of "idiopathic" oligospermia or azoospermia. At present, they are the least understood of the conditions leading to male infertility but unfortunately constitute the largest proportions of the cases seen in infertility clinics. Most likely, there are a multitude of etiological factors that can lead to maturation arrest and hypospermatogenesis; some of these are discussed below.

In recent years, as a result of improved monitoring of health hazards, increasing numbers of cases of the so-called "idiopathic" oligospermia and azoospermia have been shown to be caused by noxious environmental or occupational exposures, which may be chemical or physical. Among the chemical agents implicated are various toxic industrial substances and pesticides.[9,66–69] Workers in dry battery plants with long-term exposures to lead compounds have been shown to suffer from oligospermia, teratospermia, decreased sperm motility, and reduced fertility due to direct toxic effects of the lead compounds on the germinal epithelium; Leydig cell function in such men is not impaired, and there is usually no evidence of pituitary hypofunction.[70] Exposures to petroleum products and coal tar similarly have been reported to have a deleterious effect on spermatogenesis.[68] Pesticides constitute another major group of chemicals that can adversely affect the testis. The nematocide dibromochloropropane (DBCP) has attracted considerable attention because of its selective toxic effect on the germinal epithelium.[71] Testicular biopsies performed on workers exposed to DBCP in manufacturing plants and farmers involved in its application revealed abnormalities ranging from severe hypospermatogenesis to near absence of germ cells, depending on the level and duration of exposure.[72,73] Plasma FSH was increased in such patients, reflecting the loss of germ cells, but plasma LH and testosterone were normal, indicating intact Leydig cell function.[73,74] Follow-up studies have revealed varying degrees of recovery.[74]

A large variety of medications have also been shown to adversely affect spermatogenesis. Among the better known clinical drugs that may reduce the number of germ cells are the alkylating agents, cytotoxic agents, and antimetabolites used in treatment of malignancies.[49–56,66] Less well-known medications with documented ability to induce male infertility include the sulfa drugs used in chronic ulcerative colitis, which appear to cause maturation arrest at the spermatid stage, both experimentally and clinically;[75,76] the infertility has been shown to be reversible upon withdrawal of the sulfa drugs.[75,76]

Prominent among the harmful physical agents is heat. That heat has a detrimental influence on spermatogenesis is undoubted,[77] as attested to by the degeneration of germ cells associated with experimental cryptorchidism or scrotal insulation,[78] the temporary or permanent sterility following prolonged febrile illness,[79] the reduction of sperm counts in normal men subjected to artificial fever,[80] and the improvement of sperm counts in oligospermic men following scrotal hypothermia treatment.[81] Histologically, maturation arrest, as well as hypospermatogenesis of varying severity, has been reported as a consequence of exposure to elevated temperatures.[77] It is of interest that a number of patients in our series suffering from maturation arrest or hypospermatogenesis were steel mill workers or bakers whose occupations caused them to be exposed daily to the high-temperature environment of blast furnaces or baking ovens; a few other patients had well-documented severe and prolonged antecedent febrile illness.[9]

Other important physical agents that have a deleterious effect on spermatogenesis are radiation and microwaves.[82–84] High-energy beta rays from such radioisotopes as ^{32}P, ^{144}Ca, and ^{90}Sr, used widely in laboratory research, are apparently more dangerous to the gonads than previously assumed.[82] Men exposed professionally to ionizing radiation (x-rays and gamma rays) tend to have a lower fertility rate than age-matched controls.[83] Long-term exposure to microwaves has been reported to lead to oligospermia and azoospermia.[84]

Certain instances of hypospermatogenesis are associated with varicocele,[85,86] and a proportion of the cases of maturation arrest are caused by either mitotic or meiotic chromosome anomalies.[15–19]

Excluding all of the above examples, however, there still remains a vast number of cases in which the maturation arrest or hypospermatogenesis has no obvious cause. Recent reports indicate that as many as 40% of the phenotypically normal men diagnosed as having idiopathic oligospermia or azoospermia and without apparent clinical endocrine abnormalities may nonetheless have partial androgen insensitivity due to a deficiency of androgen receptors;[34,39,40] these subtle abnormalities may well prove to be important in a significant portion of the heretofore undiagnosable defects in spermatogenesis.[34,39,40]

The Sertoli-cell-only syndrome, despite having been recognized for four decades, has remained an enigma. Failure of migration of germ cells into the gonads during embryogenesis was initially proposed as the cause of this condition.[87] This theory, while attractive, lacks proof. Recently, the Sertoli cells in some of the patients afflicted with this syndrome have been reported to be immature and potentially abnormal developmentally,[24] but whether these changes are responsible for the loss of germ cells is not known.

In our classification, Klinefelter's syndrome and other chromosomal disorders have been placed under the testicular category of infertility (Table 16–1). The reason for this is twofold: 1. The plasma gonadotropins in these patients are generally high, indicating that the primary defects are in the testes. 2. Mosaic forms of Klinefelter's syndrome are now known, in which there is more than one stem cell line, as for example the coexistence of 46,XY and 47,XXY chromosomal patterns in the same individual.[28,29] The clinical and pathological manifestations in these instances depend largely on which tissue or tissues contain the abnormal cell line. Chromosome analysis of skin fibroblasts and peripheral lymphocytes from such mosaic patients may reveal a normal sex chromosome pattern, but if the testes contain a supernumerary X chromosome complement, testicular dysgenesis typical for Klinefelter's syndrome will develop.[28,29] Such observations indicate that the presence of abnormal numbers of X chromosomes in the testicular tissue is responsible for the changes observed in the seminiferous tubules and Leydig cells in Klinefelter's syndrome. The grouping of Klinefelter's syndrome under the testicular causes of infertility is therefore justified. The same may be said of other chromosome anomalies with testicular involvement.

As a group, the testicular causes of infertility offer little hope for treatment at present, because the loss of germ cells accompanying most of these disorders is primarily irreversible. Maturation arrest and hypospermatogenesis, the two conditions in which the germ cells are by comparison far better preserved, have been treated empirically with hormone therapy. But the incidence of success is relatively low,[21,64] which is probably a reflection of the fact that the etiological mechanisms underlying most of these cases are not known; hence rational design of therapy is not possible. An exception to this pessimistic outlook is the hypospermatogenesis observed in patients with varicocele. While the mechanism by which varicocele exerts its deleterious effect on spermatogenesis is still open to question, it is well documented that varicocelectomy leads to improved sperm counts and testicular histology in a high proportion of the cases,[88–90] although the incidence of restored fertility is lower, and there are no reliable ways at present to predict which patients would benefit from the surgical treatment.[90–92]

In regard to cryptorchidism, two types of treatment are available: the administration of chorionic gonadotropin and orchiopexy. It is now recognized that gonadotropins only promote the descent of those testes that would ultimately descend spontaneously.[29,44,45] Patients who do not respond to gonadotropin administration and who subsequently undergo orchiopexy seldom exhibit normal spermatogenesis following the surgical procedure, even when the orchiopexy is performed well before puberty.[42,44,45] The reasons seem to be that a significant percentage of such cryptorchid testes are hypoplastic and that this hypoplasia is in large measure responsible for the maldescent. Biopsies of such testes at orchiopexy often show the seminiferous tubules to be sparsely populated by germ cells in comparison to normal controls of the same age;[42–44] the germ cells present frequently have abnormally large nuclei and deoxyribonucleic acid contents above the normal diploid range.[93] It is this underpopulation of germ cells and the nuclear abnormalities that are responsible for the lack of success with orchiopexy in such patients, as has been pointed out repeatedly.[42–44,93]

PRETESTICULAR CAUSES OF INFERTILITY

As shown in Table 16–2, 8.0% of the cases of male infertility in our series belong to the pretesticular category. The various conditions included in the pretesticular causes of infertility are listed in Table 16–1.

Hypogonadotropism

Paramount among the pretesticular causes of infertility is insufficiency of pituitary gonadotropins or hypogonadotropism. Although the end result is testicular failure regardless of the cause of the gonadotropin insufficiency, it is important to separate cases of hypogonadotropism into those of prepubertal onset versus those of postpubertal onset, since the two types of cases have entirely different morphological characteristics on testicular biopsies, depending on whether the gonads have undergone the normal development associated with proper gonadotropin stimulation at the time of puberty. As expected, the two types of cases also have different clinical presentation and prognosis.

Prepubertal Hypogonadotropism

Patients with hypogonadotropism of prepubertal onset have small, immature seminiferous tubules resembling those seen in a prepubertal testis (Figures 16–11 and 16–12). They are lined by essentially undifferentiated germinal elements and immature Sertoli cells. There is little evidence of maturation of germ cells beyond the stage of spermatogonia or primary spermatocytes. The tunica propria of the tubules is thin and delicate. As in the prepubertal testis, there are no peritubular elastic fibers demonstrable with special stains, since the development of such elastic fibers occurs only with proper stimulation by pituitary gonadotropins at puberty.[94] The Leydig cells are immature and poorly developed. They resemble undifferentiated mesenchymal cells.

Clinically, the gonadal failure arising from prepubertal hypogonadotropism may be caused by organic lesions in or adjacent to the pituitary, or due to genetic defects in gonadotropin secretion (Table 16–1).

The organic lesions include tumors, cysts, or trauma of the sella turcica or suprasellar area. Patients with such lesions eventually suffer from panhypopituitarism and exhibit sexual infantilism, lack of somatic growth, and varying degrees of thyroid and adrenal dysfunction.

By contrast, patients with genetic defects in gonadotropin secretion are generally tall and eunuchoid, and exhibit no signs of deficiency of growth hormone, thyrotropin, or adrenocorticotropin. Hence the clinical syndrome embodied by such patients is referred to as hypogonadotropic eunuchoidism.[29,95,96] In the classical and most common form of this syndrome, there is an insufficiency of GnRH production by the hypothalamus.[97] In consequence, the patients have a deficiency of both FSH and LH, and give a history of never having undergone a normal puberty. Their testicular biopsies present a picture

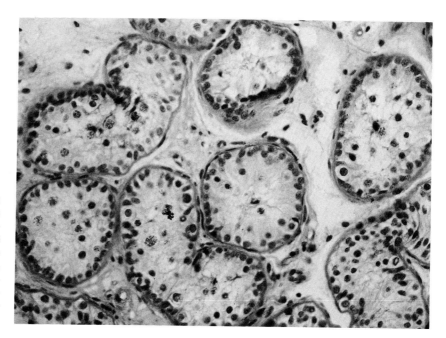

Figure 16–11. Testicular biopsy specimen from a 29-year-old man who had failed to mature sexually because of a suprasellar craniopharyngioma present since childhood. Note small and immature seminiferous tubules resembling those seen in a prepubertal testis. They are lined by Sertoli cells and spermatogonia, with some maturation to the primary spermatocyte stage. Leydig cells are poorly developed or wizened. H & E (X250).

reminiscent of a prepubertal testis.[11,29] Less common, variant forms of the syndrome consisting of isolated LH deficiency[11,29,98] or isolated FSH deficiency[99] are also known. For a more detailed discussion of congenital hypogonadotropic hypogonadism, see Chapter 17.

Postpubertal Hypogonadotropism

If hypogonadotropism occurs in the postpubertal period, the seminiferous tubules, having once attained the full development associated with normal puberty, do not revert to the prepubertal state. Instead, they show in succession maturation arrest, loss of germ cells, reduction in diameter, and progressive thickening and hyalinization of

the tunica propria (Figure 16–13). In time, the tubules are transformed into hyalinized collagenous cords. Special stains show that elastic fibers are present around these sclerotic tubules (Figure 16–14), indicating that the tubules have been subjected previously to the normal stimulation by pituitary gonadotropins. The Leydig cells are generally shrivelled and inconspicuous; they often contain lipochrome pigment in their cytoplasm.

Clinically, the gonadal failure resulting from postpubertal hypogonadotropism may be due to space-occupying lesions in or near the pituitary, such as chromophobe adenomas and craniopharyngiomas. Acidophilic adenomas, which are generally accompanied by decreased gonadotropin secretion, similarly lead to hypogonadism

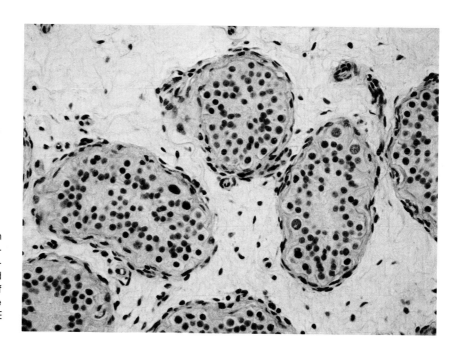

Figure 16–12. Testicular biopsy specimen from a 30-year-old man with hypogonadotropic eunuchoidism. The seminiferous tubules are small and immature. They are lined by Sertoli cells and spermatogonia; some of the latter are of giant size. Leydig cells are scarce and appear undeveloped. H & E (X250).

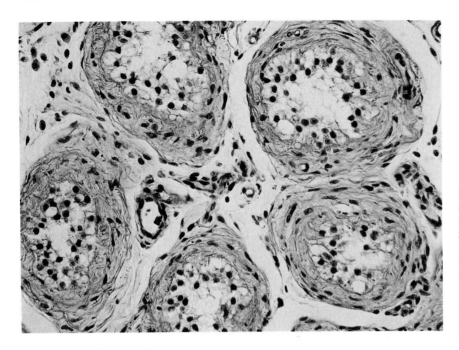

Figure 16–13. Testicular atrophy in a 51-year-old man with an acidophilic adenoma of the pituitary, first discovered at age 39, treated by x-irradiation, following which he developed panhypopituitarism. This patient was not from our biopsy series, but is included here to illustrate the extent of loss of germ cells, tubular sclerosis, and Leydig cell atrophy which postpubertal hypopituitarism is capable of causing. Only Sertoli cells persist in the tubules. H & E (X250).

(Figures 16–13 and 16–14). Trauma to the pituitary fossa, as in basal fracture of the skull, can also lead to hypopituitarism and gonadal failure.

Estrogen Excess

Chronic estrogen excess acts primarily by inhibiting the hypothalamus and the pituitary, leading to suppressed pituitary gonadotropin secretion and secondary testicular failure.[100]

Endogenous estrogen excess may be associated with hepatic cirrhosis.[101–103] The excess may also be due to an estrogen-producing tumor, such as that originating in the adrenal cortex.[11] A Sertoli-cell tumor or interstitial-cell tumor of the testis may also be estrogen-secreting on occasions. Finally, administration of exogenous estrogen, as in patients with carcinoma of the prostate, similarly leads to testicular failure (Figure 16–15), although such patients are seldom seen in infertility clinics.

Pathologically, the above disorders of estrogen excess, which occur predominantly in the postpubertal period, lead initially to failure of germ cell maturation, followed by progressive thinning of the germinal epithelium, decrease in diameter of the seminiferous tubules, and thickening and hyalinization of the tunica propria. In time, there is complete sclerosis of the tubules. The Leydig cells are atrophied. These findings are identical to those

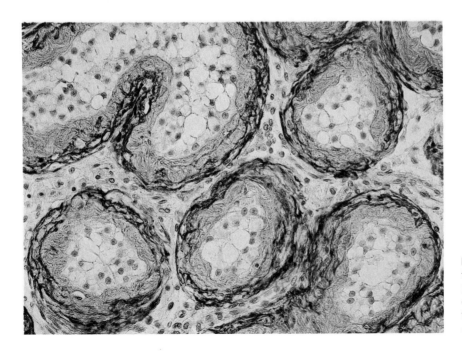

Figure 16–14. Weigert-Van Gieson stain of the testis shown in Figure 16–13. Elastic fibers (appearing as wavy black lines) are present around the sclerotic tubules, indicating that the tubular changes are postpubertal in onset. (X250).

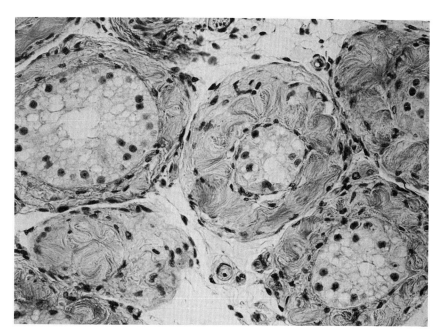

Figure 16–15. The extent of damage that can be caused by estrogen excess is illustrated in this orchiectomy specimen from a 68-year-old man treated with stilbestrol for carcinoma of the prostate. The loss of germ cells, tubular sclerosis, and Leydig cell atrophy are similar to those caused by postpubertal hypopituitarism as illustrated in Figure 16–13. This patient was not from our biopsy series. H & E (X250).

caused by postpubertal hypogonadotropism, as anticipated from the mode of pathogenesis.

Androgen Excess

Androgen excess, like estrogen excess, acts by suppression of pituitary gonadotropin secretion, leading to secondary testicular failure.[104,105]

Endogenous excess of androgen may be associated with the different biochemical variants of adrenogenital syndrome. In one such variant, a defect in 21-hydroxylation of adrenal steroids leads to reduced cortisol synthesis. The pituitary is thereby stimulated to produce an excess of ACTH, which in turn causes overproduction of 17-hydroxyprogesterone, a precursor for both cortisol and androgens. Since the biosynthesis of androgens does not require 21-hydroxylase, the end result of the precursor excess is an increased output of androgenic steroids by the adrenal cortex.[30] Such a surfeit of androgens results in premature development of the secondary sex characteristics and abnormal enlargement of the phallus (virilism). The testes, however, do not mature and remain in the prepubertal state because of inhibition of the hypothalamus and the pituitary by the excess androgens, leading to suppression of gonadotropin secretion; a deficiency of FSH leads to an inability to initiate normal spermatogenesis, while a deficiency of LH makes it impossible for the Leydig cells to develop. A much rarer biochemical variant of the adrenogenital syndrome, 11-hydroxylase deficiency, leads to virilism and hypogonadism by the same mechanism.[30] Treatment of the gonadal problems in both disorders consists of suppression of the excess ACTH secretion by administration of cortisol.

Endogenous excess of androgen may also be due to an androgen-producing tumor of the adrenal cortex or the testis. The pathological findings in the testes depend on whether the tumor exists before or after puberty. If it is present prepubertally, virilism and failure of the testes to mature are the results. On the other hand, if the tumor develops postpubertally, the testes will undergo progressive loss of germ cells and tubular sclerosis; unless the androgenic tumor is eradicated before all spermatogonia are lost, no recovery is possible.

Exogenous excess of androgen behaves in a similar fashion as endogenous excess by inhibiting the pituitary, both directly and via the hypothalamus.[104,105]

Hyperprolactinemia

Hyperprolactinemia has been reported in patients with hypothalamic, pituitary, or suprasellar tumors,[106–108] in patients taking certain medications (among which are some commonly prescribed tranquilizers, neuroleptics, and antihypertensives) that have the ability to elevate prolactin secretion,[108] and in men with idiopathic oligospermia and infertility.[109–111] The precise way in which hyperprolactinemia adversely affects male reproductive function is not completely understood.[29] Clinically, regardless of the cause, hyperprolactinemia is usually accompanied by a decrease in plasma LH and a slight lowering of plasma testosterone levels.[29] Treatment with bromocriptine, a substance that inhibits the release of prolactin by the pituitary, has been reported to alleviate the impotence and loss of libido often experienced by such patients, but the effect on spermatogenesis is less clear.[107,109–111] Reports concerning testicular biopsy findings in men with idiopathic hyperprolactinemia and infertility have been few, but seem to indicate a varied pattern of changes including maturation arrest, hypospermatogenesis, near absence of germ cells, and occasional sclerotic tubules.[109–111] Despite the slight decrease in plasma testosterone often observed in such patients, the Leydig cells in their testicular biopsies often show no obvious abnormalities on light microscopy.[109-111]

Glucocorticoid Excess

Glucocorticoid excess, whether endogenous as in Cushing's syndrome, or exogenous as in treatment for ulcerative colitis, rheumatoid arthritis, or bronchial asthma, can lead to decreased fertility, which is manifested by oligospermia on semen analysis and maturation arrest or hypospermatogenesis on testicular biopsy.[11,112,113] Improvement in sperm counts and fertility is observed when the glucocorticoid excess is corrected.

Hypothyroidism

Patients with proven hypothyroidism may have reduced fertility.[45] On testicular biopsy, the only abnormality appears to be hypospermatogenesis.[11] When thyroxine is supplied, fertility is often restored in such cases.[11]

Hyperthyroidism

Thyrotoxicosis has been reported to be associated with decreased sperm counts on semen analysis and maturation arrest on testicular biopsy.[114,115] When the thyrotoxicosis is corrected, the sperm counts return to normal. The suppressed spermatogenesis appears to be due to a combination of endocrine abnormalities accompanying the hyperthyroid state, including increased conversion of androgens to estrogens, partial Leydig cell failure, and subtle alterations in the sensitivity of the hypothalamic-pituitary axis to the feedback effects of sex steroids.[115]

Diabetes Mellitus

Patients with diabetes mellitus may have diminished fertility because of arteriosclerosis of the testicular arteries or their tributaries, leading to thinning of the germinal epithelium and thickening of the tunica propria of the seminiferous tubules. More commonly, however, the problem is one of impotence or retrograde ejaculation due to autonomic neuropathy associated with diabetes.

Comments on Pretesticular Causes of Infertility

The pretesticular causes of infertility are endocrine disorders primarily; hence any effective treatment must aim at removing such endocrine abnormalities. In a proportion of the patients afflicted with genetic hypogonadotropic eunuchoidism, full spermatogenesis and fertility can be brought about by sustained treatment with chorionic gonadotropin and human menopausal gonadotropin.[11,116] Testicular biopsy is of particular value in selecting those

patients who are likely to respond to such therapy. Other pretesticular causes of infertility, such as tumors in or about the pituitary, can be treated by surgery or radiation, and the accompanying hypopituitarism or hypogonadism may be remedied by hormone replacement therapy.[116]

POSTTESTICULAR CAUSES OF INFERTILITY

As shown in Table 16–2, 12.3% of the cases of male infertility in our series belong to the posttesticular category. The various conditions which make up the posttesticular causes of infertility are listed in Table 16–1.

Block of Ducts Leading away from the Testes

Foremost in importance among the posttesticular causes of infertility is obstruction of the ducts leading away from the testes. The obstruction may be congenital or acquired (see Chapter 18).

Congenital Block

Congenital block is usually due to aplasia of the vas deferens or the epididymis (Table 16–1).[117-119] When bilateral, the aplasia leads to azoospermia and sterility. Such aplasia could have a genetic basis, with the disorder inherited as an autosomal recessive trait.[118] Failure of anatomical union between the vas and the epididymis or between the epididymis and the testis has also been reported by others[117,119] but has not been observed in our series.

Acquired Block

The acquired obstructions are either due to infection or due to surgical interruption (Table 16–1).

Among the infectious causes, gonorrheal epididymitis is the most common; obstruction in such instances occurs most frequently in the tail of the epididymis and the adjacent portion of the vas. Because of its tendency to be bilateral, azoospermia and sterility are frequent sequelae. Tuberculous epididymitis is another infectious disorder which may lead to sterility; the epididymal involvement usually follows a prostatic or seminal-vesicle lesion, and scarring is apt to involve the vasa, seminal vesicles, and ejaculatory ducts besides the epididymides; in addition, a certain degree of orchitis, with scarring and destruction of the seminiferous tubules, may also be present.[2] Nonspecific pyogenic infections, often originating from a recalcitrant bacterial prostatitis, can also lead to scarring of the vas deferens and epididymis.[119]

Surgical occlusion of the vas may be voluntary, as for contraceptive purposes, or iatrogenic, in which case the vas is inadvertently ligated during such surgical procedure as inguinal herniorrhaphy or correction of hydrocele or varicocele.[117,119] Inadvertent bilateral vas ligation leads to sterility.

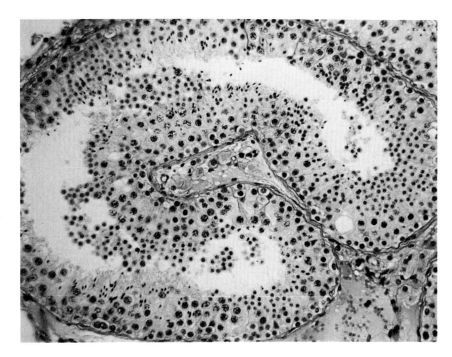

Figure 16–16. Testicular biopsy specimen from a 27-year-old man who had undergone unilateral nephrectomy 13 years earlier for renal tuberculosis. Later, tuberculous involvement of the prostate and seminal vesicles was arrested by chemotherapy. When seen in the infertility clinic, he was azoospermic. Exploration revealed postinflammatory obstructions of the epididymides and vasa deferentia. Despite such obstructions, the testicular biopsy specimen showed normal spermatogenesis. H & E (X200).

On testicular biopsy, regardless of the etiology, obstruction of the vas deferens or epididymis *per se* has no adverse effect on the germinal epithelium or the Leydig cells, as observed repeatedly by others[120,121] and ourselves.[10,12,13] In cases of obstruction due to infection, if there is no accompanying orchitis, the germinal epithelium is preserved (Figure 16–16). Similarly, in patients with surgical occlusion of the vas, unless some vasculature of the testis is ligated or transected simultaneously, the germinal epithelium is unaffected (Figure 16–17). The preservation of the germinal epithelium appears to be due to the remarkable ability of the epididymis to become enlarged to accommodate the products of germ cell activity and its capacity in phagocytizing and resorbing disintegrated spermatozoa.[120,122] Clinically, the epididymal tubules are characteristically dilated proximal to a congenital or postinflammatory obstruction or following surgical interruption of the vas. An equilibrium is apparently established between the rate of spermatogenesis on the one hand, and epididymal enlargement, sperm flow, storage, and resorption on the other. Occasionally, slight dilatation of the seminiferous tubules and hypospermatogenesis are observed in the testicular biopsies obtained from patients with known obstruction of

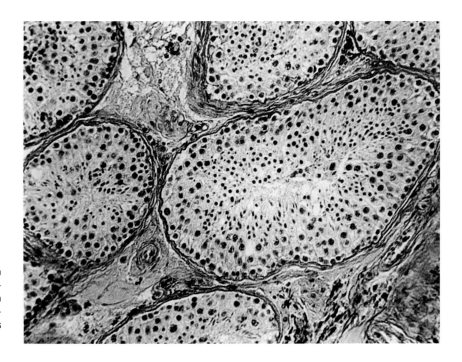

Figure 16–17. Normal germinal epithelium and Leydig cells in a biopsy specimen obtained prior to bilateral vasovasostomy, from a 35-year-old man who had undergone bilateral vasectomy for contraception 6 years previously. H & E (X200).

the excurrent ducts of the testes; such findings appear to represent mild pressure atrophy of the seminiferous tubules when the rate of sperm production exceeds the rate of sperm resorption.

Impaired Sperm Motility

Reduced sperm motility is a frequent accompaniment of oligospermia, but in these instances, the overriding problem is the low sperm count, due to faulty spermatogenesis in the testes. As used here, the term impaired motility refers specifically to those cases in which the sperm counts are adequate and the testicular biopsies are normal, yet the motility of the spermatozoa in the semen specimens is greatly reduced or absent (Table 16–1). An example of the testicular biopsies from such patients is shown in Figure 16–18, in which the germinal epithelium, the Sertoli cells, the tunica propria, the size of the tubules, and the Leydig cells are apparently normal.

It is now recognized that mammalian spermatozoa are not entirely mature when they leave the testis and are not capable of fertilization, but during their slow journey from the head to the tail of the epididymis, which takes an average of 12 days in man, they gradually gain the ability to fertilize.[123] In part, the fertilizing ability of spermatozoa in the tail of the epididymis is related to their acquired capacity for motility. Sperm in the proximal epididymis are essentially immotile or at best exhibit a circular or quivering motion, but those in the distal epididymis are capable of decisive, forward, and purposeful movements. The development of motility appears to depend on intrinsic alterations of the sperm as well as extrinsic factors produced by the epididymis.[123,124] In addition to fostering sperm maturation, the epididymis is also the organ for sperm storage. The mature sperm are housed in the tail of the epididymis, where their viability is preserved until ejaculation.[123] While passage through

the epididymis endows the maturing sperm with the capacity for motility, this motility is not expressed until the sperm are mixed with secretions of the male accessory sex glands at the time of ejaculation.

Based on such knowledge, a portion of the cases of impaired motility are believed to be due to faulty maturation or improper preservation of the spermatozoa during their sojourn in the epididymides,[45] or due to biochemical abnormalities of the seminal plasma,[125] the bulk of which is made up of secretions from the prostate and seminal vesicles, with minor contributions from the epididymides, vasa deferentia, ampullae, and bulbourethral glands. However, with the exception of bacterial infections involving the accessory sex glands, which are known to alter the biochemical composition of the seminal plasma,[125,126] the exact mechanism by which impaired sperm motility is brought about is not well understood in the majority of the cases. With respect to mycoplasma infections, the impaired motility appears to be brought about by adherence of the organisms to spermatozoa.[127]

Recently, patients with normal sperm counts but completely immotile sperm in the ejaculates have been reported, in whom there is also a prominent history of chronic respiratory infections.[128,129] Electron microscopy of the spermatozoa from such patients indicates that the lack of motility is due to a defect of the sperm tails, which have no dynein arms on their microtubules.[128] Since the respiratory cilia and the sperm tails have virtually identical microtubular structures, the nasal and bronchial epithelia of such patients have also been examined and found to show the same structural defect, an absence of dynein arms in the cilia.[128] Dynein arms are protein macromolecules which play both an enzymatic and a mechanical role in motility. They not only possess ATPase activity necessary for breakdown of ATP to produce energy for motility, but as structural molecules, they also participate in the sliding movements of the microtubules

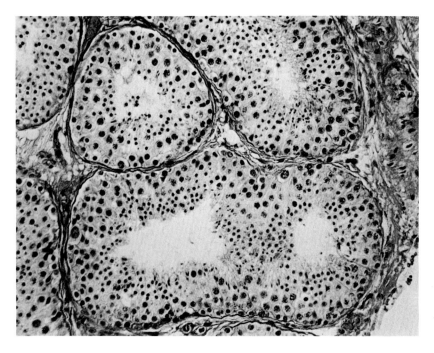

Figure 16–18. Testicular biopsy specimen from a 25-year-old man with normal sperm counts but greatly impaired sperm motility. The sperm counts consistently ranged from 60 to 80 million/ml, but only 10% to 20% of the spermatozoa were motile, and the motility was rated as 1 to 2+ on a scale of 1 to 4+. Note normal seminiferous tubules and Leydig cells. H & E (X200).

responsible for the propelling motion of sperm tails and cilia.[130] In the absence of dynein arms, the spermatozoa are immotile, and mucociliary clearance in the respiratory tract is defective, leading to sinusitis, bronchitis, and bronchiectasis. The disorder in such patients has since been named the immotile-cilia syndrome,[128] which is a genetic condition characterized by chronic respiratory tract infections and infertility. About half of the patients also have situs inversus and were formerly classified under Kartagener's syndrome (which consists of the triad of situs inversus, chronic bronchitis, and bronchiectasis).[131] Since the first reports of such cases, multiple other ultrastructural defects of the tail and midpiece of spermatozoa have been described which also result in immotility.[129] Considering the complexities of the locomotor apparatus in spermatozoa, the varieties of defects which can lead to sperm immotility seem inexhaustible. Recently, an infertile man was reported who had no dynein arms in the sperm tails but possessed structurally normal respiratory cilia.[132] Conversely, a young man with recurrent bronchitis and sinusitis since birth was found to exhibit the characteristic absence of dynein arms in the respiratory cilia, but his spermatozoa were structurally normal.[133] The occurrence of such cases adds to the difficulty of clinical detection.

More recently, acquired abnormalities leading to sperm immotility have been described in infertile men, in whom the sperm tails exhibit a vast array of microtubular anomalies; in contrast to the genetically determined cases, not all spermatozoa in the semen are immotile, and the abnormalities present in one spermatozoon may be different from those present in another spermatozoon of the same patient.[134] Increased antisperm antibodies due to previous genitourinary infection or testicular injury have been implicated in the pathogenesis of the acquired sperm immotility.[134] Since infection and injury to the respiratory tract have been reported to lead to acquired ultrastructural abnormalities and immotility of the bronchial cilia,[135,136] analogous findings in the sperm tails are not unexpected. The existence of such cases stresses the importance of examining the spermatozoa ultrastructurally in a complete semen analysis.

Comments on Posttesticular Causes of Infertility

The two dominant problems in the posttesticular causes of infertility are obstruction and impaired sperm motility.

The treatment for obstruction is surgical correction. This treatment is feasible because the spermotogenic potential of the testis is preserved indefinitely despite obstruction of its excurrent ducts. Congenital blocks due to aplasia, whether present in the vas deferens or the epididymis, are generally difficult to repair surgically; the absence of large segments of such structures makes anastomosis mechanically impossible.[137] Of the acquired blocks, those caused by gonorrheal epididymitis, tuberculous epididymitis, or other infections leading to multiple points of scarring in the epididymis, are also difficult to repair, because the epididymis is essentially a single continuous tubule despite its highly serpentine and winding course, so that a block at any one point in effect presents a complete barrier to sperm transport. Results of epididymovasostomy in such patients have not been encouraging.[117,137] Added to the difficulty is the accompanying orchitis in some of the cases. Instances of vasectomy performed for contraceptive purposes, because of their comparatively tidy nature and circumscription, are generally far more amenable to surgical repair. Using microsurgical techniques, successful vasovasostomy in terms of reappearance of motile spermatozoa in the semen has been achieved in over 90% of the cases,[138] although the rate of restored fertility in terms of the ability to induce pregnancy is generally much lower and averages around 35% of the cases in the larger series reported,[139] in part due to the development of antisperm antibodies.[121,139]

As for patients with normal testicular biopsies but greatly impaired sperm motility, the problem may be divided into several broad categories: 1. abnormalities in the epididymis, 2. abnormalities in the accessory sex glands and the seminal plasma, and 3. abnormalities in the locomotor apparatus of spermatozoa.

The pivotal role of the epididymis in sperm maturation and the acquisition of sperm motility is well recognized.[123] Because of the varieties of drugs that can exert a deleterious effect on the epithelium of the epididymis,[140] the role of this organ in posttesticular male infertility is destined to become more prominent.

The importance of the seminal plasma in regulating sperm motility is also well known.[125] Biochemical abnormalities of the seminal plasma can be acquired or inherent. The acquired abnormalities are often due to bacterial infections of the prostate and seminal vesicles,[125,126] which are amenable to treatment. In addition, certain drugs and toxic substances that impair sperm motility are known to be excreted in the seminal plasma.[67] By contrast, the inherent abnormalities of the seminal plasma are complex and poorly understood.[125] Based on the physiological fact that the accessory sex glands are hormone-dependent, empirical endocrine therapy has been tried in such cases, but the results have been disappointing.[141]

Structural abnormalities in the locomotor apparatus of spermatozoa, whether congenital[128,129] or acquired,[134] can lead to sperm immotility and infertility. Theoretically, the congenital defects should be included under the testicular causes of infertility, since the abnormalities in the dynein arms and other microtubular structures observed in such cases are the results of genetic disorders in spermatozoa formation. In contrast, the acquired defects are often associated with infection of the excurrent ducts and therefore rightly belong with the post-testicular causes of infertility. The inclusion of the congenital defects of sperm motility in the posttesticular category is for convenience of presentation only.

CONCLUSION

In this chapter, testicular biopsies from patients with different causes of infertility were presented. The causes of infertility were divided into three categories: pretesticular, testicular, and posttesticular. On theoretical grounds, the pretesticular cases would be expected to be associated with decreased gonadotropin secretion. The decrease may be the consequence of primary hypothalamic or pituitary disease, or the result of feedback inhibition of the hypothalamus or the pituitary as in disorders of estrogen or androgen excess. The testicular cases, being due to primary defects of the testes, would be expected to have increased gonadotropin secretion (especially FSH) as a compensatory response to defective spermatogenesis. Lastly, the posttesticular cases, which consist primarily of obstructions of the excurrent ducts of the testes, would be expected to have normal gonadotropin secretion, since obstructions *per se* do not affect the germinal epithelium.

The above correlations for the most part hold true in our series.[9-13] The important exceptions are the cases of maturation arrest and hypospermatogenesis. The majority of patients with either of these two testicular causes of infertility generally have normal gonadotropin levels, apparently because the extents of testicular damage are not sufficiently great to cause an increase in gonadotropin secretion. Only in those patients with severe hypospermatogenesis or maturation arrest involving the spermatogonial or primary spermatocyte stage are the FSH levels elevated.[20,21] A rise of plasma FSH in patients with idiopathic oligospermia therefore portends extensive germ cell damage and a guarded prognosis for fertility.

Recently, various abnormalities in the hormone receptors or in the hormones themselves have been detected. The frequent occurrence of partial deficiencies of androgen receptors in phenotypically normal men with so-called idiopathic oligospermia has already been mentioned previously.[34,39,40] A decrease in high-affinity binding for FSH by the testicular tissue, either due to loss of high-affinity FSH-binding receptors, or due to the presence of structurally abnormal FSH receptors, has also been reported recently as a cause of male infertility.[142] Similarly, secretion of an abnormal LH molecule which is immunoreactive but biologically inactive has been implicated in a patient with male pseudohermaphroditism.[143] These cases signal another new direction in which future investigations of male infertility may be forged.

Along with the advances in hormone and receptor studies, the increasing application of chromosome analysis is contributing greatly to our understanding of the complex process of spermatogenesis. Both somatic chromosome abnormalities in lymphocytes of peripheral blood and meiotic chromosome abnormalities in testicular tissue occur in significantly greater frequencies in infertile men than in normal men.[15,16] Some of the meiotic chromosome anomalies are due to genetic mutations affecting meiosis.[15-18] Because a significant portion of the meiotic chromosome anomalies responsible for male infertility can only be detected in the germ cells, cytogenetic and ultrastructural studies must be performed directly on testicular tissue obtained by biopsy to uncover such abnormalities (see Chapter 15, Chromosome Anomalies and Male Infertility).

In the past decade, there has been increasing aware-ness of the adverse effects of environmental chemicals and drugs on fertility.[66,67] Most of the incriminated agents have a direct toxic effect on the germ cells of the testis. But some of them have a pretesticular effect due to their inhibition of the hypothalamus or the pituitary. Other agents have a posttesticular effect on fertility; these substances either are toxic to the epididymal epithelium and interfere with posttesticular sperm maturation and storage, or are excreted into the seminal plasma, where they have the ability to inhibit the motility of ejaculated sperm. Still other agents have an extremely broad influence on the male reproductive tract which blurs the separation of pretesticular, testicular, and posttesticular infertility. For example, men exposed to estrogen (in the form of diethylstilbestrol) *in utero* are found to have elevated plasma FSH, hypoplastic testes with diminished germ cells, an increased incidence of cryptorchidism, and epididymal cysts in postnatal life, indicating that the final defects are both testicular and posttesticular in character.[144] However, in men exposed to estrogen in adult life, the defects are pretesticular in nature, in that the testicular failure is accompanied by decreased FSH and LH due to suppression of the hypothalamus and pituitary by the exogenous estrogen.[13] Similarly, the pesticide DBCP, aside from reducing the number of germ cells in the testis due to direct toxicity on the germinal epithelium, also has an adverse effect on epididymal and ejaculated sperm, apparently because DBCP has the ability to inhibit the glucose metabolism of spermatozoa, thereby rendering them immotile.[145] The action of alcohol is equally complex. It not only is toxic to the germinal epithelium, but also inhibits testosterone production by the Leydig cells directly;[146,147] aside from these primary gonadal effects, alcohol suppresses the hypothalamic-pituitary axis independently.[146,147] Finally, psychodelic drugs such as marihuana and related compounds may also have a testicular as well as a pretesticular effect. Besides damaging the germinal epithelium directly,[148] marihuana decreases plasma testosterone levels by suppressing the hypothalamic-pituitary axis.[149] These examples point to the widening role of environmental agents and drugs (both medical and illicit) in the pathogenesis of the so-called idiopathic male infertility. In addition, the rising incidence of malformation of the male reproductive system in recent years has been attributed to the ubiquitous presence or use of such noxious substances.[149,150-152]

In conclusion, testicular biopsy is an important tool in the diagnosis and management of male infertility. As radioimmunoassays of plasma hormones have become increasingly precise in recent years, the measurement of FSH has to some extent supplanted testicular biopsy as a diagnostic procedure in the investigation of men with severe oligospermia and azoospermia. Nonetheless, when used judiciously and intelligently, testicular biopsy still yields a more accurate assessment of the state of the germinal epithelium than determination of plasma FSH levels, particularly when microscopic examination of the biopsy is coupled with quantitative evaluation of the germ cells and Leydig cells.[86,90,153] In common clinical settings, testicular biopsy has been particularly useful in a number of situations. First, it can distinguish with certainty the azoospermia due to obstruction from that due to primary testicular failure. Second, in patients about to undergo surgical correction of obstruction of excurrent ducts, a biopsy is essential for assessing the possibility of success, since in cases of postinflammatory obstruction, there may be unsuspected damage to the germinal epithelium due to concomitant orchitis, which could substantially reduce the chances for restored fertility. Third, a proportion of the infertile men, particularly those with low sperm counts, have chromosome anomalies as the basis of their infertlity;[15] often, these chromosome anomalies are detectable only in testicular tissue obtained by biopsy.[15,154] Fourth, in instances of hypogonadotropism, testicular biopsy is of particular value in selecting those patients who are likely to respond prior to institution of the lengthy and costly gonadotropin therapy.[116] Fifth, in selected circumstances, such as acute lymphocytic leukemia of childhood, testicular biopsy is necessary for evaluating the efficacy or the toxic effect of a particular mode of treatment.[52,57] Finally, in those cases with a hopeless prognosis for fertility, testicular biopsy provides the necessary justification for withholding therapy.

As a research tool, testicular biopsy is equally important. Electron microscopic examination of the biopsy specimens, when carried out diligently, may provide information on the structural basis of male infertility. Cell sorting[155,156] and flow cytometry[157] carried out on testicular tissue promise to provide better quantitation on the different stages of maturing germ cells, and give a more accurate assessment of the point of maturation arrest as well as any abnormality in the DNA contents of the germ cells.[157] In addition, the ability to separate individual chromosomes by these procedures,[158] along with gene-mapping, may in time lead to a better understanding of the chromosomal and genic control of the complex process of spermatogenesis. Finally, biochemical investigations on the synthesis and action of hormones, coupled with studies on the structure and function of hormone receptors, when performed directly on testicular tissues derived from biopsies, may ultimately yield fundamental answers to the problem of deranged spermatogenesis, and provide explanations, if not solutions, for the plight of male infertility.

References

1. MacLeod J: Human male infertility. Obstet Gynecol Surv 26:335–351, 1971.
2. Amelar RD, Dubin L, Walsh PC: Male Infertility, 258 pp. Philadelphia, WB Saunders, 1977.
3. Nelson CMK, Bunge RG: Semen analysis: evidence for changing parameters of male fertility potential. Fertil Steril 25:503–507, 1974.
4. Smith KD, Steinberger E: What is oligospermia? In P Troen, HR Nankin (eds) The Testis in Normal and Infertile Men, p489–503. New York, Raven Press, 1977.
5. Dougherty RC, Whitaker MJ, Tang SY, et al.: Sperm density and toxic substances: a potential key to environmental health hazards. In JD McKinney (ed) Environmental Health Chemistry: The Chemistry of Environmental Agents as Potential Human Hazards, p263–278. Ann Arbor, Ann Arbor Science Publishers, 1981.
6. Osser S, Liedholm P, Ranstam J: Depressed semen quality: a study over two decades. Arch Androl 12: 113–116, 1984.
7. Nelson WO: Interpretation of testicular biopsy. JAMA 151:449–454, 1953.
8. Rowley MJ, Heller CG: The testicular biopsy: surgical procedure, fixation, and staining technics. Fertil Steril 17:177–186, 1966.
9. Wong TW, Straus FH, Warner NE: Testicular biopsy in the study of male infertility. I. Testicular causes of infertility. Arch Pathol 95:151–159, 1973.
10. Wong TW, Straus FH, Warner NE: Testicular biopsy in the study of male infertility. II. Posttesticular causes of infertility. Arch Pathol 95:160–164, 1973.
11. Wong TW, Straus FH, Warner NE: Testicular biopsy in the study of male infertility. III. Pretesticular causes of infertility. Arch Pathol 98:1–8, 1974.
12. Wong TW, Straus FH, Jones TM, et al.: Pathological aspects of the infertile testis. Urol Clin North Am 5:503–530, 1978.
13. Wong TW, Jones TM: Evaluation of testicular biopsy in male infertility studies. In LI Lipshultz, SS Howards (eds) Infertility in the Male, p217–248. New York, Churchill Livingstone, 1983.
14. Heller CG, Clermont Y: Kinetics of the germinal epithelium in man. Recent Prog Horm Res 20:545–571, 1964.
15. Chandley AC: The chromosomal basis of human infertility. Br Med Bull 35:181–186, 1979.
16. Chandley AC: Chromosomes and infertility. In GD Chisholm, DI Williams (eds) Scientific Foundations of Urology, 2nd ed, p564–572. London, AW Heinemann, 1982.
17. Chaganti RSK, German J: Human male infertility, probably genetically determined, due to defective meiosis and spermatogenic arrest. Am J Hum Genet 31:634–641, 1979.
18. Chaganti RSK, Jhanwar SC, Ehrenbard LT, et al.: Genetically determined asynapsis, spermatogenic degeneration, and infertility in men. Am J Hum Genet 32:833–848, 1980.
19. Söderström KO, Suominen J: Histopathology and ultrastructure of meiotic arrest in human spermatogenesis. Arch Pathol Lab Med 104:476–482, 1980.
20. de Kretser DM, Burger HG, Hudson B: The relationship between germinal cells and serum FSH levels in males with infertility. J Clin Endocrinol Metab 38:787–793, 1974.
21. de Kretser DM: Endocrinology of male infertility. Br Med Bull 35:187–192, 1979.
22. de Kretser DM, Burger HG, Fortune D, et al.: Hormonal, histological and chromosomal studies in adult males with testicular disorders. J Clin Endocrinol Metab 35:392–401, 1972.
23. Chemes HE, Dym M, Fawcett DW, et al.: Patho-physiological observations of Sertoli cells in patients with germinal aplasia or severe germ cell depletion. Ultrastructural findings and hormone levels. Biol Reprod 17:108–123, 1977.
24. Nistal M, Paniagua R, Abaurrea MA, et al.: Hyperplasia and the immature appearance of Sertoli cells in primary testicular disorders. Hum Pathol 13:3–12, 1982.
25. Mecklenburg RS, Sherins RJ: Gonadotropin response to luteinizing hormone-releasing hormone in men with germinal aplasia. J Clin Endocrinol Metab 38:1005–1008, 1974.
26. Ferguson-Smith MA: The prepubertal testicular lesion in chromatin-positive Klinefelter's syndrome (primary

micro-orchidism) as seen in mentally handicapped children. Lancet 1:219–222, 1959.

27. Laron Z, Hochman IH: Small testes in prepubertal boys with Klinefelter's syndrome. J Clin Endocrinol Metab 32:671–672, 1971.

28. Paulsen CA, Gordon DL, Carpenter RW, et al.: Klinefelter's syndrome and its variants: a hormonal and chromosomal study. Recent Prog Horm Res 24:321–353, 1968.

29. Bardin CW, Paulsen CA: The testes. In RH Williams (ed) Textbook of Endocrinology, 6th ed, p293–354, Philadelphia, WB Saunders, 1981.

30. Grumbach MM, Conte FA: Disorders of sex differentiation. In RH Williams (ed) Textbook of Endocrinology, 6th ed, p423–514. Philadelphia, WB Saunders, 1981.

31. Baghdassarian A, Bayard F, Borgaonkar DS, et al.: Testicular function in XYY men. Johns Hopkins Med J 136:15–24, 1975.

32. Skakkebaek NE, Hultén M, Jacobsen P, et al.: Quantification of human seminiferous epithelium. II. Histological studies in eight 47,XYY men. J Reprod Fertil 32:391–401, 1973.

33. Imperato-McGinley J, Peterson RE: Male pseudohermaphroditism: the complexities of male phenotypic development. Am J Med 61:251–272, 1976.

34. Wilson JD, Griffin JE, Leshin M, et al.: The androgen resistance syndromes: 5α-reductase deficiency, testicular feminization, and related disorders. In JB Standbury, JB Wyngaarden, DS Fredrickson, et al. (eds) The Metabolic Basis of Inherited Disease, 5th ed, p1001–1026. New York, McGraw-Hill, 1983.

35. Berthezène F, Forest MG, Grimaud JA, et al.: Leydig-cell agenesis: a cause of male pseudohermaphroditism. N Engl J Med 295:969–972, 1976.

36. Rogers RM, Garcia A, van den Berg L, et al.: Leydig cell hypogenesis: a rare cause of male pseudohermaphroditism and a pathological model for the understanding of normal sexual differentiation. J Urol 128:1325–1329, 1982.

37. Pérez-Palacios G, Scaglia H, Kofman S, et al.: Inherited deficiency of gonadotropin receptors in Leydig cells: a new form of male pseudohermaphroditism. Am J Hum Genet 27:71A, 1975.

38. Okon E, Livni N, Rösler A, et al.: Male pseudohermaphroditism due to 5α-reductase deficiency. Ultrastructure of the gonads. Arch Pathol Lab Med 104:363–367, 1980.

39. Aiman J, Griffin JE, Gazak JM, et al.: Androgen insensitivity as a cause of infertility in otherwise normal men. N Engl J Med 300:223–227, 1979.

40. Aiman J, Griffin JE: The frequency of androgen receptor deficiency in infertile men. J Clin Endocrinol Metab 54:725–732, 1982.

41. Migeon CJ, Brown TR, Lanes R, et al.: A clinical syndrome of mild androgen insensitivity. J Clin Endocrinol Metab 59:672–678, 1984.

42. Charny CW: The spermatogenic potential of the undescended testis before and after treatment. J Urol 83:697–705, 1960.

43. Farrington GH: Histologic observations in cryptorchidism: the congenital germinal-cell deficiency of the undescended testis. J Pediatr Surg 4:606–613, 1969.

44. Lipshultz LI: Cryptorchidism in the subfertile male. Fertil Steril 27:609–620, 1976.

45. Charny CW: Treatment of male infertility. In SJ Behrman, RW Kistner (eds) Progress in Infertility, p649–671. Boston, Little Brown, 1968.

46. Rowley MJ, Leach DR, Warner GA, et al.: Effect of graded doses of ionizing radiation on the human testis. Radiat Res 59:665–678, 1974.

47. Hahn EW, Feingold SM, Nisce L: Aspermia and recovery of spermatogenesis in cancer patients following incidental gonadal irradiation during treatment: a progress report. Radiology 119:223–225, 1976.

48. Clarke SJ, Resnick MI: Infertility following radiation and chemotherapy. Urol Clin North Am 5:531–535, 1978.

49. Sherins RJ, DeVita VT: Effect of drug treatment for lymphoma on male reproductive capacity. Studies of men in remission after therapy. Ann Intern Med 79:216–220, 1973.

50. Sieber SM, Adamson RH: Toxicity of antineoplastic agents in man: chromosomal aberrations, antifertility effects, congenital malformations, and carcinogenic potential. Adv Cancer Res 22:57–155, 1975.

51. Lentz RD, Bergstein J, Steffes MW, et al.: Postpubertal evaluation of gonadal function following cyclophosphamide therapy before and during puberty. J Pediatr 91:385–394, 1977.

52. Lendon M, Hann IM, Palmer MK, et al.: Testicular histology after combination chemotherapy in childhood for acute lymphoblastic leukemia. Lancet 2:439–441, 1978.

53. Shalet SM: Effects of cancer chemotherapy on gonadal function of patients. Cancer Treat Rev 7:141–152, 1980.

54. Schilsky RL, Lewis BJ, Sherins RJ, et al.: Gonadal dysfunction in patients receiving chemotherapy for cancer. Ann Intern Med 93 (Part 1):109–114, 1980.

55. Whitehead E, Shalet SM, Blackledge G, et al.: The effects of Hodgkin's disease and combination chemotherapy on gonadal function in the adult male. Cancer 49:418–422, 1982.

56. Johnson DH, Hainsworth JD, Linde RB, et al.: Testicular function following combination chemotherapy with cisplatin, vinblastine, and bleomycin. Med Pediatr Oncol 12:233–238, 1984.

57. Oden OB, Rankin A, Kay HEM: Isolated testicular relapse in acute lymphoblastic leukemia of childhood. Report on behalf of the Medical Research Council's working party on leukemia in childhood. Arch Dis Child 58:128–132, 1983.

58. Brauner R, Czernichow P, Cramer P, et al.: Leydig-cell function in children after direct testicular irradiation for acute lymphoblastic leukemia. N Engl J Med 309:25–28, 1983.

59. Carrascosa A, Audi L, Ortega JJ, et al.: Hypothalamo-hypophyseal-testicular function in prepubertal boys with acute lymphoblastic leukemia following chemotherapy and testicular radiotherapy. Acta Paediatr Scand 73:364–371, 1984.

60. Shalet SM, Horner A, Ahmed SR, et al.: Leydig cell damage after testicular irradiation for lymphoblastic leukemia. Med Pediatr Oncol 13:65–68, 1985.

61. Christie AB: Infectious Diseases: Epidemiology and Clinical Practice, p424–451. Edinburgh and London, E & S Livingstone, 1969.

62. Ballew JW, Masters WH: Mumps: a cause of infertility. I. Present considerations. Fertil Steril 5:536–543, 1954.

63. Charny CW, Meranz DR: Pathology of mumps orchitis. Trans Am Soc Study Steril 3:167–168, 1947.

64. Steinberger E: Management of male reproductive dysfunction. Clin Obstet Gynecol 22:187–220, 1979.

65. Adamopoulos DA, Lawrence DM, Vassilopoulos P, et al.: Pituitary-testicular interrelationships in mumps orchitis and other virus infections. Br Med J 1:1177–1180, 1978.

66. Wyrobek AJ, Gordon, LA, Burkhart JG, *et al.:* An evaluation of human sperm as indicators of chemically induced alterations of spermatogenic function. A report of the U.S. Environmental Protection Agency Gene-Tox Program. Mutat Res 115:73–148, 1983.

67. Lockey JE, Lemasters GK, Keye WR, Jr (eds) Reproduction: The New Frontier in Occupational and Environmental Health Research, 606pp. New York, Alan R Liss, 1984.

68. Steeno OP, Pangkahila A: Occupational influences on male fertility and sexuality. Part I. Andrologia 16:5–22, 1984.

69. Steeno OP, Pangkahila A: Occupational influences on male fertility and sexuality. Part II. Andrologia 16:93–101, 1984.

70. Lancranjan I, Popescu HI, Găvănescu O, *et al.:* Reproductive ability of workmen occupationally exposed to lead. Arch Environ Health 30:396–401, 1975.

71. Whorton D, Krauss RM, Marshall S, *et al.:* Infertility in male pesticide workers. Lancet 2:1259–1261, 1977.

72. Biava CG, Smuckler EA, Whorton D: The testicular morphology of individuals exposed to dibromochloropropane. Exp Mol Pathol 29:448–458, 1978.

73. Potashnik G, Yanai-Inbar I, Sacks MI, *et al.:* Effect of dibromochloropropane on human testicular function. Isr J Med Sci 15:438–442, 1979.

74. Lantz GD, Cunningham GR, Huckins C, *et al.:* Recovery from severe oligospermia after exposure to dibromochloropropane. Fertil Steril 35:46–53, 1981.

75. Toovey S, Hudson E, Hendry WF, *et al.:* Sulphasalazine and male infertility reversibility and possible mechanism. Gut 22:445–451, 1981.

76. Ó'Moráin C, Smethurst P, Doré CJ: Reversible male infertility due to sulfasalazine: studies in man and rat. Gut 25:1078–1084, 1984.

77. VanDemark NL, Free MJ: Temperature effects. *In* AD Johnson, WR Gomes, NL VanDemark (eds) The Testis, Vol 3, p233–312. New York, Academic Press, 1970.

78. Moore CR, Oslund R: Experiments on the sheep testis—cryptorchidism, vasectomy and scrotal insulation. Am J Physiol 67:595–607, 1924.

79. Mills RG: The pathological changes in the testes in epidemic pneumonia. J Exp Med 30:505–529, 1919.

80. MacLeod J, Hotchkiss RS: The effect of hyperpyrexia upon spermatozoa in men. Endocrinology 28:780–784, 1941.

81. Mulcahy JJ: Scrotal hypothermia and the infertile man. J Urol 132:469–470, 1984.

82. Rao SM, Supe SJ: Hazards to the eye lens and gonads from hard beta rays. Med Phys 5:223–225, 1978.

83. Kitabatake T, Watanabe T, Sato T: Sterility in Japanese radiological technicians. Tohoku J Exp Med 112:209–212, 1974.

84. Lancranjan I, Măicănescu M, Rafailă, *et al.:* Gonadic function in workmen with long-term exposure to microwaves. Health Phys 29:381–383, 1975.

85. Dubin L, Hotchkiss RS: Testis biopsy in subfertile men with varicocele. Fertil Steril 20:50–57, 1969.

86. Agger P, Johnsen SG: Quantitative evaluation of testicular biopsies in varicocele. Fertil Steril 29:52–57, 1978.

87. del Castillo EB, Trabucco A, de la Balze FA: Syndrome produced by absence of the germinal epithelium without impairment of the Sertoli or Leydig cells. J Clin Endocrinol 7:493–502, 1947.

88. Dubin L, Amelar RD: Varicocelectomy: 986 cases in a twelve-year study. Urol 10:446–448, 1977.

89. Greenberg SH: Varicocele and male infertility. Fertil Steril 28:699–706, 1977.

90. Johnsen SG, Agger P: Quantitative evaluation of testicular biopsies before and after operation for varicocele. Fertil Steril 29:58–63, 1978.

91. Saypol DC, Lipshultz LI, Howards SS: Varicocele. In LI Lipshultz, SS Howards (eds) Infertility in the Male, p299–313. New York, Churchill Livingstone, 1983.

92. Comhaire FH: Varicocele infertility: an enigma. Int J Androl 6:401–404, 1983.

93. Müller J, Skakkebaek NE: Abnormal germ cells in maldescended testes: a study of cell density, nuclear size and deoxyribonucleic acid content in testicular biopsies from 50 boys. J Urol 131:730–733, 1984.

94. de la Balze FA, Bur GE, Scarpa-Smith F, *et al.:* Elastic fibers in the tunica propria of normal and pathologic human testes. J Clin Endocrinol Metab 14:626–639, 1954.

95. Santen RJ, Paulsen CA: Hypogonadotropic eunuchoidism. I. Clinical study of the mode of inheritance. J Clin Endocrinol Metab 36:47–63, 1973.

96. Kallmann FJ, Schonfeld WA, Barrera SE: The genetic aspects of primary eunuchoidism. Am J Ment Defic 48:203–236, 1944.

97. Yoshimoto Y, Moridera K, Imura H: Restoration of normal pituitary gonadotropin reserve by administration of luteinizing-hormone-releasing hormone in patients with hypogonadotropic hypogonadism. N Engl J Med 292:242–245, 1975.

98. McCullagh EP, Beck JC, Schaffenburg CA: A syndrome of eunuchoidism with spermatogenesis, normal urinary FSH and low or normal ICSH ("fertile eunuchs"). J Clin Endocrinol Metab 13:489–509, 1953.

99. Maroulis GB, Parlow AF, Marshall JR: Isolated follicle-stimulating hormone deficiency in man. Fertil Steril 28:818–822, 1977.

100. Kulin HE, Reiter EO: Gonadotropin and testosterone measurements after estrogen administration to adult men, prepubertal and pubertal boys, and men with hypogonadotropism: evidence for maturation of positive feedback in the male. Pediatr Res 10:46–51, 1976.

101. Gordon GC, Olivo J, Rafii F, *et al.:* Conversion of androgens to estrogens in cirrhosis of the liver. J Clin Endocrinol Metab 40:1018–1026, 1975.

102. Van Thiel DH, Lester R: Alcoholism: its effect on hypothalamic pituitary gonadal function. Gastroenterology 71:318–327, 1976.

103. Mooradian AD, Shamma'a M, Salti I, *et al.:* Hypophyseal-gonadal dysfunction in men with non-alcoholic liver cirrhosis. Andrologia 17:72–79, 1985.

104. Mauss J, Börsch G, Bormacher K, *et al.:* Effect of long-term testosterone oenanthate administration on male reproductive function: clinical evaluation, serum FSH, LH, testosterone, and seminal fluid analyses in normal men. Acta Endocrinol 78:373–384, 1975.

105. Caminos-Torres R, Ma L, Snyder PJ: Testosterone-induced inhibition of the LH and FSH responses to gonadotropin-releasing hormone occurs slowly. J Clin Endocrinol Metab 44:1142–1153, 1977.

106. Boyar RM, Kapen S, Finkelstein JW, *et al.:* Hypothalamic-pituitary function in diverse hyperprolactinemic states. J Clin Invest 53:1588–1598, 1974.

107. Carter JN, Tyson JE, Tolis G, *et al.:* Prolactin-secreting tumors and hypogonadism in 22 men. N Engl J Med 299:847–852, 1978.

108. Thorner MO: Clinical physiology and the significance and management of hyperprolactinemia. *In* L Martin, GM

Besser (eds) Clinical Neuroendocrinology, p320–361. New York, Academic Press, 1977.

109. Jequier A, Crich JC, Ansell ID: Clinical findings and testicular histology in three hyperprolactinemic infertile men. Fertil Steril 31:525–530, 1979.

110. Segal S, Yaffe H, Laufer N, et al.: Male hyperprolactinemia: effects on fertility. Fertil Steril 32:556–561, 1979.

111. Wong TW, Jones TM: Hyperprolactinemia and male infertility. Arch Pathol Lab Med 108:35–39, 1984.

112. Mancini RE, Lavieri JC, Muller F, et al.: Effect of prednisolone upon normal and pathologic human spermatogenesis. Fertil Steril 17:500–513, 1966.

113. Gabrilove JL, Nicols GL, Sohval AR: The testis in Cushing's syndrome. J Urol 112:95–99, 1974.

114. Clyde HR, Walsh PC, English RW: Elevated plasma testosterone and gonadotropin levels in infertile males with hyperthyroidism. Fertil Steril 27:662–666, 1976.

115. Kidd GS, Glass AR, Vigersky RA: The hypothalamic-pituitary-testicular axis in thyrotoxicosis. J Clin Endocrinol Metab 48:798–802, 1979.

116. Rosemberg E: Gonadotropin therapy of male infertility. In ESE Hafez (ed) Human Semen and Fertility Regulation in Men, p464–475. St Louis, CV Mosby, 1976.

117. O'Conor VJ: Surgical correction of male sterility. Surg Gynecol Obstet 110:649–657, 1960.

118. Schellen TMCM, van Straaten A: Autosomal recessive hereditary congenital aplasia of the vasa deferentia in four siblings. Fertil Steril 34:401–404, 1980.

119. Lipshultz LI, Cunningham GR, Howards SS: Differential diagnosis of male infertility. In LI Lipshultz, SS Howards (eds) Infertility in the Male, p249–263. New York, Churchill Livingstone, 1983.

120. Moore CR: Biology of the testes. In E Allen, CH Danforth, EA Doisy (eds) Sex and Internal Secretions, 2nd ed, p353–451. Baltimore, Williams and Wilkins, 1939.

121. Alexander NJ: Vasectomy: morphological and immunological effects. In ESE Hafez (ed): Human Semen and Fertility Regulation in Men, p308–317. St Louis, CV Mosby, 1976.

122. Phadke AM: Fate of spermatozoa in cases of obstructive azoospermia and after ligation of vas deferens in man. J Reprod Fertil 7:1–12, 1964.

123. Bedford JM: Evolution of the sperm maturation and sperm storage functions of the epididymis. In DW Fawcett, JM Bedford (eds) The Spermatozoon: Maturation, Motility, Surface Properties and Comparative Aspects, p7–21. Baltimore, Urban and Schwarzenberg, 1979.

124. Hoskins DD, Johnson D, Brandt H, et al.: Evidence for a role for a forward motility protein in the epididymal development of sperm motility. In DW Fawcett, JM Bedford (eds) The Spermatozoon: Maturation, Motility, Surface Properties and Comparative Aspects, p43–53. Baltimore, Urban and Schwarzenberg, 1979.

125. Eliasson R, Lindholmer C: Functions of male accessory genital organs. In ESE Hafez (ed): Human Semen and Fertility Regulation in Men, p44–50. St Louis, CV Mosby, 1976.

126. Caldamone AA, Emilson LBV, Al-Juburi A, et al.: Prostatitis: prostatic secretory dysfunction affecting fertility. Fertil Steril 34:602–603, 1980.

127. Fowlkes DM, Dooher GB, O'Leary WM: Evidence of scanning electron microscopy for an association between spermatozoa and T-mycoplasmas in men of infertile marriage. Fertil Steril 26:1203–1211, 1975.

128. Eliasson R, Mossberg B, Camner P, et al.: The immotile-cilia syndrome: a congenital ciliary abnormality as an etiologic factor in chronic airway infections and male sterility. N Engl J Med 297:1–6, 1977.

129. Afzelius BA, Eliasson R: Flagellar mutants in man: on the heterogeneity of the immotile-cilia syndrome. J Ultrastruct Res 69:43–52, 1979.

130. Gibbons IR: Cilia and flagella of eukaryotes. J Cell Biol 91:107s–130s, 1981.

131. Kartagener M, Stucki P: Bronchiectasis with situs inversus. Arch Pediatr 79:193–207, 1962.

132. Walt H, Campana A, Balerna M, et al.: Mosaicism of dynein in spermatozoa and cilia and fibrous sheath aberrations in an infertile man. Andrologia 15:295–300, 1983.

133. Jonsson MS, McCormick JR, Gillies CG, et al.: Kartagener's syndrome with motile spermatozoa. N Engl J Med 307:1131–1133, 1982.

134. Williamson RA Koehler JK, Smith WD, et al.: Ultrastructural sperm tail defects associated with sperm immotility. Fertil Steril 41:103–107, 1984.

135. Cornillie F, Lauweryns J, Corbeel L, et al.: Acquired ultrastructural abnormalities of bronchial cilia in recurrent airway infections and bronchiectases as compared with the findings in Kartagener's syndrome. Pediatr Res 14:168–169, 1980.

136. Afzelius BA: "Immotile-cilia" syndrome and ciliary abnormalities induced by infection and injury. Am Rev Respir Dis 124:107–109, 1981.

137. Schmidt SS, Schoysman R, Stewart BH: Surgical approaches to male infertility. In ESE Hafez (ed) Human Semen and Fertility Regulation in Men, p476–493. St Louis, CV Mosby, 1976.

138. Silber SJ: Vasectomy and vasectomy reversal. Fertil Steril 29:125–140, 1978.

139. Amelar RD, Dubin L: Vasectomy reversal. J Urol 121:547–550, 1979.

140. Glover TD: Investigations into the physiology of the epididymis in relation to male contraception. J Reprod Fertil, suppl 24:95–114, 1976.

141. Amelar RD, Dubin L, Schoenfeld C: Sperm motility. Fertil Steril 34:197–215, 1980.

142. Namiki M, Koide T, Okuyama A, et al.: Abnormality of testicular FSH receptors in infertile men. Acta Endocrinol 106:548–555, 1984.

143. Park IJ, Burnett LS, Jones HW Jr, et al.: A case of male pseudohermaphroditism associated with elevated LH, normal FSH and low testosterone possibly due to the secretion of an abnormal LH molecule. Acta Endocrinol 83:173–181, 1976.

144. Gill WB, Schumacher GFB, Bibbo M, et al.: Association of diethylstilbestrol exposure in utero with cryptorchidism, testicular hypoplasia and semen abnormalities. J Urol 122:36–39, 1979.

145. Kluwe WM, Lamb JC IV, Greenwell A, et al.: 1,2-Dibromo-3-chloropropane (DBCP)-induced infertility in male rats mediated by a post-testicular effect. Toxicol Appl Pharmacol 71:294–298, 1983.

146. Morgan MY: Sex and alcohol. Br Med Bull 38:43–48, 1982.

147. Van Thiel DH, Lester R, Sherins RJ: Hypogonadism in alcoholic liver disease: evidence for a double defect. Gastroenterology 67:1188–1199, 1974.

148. Hembree WC III, Nahas GG, Zeidenberg P, et al.: Changes in human spermatozoa associated with high dose mari-

huana smoking. *In* GG Nahas, WDM Paton (eds) Marihuana: Biological Effects, p429–439. New York, Pergamon Press, 1979.

149. Kolodny RC, Masters WH, Kolodner RM, *et al.:* Depression of plasma testosterone levels after chronic intensive marihuana use. N Engl J Med 290:872–874, 1974.

150. Aarskog D: Maternal progestins as a possible cause of hypospadias. N Engl J Med 300:75–78, 1979.

151. Chilvers C, Pike MC, Forman D, *et al.:* Apparent doubling of frequency of undescended testis in England and Wales in 1962–81. Lancet 2:330–332, 1984.

152. Depue RH: Maternal and gestational factors affecting the risk of cryptorchidism and inguinal hernia. Int J Epidemiol 13:311–318, 1984.

153. Zukerman Z, Rodriguez-Rigau LJ, Weiss DB, *et al.:* Quantitative analysis of the seminiferous epithelium in human testicular biopsies, and the relation of spermatogenesis to sperm density. Fertil Steril 30:448–455, 1978.

154. Koulischer L, Schoysman R, Gillerot Y, *et al.:* Meiotic chromosome studies in human male infertility. *In* PG Crosignani, BL Rubin, M Fraccaro (eds) Genetic Control of Gamete Production and Function, p239–260. New York, Grune and Stratton, 1982.

155. Romrell LJ: Separation of male germ cells by sedimentation velocity. *In* DW Fawcett, JM Bedford (eds) The Spermatozoon: Maturation, Motility, Surface Properties and Comparative Aspects, p375–378. Baltimore, Urban and Schwarzenberg, 1979.

156. Bellvé AR, O'Brien DA: Isolation of mammalian spermatogenic cells and characterization of chromosomal proteins. *In* DW Fawcett, JM Bedford (eds) The Spermatozoon: Maturation, Motility, Surface Properties and Comparative Aspects, p379–385. Baltimore, Urban and Schwarzenberg, 1979.

157. Chan SL, Lipshultz LI, Schwartzendruber D: Deoxyribonucleic acid (DNA) flow cytometry: a new modality for quantitative analysis of testicular biopsies. Fertil Steril 41:485–487, 1984.

158. Fantes JA, Green DK, Cooke HJ: Purifying human Y chromosomes by flow cytometry and sorting. Cytometry 4:88–91, 1983.

17. Hypothalamic-Pituitary Disorders in Male Infertility

Ronald S. Swerdloff and Shalender Bhasin

Infertility is a common problem (10%–15% of the population) and is defined as the failure to conceive during a year of normal coital frequency. In approximately one-third of the couples so affected, a specific defect can be determined in the male partner. Of these, less than 1% can be ascribed to hypothalamic or pituitary hormonal dysfunction. Despite the relative infrequency of hypothalamic-pituitary disorders as a cause of male infertility, these disorders are of interest because of their value in understanding the regulation of spermatogenesis and testicular steroidogenesis, and because the patients so affected are usually responsive to medical management.

The testes serve the dual function of providing the mature haploid zygotes that constitute the male contribution to fertilization, as well as the endocrine secretion of androgens and other steroids. These androgenic hormones affect sex hormone responsive organs and have anabolic effects on the body as a whole. The testes are under the regulation of the pituitary gonadotropic hormones (LH and FSH) and the hypothalamic gonadotropic releasing hormone (GnRH). This chapter will review current understanding of the normal physiology of the hypothalamic-pituitary-gonadal axis and relate this information to sexual dysfunction due to hypothalamic-pituitary disease.

NORMAL PHYSIOLOGY OF THE HYPOTHALAMIC-PITUITARY-TESTICULAR AXIS

The hypothalamic-pituitary-testicular (HPT) axis is a complex, integrated system that is responsible for the regulation of the reproductive system. Multiple factors, particularly extrahypothalamic central nervous system factors, influence the hypothalamic-pituitary-testicular axis. Since the system is to a great extent self-regulating, it is often referred to as a "closed loop system." A schematic representation of the male reproductive axis is provided in Figure 17–1.[1] In this system, hypothalamic secretion of gonadotropin-releasing hormone (GnRH) is regulated by neurotransmitters. GnRH is released in a pulsatile fashion into the hypophyseal portal blood system; GnRH stimu-

lates the synthesis and secretion of LH and FSH which stimulate steroidogenesis and spermatogenesis; sex steroids act on androgen-sensitive end organs to produce and maintain sexual development and anabolic effects; and sex steroids and other testicular products (inhibin) regulate GnRH, LH, and FSH secretion through effects on the hypothalamus and pituitary.

Physiologic Regulation of Hypothalamic GnRH Secretion

The hypothalamus is the integrating center for stimulating and inhibiting signals from the central nervous system and testes that influence the synthesis and secretion of gonadotropin-releasing hormone (GnRH). Neurotransmitters such as norepinephrine, dopamine, endorphins, and melatonin serve as regulators of GnRH synthesis and pulsatile release into the hypophyseal portal veins.[2]

Considerable controversy exists regarding the precise role of individual neurotransmitters in the regulation of hypothalamic GnRH secretion. A large body of evidence suggests that norepinephrine stimulates and endorphins inhibit GnRH release from the hypothalamus.[3] The role of dopamine as a regulator of GnRH secretion is more controversial. While considerable evidence suggests that dopamine may act to inhibit GnRH release, recent data from our laboratory suggest that dopamine may serve as a second stimulator of GnRH.[4] The hypothalamus, especially the supraoptic and arcuate nuclei, has androgen and estrogen receptors and responds to differences in circulating concentrations of sex steroid hormones by changing its rate of synthesis and/or release of GnRH. Sex steroids and neurotransmitters may modulate the frequency and amplitude of GnRH pulses.[5,6] Androgens and estrogens regulate gonadotropin secretion differently. Administration of estradiol at physiologic concentrations results in decreases in circulating LH concentrations. The decrease in LH concentrations is associated with a decrease in LH pulse amplitude, while LH pulse frequency remains unaltered.[6] The feedback effects of testosterone are complex since it acts both as an androgen and a precursor for estradiol. "Pure androgens" (i.e., nonaro-

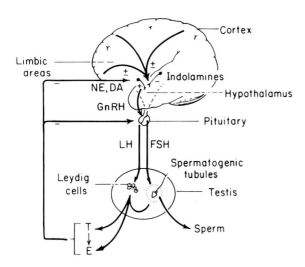

Figure 17–1. A schematic diagram of the hypothalamic-pituitary-gonadal axis in the male. Testicular function is regulated by a series of closed loop feedback systems involving the higher centers in the central nervous system, the hypothalamus, the pituitary and testicular endocrine and germinal compartments. Products of Leydig cells (steroids) as well as the tubules (inhibin) in turn regulate gonadotropin secretion. (*Adapted with permission from Swerdloff and Bhasin*[1]).

matizable androgens such as dihydrotestosterone) decrease the frequency of LH secretory pulses.[5]

Aromatization of testosterone to estradiol appears to be important in regulating gonadotropin secretion. In men pretreated with an antiestrogen such as clomiphene or with selective inhibitors of aromatization, testosterone fails to suppress LH and FSH.[5,6] It remains unclear whether this feedback control of gonadotropin secretion occurs at the hypothalamic or the pituitary level or both.

In a large number of mammalian species, the hypothalamus, the anterior pituitary, hippocampus, and amygdala can convert testosterone to dihydrotestosterone, a 5α-reduced androgen.[2,5] Reduction of the keto group at C-3 of dihydrotestosterone also occurs, to yield 5α, androstane, 3β, 17β-diol. These conversions occur under the influence of an enzymatic complex that includes a 5α reductase and two hydroxysteroid dehydrogenases (3α- and 3β-). These 5α-reduced metabolites may act as intracellular mediators for the inhibitory control of LH secretion by testosterone.[7]

Physiologic Significance of Pulsatile Release of GnRH

The importance of pulsatile secretion of GnRH was highlighted by studies done by Knobil *et al.* in a primate model.[8,9] These authors reported that in rhesus monkeys with hypothalamic lesions that abolish gonadotropin release by the pituitary gland, constant infusion of exogenous GnRH failed to restore sustained gonadotropin secretion. In marked contrast, intermittent administration of the synthetic peptide once an hour, the physiologic frequency of gonadotropin release in the monkey, rees-

tablished pituitary gonadotropin secretion. Initiation of continuous GnRH administration in animals with lesions in which gonadotropin secretion had been reestablished by pulsatile GnRH administration resulted in progressive decline in circulating gonadotropins.[8,9] These pioneering observations pointed out the importance of pattern of GnRH signal in regulating pituitary LH and FSH secretion. Continuous infusion of GnRH has been shown to result in pituitary refractoriness in rats, sheep, monkeys, and humans.

It has now become clear that LH and FSH are secreted by the pituitary gland in response to episodic stimulation by GnRH, which originates as a pulsatile signal from the hypothalamus. This signal is then amplified and modulated at the pituitary level, at least in part by the sex steroids. LH and FSH are released at a frequency of 90 to 120 minutes in the human male.[10]

FSH pulses are harder to detect because of the longer half-life of FSH. Using a regimen of more frequent blood sampling, Filicori *et al.* have reported FSH pulses throughout the menstrual cycle.[11] The LH and FSH pulsations did not always coincide but approximately 70% of LH pulses were accompanied within 20 minutes by a concomitant FSH increment.

It is becoming apparent that the pattern of hypothalamic GnRH signal may determine the relative secretion of LH and FSH. An increased GnRH pulse frequency could alter the ratio of circulating LH to FSH. The importance of abnormal patterns of GnRH secretion as a cause of gonadotropin hypo-secretion is currently being investigated.[12]

Hormonal Regulation of Testicular Function

Leydig Cell Function

Leydig cells occur as groups of polygonal cells scattered in the intertubular (interstitial) tissues and constitute about 1%–10% of total testicular volume. Leydig cells are freely exposed to the extracellular fluids and are principally under the control of pituitary LH. Knowledge of the regulation of Leydig cell function at the subcellular level has been greatly advanced by the development of highly sensitive and specific methods for characterizing LH receptor binding at the Leydig cell surface and the postreceptor intracellular events that follow.[13] LH binding to its highly specific membrane receptor causes conformational changes in the receptor and the adjacent membrane and, ultimately, these changes induce activation of a cascade of postreceptor events, including increases in intracellular cyclic AMP and GMP levels, increased phosphorylation of intracellular proteins, accelerated membrane phospholipid turnover, and rapid calcium channel flux. The net result of these changes is the activation of the rate-limiting steps of testicular steroidogenesis. The highly specific interaction of LH with its membrane receptor protein also induces changes in the normal turnover of cell surface LH receptors and at other undefined intracellular postreceptor sites that act to limit Leydig cell responses to prolonged or excessive exposure to LH.

These coordinated changes include decreases in the number of remaining LH receptors (down-regulation) and sensitivity of the Leydig cell (desensitization) to further stimulation.

LH receptor stimulation ultimately leads to increased secretion of testosterone, the principal steroidal product of the testis and major androgen in the body.[14] Testosterone is secreted into the bloodstream, where it circulates bound to plasma proteins, principally sex-hormone binding globulin (SHBG), and into the seminiferous tubules where it is bound to androgen-binding protein (ABP), a Sertoli cell product. The roles of the gonadal and circulating steroid binding proteins are not fully understood but these binding proteins may modulate androgen actions. The physiologically active androgen moiety has been identified as the nonprotein bound "free" testosterone. The SHBG-bound testosterone may function as a reservoir that buffers the "free" fraction with other steroid-binding proteins with less avid binding, such as albumin and α-1 acid glycoprotein, serving intermediate roles. Androgen effects are exerted on the appropriate target organs which are distinguished by the presence of the specific, high-affinity, androgen-receptor protein in the cell nucleus. Biologically active androgens can bind reversibly to the androgen receptor with relative affinities that reflect their biopotency as androgens in vivo. Such binding events are followed by transformation of the androgen-receptor complex into an activated state, and binding to nucleoproteins.

The interaction of the activated nuclear androgen receptor initiates a cascade of DNA transcription, RNA translation, and protein synthesis, leading to expression of the characteristic spectrum of effects of androgens on general anabolism and induction of specific androgenic effects in the appropriate target tissues.

Although testosterone is the major testicular androgen product, it is converted to an even more potent androgen, dihydrotestosterone (DHT), by the action of the enzyme 5α reductase found specifically in many androgen-responsive target tissues. Since the metabolite DHT is several times more potent than testosterone as an androgenic ligand at the androgen receptor, it has been suggested that testosterone is a circulating prohormone for the active androgen, DHT. Tissues embryologically derived from the urogenital sinus (and from which ultimately the external and internal genitalia are formed) are particularly dependent on the actions of DHT as an androgen. Apart from the urogenital tissues which appear more responsive to DHT, the more general anabolic actions of androgens on bone, marrow, muscle, skin, and brain may be subserved by either DHT or T.

Role of the Testis in Control of LH and FSH Secretion

It is generally accepted that testicular products are important factors in the determination of LH and FSH levels. As indicated above, sex steroids (testosterone and estrogens) have inhibitory effects on the secretion of these gonadotropic hormones. The primary modulators of both LH and FSH secretion appear to be the sex steroids. In addition, the spermatogenic compartment influences the secretion of FSH through the production and release of inhibin (see above). Knowledge of the normal testicular regulation of LH and FSH secretion is important in diagnosing the site of abnormality in patients with hypogonadism and infertility. Patients with low testosterone due to primary damage of the testes will have elevated blood concentrations of LH and FSH. Patients with isolated damage to the germinal compartment often have elevation of blood FSH levels, while LH concentrations are normal. Testicular insufficiency (sex steroid and germ cell damage) associated with low gonadotropin levels indicates a primary abnormality at the hypothalamic and/or pituitary level.

CLINICAL MANIFESTATIONS OF HYPOGONADISM AND INFERTILITY

The clinical manifestations of androgen deficiency depend on the age of onset, degree of deficiency, and the anatomical site of the abnormality.[15] Most patients with androgen deficiency will have associated infertility. By contrast, many patients with infertility due to primary damage at the germ cell level will have normal Leydig cell function. Since most patients with hypothalamic or pituitary cause of infertility have impaired secretion of both LH and FSH, they usually have pangonadal insufficiency (androgen deficiency and infertility).

Hypogonadism or impaired testicular function may be reflected clinically as decreased androgenization, infertility, or a combination of the two. The clinical features of decreased testosterone secretion depend on the degree of deficiency and the age of onset of the disorder. Deficiencies occurring during early fetal development result in pseudohermaphroditism; those first becoming manifest during late gestation may result in micropenis.

The clinical onset of testosterone deficiency prior to puberty will result in eunuchoid features and female hair distribution. Eunuchoid features include an arm span two inches greater than height and an upper-lower body ratio of less than one. (These proportions may be normal for black men of east African derivation.) Patients with hypogonadism acquired after puberty have normal body proportions and male temporal hair recession, but show other clinical signs of hypogonadism.

The distribution of facial beard in normal males depends on the individual's racial background. Deviations from the racially determined norm indicate the presence of hypogonadism. Normal hair distribution varies from that on the cheek, mustache, chin, and neck requiring shaving at least once a day to that on the upper lip and chin requiring shaving every two to three days. The former is normal for most Caucasian sub-races while the latter may be normal for men of Black, Oriental, or American Indian extraction. Detailed questioning of other male family members is helpful in assessing the clinical status of a suspected hypogonadal patient. Hypogonadism is also associated with increased fine wrinkling of the skin about the mouth and eyes.

Body hair distribution also varies with racial background. Many normal Black, Oriental, and Indian men have body hair limited to the axillary, pubic, and sternal areas while many Caucasian men have additional pectoral, back, and flank hair. The male pubic hair distribution is diamond-shaped with hair extending up toward the umbilicus. When the pubic hair has an inverted triangle appearance, it is described as a female escutcheon. Severe longstanding hypogonadism results in absence of chest hair and sparseness of pubic hair. Less severe defects produce more subtle changes which should be evaluated with the patient's racial and family hair patterns as a guide.

Ninety percent of the normal volume of the testis consists of spermatogenic tubules. The testes should be measured in all patients; testes greater than 4.0 cm in length or greater than 15 ml in volume (measured with a Prader orchidometer) are normal in size. Hypogonadism beginning after puberty results in testicular size varying from small, soft organs to those that are near normal. Severe tubular injury not associated with decreased androgenization may result in small testes and normal Leydig cell function.

Causes of Hypothalamic Hypogonadism

These disorders can be generally divided into acquired and congenital causes (Table 17–1).

Congenital Disorders

Kallman's Syndrome. This syndrome was first described in the human male by Kallman, Schoenfeld, and Barrera and is characterized by hypogonadotropic hypogonadism due to a congenital defect in hypothalamic GnRH secretion.[16] It may occur in both sexes, but is more common in men. A positive family history is present in about 50% of the cases; relatives may have hypogonadism or may only manifest one of the associated defects.[17] More severe forms may show sexual infantilism while those with partial defect may have delayed sexual maturation. A number of midline defects may occur. More common associations include anosmia, color blindness, and eighth nerve deafness. Men with this syndrome have azoospermia, and women, primary amenorrhea.[18]

In a child of prepubertal age, it is often difficult to distinguish hypogonadotropism from constitutional delay of puberty. Serum gonadotropins in both conditions are low and show a prepubertal response to GnRH.[19] Progressive testicular growth and onset of virilizing signs provide the only reliable method for determining that puberty is progressing normally. The presence of nocturnal LH release in early pubertal boys may help to establish that puberty has been initiated. Release of prolactin following administration of chlorpromazine has been reported to be useful in differentiating normal from hypogonadotropic males, since recent studies have shown that the release of prolactin in normal pubertal boys is brisk (greater than 15 ng/ml), while among hypogonadotropic

Table 17–1. Causes of Hypothalamic Hypogonadotropic Hypogonadism (GnRH Deficiency)

Congenital
  Isolated GnRH deficiency
  Kallman's syndrome (anosmia)
  Fertile eunuch syndrome
  Prader-Willi syndrome
  Laurence-Moon-Biedl syndrome
Acquired
  Functional
    Anorexia nervosa
    Malnutrition
    Drug-related
      Marijuana
      Steroids (androgens, estrogens, progestogens)
    Systemic disease (uremia, liver failure)
    Functional hyperprolactinemia (drug-induced, idiopathic)
  Organic
    Trauma
    Infiltrative disease (sarcoid, tuberculosis, fungal, histiocytosis X)
    Neoplasms (craniopharyngioma, hypothalamic tumors, extension from pituitary and meningeal neoplasms, metastatic tumors)

individuals it is virtually nonexistent. In isolated hypogonadotropism levels of adrenal steroids (DHAS) are usually normal relative to chronologic age, while in constitutional delay both are delayed.

A careful analysis of the growth chart can be useful. Patients with constitutional delay in puberty have a history of slow growth velocity while in those with Kallman's syndrome growth velocity is normal or slightly slower during the prepubertal growth spurt even though they may eventually be taller with eunuchoidal proportions.

In the final analysis, none of these tests alone provides a definitive diagnosis. Only progression of virilization and testicular size (greater than 2.5 cm in longitudinal diameter) provide assurance that puberty is advancing normally.

Fertile Eunuch Syndrome. This term has been used to describe patients with eunuchoidism and delayed sexual development who have large testes. Such individuals appear to have sufficient gonadotropin to stimulate high intratesticular testosterone levels and to initiate spermatogenesis, but not enough testosterone secretion into the blood to adequately virilize the peripheral tissues; they are in fact partially gonadotropin-deficient.[20]

Prader-Willi Syndrome. A syndrome consisting of obesity, hypotonic musculature, mental retardation, hypogonadism, short stature, and small hands and feet was originally described in 1956 by Prader, Labhart, and Willi.[21] An updated review of this syndrome has been presented recently.[22] Hypogonadism and cryptorchidism are characteristic features, and micropenis is common. Histologic examination shows that the testes are immature without germ cells, but with Sertoli cells and diminutive tubules.[23] The LH response to a single bolus of GnRH is subnormal in comparison to obese controls.[24] Clomiphene has been shown to "turn on" the pituitary gonadal axis of individuals of either sex with the Prader-Willi syndrome to secrete gonadotropins and gonadal steroids.[25]

Laurence-Moon-Biedl Syndrome. This condition is characterized by obesity, hypogonadism, mental retardation, polydactyly, and retinitis pigmentosa.[26,27] Renal abnormalities are common and include glomerular sclerosis, mesangial proliferation, and cyst formation.[28] The syndrome is inherited as an autosomal recessive disorder.

Basal Encephalocele. A rare cause of hypothalamic failure is a basal encephalocele with midfacial anomalies including a broad nasal root, hypertelorism, and cleft-lip.[29] In these patients, the pituitary may herniate through the floor of the sella turcica, and the secretion of growth hormone, FSH, LH, and prolactin, is altered.

Acquired Disorders

Functional Disorders of Hypothalamic GnRH Secretion

Anorexia Nervosa. This is a disorder predominantly of adolescent girls characterized by excessive weight loss, a result of voluntary dietary restriction. The topic has been extensively reviewed elsewhere.[30,31] Occurring almost exclusively in young, white, middle-to-upper class women under the age of 25,[32] the syndrome includes a distorted body image accompanied by self-imposed restriction on food intake.[33] This disorder may occasionally appear in young men and include infertility in its manifestations. The term anorexia nervosa is a misnomer since there is no loss of appetite; on the contrary, these patients are preoccupied with food. Some of the patients with this disorder may manifest bizarre eating-related habits such as hiding of food, mastication and spitting, self-induced vomiting, and hyperactivity (running, jogging, gymnastics).[34,35]

Malnutrition. Females seem to be more susceptible to loss of normal reproductive capacity at times of severe dietary restriction than males. While considerable data are available on the pathophysiology of undernutrition in male laboratory animals,[36,37] less is known about the condition in men. Smith *et al.*[38] described reproductive function in severely malnourished Pakistani men and noted that they seemed to have a mixed pattern of androgen deficiency. Some patients had the anticipated pattern of hypogonadotropic hypogonadism (low testosterone, low LH), while others had depressed testosterone and elevated gonadotropins. Spermatogenic function appeared to be relatively well preserved.

Athletes, Joggers, and Marathon Runners. Unlike their female counterparts,[39-41] competitive male athletes who are not drug abusers seem to have minimal changes in sex steroid and reproductive function. Male athletes receiving anabolic androgens may have severe suppression of gonadotropin secretion and marked inhibition of spermatogenesis with infertility.

Drug-induced Hypothalamic Dysfunction.

1. Marijuana: Marijuana decreases gonadotropin secretion when administered to ovariectomized monkeys.[42] It blocks reflex ovulation in the rabbit and prevents ovulation in the rhesus monkey. Delayed puberty, primary amenorrhea, and secondary amenorrhea may be seen in preadolescent, adolescent, and young adult marijuana users. Normal menstrual cycles resume within 3 to 6 months after discontinuation of marijuana use.

Men who are heavy users of marijuana have decreased sex hormone secretion and sperm production. Gynecomastia in some of the marijuana users is believed to be due to the plant estrogens in the crude preparations. The mechanism of marijuana-induced hypogonadism appears to be due to decreased GnRH secretion.[43]

2. Androgens, Progestogens, Anabolic Steroids, and Estrogens: These steroids all suppress LH and FSH secretion by inhibition at the hypothalamic and pituitary levels.[44,45]

Organic Causes of GnRH Deficiency

Neoplastic. The most common neoplasm is craniopharyngioma. The tumor usually has its onset before age 15 and may produce GnRH deficiency, anterior pituitary failure, and diabetes insipidus. Suprasellar calcification is characteristic. Hypothalamic hamartomas represent a much less frequent cause of similar changes.

Non-neoplastic. Hypothalamic involvement may be seen in sarcoidosis and Hand-Schuller-Christian disease. Some of these patients may show bizarre behavioral problems, fever of unknown origin, bradycardia, sleep disturbances, episodes of uncontrolled laughter or rage, and eating disorders.

Causes of Pituitary Hypogonadotropic Hypogonadism

These disorders have congenital and acquired causes (Table 17-2) with the latter accounting for many of the abnormalities.

Congenital Pituitary Deficiency of LH and/or FSH Secretion

Primary disorders of synthesis and secretion of LH/FSH do occur, but they are considerably less common than GnRH deficiency.

Acquired Pituitary Diseases

Pituitary Tumors. Patients may evidence androgen deficiency, impaired potency, and infertility.

Prolactinomas are much less common in men than women and usually present as macroademonas, manifesting both hormone symptoms and features of a space-occupying mass (headaches, visual field defects, and hypothalamic syndrome).

The manifestations of gonadotropin insufficiency are usually the result of hyperprolactinemia rather than anatomical damage to the gonadotropic cells. Hyperprolac-

Table 17–2. Causes of Pituitary Hypogonadotropic Hypogonadism

Congenital
  Isolated LH and/or FSH deficiency
  Pituitary aplasia
Acquired
  Pituitary Tumor
    Prolactin-secreting (macro- or microadenoma)
    Other hormone or nonsecreting tumor
  Infiltrative Pituitary Disease
    Hemochromatosis
    Congenital
    Acquired transfusional iron overload
      Thalassemia
      Other blood disease
    Granulomatous disease (sarcoid, tuberculosis, syphilis)
  Autoimmune hypophysitis

tinemia inhibits gonadotropic secretion by inhibiting GnRH release and pituitary responsiveness to GnRH. An inhibitory action of prolactin directly on the testes may represent a third pathogenetic mechanism of hypogonadism in this disorder.

Prolactin measurements are of great importance in the diagnosis of prolactin-secreting adenomas of the pituitary.[46] Prolactin levels over 200 ng/ml are virtually diagnostic of macroadenoma whereas levels of 50–200 ng/ml are consistent with either structural (macroadenoma, microadenoma) or functional (drug ingestion, renal or hepatic failure) disorders of prolactin regulation.

Suppression of prolactin levels with bromergocryptine therapy is associated with marked reduction in pituitary tumor size and improvement in potency, although testicular function does not improve readily. Prolactin levels in the range between the upper limit of the normal range (10–15 ng/ml) but under 50 ng/ml are most commonly due to the stress associated with venipuncture or cannulation and typically do not remain elevated during serial sampling or on repeated sampling on another occasion. Minor elevations of prolactin levels (15–50 ng/ml) are common in men with primary testicular dysfunction, possibly because of estrogen-induced hyperprolactinemia, since estradiol levels may be elevated in some men with hypergonadotropic hypogonadism. Suppression of minor elevations of prolactin levels (15–50 ng/ml) by administration of bromergocryptine is ineffective in improving depressed spermatogenesis so that the diagnostic importance of prolactin levels is restricted to marked elevations (>50 ng/ml).

Nonprolactin secreting adenomas, local invasion from meningiomas, craniopharyngiomas, and metastatic cancers may present with gonadotropin insufficiency or as panhypopituitarism.

Infiltrative and Infectious Causes of Hypopituitarism. Hemochromatosis (congenital and acquired); syphilitic, tuberculous, and fungal granulomas; and abscesses of the pituitary may be occasional causes of hypogonadism.

Autoimmune Hypophysitis. The syndrome of multiple endocrine end-organ failure is the result of production of antibodies directed at various endocrine tissues. Hypothyroidism, adrenal insufficiency, and diabetes occur more commonly than either primary or secondary gonadal insufficiency.[47,48]

Evaluation and Treatment of Patients with Hypothalamic and Pituitary Hypogonadism

Conventional Management

Men with hypothalamic hypogonadism are characterized by low serum testosterone and inappropriately low serum concentrations of LH and FSH. The distinction between hypothalamic and pituitary causes of hypogonadotropic hypogonadism is often difficult, but may be suggested if hypogonadotropism is accompanied by anosmia or diabetes insipidus (hypothalamic) or bitemporal upper quadrant visual defects (pituitary). Further resolution will usually require radiographs of the pituitary fossa and CT scans, which may be combined with angiography or pneumoencephalography to determine the extent of the lesions.

Hyperprolactinemia of any cause may produce hypogonadotropic hypogonadism, primarily by suppressing LH secretion, and must be excluded by serum prolactin determination. Laboratory confirmation sometimes requires stimulation tests, since the distinction between subnormal and low normal levels of LH and FSH may be difficult. An absent or subnormal response of FSH and LH (less than a doubling) to clomiphene citrate (100 mg/day for 7–10 days) confirms impaired gonadotropic secretory reserve. Since both hypothalamic and pituitary disease may result in a blunted or absent response of LH and FSH to an acute bolus of gonadotropin-releasing hormone (GnRH), this test is not of use in distinguishing these two pathologic anatomical sites. However, continued pulsatile administration of GnRH will restore LH secretion in patients with hypothalamic GnRH deficiency and could be of value, not only in separating such patients from those with pituitary disease, but also in providing a therapeutic modality.

Difficulty also exists in separating delayed sexual maturation from incomplete hypogonadotropic hypogonadism because basal LH and FSH levels may be similarly low in both circumstances.[44] Since normal children prior to the second and third stages of puberty do not produce increases in serum gonadotropins in response to administered clomiphene, this test is of little value in separating the two disorders.[49] GnRH testing may be of somewhat greater potential value, but is limited by the smaller LH response in normal prepubertal children that can overlap with the response of patients with incomplete hypogonadotropic hypergonadism. Better resolution now seems possible by testing such patients with either clomiphene[50] or metaclopramide and assessing the prolactin response. Patients with delayed sexual maturation respond with an increase in serum prolactin (15 ng/ml) while those with hypogonadotropic hypogonadism do not. Newborns with hypogonadotropic hypogonadism may be detected by measuring testicular volume sequentially during the first 3 months of life. Normal children will apparently double their testicular volume during this period.[51]

Once hyperprolactinemia, primary pituitary disease, and neoplastic, infiltrative, and infectious etiologies of hypothalamic dysfunction have been separated from congenital GnRH deficiency, the choice of therapy depends on whether fertility is desired or not. If the patient does not immediately desire restoration of fertility, replacement therapy with testosterone may be adequate. However, restoration of fertility requires therapy with gonadotropins or pulsatile administration of GnRH as outlined below.

Androgen Therapy

If spermatogenesis is not considered an important endpoint, therapy with androgens can be initiated to stimulate development of secondary sex characteristics, libido, and potency, and promote appropriate somatic development. Although androgen therapy in man does not restore spermatogenic function, even long-term androgen treatment does not impair subsequent response to gonadotropins.

A more detailed review of androgen therapy has been recently published.[52] The main points are summarized below:

Treatment commences with intramuscular injection of long-acting ester (e.g. enanthate or cypionate) of testosterone in doses of 150–200 mg, given every 10 days for 4–6 weeks. Once the patient has experienced the effects of the androgens, the interval between injections is increased until the patient experiences symptoms of androgen withdrawal (tiredness, loss of libido, mood swings, and hot flushes). The next injection is then given and the interval between injections is shortened to prevent recurrence of symptoms.

The optimum time interval for injections varies considerably, but 14–17 days is usual except in patients with Klinefelter's syndrome who tend to require more frequent injection (10–14 days). Occasionally, patients respond to these doses by an increased red cell mass and may become symptomatically polycythemic. Hence, it is important to measure the hematocrit at intervals of 3–6 months. Other side effects are rare, although fluid retention may sometimes occur.

The criteria for successful therapy are: 1. development of normal secondary sex characteristics, 2. increased frequency of shaving, 3. restoration of libido and potency, 4. increased muscle mass, and 5. decreased tiredness.

Synthetic oral androgens, such as methyl testosterone, fluoxymesterone and oxymethalone, are available but not recommended since they produce only partial androgenization and have been associated with several hepatic disorders including cholestatic jaundice, liver cell carcinoma, and a rare vascular disorder, peliosis hepatis.

Treatment with Gonadotropins

When fertility is desired, testosterone is withdrawn and injections of human chorionic gonadotropin (hCG) 3000 I.U. can be given weekly for a period of approximately 6 months. If sperm production has not commenced, or is less than 7–10 million/ml, FSH as hMG in a dose of 75 I.U. three times a week is added to the hCG regimen. Combined therapy is often needed for 12–15 months.[53–55]

Pulsatile Administration of GnRH

This form of therapy has been utilized in several research centers as a therapeutic approach for patients with GnRH deficiency.[12,56] This therapy is not useful in patients with primary dysfunction of the gonadotropic cells.

Studies of Knobil et al. clearly demonstrated that continuous administration of GnRH was ineffective in evoking the desired pattern of gonadotropin discharge, and that the synthetic decapeptide could stimulate appropriate gonadotropin secretion only when the hormone was administered in an episodic mode and at a physiologic frequency.[57,58] These physiologic principles have been exploited in treatment of a number of clinical conditions characterized by hypothalamic hypogonadism.

Hoffman et al. used long term low dose subcutaneous GnRH in two-hour pulses to six men with delayed puberty due to idiopathic hypogonadotropism.[59] The dose used was 25 ng/kg/pulse and was administered by a portable infusion device (Autosyringe). All six subjects noted spontaneous erections, nocturnal emissions, and breast tenderness which were associated with elevations of serum testosterone levels (77 ± 13 ng/dl before therapy vs. 520 ± 182 ng after one month of treatment). Serum LH and FSH concentrations rose to normal adult levels within one week of therapy and to supraphysiologic levels by 14 days. Testis size increased in four patients and spermatogenesis was achieved in three patients by 43 weeks of therapy. These results suggest that long-term pulsatile administration of GnRH can reverse hypogonadotropic hypogonadism.

Others have been less successful in reinstituting spermatogenesis with the pulsatile GnRH approach.[60] While the approach has provided exciting new data on pituitary responses to different regimens of GnRH, there seems to be little advantage of this modality over simple treatment with hCG and hMG.

References

1. Swerdloff RS, Bhasin S: Male reproductive physiology. In EJ Aiman (ed) Infertility—Diagnosis and Management. Springer-Verlag, pp 177–184, 1984.
2. Raum WJ, Swerdloff RS: Neuroendocrine control of reproduction. In G Adelman (ed) Encyclopedia of Neuroscience. Boston, WB Saunders, 1986.
3. Barraclough CA, Wise PM: The role of catecholamines in the regulation of pituitary LH and FSH secretion. Endocrin Rev 3:91–120, 1982.
4. Jarjour LT, Handelsman DJ, Raum WJ, et al.: Mechanism of action of dopamine on the in vitro release of gonadotropin-releasing hormone. Endocrinology (to be published).
5. Santen RJ: Is aromatization of androgens to estradiol required for inhibition of LH secretion in men? J Clin Invest 56:1555–1563, 1975.
6. Winters RJ, Jannick JJ, Loriaux DL, et al.: Studies on the role

of sex steroids in the feedback control of gonadotropin concentrations in men. II: Use of the estrogen antagonist clomiphene citrate. J Clin Endocrinol Metab 48:222–227, 1979.

7. Martin L: The 5 α-reduction of testosterone in the neuroendocrine structures. Biochemical and physiological implications. Endocrinol Rev 3:1–25, 1982.

8. Wildt L, Hausler A, Marshall G, et al: Frequency and amplitude of GnRH stimulation and gonadotropin secretion in the rhesus monkey. Endocrinol 109:376–385, 1981.

9. Belchetz PE, Plant TM, Nakai Y, et al.: Hypophysial responses to continuous and intermittent delivery of hypothalamic gonadotropin-releasing hormone. Science 202:631–633, 1978.

10. Santen RJ, Bardin CW: Episodic LH secretion in man. J Clin Invest 52:2617–2628, 1973.

11. Filicori M, Hoffman AR, Mansfield MJ, et al.: Discernible FSH pulsations in the human menstrual cycle: their concordance with LH pulsations and the critical nature of sampling frequency in their demonstration. Clin Res 30:270A, 1982(a).

12. Crowley Jr, WF, Filicori M, Spratt DI, et al.: The physiology of gonadotropin-releasing hormone (GnRH) secretion in men and women. Recent Prog Horm Res 41, 473–531, 1985.

13. Catt KJ, Harwood JP, Clayton RC, et al: Regulation of peptide hormone receptors and gonadal steroidogenesis. Recent Prog Horm Res 36:557–622, 1980.

14. Handelsman DJ, Swerdloff RS: Male gonadal dysfunction. Clin Endocrinol Metab 14:89–124, 1985.

15. Swerdloff RS, Glass AR: Male reproductive abnormalities. In J Hershman (ed) Endocrine Pathophysiology. Philadelphia, Lea and Febiger, 1982.

16. Kallman FJ, Schoenfeld WA, Barrera SE: The genetic aspects of primary eunuchoidism. Am J Ment Defic 68:203–236, 1944.

17. Santen JR, Paulsen CA: Hypogonadotropic eunuchoidism. I. Clinical study of the mode of inferitance. J Clin Endocrinol Metab 36:47–54, 1973.

18. Bardin CW, Ross GT, Rifkind AB, et al.: Studies of the pituitary-Leydig cell axis in young men with hypogonadotropic hypogonadism and hyposmia: comparison with normal men, prepuberal boys and hypopituitary patients. J Clin Invest 48:2046–2056, 1969.

19. Bell J, Spitz I, Perlman A, et al.: Heterogeneity of gonadotropin response to LHRH in hypogonadotropic hypogonadism. J Clin Endocrinol Metab 36:791–794, 1973.

20. Boyar RM, Wu RHK, Kapen S, et al.: Clinical and laboratory heterogeneity in idiopathic hypogonadotropic hypodonadism. J Clin Endocrinol Metab 43:1268–1275, 1977.

21. Prader A, Labhart A, Willi H: Ein Syndrom von Adipositas, Kleinwuchs, Kryptorchismus, und Oligophrenie nach myotoniertigen Zustand im Neugeborenenalter. Schweiz Med Wochenschr 86:1260–1261, 1956.

22. Bray GA, Dahms WT, Swerdloff RS, et al.: The Prader-Willi syndrome: a study of 40 patients and a review of the literature. Medicine 62:59–80, 1983.

23. Katcher ML, Bargman GJ, Gilbert EF, et al.: Absence of spermatogonia in the Prader-Willi syndrome. Eur J Pediatr 124:257–260, 1977.

24. Zarate A, Soria J, Canales ES, et al.: Pituitary response to synthetic luteinizing hormone-releasing hormone in Prader-Willi syndrome, prepubertal and pubertal children. Neuroendocrinology 13:321–326, 1973/1974.

25. Hamilton CR, Scully RE, Kliman B: Hypogonadotropinism in Prader-Willi syndrome. Induction of puberty and spermatogenesis by clomiphene citrate. Am J Med 52:322–329, 1972.

26. McLoughlin TG, Shanklin DR: Pathology of Laurence-Moon-Bardet-Biedl syndrome. J Pathol Bacteriol 93:65–79, 1967.

27. Nadjmi B, Flanagan MJ, Christian JR: Laurence-Moon-Biedl syndrome: associated with multiple genitourinary tract anomalies. Am J Dis Child 117:352–356, 1969.

28. Hurley RM: The renal lesion of the Laurence-Moon-Biedl Syndrome. J Pediatr 87:206–209, 1975.

29. Ellyin F, Khatir AH, Singh SP: Hypothalamic-pituitary functions in patients with transsphenoidal encephalocele and mid-facial anomalies. J Clin Endocrinol Metab 51:854–856, 1980.

30. Drossman DA: Anorexia nervosa: a comprehensive approach. Adv Intern Med 339–361, 1983.

31. Boyar, RM: Endocrine changes in anorexia nervosa. Med Clin North Am 62:297–303, 1978.

32. Crisp AH, Palmer RL, Kalney RS: How common is anorexia nervosa? a prevalence study. Br J Psych 128:549–554, 1976.

33. Slade PD, Russell GFM: Awareness of body dimensions in anorexia nervosa: cross-sectional and longitudinal studies. Psychol Med 3:188–199, 1973.

34. Garfinkel PE, Moldowsky H, Garner DM: The heterogeneity of anorexia nervosa. Bulimia as a distinct subgroup. Arch Gen Psychiatry 37:1036–1040, 1980.

35. Stonehill E, Crisp AH: Psychoneurotic characteristics of patients with anorexia nervosa before and after treatment and at follow-up 4–7 years later. J Psychosom Res 21:187–193, 1977.

36. Glass AR, Mitt R, Burman KD, et al.: Serum triiodothyronine in undernourished rats: dependence on dietary composition rather than total calorie or protein intake. Endocrinology 102:1925–1928, 1978.

37. Glass AR, Swerdloff RS: Nutritional influences on sexual maturation in the rat. Fed Proc 39:2360–2364, 1980.

38. Smith SR, Chhetri MK, Johanson AJ, et al.: The pituitary-gonadal axis in men with protein-calorie malnutrition. J Clin Endocrinol Metab 41:60–80, 1975.

39. Frisch RE, Wyshak G, Vincent L: Delayed menarche and amenorrhea in ballet dancers. N Engl J Med 303:17–19, 1980.

40. Dale E, Gerlach DH, Wilhite AL: Menstrual dysfunction in distance runners. Obstet Gynecol 54:47–52, 1979.

41. Feicht CB, Johnson TS, Martin BJ, et al.: Secondary amenorrhea in athletes. Lancet 2:1145–1156, 1978.

42. Asch RH, Smith CG, Siler-Khodr TM, et al.: Effects of Δ⁹-tetrahydrocannabinol during the follicular phase of the rhesus monkey (Macaca mulatta). J Clin Endocrinol Metab 52:50–55, 1981.

43. Charavarty I, Sheth PR, Sheth AR, et al.: Delta-9-tetrahydrocannabinol: Its effects on hypothalamo-pituitary system in male rats. Arch Androl 8:25–27, 1982.

44. Swerdloff RS: Physiology of Male Reproduction: hypothalamic-pituitary function. In PC Walsh, RF Gittes, AD Perlmutter, et al. (eds) Campbell's Urology (5th ed). Philadelphia, WB Saunders, 1986.

45. Swerdloff RS, Sokol RZ: Manifestations of androgen deficiency and effects of androgen therapy. In Serono Symposia, International Symposium on Reproductive Medicine. New York, Raven Press (to be published).

46. Perryman RL, Thorner MO: Effects of hyperprolactinemia on sexual and reproductivce function in men. J Andrology 2:233–242, 1981.

47. Scheithauer BW: Pathology of the pituitary and sellar region: exclusive of pituitary adenoma. Pathol. Ann. 20, Part I: 67–155, 1985.

48. Boyar RM, Finkelstein JW, Witkin M, *et al.*: Studies of endocrine function in "isolated" gonadotropin deficiency. J Clin Endocrinol Metab 36:64–72, 1973.

49. Marshall JC: Investigative procedures. Clin Endocrinol Metabol 4:545–567, 1975.

50. Winters SJ, Johnsonbaugh RE, Sherins RJ: The response of prolactin to chlorpromazine stimulation in men with hypogonadotropic hypogonadism and in early pubertal boys: relationship to sex steroid exposure. Clin Endocrinol 16:321–330, 1982.

51. Cassorla RG, Golden SM, Johnsonbaugh RE, *et al:* Testicular volume during early infancy. J Pediatr 99:742–745, 1981.

52. Sokol RZ, Swerdloff RS: Practical considerations in the use of androgen therapy. In: RJ Santen, RS Swerdloff (eds) Male Sexual Dysfunction. New York, Marcel Dekker, 211–225, 1986.

53. Johnsen SG: Maintenance of spermatogenesis induced by HMG treatment by means of continuous HCG treatment in hypogonadotropic men. Acta Endocrinol 89:763–769, 1978.

54. Schill WB: Recent progress in pharmacologic therapy in male subfertility; a review. Andrologia 11:77–107, 1979.

55. Sherins RJ: Evaluation and management of men with hypogonadotropic hypogonadism. *In* CR Garcia, L Mastroianni, RD Amelar (eds) Current Therapy of Infertility. New Jersey, BC Decker, p 10–14, 1982.

56. Handelsman DJ, Swerdloff RS: Pharmacokinetics of gonadotropin-releasing hormone and its analogs. Endocrine Rev 7:95–105, 1986.

57. Knobil E: Patterns of hypophysiotropic signals and gonadotropin secretion in the rhesus monkey. Biol Reprod 24:44–49, 1981.

58. Hausler A, Wildt L, Marshall G, *et al.:* Modulation of pituitary gonadotropin secretion by frequency of GnRH input. Fed Proc 38:1107–1112, 1979.

59. Hoffman AR and Crowley WF: Induction of puberty in men by long-term pulsatile administration of low-dose GnRH. N Engl J Med 307:1237–1241, 1982.

60. Handelsman DJ: GnRH treatment of hypogonadotropic hypogonadal men (personal communication).

18. Varicocele and Obstructive Disorders of the Male Genital Tract

Peter T. Nieh

The most common, and fortunately most treatable, cause of male infertility is the varicocele. Between 8% and 22% of all males will harbor such varicosities of the spermatic veins. Yet only a minority may suffer from infertility.[1,2] Of males being evaluated for infertility, up to 39% will be found to have varicoceles.[3] The presence of the varicosity does not invariably lead to impaired spermatogenesis, but the association, and response to therapy, are impressive enough to concern pediatric urologists with the problem of the asymptomatic varicocele in preadolescent and adolescent males where incidence increases with age.[4,5]

Another group of infertile patients, which is rapidly growing, consists of males with obstructive disorders. While those with congenital abnormalities may be relatively constant, the number of evaluations for acquired obstructive lesions has exploded with the prevalence of sexually transmitted diseases, the wide acceptance of vasectomy for birth control, the high divorce and remarriage rates, and the success of the exquisitely delicate microscopic anastomoses of vas deferens and epididymis.

This chapter will discuss the current status of varicoceles and obstructive disorders of the male genital tract, highlighting the variety of histologic patterns encountered, as well as some aspects of treatment.

VARICOCELE

Anatomic Aspects and Diagnosis

Embryologically, the testes derive their arterial supply from the aorta just below the renal vessels. However, there are different venous drainage pathways for the right and left testes. While the right internal spermatic vein drains into the vena cava below the renal vein, the left enters directly into the left renal vein. The valves within these veins normally prevent retrograde flow. Failure of

these valves, from congenital hypoplasia or high pressures from relative obstruction of the left renal vein by the superior mesenteric artery and aorta (the "nutcracker phenomenon"), results in retrograde flow down toward the left testis. The collateral venous drainage via the external spermatic (cremasteric) vein to the deep epigastric vein and via the deferential vein to the superior vesical vein is usually unaffected. The upright posture and any increase in intra-abdominal pressure permit the column of venous blood to gradually dilate the plexus of tiny veins surrounding the spermatic cord and testicle to produce the typical "bag of worms" palpable, and sometimes visible, superior and lateral to the testicle. While the majority of varicoceles are left-sided (70% to 100%) up to 9% of varicoceles may be on the right side from renal vein insertion and 20% may be bilateral from cross-circulation via suprapubic veins or pampiniform plexus.[6] Patients with small varicoceles are usually asymptomatic. The moderate to large varicocele may result in scrotal discomfort, sometimes a vague "pulling" sensation from the groin into the testicle, sometimes an "itching" pain which is poorly defined. The testicle may be smaller on the affected side. Since the seminiferous tubules account for over 85% of testicular volume, this atrophy represents loss of germinal epithelium.[7]

The diagnosis of the moderate to large varicocele is readily made in the standing position, accentuated by Valsalva maneuver. The small varicocele may require selective venography, Doppler stethoscope, or thermography.

Pathophysiology

The mechanism by which the varicocele produces infertility is still debated. The various theories are summarized below, with hyperthermia and toxic metabolite theories dominating the literature.

Scrotal Thermoregulatory Disturbance

With increased venous pressure, the resultant stagnation leads to elevation of the testicular temperature, which is around 2.8°C below intra-abdominal temperature.[8] An in-

The author is especially grateful for the assistance of Drs. Harold T. Yamase and Thomas Ciesielski in preparing the photomicrographs for this chapter.

crease of 0.6° to 0.8° C is sufficient to produce the changes in semen analysis which characterize the infertile varicocele patient.[8]

While there have been some conflicting data,[9] most work points to hyperthermia as a major factor. Impaired amino acid incorporation and protein synthesis has been reported in rat spermatids incubated at 37°C compared with 34°C.[10] Animal models have supported the concept of varicocele-induced increase in testicular blood flow, intratesticular temperature, and impaired spermatogenesis.[11,12]

Toxic Adrenal/Renal Metabolite Theory

This postulates that it is the reflux of toxic metabolites down the internal spermatic vein that bathes the testes, causing impaired spermatogenesis. Adrenal steroids have not been detected in higher concentration in the spermatic vein of varicocele patients, but elevated catecholamine[13] and serotonin[14] levels over peripheral blood levels have been identified. Chronic exposure to such agents would produce vasoconstriction and testicular injury. In addition, serotonin may inhibit testosterone synthesis to further damage spermatogenesis.[14] Renal metabolites, particularly prostaglandins, have also been studied.[15]

Testicular Hypoxia

With venous pooling, a low pO_2 would result in chronic hypoxia. However, pO_2 is usually higher in the internal spermatic vein of varicocele patients.[16]

Intratesticular Mechanical Obstruction

This obstruction could occur as follows: As intratesticular veins dilate, compression of seminiferous tubules and efferent tubules results in atrophy and sclerosis.[17]

Hormonal Dysfunction

Hormonal dysfunction is an unlikely possibility. Leydig cell dysfunction and gonadotropin impairment have not been documented in varicocele patients.[18]

Whichever theory is correct, chronic exposure eventually results in unilateral testicular atrophy and histologic changes in the contralateral testis.[7]

Semen Analysis

The stress pattern was described by MacLeod in 1965 in over 85% of patients with varicocele.[19] It is characterized by markedly impaired sperm motility, decrease in the

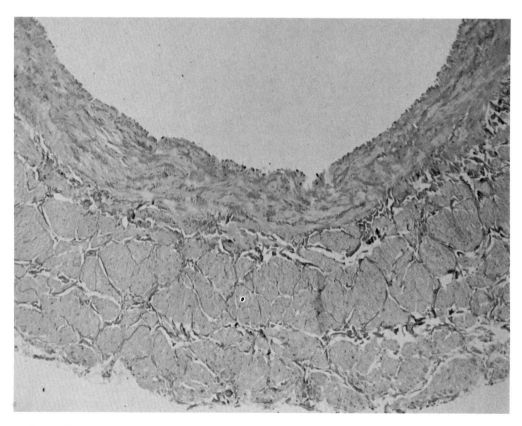

Figure 18–1. Varicocele—the involved spermatic vein shows marked dilatation with hypertrophy of the elastica and muscular layers. Masson trichrome (×40).

percentage of normal oval-shaped heads (less than 60%) with increase in the numbers of tapering (>10%) and/or immature forms (>4%), and varying degrees of oligospermia. The pattern is not exclusively associated with varicocele, as a similar picture is seen with exposure to antispermatogenic drugs, following severe viral illnesses, acute allergic reactions, and severe environmental changes.[19]

Following varicocele repair, sperm motility is the first parameter to improve, followed by sperm morphology and sperm count.[20] While there is often improvement in the stress pattern following varicocele repair, the semen analysis usually does not return completely to normal.[19]

Histology

The internal spermatic veins may be impressively dilated with marked thickening of the muscular layers (Figure 18–1).

The various histologic findings in both testes of varicocele patients have been reported and confirmed by numerous investigators.[21–25] Usually the ipsilateral testis displays the more severe derangements, with milder changes in the contralateral testis. However, there are some instances where the only histologic damage is detectable in the contralateral testis, with a normal testis on the involved side. As significant differences in histology of the testes occur in 10% of cases, bilateral biopsies are recommended.[22] Testis biopsies obtained at the time of internal spermatic vein ligation are fixed in Bouin's or Zenker's solution and stained with hematoxylin and eosin.

The major findings in infertile patients with varicocele are germinal hypoplasia, premature sloughing of immature cells, interstitial hyperplasia, and tubular thickening. Less commonly, maturation arrest, Sertoli-cell-only, and atrophic fibrosis may be seen. Significant improvement in testis histology occurs after varicocelectomy, but complete resolution is rare.[24]

Germinal cell hypoplasia is the most common histologic change in varicocele patients, reported in 50% to 80% of cases. It is often a mixed picture, with normal-appearing tubules interspersed with tubules displaying decreased spermatogenesis (Figure 18–2). In more advanced cases, the homogeneous pattern will be evident. In contrast to maturation arrest, spermatogenesis progresses to mature spermatozoa but with an overall reduction in germinal cells. The quantitative method of measuring mature spermatids per tubule has been used to

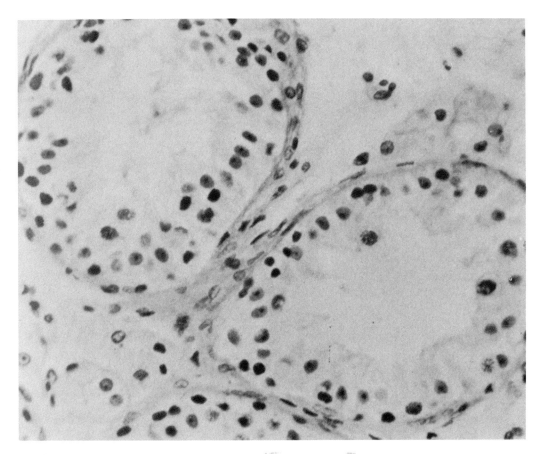

Figure 18–2. Varicocele—germ cell hypoplasia or hypospermatogenesis. The various levels of spermatogenesis are present, but in diminished numbers. (Reproduced from McFadden and Mehan[25] with permission.)

correlate spermatogenesis with mean ejaculatory sperm counts to differentiate partial obstruction from hypospermatogenesis.[26] At least 10 seminiferous tubules are studied from each side, counting only the mature spermatids. Using an exponential graph (Figure 18–3) the expected sperm count in the unobstructed patient can be estimated. Thus, with at least 20 spermatids per tubule, there should be over 10,000,000 per cc. The patient with "normal" spermatids per tubule, yet with severe oligospermia, probably has an obstructive defect distal to the rete testis.

In premature sloughing, progressively immature cells are seen in the ejaculate as tapering heads and amorphous forms. These changes are reflected in the testis biopsy with increasing numbers of immature spermatids and secondary spermatocytes sloughing into the tubular lumen (Figure 18–4). Caution should be exercised in applying this description, as crush injury from careless handling of the biopsy tissues may produce a similar picture.

Electron microscopy has demonstrated the importance of the Sertoli-Sertoli junctional complexes in maintaining the blood-testis barrier and protecting the basal compartment with its associated progenitor germ cells.[27] With increasing vacuolization within the Sertoli cell, the apical or adluminal portion is involved, resulting in breaks in the plasma membrane and release of immature germ cells.[28]

Another common finding is the presence of increased numbers of Leydig cells in the interstitium, presumably a response to decreased spermatogenesis (Figure 18–5).

Tubular thickening with progressive hyalinization of the basement membrane is indicative of chronic injury (Figure 18–6), but scattered tubules with such thickening may be seen in normal testes.

While most often reported in patients with idiopathic oligospermia, maturation arrest may be seen in patients with varicocele (Figure 18–7). The biopsy will display homogenous arrest, but the level of arrest will vary from individual to individual.

Complete absence of germ cells has been reported in a small percentage of varicocele patients (Figure 18–8).[18] Plasma FSH is usually elevated in response to the lack of germinal cells.

Fibrotic atrophy, characterized by extensive hyalinization of the seminiferous tubules, peritubular fibrosis, and preservation of interstitial cells (Figure 18–9), may occasionally occur.

The indications for testis biopsy in patients with varicocele have been better defined by the above-cited studies (Table 18–1).[21-25] The biopsy should be limited to patients in whom the histology will affect treatment or prognosis. Those varicocele patients who will not benefit from biopsy include the azoospermic patient with bilaterally small atrophic testis and the severely oligospermic patient with significantly elevated FSH (more than two

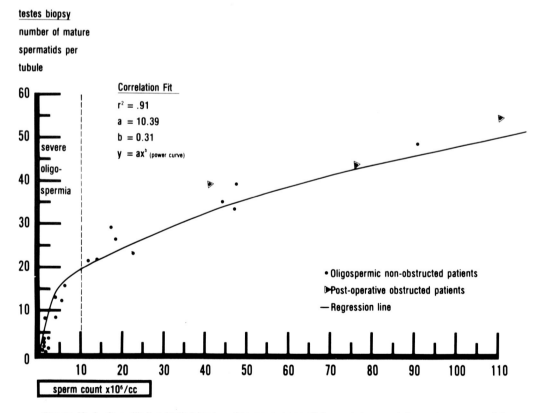

Figure 18–3. Quantitative testis biopsy, using an exponential graph to correlate mature spermatid count per tubule with estimated sperm count, is helpful in differentiating the obstructed ductal system from hypospermatogenesis. (Reproduced from Silber[34] with permission.)

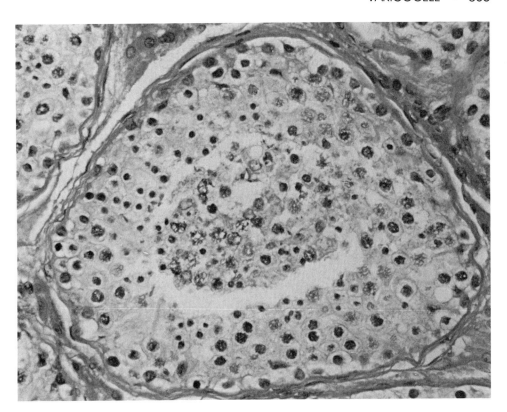

Figure 18–4. Varicocele—prematurely sloughed spermatids and spermatocytes can be seen clumped in the tubular lumen. H & E (×250).

times normal), for both will have irreversible germinal cell damage.

In those patients with less severe germinal cell loss, the severity of histologic changes does not correlate consistently with prognosis. The oligospermic patient with multiple histologic defects, but minimal testicular atrophy, may have remarkable improvement in semenogram after internal spermatic vein ligation. The histologic patterns of responders for internal spermatic vein ligation are similar to nonresponders.[22] Thus, the role of testis biopsy

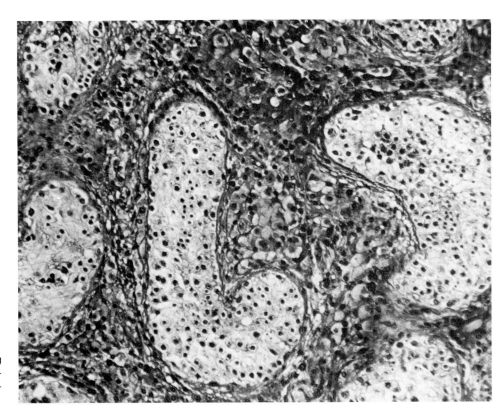

Figure 18–5. Varicocele—Leydig cell hyperplasia may be prominent in various areas of the biopsy. H & E (×100).

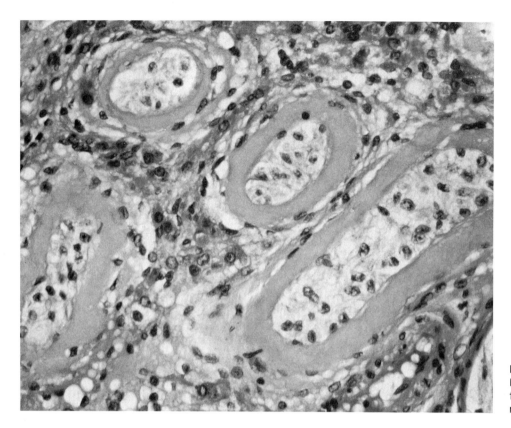

Figure 18–6. Varicocele—peritubular fibrosis is depicted, with extensive thickening of the basement membrane. H & E (×250).

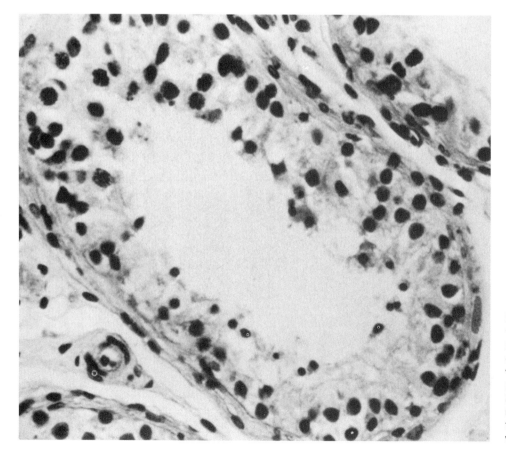

Figure 18–7. Varicocele—a uniform level of maturation arrest may be seen throughout the biopsy, but the level of arrest will vary from patient to patient. In this particular biopsy, progression has been halted at the primary spermatocyte level. (Reproduced from McFadden and Mehan[25] with permission).

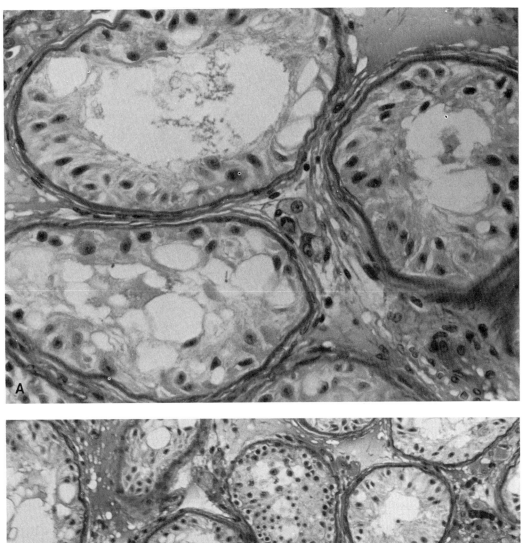

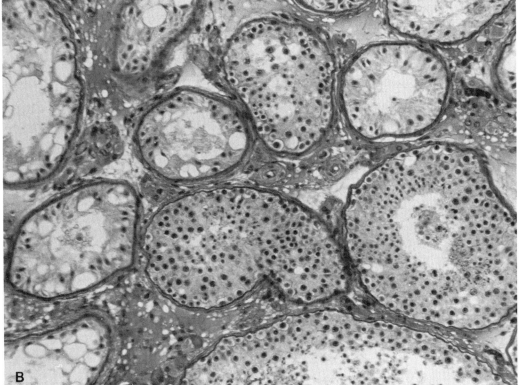

Figure 18–8. Varicocele—A. Absence of germ cells is an unusual finding with varicoceles. H & E (×250). B. The segmental nature of the testicular abnormality is reflected in this view in which tubules containing only Sertoli cells abut with tubules exhibiting normal spermatogenesis. H & E (×100).

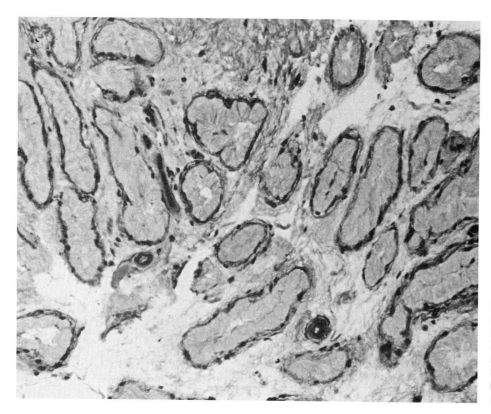

Figure 18–9. Varicocele—progressive injury from the varicocele will result in fibrous atrophy seen in this 35-year-old patient with progressively severe oligospermia. Extensive hyalinization of tubules with negligible interstitial cells is seen. Trichrome (×100).

in the varicocele patient is limited to the azoospermic, and possibly the severely oligospermic, individual with normal or borderline elevated FSH. If the biopsy shows normal spermatogenesis, the primary problem is obstruction and not the varicocele. If there were significant histologic abnormalities, such as fibrosis, severe hypoplasia, or maturation arrest, the prognosis is poor. However, the varicocele will often be repaired regardless because of the low morbidity of the procedure and the desperation of the infertile couple.

Treatment

Current management of varicoceles is focused on either occluding the retrograde flow through the spermatic veins or lowering the scrotal temperature. Surgical approaches to ligate the spermatic veins in the inguinal canal or just proximal to the internal inguinal ring have been popular. Improvement in sperm counts, motility, and morphology in 88%, and subsequent pregnancies in 68%, of patients with preoperative sperm counts over 10,000,000 per cc have been reported.[29] Radiographic occlusion of the internal spermatic vein by injection with a sclerosing agent or with a detachable balloon has yielded similar initial success rates. Scrotal hypothermia devices have recently been marketed, with limited clinical experience to date.[30]

OBSTRUCTIVE DISORDERS

Obstruction beyond the efferent ductules, whether congenital or acquired, impairs sperm transport. Such ductal obstruction accounts for as little as 7% of male infertility cases,[3] but will steadily increase, as has the demand for vasectomy. If the lesion occurs within the epididymis or

Table 18–1. Indications for Testis Biopsy in Varicocele Patients

FSH	Azoospermia	Severe Oligospermia	Mild to Moderate Oligospermia
Normal	Yes	±	No
Borderline elevated	Yes	±	No
Severely elevated (>2× nl)	No	No	No

beyond, as is often the case, the testicular histology is favorable if reversal is pursued within 10 years. However, when the obstruction is at the level of the caput epididymis or efferent ducts, damage is severe with atrophy and sclerosis of seminiferous tubules.

Congenital Obstruction

The male genital duct system derives embryologically from the wolffian or mesonephric duct. Where the mesonephros is closely approximated to the primitive gonad, the mesonephric tubules fuse with the rete testis forming the efferent ducts by 6 to 8 weeks, becoming the caput epididymis. The mesonephric duct just beneath the gonad then becomes the corpus and cauda epididymis, and vas deferens. The caudal end of the mesonephric duct provides for the ureteral bud, trigone of the bladder, and seminal vesicles. Thus, a defect in the development of the pronephros, the precursor to the mesonephric duct, will result in absence of the kidney, seminal vesicle, vas, and epididymis. An insult to the mesonephric duct cephalad to the ureteral bud may result in absence or atresia of the vas and/or epididymis only with preservation of the kidney, and possible absence of the seminal vesicle or obstruction of the ejaculatory ducts. Bilateral seminal vesicle agenesis or ejaculatory duct obstruction results in azoospermia. These patients will have sparse ejaculate with absence of fructose, which is produced exclusively by the seminal vesicle. However, if there is bilateral vas deferens atresia or agenesis, the patient will have azoospermia with almost normal ejaculate volume and presence of seminal fructose.

When only one or two efferent ducts fail to fuse with the epididymis, cysts within the caput will occur. These are lined by flat, cuboidal, or pseudostratified epithelium (Figure 18–10). If the cyst contains sperm, it is termed a spermatocele. With more defects in the 5 to 30 efferent ducts fusing with the epididymis, varying degrees of nonunion will occur. Such epididymal cysts or nonunion may impair sperm transport. One particular problem receiving attention involves the young males exposed to diethylstilbestrol (DES) *in utero* during the early 1940s to late 1960s. Many such males have impaired spermatogenesis (Figure 18–11) but also epididymal cysts which may contribute to their infertility.[31,32]

Congenital absence or atresia of the vas, in association with absence of both corpus and cauda epididymis or absence of only the cauda epididymis, is seen in patients with cystic fibrosis.[33] Testis biopsies in infancy will be normal, but postpubertal biopsy will show varying degrees of hypospermatogenesis and immature spermatozoa.

In general, post-testicular obstruction may produce some tubular dilation but normal spermatogenesis, as is illustrated in the testis biopsy of a 30-year-old man with congenital absence of the right vas and cauda epididymis (Figure 18–12).

Acquired Obstruction

With couples delaying their family-raising years, the increased incidence of sexually transmitted disease, and the high divorce and remarriage rate, infertility workups are revealing more males with acquired obstructive dis-

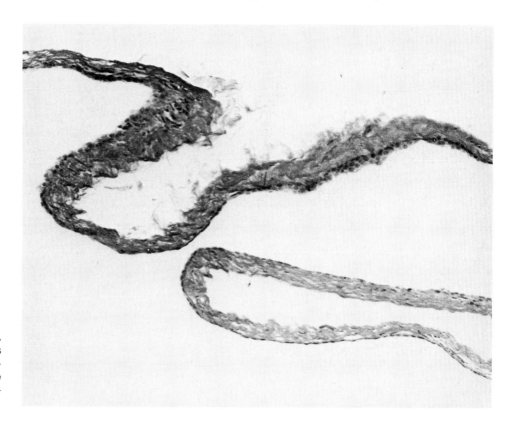

Figure 18–10. Epididymal cyst, filled with clear fluid, which was excised from the caput epididymis, demonstrating a delicate thin wall lined by cuboidal epithelium. H & E (×100).

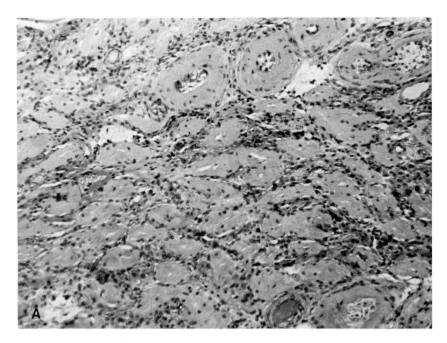

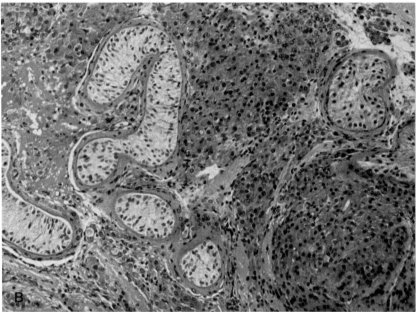

Figure 18–11. DES exposure *in utero* may produce defects in the genital tract, including epididymal cysts, testicular hypoplasia, and abnormal semen analysis. This 30-year-old man was seen because of severe oligospermia and somewhat small testes. Biopsy shows (A) extensive hyalinization of the tubules. H & E (×100) and (B) prominent Leydig cell hyperplasia with only Sertoli cells surviving in the tubules. H & E (×100).

orders. Vasectomy accounts for a large percentage of patients with acquired obstruction, but postinfection scarring continues to be a difficult problem. The advances in microsurgery have offered hope to many patients who, just a few short years ago, were considered untreatable.

Postvasectomy

Whether performed by simple ligature, fulguration, or surgical clip occlusion, vasectomy results in formation of a palpable inflammatory nodule in more than 30% of patients.[34] This sperm granuloma is seen in patients undergoing vasovasostomy representing the site of ongoing spermatic fluid leakage. Histology of the early granuloma reveals sperm heads within a central area of debris surrounded by leukocytes, epithelioid cells, phagocytizing histiocytes, and giant cells (Figure 18–13A).[35] The histiocytes fill with fatty acids, which eventually oxidize, forming yellowish pigment within the cytoplasm (ceroid granuloma). The late stages of the granuloma may show extensive fibrosis and even calcification.

A variant of sperm granuloma is vasitis nodosum, in which numerous narrow interconnected channels filled with sperm fragments are seen (Figure 18–13B).[35] Failure of vasectomy is often related to establishment of microanastomoses through this lesion.

While the one-month postvasectomy testis biopsy will show widespread disruption of spermatogenesis with spermatogenic arrest and basement membrane thickening, in 2.5 to 3 years there will be complete recovery.[36]

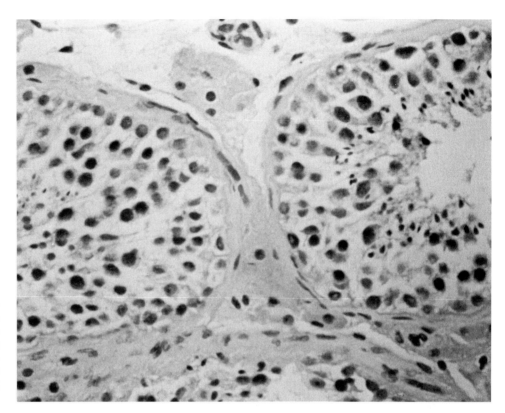

Figure 18-12. Obstruction beyond the caput epididymis will often be associated with preservation of spermatogenesis, as is depicted by this biopsy in a 30-year-old man with oligospermia and agenesis of the vas and cauda epididymis. H & E (×250).

Biopsy demonstrates no significant abnormality in spermatogenesis, similar to those patients with agenesis of the vas or epididymis. Compared to vasa without sperm granuloma, those vasa with sperm granuloma had less dilatation of the vas lumen proximal to the vasectomy site and produced better quality sperm at time of vasovasostomy.[34] The abnormalities in sperm quality must be related to epididymal injury. The back pressure produced by vasectomy is transmitted to the delicate epididymal tubules where dilatation and epithelial rupture occur. This leads to sperm extravasation, granuloma formation, and tubular obstruction, usually in the region of the junction of the corpus and cauda epididymis. Thus, in those patients with sperm granuloma at the vasectomy site, the continued leakage prevents significant back pressure, sparing the epididymal tubules from scarring. The greater the time lapse after vasectomy without sperm granuloma, the more epididymal damage occurs, so that after ten years there is a significant drop-off in successful microsurgical repair.[34]

Traumatic or iatrogenic injury to the vas will impair sperm counts, and bilateral involvement will lead to azoospermia. Such damage may occur during inguinal herniorrhaphy, orchidopexy, varicocele repair, hydrocelectomy, and complicated ureteral reimplantation. In particular, children are more at risk for injury because of the delicate vas.

Postinfectious Obstruction

Organisms ascending from the ejaculatory ducts may result in epididymitis and even orchitis. Resolution of the inflammatory response yields scarring of the epididymal tubules, resulting in a drop in ejaculatory sperm counts. While gonorrhea was the major disease in the preantibiotic era, Chlamydia trachomatis has recently been recognized as the leading agent in epididymitis in males under age 35, and E. coli as the usual organism in males over age 35.[37] Chronic prostatitis, bacterial or nonbacterial, may also produce epididymitis. In patients with infertility and prior epididymitis, histology of the epididymis will demonstrate interstitial inflammatory infiltrates, dilated tubules filled with spermatozoa, and oftentimes phagocytizing macrophages (Figure 18-14).

Another route of infection is the hematogenous or descending route, exemplified by tuberculosis. This results in granulomatous scarring in the prostate, vas, and epididymis (Figure 18-15). Other forms of granulomatous epididymitis have been reported from leprosy, filariasis or schistosomiasis, brucellosis, fungi, or malakoplakia.[16]

Ejaculatory Duct Obstruction

This may occur from traumatic urethral instrumentation, inflammatory scarring from indwelling urethral catheter, or overzealous cauterization for congenital posterior urethral valves. Patients complain of scant volumes of ejaculate, a condition which will reveal azoospermia. Seminal fluid fructose will be absent and the testis biopsy will demonstrate normal spermatogenesis as the epididymal tubules will be a buffer from back pressure.

Treatment of these obstructive states has advanced with the evolution of microsurgery. For lesions confined to the vas, high success rates are achieved with microscopic vasovasostomy.[34] As the obstruction moves more proximally into the epididymis, the difficulty of repair

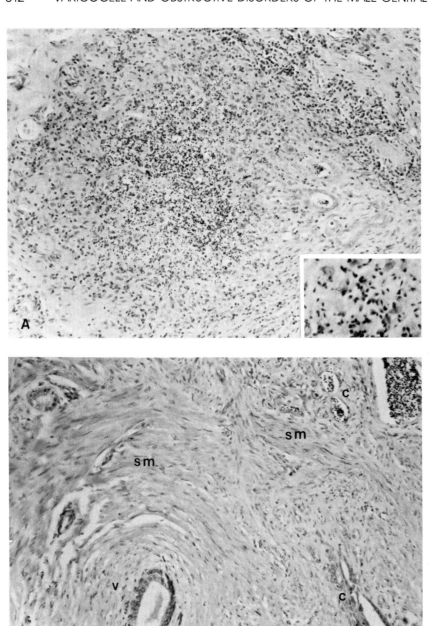

Figure 18–13. Postvasectomy leakage results in sperm granuloma formation. A. The central necrosis is encircled by extensive chronic inflammatory cells. H & E (×100). Numerous sperm heads may be seen within the debris. Inset, H & E (×250). B. Vasitis nodosum, a variant of sperm granuloma, consists of smooth muscle bundles (sm) surrounding the vas (v) and multiple epithelial-lined channels (c) filled with sperm. H & E (×100).

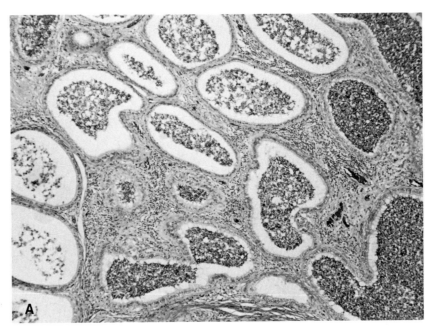

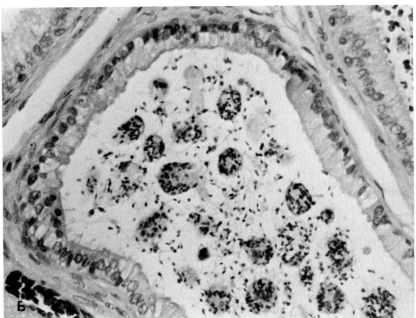

Figure 18–14. Resolution of epididymitis results in tubular obstruction. Often there will be persistent chronic interstitial infiltrates surrounding the ducts (A: H & E, ×40) which are dilated and filled with numerous sperm fragments and macrophages (B: H & E, ×250).

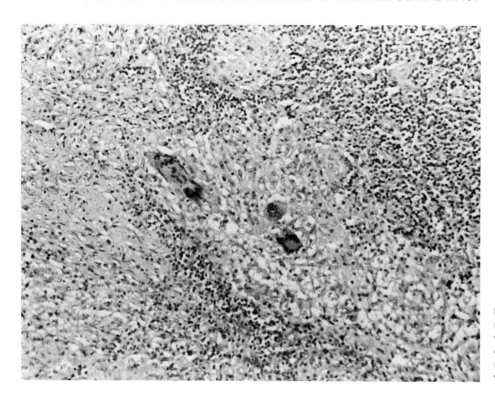

Figure 18–15. Tuberculous epididymitis produces typical granulomas with epithelioid cells and multinucleated giant cells. Similar granulomas may occur along the vas or within the prostate. H & E (×100).

increases and sperm maturation may be compromised by the shortening in epididymal transport. Thus, a microscopic vasoepididymostomy has a lower technical success rate as well as lower likelihood of producing motile sperm.

If there is no obvious obstruction in the epididymis or vas, a vasogram will define the drainage into the prostatic urethra. The obstructed ejaculatory duct may be relieved by superficial transurethral resection of the duct.

If the vas is unusable, the efforts to create an alloplastic spermatocele meet with limited success. Such a reservoir for sperm collection within the epididymis might be aspirated periodically for insemination. Testicular transplantation has also been successful using microsurgical techniques.

Young's Syndrome

This is a progressive obstructive disorder of the epididymis by inspissated secretions associated with mild chronic sinopulmonary infections.[38] The respiratory difficulties, manifested by recurrent cough and sputum production, begin in early childhood but become quiescent after adolescence. Paternity prior to development of infertility and azoospermia suggests that the obstruction is partial and progresses after puberty. Amorphous yellowish secretions in the mid-epididymis with normal spermatogenesis and a dilated caput epididymis filled with abundant spermatozoa characterized the surgical findings. Young's syndrome may be differentiated from immotile-cilia syndrome by the azoospermia and absence of ultrastructural defects of cilia and sperm, and from cystic fibrosis by the palpably normal vas and cauda epididymis with normal sweat and pancreatic functions. Microsurgi-

cal epididymovasostomy may bypass the obstruction, but results have been poor.

References

1. Clarke BG: Incidence of varicocele in normal men and among men of different ages. JAMA 198:1121–1122, 1966.

2. Greenberg SH: Varicocele and male fertility. Fertil Steril 28:699–706, 1977.

3. Dubin L, Amelar RD: Etiologic factors in 1,294 consecutive cases of male infertility. Fertil Steril 22:469–474, 1971.

4. Lyon RP, Marshall S, Scott MP: Varicocele in childhood and adolescence: implication in adulthood infertility? Urology 19:641–644, 1982.

5. Pozza D, D'Ottavio G, Masci P, et al.: Left varicocele at puberty. Urology 22:271–274, 1983.

6. Belker AM: The varicocele and male infertility. Urol Clin North Am 8:41–51, 1981.

7. Lipshultz LI, Corriere JN: Progressive testicular atrophy in the varicocele patient. J Urol 117:175–176, 1977.

8. Zorgniotti AW, MacLeod J: Studies in temperature, human semen quality, and varicocele. Fertil Steril 24:854–863, 1973.

9. Tessler AN, Krahn HP: Varicocele and testicular temperature. Fertil Steril 17:201–203, 1966.

10. Nakamura M, Hall PF: The mechanism by which body temperature inhibits protein biosynthesis in spermatids of rat testes. J Biol Chem 255:2907–2913, 1980.

11. Saypol DC, Howards SS, Turner TT, et al.: Influence of surgically induced varicocele on testicular blood flow, temperature, and histology in adult rats and dogs. J Clin Invest 68:39–45, 1981.

12. Green KF, Turner TT, Howards SS: Varicocele: reversal of

the testicular blood flow and temperature effects by varicocele repair. J Urol 131:1208–1211, 1984.

13. Comhaire F, Vermeulen A: Varicocele sterility: cortisol and catecholamines. Fertil Steril 25:88–95, 1974.

14. Caldemone AA, Al-Juburi A, Cockett ATK: The varicocele: elevated serotonin and infertility. J Urol 123:683–685, 1980.

15. Ito H, Fuse H, Minagawa H, *et al.*: Internal spermatic vein prostaglandins in varicocele patients. Fertil Steril 37:218–222, 1982.

16. Nistal M, Paniagua R: Testicular and epididymal pathology. New York, Thieme-Stratton, 1984.

17. Nistal M, Paniagua R, Regadera J, *et al.*: Obstruction of the tubuli recti and ductuli efferentes by dilated veins in the testes of men with varicocele and its possible role in causing atrophy of the seminiferous tubules. Int J Androl 7:309–323, 1984.

18. Swerdloff RS, Walsh PC: Pituitary and gonadal hormones in patients with varicocele. Fertil Steril 26:1006–1012, 1975.

19. MacLeod J: Seminal cytology in the presence of varicocele. Fertil Steril 16:735–757, 1965.

20. Glezerman M, Rakowszczyk M, Lunenfeld B, *et al.*: Varicocele in oligospermic patients: pathophysiology and results after ligation and division of the internal spermatic vein. J Urol 115:562–565, 1976.

21. Charny CW: Effect of varicocele on fertility: results of varicocelectomy. Fertil Steril 13:47–56, 1962.

22. Dubin L, Hotchkiss RS: Testis biopsy in subfertile men with varicocele. Fertil Steril 20:50–57, 1969.

23. Ibrahim AA, Awad HA, El-Haggar S, *et al.*: Bilateral testicular biopsy in men with varicocele. Fertil Steril 28:663–667, 1977.

24. Johnsen SG, Agger P: Quantitative evaluation of testicular biopsies before and after operation for varicocele. Fertil Steril 29:58–63, 1978.

25. McFadden MR, Mehan DJ: Testicular biopsies in 101 cases of varicocele. J Urol 119:372–374, 1978.

26. Silber SS, Rodriguez-Rigau LJ: Quantitative analysis of testicle biopsy: determination of partial obstruction and prediction of sperm count after surgery for obstruction. Fertil Steril 36:480–485, 1981.

27. Cameron DF, Snydle FE: The blood-testis barrier in men with varicocele: a lanthanum tracer study. Fertil Steril 34:255–258, 1980.

28. Terquem A, Dadoune J-P: Morphological findings in varicocele: an ultrastructural study of 30 bilateral testicular biopsies. Int J Androl 4:515–531, 1981.

29. Dubin L, Amelar RD: Varicocelectomy as a therapy in male infertility: a study of 504 cases. Fertil Steril 26:217–220, 1975.

30. Zorgniotti AW, Sealfon AI, Toth A: Further clinical experience with testis hypothermia for infertility due to poor semen. Urology 19:636–640, 1982.

31. Gill WB, Shumacher GFB, Bibbo M, *et al.*: Association of diethylstilbestrol exposure *in utero* with cryptorchidism, testicular hypoplasia, and semen abnormalities. J Urol 122:36–39, 1979.

32. Whitehead ED, Leiter E: Genital abnormalities and abnormal semen analysis in male patients exposed to diethylstilbestrol *in utero*. J Urol 125:47–50, 1981.

33. Kaplan E, Schwachman H, Perlmutter AD, *et al.*: Reproductive failure in males with cystic fibrosis. N Engl J Med 279:65–69, 1968.

34. Silber SJ: Microsurgery for vasectomy reversal and vasoepididymostomy. Urology 23:505–524, 1984.

35. Schmidt SS, Morris RR: Spermatic granuloma: the complication of vasectomy. Fertil Steril 24:941–947, 1973.

36. Gupta AS, Kothari LK, Dhruva A, *et al.*: Surgical sterilization by vasectomy and its effect on the structure and function of the testis in man. Br J Surg 62:59–63, 1975.

37. Berger RE, Alexander ER, Harnisch JP, *et al.*: Etiology, manifestations, and therapy of acute epididymitis: prospective study of 50 cases. J Urol 121:750–754, 1979.

38. Handelsman DJ, Conway AJ, Boylan LM, *et al.*: Young's syndrome: obstructive azoospermia and chronic sinopulmonary infections. N Engl J Med 310:3–9, 1984.

19. Regulation of Immune Responsiveness to Sperm Antigens

Nancy J. Alexander, Thomas H. Tarter, and Mohamed Isahakia

ANTIGENICITY OF SPERM AND TESTES

During spermatogenesis, dynamic cellular interactions take place. These are governed partly by initial recognition events involving plasma membranes of cells within the seminiferous tubules. This feature is thought to result in the overall regulation of spermatogonial proliferation and spermatocyte meiotic division. Many alterations in somatic cell surfaces have been shown to be correlated with the cell cycle,[1] and thus perhaps directly related to changes in cell surfaces. These events are highly orchestrated with respect to the number, timing, and positioning of successive cell divisions.[2,3]

Mature human and other mammalian spermatozoa exhibit a polar distribution of some glycoproteins and cell surface antigens.[4] Lectin binding sites,[5] lipid distribution,[6] and the sperm surface membrane change[7] are all polarized into five major regions: the acrosome, equatorial segment, postacrosome, midpiece, and tail.[8] Spermatozoa in transit down the male reproductive tract lack any lateral mobility of cell surface molecules.[4] The molecular mechanism limiting the fluidity of human sperm membrane proteins has not been described, but it is thought that the appearance of most sperm surface domains is not established until late spermiogenesis[9] or, even later, during epididymal maturation.[10,11] We as well as others[12] have shown that this localized distribution of membrane components on spermatozoa is maintained at least until capacitation.

Spermatozoa are distinguished from many somatic cells not only by the fluid mobility of membrane constituents but also by particular molecules of the sperm membrane itself. The expression of many sperm surface macromolecules occurs during a precise time in spermatogenesis. In the mouse, testis-specific autoantigens first appear on late pachytene spermatocytes and persist throughout spermiogenesis.[13] However, some antigens, which appear first on B spermatogonia, are found at all stages of spermatogenesis, on spermatids, and even on residual bodies, but not on mature sperm.[14] By comparing antitestis cell and antisperm autoantisera, Romrell and O'Rand[14] found that the majority of autoantigens predominating on the sperm surface are inserted into the plasma membrane after the midspermatid stage. Many of these testis-specific autoantigens readily elicit antibody production, cell-mediated immune responses, or both, in males and females. These antigens may be termed *aspermatogenic antigens* if capable of inducing experimental allergic orchitis (EAO).[15]

Although semen autoantibodies against Leydig cells[16] and Sertoli cells[17] have been detected in human autoimmune disease, antigens associated with these cells do not elicit an autoimmune response in normal experimental animals even when the antigen is incorporated into Freund's complete adjuvant. By contrast, sperm and their progenitor cells readily induce an autoantibody response and EAO. The existence of immunologic foreignness of testis-specific autoantigens is supported by data on the age-related incidence of antibodies to sperm antigens.[18] Large numbers of serum samples from different age groups of both sexes were studied for the age-related prevalence of antisperm antibodies to foreign antigens. The number of testis-specific autoantigens capable of autoantibody induction was greater than the number present on other organs; in serum from vasectomized men, as many as eight internal antigens to sperm were identified with the indirect immunofluorescence test.[19] Unlike the immune responses to most autoantigens, the responses to sperm resemble responses to foreign antigens (Figure 19–1,2,3).

Most attempts at isolating human sperm membrane autoantigens have not yet resulted in direct, detailed information about the antigens, except for those involving lactate dehydrogenase C_4 (LDH-C_4). However, indirect evidence of the multiplicity of sperm autoantigens has come from the use of autoimmune sera. These sperm-specific autoantibodies, found in serum of some naturally

The work described in this chapter, Publication No. 1412 of the Oregon Regional Primate Research Center, was supported by National Institutes of Health grants HD-14572, HL-14164, and RR-00163.

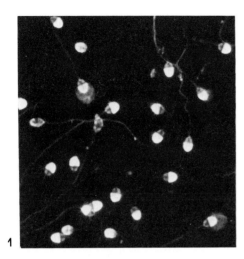

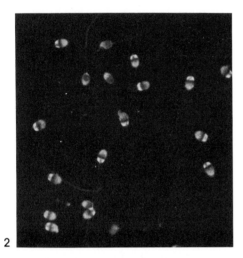

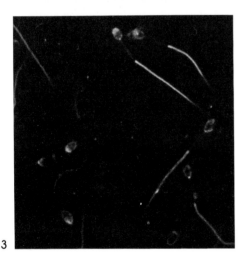

Figures 19–1,2,3. Many antigenic sites are on the spermatozoon. When antisperm antibodies develop after vasectomy, different antigen-antibody patterns can be observed by immunofluorescence. Serum samples from 3 vasectomized monkeys revealed different antigenic specificities. Figure 19–1 depicts antibodies that are bound to the acrosome. Figure 19–2 reveals antibodies that are bound to the acrosome and postacrosomal region. Figure 19–3 demonstrates some reaction with the acrosome and tail antibodies, but no binding in the midpiece region (×750).

infertile and vasectomized men, produce different patterns of agglutination that suggest that distinct surface antigens occur on the head (Figure 19–4), the tail, and the tip of the tail.[20,21] Poulsen and Hjort,[22] using human sera containing agglutinating and immobilizing antibodies, isolated 2 polypeptides from human sperm membranes (65,000 K and 75,000 K mol wt). More recently, monoclonal antibodies have been used to study surface sperm antigens (Figure 19–5).[23]

A number of sperm surface molecules seem to be unique to spermatozoa, while others of them are found also on certain types of somatic cells, especially those of the central nervous system. The FA teratocarcinoma antigen,[24] H-Y antigen,[25] and NS antigens[26] are examples of such surface components. In humans, the presence of ABO blood group substances was demonstrated by Landsteiner and Levine[27] in 1926 and confirmed more recently by Kerek.[28] There is continuing controversy about whether these alloantigens are intrinsic to sperm with haploid expression or are sperm-coating; a majority of the evidence favors the latter hypothesis. Human sperm appear also to share antigenic determinants with lymphocytes,[29,30] but the significance of this finding is uncertain. Early serologic studies suggested the haploid expression of major histocompatibility complex (MHC) antigens on sperm of several species including human and mouse, but recent studies with better defined monoclonal reagents have failed to detect class I or class II MHC determinants on postmeiotic human testicular germ cells and sperm.[31,32]

FUNCTIONS OF THE EPIDIDYMIS

The epididymides perform absorptive and secretory functions, including transportation of spermatozoa from the testes to the ejaculatory ducts. The existence of intraepithelial lymphocytes and macrophages in the human epididymis has been reported,[33] and they may be an important component of the immunologic barrier of the male reproductive duct. Intraepithelial lymphocytes are more numerous in the caudal epididymis, where spermatozoa degenerate, than elsewhere in the male reproductive tract.

Development of the fertilizing capacity of mammalian spermatozoa in the epididymis was first recognized over fifty years ago by Young, who made a study of guinea pigs.[34] In men, epididymovasovasostomies between the caput region of the epididymis and the vas deferens result in infertile semen.[35] This suggests that part of the proximal human epididymis contributes to sperm maturation. Confirmation has come from an *in vitro* assay of zona-free hamster ovum penetration.[36]

The most important functional change associated with the development of sperm fertilizing ability is the acquisition of forward motility. In all mammals spermatozoa recovered from the proximal epididymis exhibit characteristic circular or twitching motions with little progression.[37,38] By contrast, spermatozoa released from the cauda epididymidis possess forward motility. This has been attributed to the secretion of a forward motility

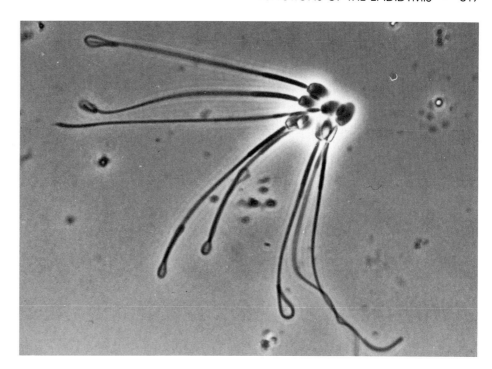

Figure 19–4. Agglutinated sperm are commonly observed in cervical mucus or semen of individuals with immunologically mediated infertility.

protein coupled with an increase in cyclic AMP levels within the spermatozoa.[38,39] Other biochemical changes in the sperm-tail organelles during maturation also influence sperm movement. These changes include formation of stabilizing sulfhydryl double bonds in the dense fibers of the principal piece[40] and phosphorylation of microtubules.[41]

Mammalian spermatozoa also undergo ultrastructural modifications within the epididymis. The most striking morphological change involves the cytoplasmic droplet, a remnant of spermatid cytoplasm that migrates caudally from the neck of the spermatozoon to the end of the midpiece.[42] Fine structural alterations involving the acrosome have been observed in several species. Both intracellular and surface changes are thought to occur. The distribution and density of carbohydrate moieties over various regions of the sperm surface change during maturation.[4,43] This changing character of the sperm surface parallels development of the ability to fertilize.[44,45]

Spermatozoa passing along the lumen of the epididymis are continuously suspended in the complex epididymal plasma. This milieu, derived from rete testis fluid and modified by secretory and absorptive activities of the epididymal epithelium, is therefore critical for sperm maturation and survival.[46] Specific glycoproteins secreted by the epithelium are known to bind to the sperm surface.[47–49] Most of these secretions are androgen-dependent and hence decline rapidly upon androgen withdrawal, as, for instance, after castration.[50] Recent investigators have employed conventional and monoclonal antibodies to isolate membrane components of the maturing sperm surface.[51,52]

Sperm transit through the epididymis takes about 12 to 21 days in men; the time is influenced by both sexual activity and androgen levels.[53] Intraluminal pressure action of catecholamines and neurohypothalamic hormones (oxytocin and vasopressin) stimulate contractions of smooth muscle in the epididymis. Certain pathologic

 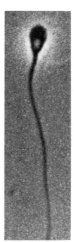 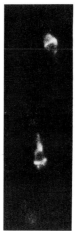 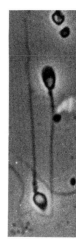

Figure 19–5. Monoclonal antibodies allow localization of antigenic determinants. The left pair of photomicrographs are a fluorescence micrograph of an antihuman sperm monoclonal that reacts to the acrosome and a phase picture of the same spermatozoon. The right pair depicts antibody that reacts mainly to the equatorial region and the companion phase micrograph.

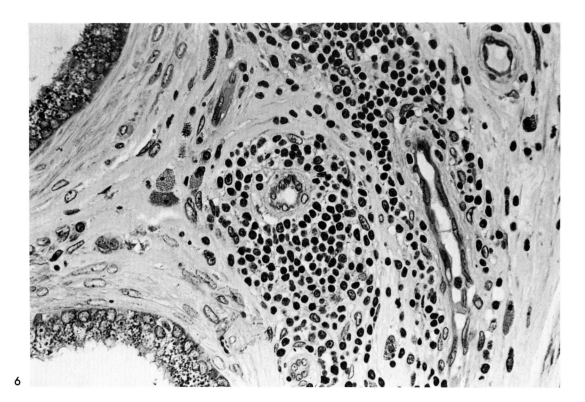

6

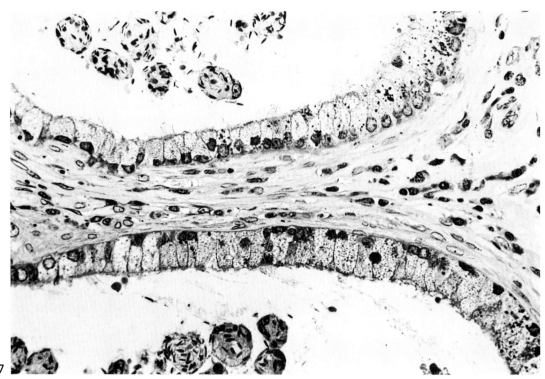

7

Figure 19–6,7. The epididymis may be a site of immune interaction with reproductive antigens. Figure 19–6. Lymphocytic infiltrates in the interstitium of the epididymis (×560). Figure 19–7. Macrophages traverse the epididymal epithelium and ingest spermatozoa (×560).

conditions in the epididymis may interfere with the transit time of sperm (Figures 19–6, 7). Obstructions in the epididymal duct may increase pressure in the lumen and thus cause rupture of the tubules. Obstruction can occur in cases of infectious diseases such as tuberculosis and schistosomiasis.

Approximately half the spermatozoa that enter the epididymis disintegrate before reaching the caudal region. This region, in which mature spermatozoa are stored, contains about 70% of the spermatozoa in the male; only 2% are stored in the vas deferens. Increased epididymal temperature, as in cryptorchidism, promotes disintegration of spermatozoa in the caudal region.

Seminal plasma, the liquid portion of semen, is composed of exocrine secretions from the prostate gland and seminal vesicles; the epididymides and bulbourethral glands make minor contributions. Mucinous secretions of the bulbourethral glands are emitted prior to ejaculation and serve as lubricants during sexual intercourse. Semen is formed by the sequential emission of prostatic fluid, sperm-rich epididymal fluid, and vesicular fluid during ejaculation. Greater than 95% of semen volume is seminal plasma, which comprises a complex mixture of organic and inorganic molecules that contribute to sperm function and thus to the events leading to fertilization. Among body fluids, seminal plasma has unusual properties. For example, its osmolarity is determined by high concentrations of organic rather than inorganic molecules. Also, seminal plasma contains uniquely high concentrations of zinc, fructose, citric acid, prostaglandins, polyamines, iron-binding proteins, phosphatases, nucleolytic enzymes, glycosidases, proteinases, proteinase inhibitors, small peptides, and amino acids. Whether all of these constituents have functional roles to play in fertilization is unknown.

SEMINAL PLASMA

In general, seminal plasma is thought to aid in the transport of sperm to the site of fertilization. Activating substances, such as prostaglandins[54] and forward motility protein,[55] have been shown to enhance the forward progression of sperm. Fructose is utilized as a nutrient substrate by sperm in the anaerobic environment of the upper vagina. After insemination, uterine contractions propel the sperm toward the uterotubal junction; the myometrium is thought to be stimulated by prostaglandins that enter the systemic circulation through the vagina.[56]

The importance of seminal plasma in human reproduction has been questioned because artificial insemination has been successful with sperm obtained directly from the epididymis.[57] However, this argument ignores two of the more obvious functions of seminal plasma as 1. a diluent, and 2. a transport vehicle. Tightly packed, immotile spermatozoa become motile only after their concentration is reduced with a diluent, and artificial insemination medium, like seminal plasma, serves this function as well as a means of transport.

An obvious functional characteristic of seminal plasma is coagulation; however, the physiological relevance of a seminal clot in humans is unclear since liquefaction normally occurs within 20 minutes.

Recent studies have indicated that another important physiological role of seminal plasma might be to minimize immunologic sensitization to sperm in the female after insemination. Investigators have used a variety of antigens in several mammalian species to show that the female reproductive tract does not have a privileged immune status.[58–61] The antigenic nature of sperm is clinically relevant in that high serum titers of sperm-agglutinating and sperm-immobilizing antibodies are correlated with infertility.[62–64] Because reproductive success would be compromised if women were immunized against sperm with each insemination, it is likely that immunosuppressive components of seminal plasma protect sperm from immunologic consequences in the female reproductive tract.

Likewise, the microenvironment of the sperm compartment and accessory organs of the male reproductive tract may not be favorable for antigen recognition or lymphocyte stimulation. In view of the immunosuppressive effects of its exocrine secretions, the male reproductive tract may be a particularly hospitable environment for the growth of neoplasms and replication of certain viruses.

Prostatic carcinoma accounts for 10% of cancer mortality and is the second most common cancer in men.[65] Autopsies have revealed that more than 40% of men in their 70s and 50% of men in their 80s have microscopic areas of cancer in their prostates. To explain this unusually high incidence of occult cancer foci, Gittes and McCullough[66] have hypothesized that the prostate is an immunologically privileged site where an effective primary immune response cannot be induced.

As for viral infection, herpes-type viruses have been shown to persist in the male reproductive tract in the absence of overt disease. In a study of 190 randomly selected men with no evidence of genital herpes virus infection, 15% were positive for herpes virus type 2 in genitourinary specimens; a higher incidence was noted for specimens from deeper tissues such as the prostate and vas deferens.[67] In a study of 43 asymptomatic men, the ejaculates of 5 were positive for cytomegalovirus,[68] and 1 case report showed that cytomegalovirus persisted in high titers in the ejaculates of a man who had recovered from mononucleosis and was asymptomatic.[69] More recently, the human T cell lymphotropic virus type III was detected in, and isolated from, the semen of patients with acquired immunodeficiency syndrome and from an asymptomatic homosexual man.[70,71]

The male reproductive and immune systems appear to interact in a way that 1. eliminates infectious organisms and 2. protects sperm from autoimmune damage. Components of seminal plasma may mediate these competing requirements. Lactoferrin, zinc, lysozyme, glucosidases, polyamines, and secretory IgA are constituents of seminal plasma known to be bacteriostatic, and may provide an important barrier to infection.[72,73] Furthermore, seminal plasma contains factors that suppress a variety of immunologic functions and may protect sperm from autoimmune elimination. Human seminal plasma has been shown to suppress lymphocyte transformation and DNA synthesis induced by phytohemagglutinin mitogen,[74-78] concanavalin A and pokeweed mitogens, Candida albicans antigen, and allogeneic cells in vitro.[77] Human seminal plasma also inhibits the antibody responses of mouse plasma cells to T-dependent and T-independent antigens in vitro.[77] Suppression of mitogen-induced lymphocyte stimulation has also been reported for bovine and murine seminal plasma.[79,80] Mouse seminal plasma exerts potent immunosuppresive effects in vivo as well; it has been shown to suppress primary and secondary antibody responses in mice to low immunizing doses of antigen (bovine serum albumin, or washed epididymal sperm), and also to significantly suppress antibody responses to high doses of antigen.[80]

The effects of human seminal plasma on mononuclear phagocyte and natural killer (NK) cell responses have also been studied. There is evidence that selective inhibition of macrophage function mediates suppression of mitogen-induced lymphocyte stimulation by seminal plasma.[81] Lymphocyte cultures depleted of mononuclear phagocytes are unresponsive to mitogens, and reconstitution of these cultures with peritoneal macrophages normally restores the blastogenic response. In one study, peritoneal macrophages that were harvested from mice into which 0.2 ml of human seminal plasma had been injected a few days earlier were unable to restore the blastogenic response of lymphocytes to concanavalin A.[81] In this study in vitro treatment of Corynebacterium-parvulum-elicited peritoneal macrophages with low concentrations of human seminal plasma inhibited other macrophage functions, such as attachment and spreading on glass and phagocytosis of latex particles. In another study, human prostatic fluid inhibited spreading, motility, and O_2 consumption of thioglycolate-elicited rat peritoneal macrophages.[82] The production of reactive oxygen intermediates such as superoxide, hydrogen peroxide, and hydroxyl radical correlates with intracellular killing of microbial parasites and, under certain conditions, with the nonphagocytic lysis of tumor cells.[83] It has been reported that human seminal plasma inhibits the release of reactive oxygen intermediates from zymosan-activated human mononuclear phagocytes, as detected by a chemoluminescence method.[81]

In a study designed to investigate the influence of germ cells on cellular immune reactions, it was shown that NK cell activity against a susceptible target tumor cell line was significantly reduced in mice into which 1×10^7 syngeneic sperm had been injected 8 days earlier, and the NK cell cytotoxic activity was completely abolished 22 days after inoculation.[84] Whether or not suppression of this type is mediated by soluble products of germ cells remains to be tested. Recently, human seminal plasma was found to be a potent suppressor of human NK cell cytotoxic activity against the K562 erythroleukemia target in vitro; a strong reduction in target cell lysis was observed at a final dilution of 1/400. The suppression was mediated by the predominant prostaglandins in this fluid, 19-OH-PGE and 19-OH-PGE$_2$.[85]

In addition to suppressing lymphocyte, mononuclear phagocyte, and NK cell responses, seminal plasma inhibits complement, an important mediator of humoral immunity.[86,87] Prostatic and vesicular secretions of the mouse and rhesus macaque have also been observed to have this effect.[80,88,89] Human seminal plasma has been shown to inhibit complement-mediated killing of bacteria and lysis of sheep erythrocytes,[86,87] and to inhibit the opsonization of gram-negative bacteria and subsequent phagocytosis by leukocytes.[90] Complement activity has been measured in human midcycle cervical mucus,[91] and complement-fixing antibodies have been observed in the cervicovaginal secretions of sperm-immunized rabbits[92] and women with idiopathic infertility.[93,94] In a study on antisperm immunity in infertile couples, immobilizing and cytoxic antibodies were detected in the seminal plasma of 3 of 8 men whose serum contained these antibodies. This study first revealed that human seminal plasma inhibits the action of complement, and the investigators concluded that immune-mediated immobilization and cytotoxicity are unlikely to be observed in ejaculates.[95] The presence, in seminal plasma, of a complement inhibitor (or inhibitors) may provide a mechanism by which sperm are protected from humoral immunologically mediated immobilization.

The biochemical repertoire of seminal plasma includes components that interfere with antigen recognition in addition to those that directly inhibit immunologic effector functions. A recent study in rabbits showed that epididymal sperm lose the ability to stimulate lymphocyte DNA synthesis after incubation in transglutaminase and uteroglobin, two proteins of seminal plasma.[96] Immunofluorescence studies revealed that uteroglobin is bound to the sperm surface in the presence of transglutaminase. The "masking" phenomenon may apply only to ejaculated sperm, since transglutaminase was identified with prostatic secretions and uteroglobin with vesicular secretions. Other masking substances may be produced in the testis or epididymis. Immunoglobulins of the A class provide a barrier to absorption of food antigens from the gastrointestinal tract.[97] The antibody isotype, also produced within the male reproductive tract, is present in epididymal secretions;[98,99] it may be bound to sperm surface antigens and thereby sterically hinder the access of antigen receptors on reactive lymphocytes. Antigen recognition may also be hindered by a complement inhibitor that prevents opsonization.[90]

In summary, factors produced within the male reproductive tract suppress a variety of immunologic functions in vitro and in vivo. Seminal plasma interferes with antigen recognition, lymphocyte stimulation, mononuclear phagocyte and NK cell activities, and complement-mediated effects. Sperm are iso- and autoantigenically immunosuppesive; therefore, substances produced within the male reproductive tract probably protect sperm from immunologic elimination. An absence of certain immunosuppressive components may predispose certain men, or their partners, to immunologic infertility. An important corollary is that the microenvironment of the sperm compartment and accessory organs may not be favorable for the immunologic elimination of virus-infected cells, other infectious organisms, or spontaneous neoplasms.

IMMUNOREGULATION

The antigenic nature of sperm is probably due to the appearance of sperm-specific proteins and glycoproteins at puberty, a time when numerous mature and reactive lymphocytes are present. Two important consequences of autoimmunization to sperm are 1. production of antisperm antibodies and 2. development of immunologically mediated aspermatogenesis, or allergic orchitis.[100,101] Autoimmunity to sperm, generally confined to experimental conditions, can be traumatically induced through testicular injury or surgical ligation of the sperm duct system. Spontaneous antisperm immunity is rare in men, and immunologic causes account for, at most, 5% to 10% of male infertility.[102] After vasectomy, however, persistent antisperm antibodies develop in 50% to 60% of men.[103] Apparently, this procedure disrupts the normal mechanisms that maintain immunologic tolerance to sperm. Orchitis is a rare condition in men, and develops secondarily to mumps infection or scrotal injury. Naturally occurring orchitis of suspected immunologic origin has been observed in black mink,[101] A-line beagles,[104] mice with the T-locus haplotype t^{w18},[105] and rhesus macaques.[102] These animals may be useful models in which to study the mechanisms that induce and maintain immunologic tolerance to sperm.

In the normal male, it is likely that autoimmunization to sperm is prevented by a combination of anatomical and physiological specializations, such as the blood-testis barrier, local production of immunosuppressive factors, and antigen-mediated mechanisms.

Immunosuppressive factors may be ubiquitous throughout the sperm compartment and not unique to secretions of the accessory glands. Mouse epididymal fluid has been shown to suppress the blastogenic responses of mouse spleen lymphocytes to T and B cell mitogens in vitro.[80] Furthermore, epididymal-testicular plasma obtained from the testicular ends of vasa deferentia of men undergoing vasovasostomy has been shown to contain nearly twice the amount of complement inhibitory activity as whole human seminal plasma.[87] Finally, autologous testicular germ cells have been shown to activate suppressor T lymphocytes in vitro,[106] and when injected into a syngeneic host, they reduce various indicators of cell-mediated immunity.[84] Whether or not soluble products of germ cells mediate germ-cell-induced suppression has not been tested.

The specialized inter-Sertoli-cell attachment region known as the blood-testis barrier is one of the tightest described for an epithelium, and effectively prevents leakage of germ cell components from the seminiferous tubules, as well as passage of immunoglobulins and lymphocytes into the tubules (Figure 19–8).[107,108] Resorption of germ cells and residual bodies by Sertoli cells may create a high concentration of autoantigens in the

adluminal compartment and thus require an exceptionally tight permeability barrier. However, the luminal contents may not be completely sequestered throughout the remainder of the sperm compartment distal to the blood-testis barrier. Less than ten parallel lines of discontinuous membrane fusion constitute a weak permeability barrier for the cuboidal epithelium of the rete testis, and the single discontinuous tight junctional strand that occurs between nonciliated cells of the efferent ducts is the weakest barrier of the sperm duct epithelium. Lanthanum has been shown to permeate intercellular spaces of the efferent ducts and gain access to the lumen in the rat.[109] Sperm autoantigens may not be completely sequestered, and a small amount of sperm antigen leakage may be required for the induction and maintenance of immunologic tolerance to sperm.

Thyroglobulin was once thought to be a sequestered antigen, but, with the advent of radioimmunoassays, it has been detected in serum of normal humans[110] and in the cervical lymphatics that drain the thyroid glands of non-human primates.[111] Antigen-mediated tolerance to thyroglobulin is thought to occur in human beings[112] and has been experimentally demonstrated in rabbits.[113] Likewise, antigen-mediated mechanisms may partially maintain a state of immunologic unresponsiveness toward sperm, and it is possible that sperm antigens interact with lymphocytes in normal males. Large quantities of sperm and cytoplasmic droplets are resorbed in the epididymis by mechanisms as yet undefined; half of the caput sperm disappear before reaching the cauda.[114] Soluble sperm antigens may leak from regions of the sperm compartment distal to the blood-testis barrier, and such regions are amply served by afferent lymphatics.

Recent experimental evidence favors the notion that suppressor T lymphocytes partially mediate the normal state of immunologic unresponsiveness toward sperm and testis autoantigens. In mouse experiments, T lymphocytes were required for the induction of EAO. The disease could not be induced in athymic BALB/c mr/mr mice, but susceptibility was restored after these mice received thymus cells from BALB/c nu/+ mice.[115] Thymectomy also prevented EAO,[116] but the effects of thymectomy varied according to timing of the procedure in relation to development of the immune system.[117] Experimental allergic orchitis was not easily induced in mice, and testicular homogenate had to be injected with Freund's complete adjuvant containing pertussis organisms to override tolerance. However, severe EAO and high titers of serum antisperm antibodies spontaneously developed in mice 3 to 4 months after thymectomy had been performed on postnatal day 3. The disease did not develop in mice thymectomized either on the day of birth or on day 7 after birth. In the same study, EAO did not develop in day-3-thymectomized mice given, on day 4, adult spleen cells from normal male, orchidectomized male, or female mice. When T lymphocytes were selectively removed from the normal male spleen cell population, the ability to prevent EAO was abolished. This evidence indicates that specific suppressor T lymphocytes are present in day-7-thymectomized mice, whereas this cell population is absent from day-3-thymectomized

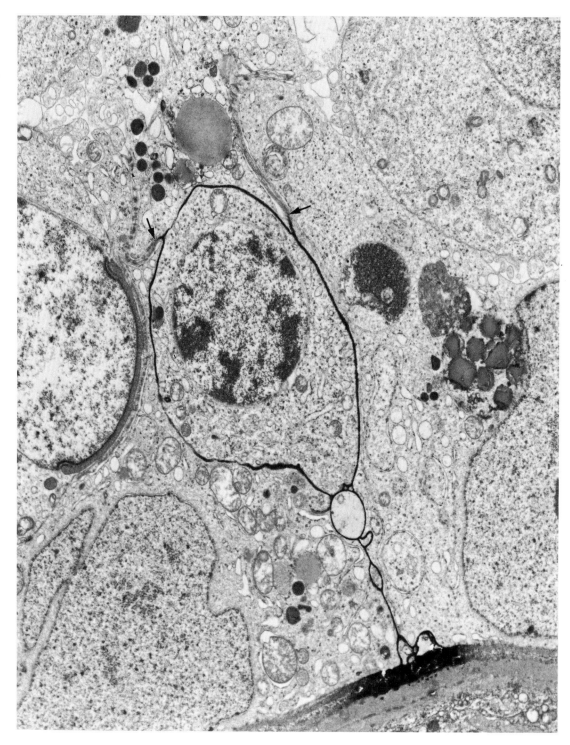

Figure 19–8. Lanthanum infiltration of a rat seminiferous tubule reveals that penetration stops at the tight junctions (arrow) (×9750).

mice; autoreactive T lymphocytes present in day-3-thymectomized mice are responsible for the EAO, and these cells are not present on the day of birth. Since the dose of adult spleen cells required to prevent EAO is ten-fold less when the cells come from normal males than when they

come from orchidectomized males and normal females, it is possible that specific suppressor T lymphocytes are activated by autoantigens of the testes.

In contrast neonatal thymectomy induces EAO in rats.[118] After vasectomy, antisperm antibodies develop in

Lewis, but not in Fisher 344 rats. However, neonatal thymectomy alone induces EAO and antisperm antibody production in both of these strains.

Further support for the role of suppressor T lymphocytes in mediating immunologic unresponsiveness to sperm and testis autoantigens has come from immunization experiments in guinea pigs. Tolerance to EAO induction resulted after injection of testis homogenate; subsequent immunization with testis homogenate in Freund's complete adjuvant did not result in EAO.[119] However, tolerance was abrogated when cyclophosphamide, which inactivates suppressor T lymphocyte precursors, was administered with the original tolerizing treatment.[120]

Finally, epididymitis is part of the natural history of the NZB mouse (unpublished observation). This fact deserves mention because 1. epididymitis is the first manifestation of EAO in 3-day-thymectomized mice[117] and 2. the major T lymphocyte defect in this autoimmune strain is in the function of suppressor T lymphocytes that express an Ly123+ phenotype and are responsible for feedback inhibition of antigen-induced helper T lymphocyte activity.[121]

Suppressor T lymphocytes are probably instrumental in the maintenance of immunologic tolerance to sperm and testis autoantigens. Because these antigens appear at puberty, they are viewed by mature and reactive lymphocytes as foreign, and suppressor T lymphocytes are likely to be partially responsible for the immunologically unresponsive state. Release of small amounts of sperm antigens from the sperm compartment may induce subclinical autoimmune responses that are accompanied by suppressor T cell activity.

IMMUNOGENETICS

Surgical ligation of the vas deferens (vasectomy) often results in autoimmunization against sperm antigens, and this widely accepted iatrogenic form of contraception provides a means of studying a persistent antibody response. There is a great amount of individual variation in the immune response to sperm after vasectomy, and results of studies on the pathophysiologic effects of vasectomy in animals have not been uniform. Through use of genetically standardized strains of laboratory animals, it has been learned that genetic factors can influence the degree of antisperm antibody responsiveness. Investigators have identified inbred strains of rats and mice in which either high or low serum titers of antibodies to sperm acrosomal antigens develop after vasectomy.[122,123] These investigators have further revealed that inbred strains of rodents can exhibit different degrees of antisperm immunity even though they may share an identical gene region that is known to control the degree of antibody responsiveness to a variety of synthetic and natural antigens. This gene region, known as the MHC, is characterized by a high degree of polymorphism, and the unique set of polymorphisms is known as the MHC haplotype for that strain. High antisperm antibody responder

DBA/1 mice and nonresponder BUB/Br mice both share the "q" MHC haplotype; Lewis and Fisher 344 rats share the MHC Ag-B1 region but differ in the postvasectomy prevalence of antiacrosomal antibodies. When congeneic rats were examined, no linkage was observed between the antiacrosomal antibody response after vasectomy and genes of either the MHC or the Y chromosome;[124] the response appeared to be controlled by more than a single gene lying outside the MHC.

In a genetic study on inbred guinea pigs, it was determined that the antibody response to testicular germ cell surface antigen (or antigens) after vasectomy is controlled by a single dominant gene.[125] A possible linkage of this response to other traits was not explored.

In a study involving 188 vasectomized men, association between the type of antisperm antibody and antigens encoded by the MHC loci was investigated. Head-to-head agglutinating antibody was found to be strongly associated with the A28 histocompatibility antigen. Production of agglutinins to the head region of sperm after vasectomy may be linked to a locus (or loci) within the human MHC.[126]

Genes that control antigen-specific antibody responsiveness could be responsible for the differences in serum antisperm antibody titers observed between inbred strains and individuals of outbred populations after vasectomy. However, in vasectomy studies one cannot control for several traits, such as the sperm production rate, route of immunization, antigenicity of sperm, and degree of acquired tolerance to sperm, that could contribute to variation in the immune response to sperm autoantigens. For example, monkeys that have high initial sperm counts exhibit sustained high levels of antisperm antibody,[127] and in men, higher preoperative sperm counts are associated with an early sperm-agglutinating antibody response.[128] The responder DBA/2 mouse strain produces about twice as many sperm as the nonresponder C57Bl/10 strain;[129] the antigen dose alone could explain differences in the antisperm antibody responses of these strains after vasectomy.

The earliest indication that antisperm antibody responses are under antigen-specific control of the immune response gene came from immunization experiments. Strain 2 and strain 13 guinea pigs showed opposite antibody responsiveness to 2 semipurified acrosomal antigens, known as P and S antigens.[130] Strain 2 responded more than strain 13 to P immunization, and strain 13 was a better responder than strain 2 to S immunization. Since these strains differ by only a single locus of the guinea pig MHC, the results indicate genetic control of the immune response gene type. In another study, a sperm immunization dose that distinguished, when 2 antigenic regions of sperm were examined, between high- and low-responder strains of genetically standardized mice was identified. Virgin females were used to eliminate concern about prior sensitization or tolerization to sperm antigens, and antibody responses were measured in parental, parental × F₁ backcross, and F₁ × F₁ inbred strains after immunization with syngeneic, allogeneic, or F₁ sperm. This study revealed that 1. antibody responsiveness to each of 2 antigenic regions of sperm is controlled through more than a single dominant gene, 2. these immune response genes are not linked to the immune response gene region of the murine MHC, and 3. acrosomal antigens differ in immunogenicity between strains, a trait linked to the Y chromosome.[131]

Genes that specifically control the degree of antisperm immunity are sufficient to explain individual differences in the development of antisperm antibodies after vasectomy. Men and women who are infertile because of high serum titers of antisperm antibodies may be genetically predisposed to this condition.

The most recent data suggest that environmental factors can influence the degree of antisperm immunity. The antiacrosomal antibody response of a single inbred rat strain was shown to vary according to the source of the animals.[124] Also, a colony of BALB/c mice that was resistant to induction of autoimmune orchitis became susceptible 4 months after it was moved to another facility (Tung, personal communication). Identification of these environmental factors may aid in our understanding of immunologically mediated infertility.

The main cause of antibodies in men is vasectomy, after which there is an apparent breakdown of certain barriers; antisperm antibodies have been detected in the serum or semen of a percentage of every mammalian species thus far studied (Figures 19–9,10,11). Spermatozoa can also cause antibody development in serum and reproductive fluids, including cervical mucus in women, but the reasons are not clear.

Two tests are commonly used to detect free antisperm antibodies: the sperm agglutination test and the sperm immobilization test. Sperm-agglutinating antibodies occur in approximately 67% of vasectomized men. Antibodies to sperm are found in less than 10% of infertile women. Sperm-immobilizing antibodies are also produced in vasectomized men (40%) and in about 8% of infertile women. As a rule the serum first is screened and then the seminal plasma or cervical mucus. Antibodies are usually of the IgG class, but IgA, and occasionally IgM, have been found in semen and cervical mucus. Recently an immunobead test involving micrometer-sized polyacrylamide beads coated with covalently-bound antiimmunoglobulin antibody for the detection of antisperm antibodies was developed. This rosette assay can provide information on the location of antibodies on the sperm surface (for instance, on the head, tail, midpiece, and tail tip). The immunoglobulin class can also be determined.

The question of how circulating antibodies affect fertility is unanswered. There may be three main anatomical levels at which antibodies have access to sperm antigens. *First,* antisperm antibodies might breach the blood-testis barrier and directly affect sperm production. Autoimmune orchitis can be induced in some men and animals by immunization with testicular tissue or spermatozoa.[132] Such an immune reaction in the testis involves the cellular immune system and perhaps the humoral system. Clinical support for this hypothesis is the demonstration of higher incidences of cellular immune responses to sperm in oligospermic men than in normal men.[133] Because of patchy seminiferous tubule degeneration, spermatogenesis is impeded but not stopped after vasectomy in some species, such as the guinea pig,[134] mouse (Figures 19–12,13),[135] and rabbit.[136,137] The humoral system may be involved in this phenomenon. Immune-complex deposition in the basal lamina surrounding the seminiferous tubules has been observed in long-term vasectomized rabbits with high levels of circulating antisperm antibodies.[136,137] Infertile men sometimes exhibit similar immune complexes in the basal lamina surround-

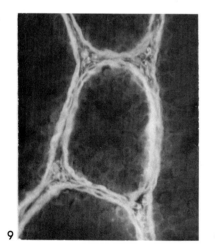 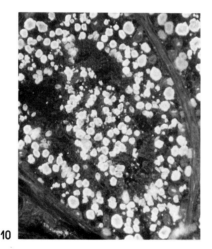 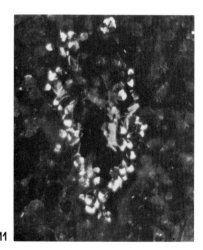

Figures 19–9,10,11. The blood-testis barrier prevents serum proteins from entering the seminiferous tubules. Blood proteins may be present around the tubules. Figure 19–9. Normal monkey testis stained with fluorescein-isothiocyanate (FITC) anti-IgG. Fluorescence appears only outside the barrier (×330). Figure 19–10. There are, however, antigenic moieties within the tubule. This testis section was exposed to serum from a vasectomized monkey and then FITC anti-IgG. The spermatocytes are entirely stained. Figure 19–11. Postvasectomy antibody types vary among individuals. This figure reveals that only mature sperm are stained when exposed to this vasectomy serum and FITC anti-IgG.

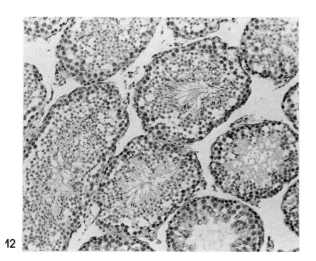
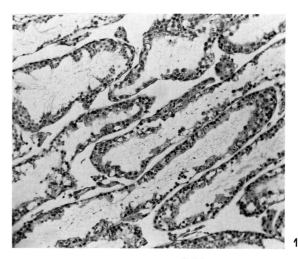

12   13

Figures 19–12,13. Allergic orchitis results in loss first of mature spermatozoa, then of spermatocytes, and finally of spermatogonia. In some species, such as the mouse, reduced spermatogenesis occurs after vasectomy. Figure 19–12 shows a testis section of a sham-operated control; Figure 19–13 is a section of testis from a mouse vasectomized 15 months earlier.

ing the seminiferous tubules.[138,139] Such deposition and associated patchy orchitis do not halt spermatogenesis but might make portions of the male reproductive duct accessible to immunoglobulins.

Second, antisperm antibodies might enter the male reproductive tract through the epididymis or the rete testis, which has long been considered a weak barrier (Figures 19–14,15).[140] Evidence includes the fact that broken and agglutinated sperm are common within the epididymal lumen in vasectomized monkeys with circulating complement-dependent antisperm antibodies.[141] Macrophages are commonly observed engulfing spermatozoa (Figure 19–16). Furthermore, immunoglobulins have been found in the luminal contents in vasectomized rabbit epididymides.[137] Such antibodies would have a long period of exposure to sperm and could aid in their degradation.

Third, antibodies to spermatozoa might enter the seminal plasma via transudation from the prostate.[98] The majority of immunoglobulin in the seminal plasma is of the G class and is contributed by the male accessory organ. In this case, spermatozoa would not be exposed to antisperm antibodies until ejaculation, when the antibodies could coat each spermatozoon. The antibody effect would depend upon the concentration, time, and contact with antigen. This hypothesis is supported by the finding that men with antibodies in their semen, as well as serum, are less fertile than men with only serum antibodies, and by the fact that there is a correlation between high levels of seminal plasma antibodies and high levels of circulating antibodies.[98]

In studies on rhesus macaques given vasectomies and subsequent vasovasostomies, antisperm antibody levels were determined. If antibodies could transude from the serum into the seminiferous tubules, spermatogenesis could be affected. In such a case, microscopic evaluation of ejaculated sperm from infertile monkeys with antibodies should reveal an increase in abnormal forms. Semen

samples were collected from fertile and subfertile monkeys that had undergone vasovasostomies, but no increase in abnormal forms proved evident.[142] If antigen-antibody reactions were occurring in the seminiferous tubules, immune-complex deposition in the basement membranes surrounding the tubules might have been expected. No evidence of immune-complex deposition was found in monkeys that had antisperm antibodies, which led to the hypothesis that the blood-testis barrier was intact in these animals. Thus, it appeared that fertility was not affected at the testicular level.

Since immunoglobulins might have had access to epididymal sperm, epididymal sperm were collected from infertile animals and stained to reveal antiimmunoglobulins. There was little indication that immunoglobulins were present within the epididymal lumen.

If spermatozoa were exposed to antisperm antibodies at the time of ejaculation, perhaps their longevity and ability to fertilize would be reduced. When the percentages of motility 30 minutes after ejaculation in fertile and infertile monkeys that had antisperm antibodies were compared, no significant difference was found. In another experiment semen samples, that is, homologous sperm and seminal plasma from fertile, subfertile, and infertile animals, were incubated, no remarkable difference in longevity was noted.

Sperm migration through the female tract, particularly through the cervical mucus, could be seriously impaired by antisperm antibodies. Such antibodies could adhere to the sperm surface and, without killing the sperm, could affect their motility and ability to penetrate cervical mucus. Kremer and Jager[143] have described such a phenomenon in which coated sperm exposed to antisperm antibodies exhibit shaking but poor forward progression through cervical mucus. In another study, when investigators took normal sperm and exposed them to serum containing antisperm antibodies, even though the initial motility was above 70%, the motility fell as the sperm

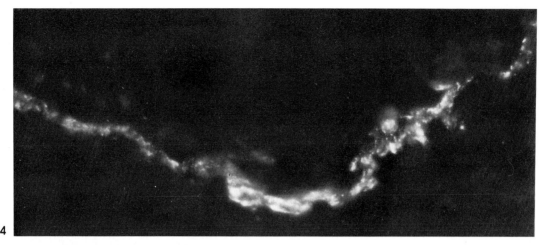

14

15

Figures 19–14,15. The immune response after vasectomy can result in immune-complex deposition, especially in the ductuli efferentes. Such complexes can be observed through the use of immuno-fluorescence and electron microscopy. Figure 9–14 reveals C3 deposits in the basement membrane (×800). Figure 9–15 is an electron micrograph of tissue from the same monkey. The immune complexes appear as electron densities in the thickened basement membrane (×16,000).

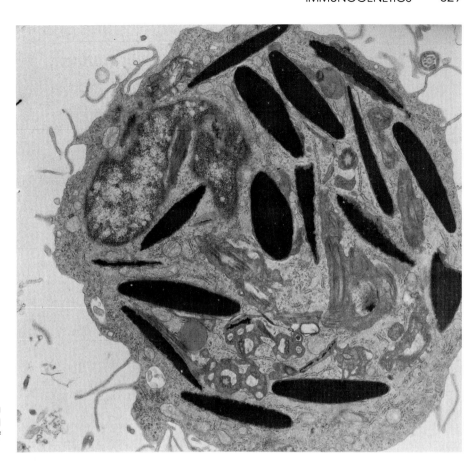

Figure 19–16. Vasectomy results in a macrophage influx into the proximal epididymis. Here the cells actively engulf and degrade sperm (×11,800).

proceeded through cervical mucus. Fewer sperm were observed in the distal portion of a capillary tube measurement system.[144] It seems that antisperm antibodies can affect sperm transit through cervical mucus. All types of antibodies tested, that is, agglutinating and immobilizing, and those revealed by immunofluorescence, affected penetration.

Antisperm antibodies develop in men as well as in animals after vasectomy. In a prospective study of 160 men, agglutinating antibodies were found in 63%, immobilizing antibodies in 37%, and antibodies in the seminal plasma in 3%.[145] Vasovasostomy did not increase serum antisperm antibody levels, although the percentage of men exhibiting such antibodies in their seminal plasma rose from 3% to 16%. This rise was most likely because of the contribution of the epididymal segment to the seminal plasma. Pregnancy rates were inversely correlated with antibody levels. No man in the study caused a pregnancy if he had a titer greater than 1 : 160 (Figure 19–17).

If antibodies to sperm can affect fertility, one might expect people with such antibodies to have their levels reduced by corticosteroids; such treatment should enhance pregnancy rates. This hypothesis was tested[146] by administration of prednisone to 24 patients; 26 patients with similar antibody levels were not treated and served as controls. Both men and women with antisperm antibodies were studied. In men, the drug did not change the sperm count, motility, or percentage of sperm with normal forms. It did, significantly, reduce the levels of circu-

lating sperm-immobilizing antibodies in both sexes (Tables 19–1,2). Fourteen pregnancies occurred in the 4-month evaluation period. It was thought that pregnancies in response to the therapy should occur within that time period. Significantly more pregnancies occurred in the treatment group than in the control group (45% versus 16%, p < 0.025) (Figure 19–18). Prednisone treatment did not always eliminate circulating antisperm anti-

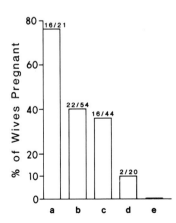

Figure 19–17. Correlation of serum sperm-agglutinating antibodies and pregnancy rates. The letters *a* through *e* indicate the titers: *a*, <1:20; *b*, ≥1:20; *c*, ≥1:40; *d*, ≥1:80; *e*, ≥1:160. The pregnancy rates drop as the husbands' serum antibody levels increase.

Table 19–1. Percentage of Patients with Sperm-agglutinating Antibodies

| Titer | Percentage | | |
	Control	Experimental before Treatment	Experimental after Treatment
1:640	23	29	10
1:160	35	46	10
1:40	73	75	33
1:10	100	96	57

Table 19–2. Percentage of Patients with Sperm-immobilizing Antibodies

| SIV[a] | Percentage | | |
	Control	Experimental before Treatment	Experimental after Treatment
	19	33	9
12	19	38	9
4	38	62	32
2	70	67	45

[a] Sperm immobilization value.

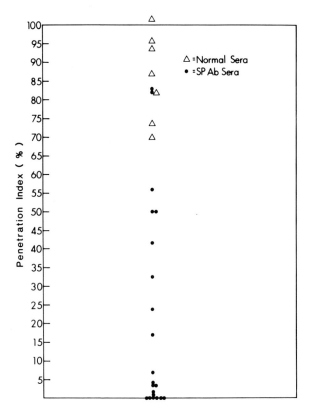

Figure 19–19. Comparison of the penetration indices of spermatozoa exposed to serum samples containing antisperm antibodies (SP Ab Sera) with those of spermatozoa not so exposed. These values are significantly different (p < 0.001).

bodies (the levels were measured 2 months after treatment). Perhaps doses other than 60 mg, or treatment periods longer than 7 days, would have been more effective. Data of Hendry and associates[147] suggest that lower levels may be effective in some patients.

In a study designed to clarify how antisperm antibodies can affect fertility, serum samples from patients with antisperm antibodies were added to sperm. Would sperm coated with antibodies penetrate hamster eggs? Six serum samples totally blocked and another 10 substantially reduced penetration (Figure 19–19). Only two samples yielded data comparable to those on the controls. The serum samples were purified and the IgG fraction was used to determine whether sperm-egg penetration was reduced because of the antibodies. This fraction caused a reduction similar to that found with whole serum, an indication that the observed effect occurred in the immunoglobulin fraction. No one antisperm antibody type was particularly associated with infertility. Agglutinating antibodies, immobilizing antibodies, and those revealed

by immunofluorescence were found in specimens affecting egg penetration.[148]

In a test of whether or not exposure of sperm to antisperm antibodies would reduce the ability of sperm to penetrate cervical mucus as well, 21% of the serum samples did reduce penetration. So antisperm antibodies affect cervical mucus penetration as well as oocyte fusion.[148]

CONCLUSION

Many proteins and other molecules associated with the reproductive tract are not produced until puberty. It is hardly surprising that the immune system recognizes them as foreign and responds. Allergic orchitis does not occur frequently in healthy men because of extremely effective mechanisms that deal with the byproducts of spermatogenesis. In the male, antisperm antibodies most commonly develop after vasectomy. Why all men do not produce antibodies is not understood. Some evidence points to sperm production rates, some to variability in sperm antigenicity, some to the presence of sperm granulomas and associated foreign body cells, and some to the hypothesis that a man's genetic make-up influences the type and intensity of his immune response. Obviously, vasectomy or testicular injury disrupts the normal mecha-

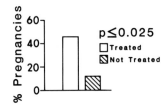

Figure 19–18. Percentage of pregnancies after prednisone treatment.

nisms that prevent responsiveness to sperm antigens. There is some experimental evidence that T cells are important mediators of immunologic tolerance to sperm antigens. This implies direct interaction of sperm components with the immune system.

Seminal plasma minimizes immunologic sensitization after insemination. Should a woman become responsive to sperm antigens, inseminated sperm would be afforded protection from cytotoxic antibodies by a potent complement inhibitor.

Immunologically mediated infertility has been difficult to define and ameliorate. Recent advances in molecular biology will surely provide us with better diagnostic approaches and therapeutic interventions.

References

1. Nicolson GL: Transmembrane control of the receptors on normal and tumor cells. II. Surface changes associated with transformation and malignancy. Acta Biochim Biophys 458:1–72, 1976.
2. Clermont Y, Leblond CP: Renewal of spermatogonia in rat. Am J Anat 93:475–501, 1953.
3. Huckins C: The spermatogonial stem cell population in adult rats. I. Their morphology, proliferation and maturation. Anat Rec 169:533–558, 1971.
4. Millette CF: Distribution and mobility of lectin binding sites on mammalian spermatozoa. In M Edidin, MH Johnson (eds): Immunobiology of Gametes. Cambridge, Cambridge University Press, pp 51–71, 1977.
5. Edelman GM: Surface modulation in cell recognition and cell growth. Science 192:218–226, 1976.
6. Elias PM, Friend DS, Goerke J: Membrane sterol heterogeneity: Freeze fracture detection with saponins and filipin. J Histochem Cytochem 27:1247–1260, 1979.
7. Koehler JK: The mammalian sperm surface: studies with specific labeling techniques. Int Rev Cytol 54:73–108, 1978.
8. Fawcett DW: The anatomy of the mammalian spermatozoon with particular reference to the guinea pig. Z Zellforsch Mikrosk Anat 67:279–296, 1965.
9. Millette CF, Bellvé AR: Selective partitioning of plasma membrane antigens during mouse spermatogenesis. Dev Biol 79:309–324, 1980.
10. Oliphant G, Singhas CA: Iodination of rabbit sperm plasma membrane: relationship of specific surface proteins to epididymal function and sperm capacitation. Biol Reprod 21:937–944, 1979.
11. Olson GE, Danzo BJ: Surface changes in rat spermatozoa during epididymal transit. Biol Reprod 24:431–443, 1981.
12. Friend DS, Orci L, Perrelet A, et al.: Membrane particle changes attending the acrosome reaction in guinea pig spermatozoa. J Cell Biol 74:561–577, 1977.
13. Millette CF, Bellvé AR: Temporal expression of membrane antigens during mouse spermatogenesis. J Cell Biol 74:86–97, 1977.
14. Romrell LJ, O'Rand MG: Capping and ultrastructural localization of sperm surface isoantigens during spermatogenesis. Dev Biol 63:76–93, 1978.
15. Brown PC, Holborow EJ, Glynn LE: The aspermatogenic antigen in experimental allergic orchitis in guinea pigs. Immunology 9:255–260, 1965.
16. Irvine WJ, Chan MM, Scarth L: The further characterization of autoantibodies reactive with extra-adrenal steroid-producing cells in patients with adrenal disorders. Clin Exp Immunol 4:489–503, 1969.
17. Wekerle H, Begemann M: Experimental autoimmune orchitis: In vitro induction of an autoimmune disease. J Immunol 116:159–161, 1976.
18. Tung KSK, Cooke WD Jr, McCarty TA, et al.: Human sperm antigens and antisperm antibodies. II. Age-related incidence of antisperm antibodies. Clin Exp Immunol 25:73–79, 1976.
19. Tung KSK: Human sperm antigens and antisperm antibodies. I. Studies on vasectomy patients. Clin Exp Immunol 20:93–104, 1975.
20. Rümke P: Sperm-agglutinating autoantibodies in relation to male infertility. Proc Roy Soc Med 61:275–278, 1968.
21. Rümke P, Hekman A: Autoimmunity to spermatozoa. Biol Reprod 25:1–8 and 113–117, 1975.
22. Poulsen F, Hjort T: Human sperm membrane antigens. II. Isolation and partial characterisation of labelled antigens. In JL Preud'homme, VAL Hawken (eds) Abstracts: 4th International Congress of Immunology of the International Union of Immunological Societies (held in Paris, July 21–26, 1980). Paris: French Society of Immunology, Abstract No. 16.1.19, 1980.
23. Isahakia M, Alexander NJ: Interspecies cross-reactivity of monoclonal antibodies directed against human sperm antigens. Biol Reprod 30:1015–1026, 1984.
24. Vitetta ES, Artzt K, Bennett D, et al.: Structural similarities between a product of the T/t-locus isolated from sperm and teratoma cells, and H-2 antigens isolated from splenocytes. Proc Natl Acad Sci USA 72:3215–3219, 1975.
25. Wachtel SS: H-Y antigen and the genetics of sex determination. Science 198:797–799, 1977.
26. Schachner M, Wortham KA, Carter LD, et al.: NS-4 (nervous system antigen-4), a cell surface antigen of developing and adult mouse brain and sperm. Dev Biol 44:313–325, 1975.
27. Landsteiner K, Levine P: On group specific substances in human spermatozoa. J Immunol 12:415, 1926.
28. Kerek G: Distribution of the blood group antigens A and B on human spermatozoa. Int J Fertil 19:181–191, 1974.
29. Jilek F, Veselský L: The occurrence of lymphocyte antigens on boar spermatozoa. J Reprod Fertil 31:295–298, 1972.
30. Mathur S, Melchers JT III, Ades EW, Williamson HO, et al.: Anti-ovarian and anti-lymphocyte antibodies in patients with chronic vaginal candidiasis. J Reprod Immunol 2:247–262, 1980.
31. Erickson RP: Differentiation and other alloantigens of spermatozoa. In M Edidin, MH Johnson (eds) Immunobiology of Gametes. Cambridge, Cambridge University Press, pp 85–114, 1977.
32. Anderson DJ, Narayan P, DeWolf WC: Major histocompatibility antigens are not detectable on post-meiotic human testicular germ cells. J Immunol 133:1962–1965, 1984.
33. Ritchie AWS, Hargreave TB, James K, et al.: Intra-epithelial lymphocytes in the normal epididymis. A mechanism for tolerance to sperm auto-antigens? Br J Urol 56:79–83, 1984.
34. Young WC: Study of function of epididymis; functional changes undergone by spermatozoa during their passage through epididymis and vas deferens in guinea pig. J Exp Biol 8:151–162, 1931.
35. Young DH: Surgical treatment of male infertility. J Reprod Fertil 23:541–542, 1970. (Abstr)

36. Hinrichsen MJ, Blaquier JA: Evidence supporting the existence of sperm maturation in the human epididymis. J Reprod Fertil 60:291–294, 1980.

37. Bedford JM: Maturation, transport, and fate of spermatozoa in the epididymis. *In* RO Greep, EB Astwood (eds) Handbook of Physiology (Sect 7). Endocrinology (Vol 5). Washington, DC, American Physiological Society, pp 303–317, 1975.

38. Hoskins DD, Casillas ER: Function of cyclic nucleotides in mammalian spermatozoa. *In* RO Greep, EB Astwood (eds) Handbook of Physiology (Sect 7): Endocrinology (Vol 5). Washington, DC. American Physiological Society, pp 453–460, 1975.

39. Hoskins DD, Johnson D, Brandt H, *et al.*: Evidence for a role for a forward motility protein in the epididymal development of sperm motility. *In* DW Fawcett, JM Bedford (eds) The Spermatozoon. Baltimore, Urban & Schwarzenberg, pp 43–53, 1979.

40. Bedford JM, Calvin HI: Changes in -S-S- linked structures of the sperm tail during epididymal maturation, with comparative observations in sub-mammalian species. J Exp Zool 187:181–204, 1974.

41. Tongkao D, Chulavatnatol M: Phosphorylation of microtubules of rat spermatozoa during epididymal maturation. *In* DW Fawcett, JM Bedford (eds) The Spermatozoon. Baltimore, Urban & Schwarzenberg, pp 129–134, 1979.

42. Hancock JL: The cytoplasmic beads of boar spermatotoa. J Endocrinol 14:xxxviii–xxxix, 1957. (Abstr)

43. Bedford JM, Cooper GW: Membrane-fusion events in fertilization of vertebrate eggs. *In* G Poste, GL Nicolson (eds) Cell Surface Reviews: Membrane Fusion (Vol 5). Amsterdam, Elsevier North Holland, pp 65–125, 1978.

44. Fournier-Delpech S, Courtens JL, Pisselet CL, *et al.*: Acquisition of zona binding by ram spermatozoa during epididymal passage, as revealed by interaction with rat oocytes. Gamete Res 5:403–408, 1982.

45. Saling PM: Development of the ability to bind to zonae pellucidae during epididymal maturation: reversible immobilization of mouse spermatozoa by lanthanum. Biol Reprod 26:429–436, 1982.

46. Jones R: Comparative biochemistry of mammalian epididymal plasma. Comp Biochem Physiol [B] 61:365–370, 1978.

47. Lea OA, Petrusz P, French FS: Purification and localization of acidic epididymal glycoprotein (AEG): A sperm coating protein secreted by the rat epididymis. Int J Androl (Suppl) 2:592–607, 1978.

48. Kohane AC, González Echeverría FMC, Piñeiro L, *et al.*: Interaction of proteins of epididymal origin with spermatozoa. Biol Reprod 23:737–742, 1980.

49. Moore HDM: Localization of specific glycoproteins secreted by the rabbit and hamster epididymis. Biol Reprod 22:705–718, 1980.

50. Orgebin-Crist M-C, Danzo BJ, Davies J: Endocrine control of the development and maintenance of sperm fertilizing ability in the epididymis. In RO Greep, EB Astwood (eds) Handbook of Physiology (Sect 7): Endocrinology (Vol 5). Washington, DC, American Physiological Society, pp 319–338, 1975.

51. Feuchter FA, Vernon RB, Eddy EM: Analysis of the sperm surface with monoclonal antibodies: topographically restricted antigens appearing in the epididymis. Biol Reprod 24:1099–1110, 1981.

52. Moore HDM, Hartman TD: Localization by monoclonal antibodies of various surface antigens of hamster spermatozoa and the effect of antibody on fertilization *in vitro*. J Reprod Fertil 70:175–183, 1984.

53. Orgebin-Crist M-C: Studies on the function of the epididymis. Biol Reprod (Suppl) 1:155–175, 1969.

54. Schlegel W, Fischer B, Beier HM, *et al.*: Effects on fertilization of rabbits of insemination with ejaculates treated with PG-dehydrogenase and antisera to PGE-2 and PGF-2α. J Reprod Fertil 68:45–50, 1983.

55. Acott TS, Hoskins DD: Bovine sperm forward motility protein partial purification and characterization. J Biol Chem 253:6744–6749, 1978.

56. Fuchs A-R: Uterine activity during and after mating in the rabbit. Fertil Steril 23:915–923, 1972.

57. Bedford JM: Development of the fertilizing ability of spermatozoa in the rabbit epididymis. J Reprod Fertil 10:286–287, 1965. (Abstr)

58. Edwards RG: Antigenicity of rabbit semen, bull semen, and egg yolk after intravaginal or intramuscular injections into female rabbits. J Reprod Fertil 1:385–401, 1960.

59. Waldman RH, Cruz JM, Rowe DS: Immunoglobulin levels and antibody to *Candida albicans* in human cervicovaginal secretions. Clin Exp Immunol 10:427–434, 1972.

60. Polakoski KL, Syner FN, Zaneveld LJD: Biochemistry of human seminal plasma. *In* ESE Hafez (ed) Human Semen and Fertility Regulation in Men. St. Louis, CV Mosby, pp 133–142, 1976.

61. Yang S-L, Schumacher GFB: Immune response after vaginal application of antigens in the rhesus monkey. Fertil Steril 28:314–315, 1977. (Abstr)

62. Ansbacher R, Manarang-Pangan S, Srivannaboon S: Sperm antibodies in infertile couples. Fertil Steril 22:298–302, 1971.

63. Isojima S, Koyama K, Tsuchiya K: The effect on fertility in women of circulating antibodies against human spermatozoa. J Reprod Fertil (Suppl) 21:125–150, 1974.

64. Mettler L, Scheidel P, Shirwani D: Sperm antibody production in female sterility. Int J Fertil 19:7–12, 1974.

65. Bouffioux CR: Prostatic cancer: epidemiology and etiology. *In* M Pavone-Macaluso, PH Smith (eds) Cancer of the Prostate and Kidney. New York, Plenum Press, pp 17–32, 1983.

66. Gittes RF, McCullough DL: Occult carcinoma of the prostate: an oversight of immune surveillance—a working hypothesis. J Urol 112:241–244, 1974.

67. Centifanto YM, Drylie DM, Deardourff SL, *et al.*: Herpes virus type 2 in the male genitourinary tract. Science 178:318–319, 1972.

68. Ulstein M, Capell P, Holmes KK, *et al.*: Nonsymptomatic genital tract infection and male infertility. *In* ESE Hafez (ed) Human Semen and Fertility Regulation in Men. St. Louis, CV Mosby, pp 355–362, 1976.

69. Lang DJ, Kummer JF: Demonstration of cytomegalovirus in semen. N Engl J Med 287:756–758, 1972.

70. Ho DD, Schooley RT, Rota TR, *et al.*: HTLV-III in the semen and blood of a healthy homosexual man. Science 226:451–453, 1984.

71. Zagury D, Bernard J, Leibowitch J, *et al.*: HTLV-III in cells cultured from semen of two patients with AIDS. Science 226:449–451, 1984.

72. Broxmeyer HE, Smithyman A, Eger RR, *et al.*: Identification of lactoferrin as the granulocyte-derived inhibitor of col-

ony-stimulating activity production. J Exp Med 148:1052–1067, 1978.

73. Polakoski KL, Kopta M: Seminal plasma. *In* LJD Zaneveld, RT Chatterton (eds) Biochemistry of Mammalian Reproduction. New York, John Wiley & Sons, pp 89–117, 1982.

74. Davis CP: Inhibition of PHA-induced lymphocyte transformation by human semen. Seventeenth Interim Congress of the South African Society of Obstetricians and Gynaecologists, Pretoria, p 45, 1974.

75. Stites DP, Erickson RP: Suppressive effect of seminal plasma on lymphocyte activation. Nature 253:727–729, 1975.

76. Pitout MJ, Jordan JH: Partial purification of an antimitogenic factor from human semen. Int J Biochem 7:149–151, 1976.

77. Lord EM, Sensabaugh GF, Stites DP: Immunosuppressive activity of human seminal plasma. I. Inhibition of *in vitro* lymphocyte activation. J Immunol 118:1704–1711, 1977.

78. Marcus ZH, Freisheim JH, Houk JL, *et al.: In vitro* studies in reproductive immunology. 1. Suppression of cell-mediated immune response by human spermatozoa and fractions isolated from human seminal plasma. Clin Immunol Immunopathol 9:318–326, 1978.

79. Prakash C, Coutinho A, Möller G: Inhibition of *in vitro* immune responses by a fraction from seminal plasma. Scand J Immunol 5:77–85, 1976.

80. Anderson DJ, Tarter TH: Immunosuppressive effects of mouse seminal plasma components *in vivo* and *in vitro*. J Immunol 128:535–539, 1982.

81. James K, Harvey J, Bradbury AW, *et al.*: The effect of seminal plasma on macrophage function—a possible contributory factor in sexually transmitted disease. AIDS Res 1:45–57, 1983.

82. Chvapil M, Stankova L, Bernhard DS, *et al.* Effect of prostatic fluid and its fractions on some functions of peritoneal macrophages. Invest Urol 15:173–179, 1977.

83. Nathan CF: Secretion of oxygen intermediates: role in effector functions of activated macrophages. Fed Proc 41:2206–2211, 1982.

84. Hurtenbach U, Shearer GM: Germ cell-induced immune suppression in mice. Effect of inoculation of syngeneic spermatozoa on cell-mediated immune responses. J Exp Med 155:1719–1729, 1982.

85. Tarter TH, Koide SS, Cunningham-Rundles S: Human seminal plasma suppression of natural killer cell activity. Clin Res 32:385A, 1984. (Abstr)

86. Peterson BH, Lammel CJ, Stites DP, *et al.*: Human seminal plasma inhibition of complement. J Lab Clin Med 96:582–591, 1980.

87. Tarter TH, Alexander NJ: Complement-inhibiting activity of seminal plasma. Am J Reprod Immunol 6:28–32, 1984.

88. Peitz B, Bennett D: Inhibition of complement-mediated cytotoxicity of antisera by fluid secreted by the seminal vesicle of the house mouse. J Reprod Immunol 3:109–116, 1981.

89. Tarter TH, Isahakia M: Inhibition of complement-mediated hemolysis by aqueous extracts of monkey prostate and seminal vesicle. J Androl 3:10, 1982. (Abstr)

90. Brooks GF, Lammel CJ, Petersen BH, *et al.*: Human seminal plasma inhibition of antibody complement-mediated killing and opsonization of *Neisseria gonorrhoeae* and other gram-negative organisms. J Clin Invest 67:1523–1531, 1981.

91. Price RJ, Boettcher B: The presence of complement in human cervical mucus and its possible relevance to infertility in women with complement-dependent sperm-immobilizing antibodies. Fertil Steril 32:61–66, 1979.

92. Carraher RP: The induction and activity of sperm immobilizing antibody in rabbit cervicovaginal secretion. Contraception 15:15–23, 1977.

93. Parrish WE, Carron-Brown JA, Richards CB: The detection of antibodies to spermatozoa and to blood group antigens in cervical mucus. J Reprod Fertil 13:469–483, 1967.

94. Cantuária AA: Sperm immobilizing antibodies in the serum and cervicovaginal secretions of infertile and normal women. Br J Obstet Gynaecol 84:865–868, 1977.

95. Husted S, Hjort T: Microtechnique for simultaneous determination of immobilizing and cytotoxic sperm antibodies. Methodological and clinical studies. Clin Exp Immunol 22:256–264, 1975.

96. Mukherjee DC, Agrawal AK, Manjunath R, *et al.*: Suppression of epididymal sperm antigenicity in the rabbit by uteroglobin and transglutaminase in vitro. Science 219:989–991, 1983.

97. Cunningham-Rundles C, Brandeis WE, Good RA, *et al.*: Milk precipitins, circulating immune complexes, and IgA deficiency. Proc Natl Acad Sci USA 75:3387–3389, 1978.

98. Rümke P: The origin of immunoglobulins in semen. Clin Exp Immunol 17:287–297, 1974.

99. Linnet L, Fogh-Andersen P, Hjort T, *et al.*: Immunoglobulin classes, secretory component, and sperm agglutinins in semen after vasovasostomy. Am J Reprod Immunol 2:13–17, 1982.

100. Shulman S: Reproduction and Antibody Response. Cleveland, CRC Press, p 12, 1975.

101. Tung KSK, Teuscher C, Meng AL: Autoimmunity to spermatozoa and the testis. Immunol Rev 55:217–255, 1981.

102. Alexander NJ, Tung, KSK: Effects of vasectomy in rhesus monkeys. *In* IH Lepow, R Crozier (eds) Vasectomy: Immunologic and Pathophysiologic Effects in Animals and Man. New York, Academic Press, pp 423–458, 1979.

103. Tung KSK: Autoimmunity of the testis. *In* DS Dhindsa, GFB Schumacher (eds) Immunological Aspects of Infertility and Fertility Regulation. New York, Elsevier North Holland, pp 33–91, 1980.

104. Fritz TE, Lombard SA, Tyler SA, *et al.*: Pathology and familial incidence of orchitis and its relation to thyroiditis in a closed beagle colony. Exp Mol Pathol 4:142–158, 1976.

105. Dooher GB, Artzt K, Bennett D, *et al.*: Observations on autoimmune orchitis in sterile mice carrying a recessive lethal mutation at the T/t complex exhibiting spontaneous allergic orchitis. J Reprod Fertil 62:505–511, 1981.

106. Hurtenbach U, Morgenstern F, Bennett D: Induction of tolerance *in vitro* by autologous murine testicular cells. J Exp Med 151:827–838, 1980.

107. Gilula NB, Fawcett DW, Aoki A: The Sertoli cell occluding junctions and gap junctions in mature and developing mammalian testis. Dev Biol 50:142–168, 1976.

108. Fawcett DW: Interpretation of the sequelae of vasectomy. *In* IH Lepow, R Crozier (eds) Vasectomy: Immunologic and Pathophysiologic Effects in Animals and Man. New York, Academic Press, pp 3–23, 1979.

109. Suzuki F, Nagano T: Regional differentiation of cell junctions in the excurrent duct epithelium of the rat testis as revealed by freeze-fracture. Anat Rec 191:503–519, 1978.

110. Torrigiani G, Doniach D, Roitt IM: Serum thyroglobulin

levels in healthy subjects and in patients with thyroid disease. J Clin Endocrinol Metab 29:305–314, 1969.

111. Daniel PM, Pratt OE, Roitt IM, et al.: The release of thyroglobulin from the thyroid gland into thyroid lymphatics; the identification of thyroglobulin in the thyroid lymph and in the blood of monkeys by physical and immunological methods and its estimation by radioimmunoassay. Immunology 12:489–504, 1967.

112. Chiller JM, Habicht GS, Weigle WO: Kinetic differences in unresponsiveness of thymus and bone marrow cells. Science 171:813–815, 1971.

113. Weigle WO: Analysis of autoimmunity through experimental models of thyroditis and allergic encephalomyelitis. Adv Immunol 30:159–273, 1980.

114. Hafez ESE, Prasad MRN: Functional aspects of the epididymis. In ESE Hafez (ed) Human Semen and Fertility Regulation in Men. St. Louis, CV Mosby, p 34, 1976.

115. Bernard CCA, Mitchell GF, Leydon J, et al.: Experimental autoimmune orchitis in T-cell-deficient mice. Int Arch Allergy Appl Immunol 56:256–263, 1978.

116. Vojtíšková M, Pokorná Z: Prevention of experimental allergic aspermatogenesis by thymectomy in adult mice. Lancet 1:644–645, 1964.

117. Taguchi O, Nishizuka Y: Experimental autoimmune orchitis after neonatal thymectomy in the mouse. Clin Exp Immunol 46:425–434, 1981.

118. Lipscomb HL, Gardner PJ, Sharp JG: The effect of neonatal thymectomy on the induction of autoimmune orchitis in rats. J Reprod Immunol 1:209–217, 1979.

119. Chutná J, Rychlíková M: Prevention and suppression of experimental autoimmune aspermatogenesis in adult guinea pigs. Folia Biol 10:177–187, 1964.

120. Chutná J: Study of mechanism of specific inhibition of delayed sensitivity and IgM antibodies in guinea pigs immunized with organ-specific antigen. Int Arch Allergy 37:278–292, 1970.

121. Cantor H, McVay-Boudreau L, Hugenberger J, et al.: Immunoregulatory circuits among T-cell sets. II. Physiologic role of feedback inhibition in vivo: Absence in NZB mice. J Exp Med 147:1116–1125, 1978.

122. Bigazzi PE, Kosuda LL, Harnick LL: Sperm autoantibodies in vasectomized rats of different inbred strains. Science 197:1282–1283, 1977.

123. Kosuda LL, Bigazzi PE: Autoantibodies to acrosomal antigens of spermatozoa in vasectomized mice. Invest Urol 16:140–141, 1978.

124. Takami T, Kunz HW, Gill TJ, III, et al.: Genetic control of autoantibody production to spermatozoa in vasectomized rats. Am J Reprod Immunol 2:5–7, 1982.

125. Tung KSK, Teuscher C, Goldberg EH, et al.: Genetic control of antisperm autoantibody response in vasectomized guinea pigs. J Immunol 127:835–839, 1981.

126. Law HY, Bodmer WF, Mathews JD, et al.: The immune response to vasectomy and its relation to the HLA system. Tissue Antigens 14:115–139, 1979.

127. Alexander NJ: Vasectomy and vasovasostomy in rhesus monkeys: the effect of circulating antisperm antibodies on fertility. Fertil Steril 28:562–569, 1977.

128. Linnet L, Hjort T: Sperm agglutinins in seminal plasma and serum after vasectomy: correlation between immunological and clinical findings. Clin Exp Immunol 30:413–420, 1977.

129. Shire JGM, Bartke A: Strain differences in testicular weight and spermatogenesis with special reference to C57BL/10J and DBA/2J mice. J Endocrinol 55:163–171, 1972.

130. Toullet F, Voisin GA: Induction d'orchi-épididymite aspermatogène autoimmune et de réponses immunes chez des cobayes des lignes consanguines S2 et S13 par immunisation avec des spermatozoides isogéniques et allogéniques et des autoantigènes extraits de spermatozoides homologues. Ann Immunol (Paris) 130C:373–384, 1979.

131. Tarter TH, Alexander NJ: Genetic control of humoral immunity to sperm acrosomal and cell surface antigens. J Reprod Immunol 6:213–226, 1984.

132. Tung KSK, Alexander NJ: Autoimmune reactions in the testis. In AD Johnson, WR Gomes (eds) The Testis (Vol 4). New York, Academic Press, pp 491–516, 1977.

133. Wall JR, Stedronska J, David RD, et al.: Immunologic studies of male infertility. Fertil Steril 26:1035–1041, 1975.

134. Alexander NJ: Autoimmune hypospermatogenesis in vasectomized guinea pigs. Contraception 8:147–164, 1973.

135. Anderson DJ, Alexander NJ: Antisperm antibody titres, immune complex deposition and immunocompetence in long-term vasectomized mice. Clin Exp Immunol 43:99–108, 1981.

136. Bigazzi PE, Kosuda LL, Hsu KC, et al.: Immune complex orchitis in vasectomized rabbits. J Exp Med 143:382–404, 1976.

137. Alexander NJ, Tung KSK: Immunological and morphological effects of vasectomy in the rabbit. Anat Rec 188:339–350, 1977.

138. Dondero F, Isidori A: Autoimmunisation antitesticularie chez l'homme. Ann Endocrinol (Paris) 33:417–425, 1972.

139. Rabin BS, Nankin HR, Troen P: Immunological studies of patients with idiopathic oligospermia. In P Troen, HR Nankin (eds) The Testis in Normal and Infertile Men. New York, Raven Press, pp 435–441, 1977.

140. Waksman BH: Experimental allergic encephalomyelitis and the "auto-allergic" diseases. Int Arch Allergy 14 (Suppl):1–87, 1959.

141. Alexander NJ: Immunologic and morphologic effects of vasectomy in the rhesus monkey. Fed Proc 34:1692–1697, 1975.

142. Alexander NJ, Fulgham DL: Antibodies to spermatozoa in male monkeys: Mode of action. Fertil Steril 30:334–342, 1978.

143. Kremer J, Jager S: The sperm-cervical mucus contact test: a preliminary report. Fertil Steril 27:335–340, 1976.

144. Alexander NJ: Evaluation of male infertility with an in vitro cervical mucus penetration test. Fertil Steril 36:201–208, 1981.

145. Fuchs EF, Alexander NJ: Immunologic considerations before and after vasovasostomy. Fertil Steril 40:497–499, 1983.

146. Alexander NJ, Sampson JH, Fulgham DL: Pregnancy rates in patients treated for antisperm antibodies with prednisone. Int J Fertil 28:63–67, 1983.

147. Hendry WF, Treehuka K, Hughes L, et al.: Cyclic prednisolone therapy for male infertility associated with autoantibodies to spermatozoa. Fertil Steril 45:249–254, 1986.

148. Alexander NJ: Antibodies to human spermatozoa impede sperm penetration of cervical mucus or hamster eggs. Fertil Steril 41:433–439, 1984.

20. Semen Analysis, Sperm Functional Abnormalities, and Enhancement of Semen Parameters

B. Jane Rogers and Lonnie D. Russell

Routine semen analyses evaluate sperm concentration, motility, and morphology. While informative, the results provide no direct information about the functional capabilities of the sperm. Many men are diagnosed as normal, based on the three major semen criteria, when, in fact, they are functionally abnormal. The reverse misdiagnosis also occurs when a patient exhibits an abnormal count, motility, or morphology, but in reality has functionally competent sperm. The focus of this chapter is to examine semen analysis parameters (Table 20–1) which can diagnose the fertilization potential and other functional aspects of sperm. Techniques for improvement of semen parameters are presented and critically evaluated.

ROUTINE SEMEN ANALYSIS

The routine semen analysis is performed with widely varying degrees of skill and sophistication. The most rudimentary semen analysis consists of a simple count. Although no consistency exists, most laboratories report values for sperm concentration, percentage motility, and percentage of sperm with normal morphology.

A brief article which appeared a few years ago referred to the semen analysis as "the neglected laboratory test."[1] These authors echo our sentiments concerning the poor quality of performance and reporting of the semen analysis. They collected data from 64 laboratories to compare the semen analyses offered and felt that there was an absolute need for adequate standardization of this important test since it is the basis of the clinician's important decision for implicating the male partner in the infertility problem. They concluded that very few laboratories update their normal values or follow the standards for semen analysis as proposed by the World Health Organization.[2]

Standards for normality vary; Table 20–2 shows the values given for normal parameters in our routine semen analysis. Chong and coworkers[1] recommend the following standards for normal semen: a. volume: 1 to 5 ml; b. liquefaction: within 20 minutes; c. sperm concentration: more than 20,000,000/ml; d. percent motility (at 37° C): more than 50% (rated 0% to 100%); e. forward progression: more than 5+ (at 37° C, rated 0 to 10+; this decreases significantly after 5 hours); f. percent normal morphology: more than 60%; g. white blood cell count: none/hpf; h. pH: 7.3 to 7.7; i. agglutination: occasionally, and in small clumps. Considerable variability in sperm output is to be expected, and more than one sample may be required to establish an adequate estimate of both sperm quantity and quality.[3] Morphology appears to be the most stable semen parameter if skillfully and correctly evaluated. Since immature forms and leukocytes are difficult to distinguish, and their improper identification and quantitation can lead to errors in semen cytology, these values should be weighted in terms of the quality of the laboratory.

Semen parameters which are clearly in the normal range allow an easy diagnosis, but equivocal analyses are common and contribute to inaccurate diagnoses of male infertility. The utilization of more sophisticated functional tests can perhaps provide better diagnosis and treatment of male infertility. In addition, since count, motility, and morphology do not correlate absolutely with fertility, even well-performed semen analyses cannot be sufficiently diagnostic in many instances. In our experience, semen samples with counts as low as 6 million/ml have been associated with pregnancies while those as high as 330 million/ml were found with fertility impairment. Motility is, in general, not a good predictor when percentage of motile sperm by itself is considered. However, more sophisticated evaluations of motility quality (see section on motility) appear to be highly diagnostic. The routine analysis generally evaluates just motility and only very low motility values are diagnostic. Morphology appears to be the best predictor of fertility potential[3,4] among the routine semen parameters.

Table 20–1. Sperm Functions Available for Potential Use in Fertility Diagnosis

Sperm Function	Assayable Parameter
Penetrate cervical mucus	Mucus Penetration
Swim to site of fertilization	Motility
Capacitation and acrosome reaction	Acrosome reaction
Penetrate cumulus matrix surrounding egg	Hyaluronidase
Penetrate zona-pellucida of egg	Acrosin
Fuse with egg	Sperm penetration assay (hamster egg)

Table 20–2. Normal Values for Routine Semen Analysis

Volume	1.5 – 5.0 ml
Concentration	Greater than 20 million/ml
Total count	Greater than 30 million
Motility	Greater than 50% motile
Activity	Greater than 2 (1 = sluggish; 4 = very active)
Forward progression	Greater than 2 (1 = slight; 4 = energetic)
Liquefaction	Liquefied within 30 minutes
Viscosity	Greater than 2 (1 = high; 4 = low)
Agglutination	Slight
Morphology	Greater than 50% normal
WBC	Less than 1 million/ml

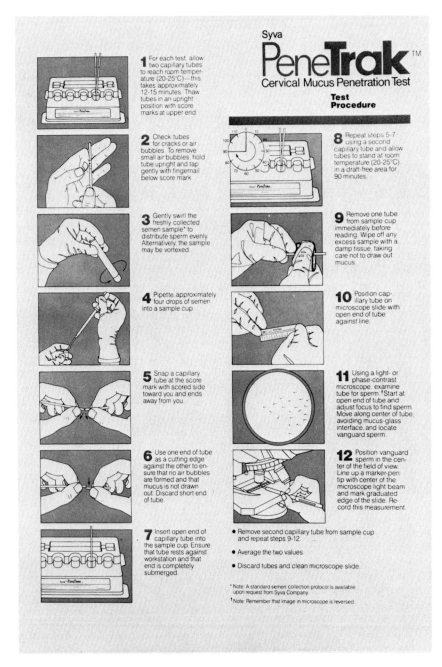

Figure 20–1. Method for the bovine cervical mucus (BCM) penetration assay. Capillary tubes containing mucus are commercially available as the PENETRAK® test from Syva Company, Palo Alto, California.

CERVICAL MUCUS PENETRATION

Penetration of mucus is one *in vitro* technique to assess the functional competence of human spermatozoa. Passage of spermatozoa through the mucus of the cervical canal *in vivo* is a critical step. In the absence of mucus penetration none of the other steps in fertilization matter since the sperm would not reach the egg. An evaluation of the interaction of spermatozoa and cervical mucus is regarded by some to be essential in the investigation of the infertile couple.[5] *In vitro* penetration tests can reveal incompatibilities within a couple, such as hostile cervical mucus and antibodies to spermatozoa, as well as information about the quality of the spermatozoa. The mucus needed for these tests is produced only during the periovulatory phase of a woman's menstrual cycle. Bovine cervical mucus is more readily obtained than human cervical mucus (HCM), and human spermatozoa can penetrate bovine cervical mucus at the same rate as human cervical mucus[6] or faster.[7] Bovine cervical mucus can be effectively substituted for human cervical mucus in laboratory testing of spermatozoa.[7–12]

A description of the procedure for the bovine cervical mucus penetration laboratory test (Figure 20–1) will indicate the ease of performance. After a period of sexual abstinence of at least 48 hours, semen samples are collected in sterile plastic containers and allowed to liquefy for 30 minutes at room temperature. Two flat, sealed capillary tubes of bovine cervical mucus are brought to room temperature by allowing them to thaw for 10 minutes in an upright position with the score marks at the top. Four drops (0.2 ml) of fully liquefied semen are pipetted into a labeled sample cup. One tube is broken cleanly at the score mark, held with the open end up, and tapped to remove any bubbles. The open end is inserted into the sample cup, and the time of insertion recorded. The second tube is inserted into the same cup following an interval of a few minutes. After incubation at room temperature for 90 minutes, the first tube is removed and wiped clean of residual semen, care being taken to avoid drawing any mucus from the open end. The tube then is placed on a calibrated microscope slide and examined at a magnification of ×100. The vanguard spermatozoa are located using either phase contrast or dark field microscopy. The second tube is examined in the same way. Mucus penetration test results are reported as the average migration distance of the vanguard spermatozoa in the two tubes. Mucus penetration from 0 to 20 mm is considered inadequate or reduced, 21 to 30 mm unclear or not discriminated, and greater than 30 mm adequate or normal. The actual technician time to do the manipulations required for this procedure is less than a half hour. Its simplicity enables the test to be used as a routine screen for spermatozoal functional competence.

Comparisons of the penetration ability of fertile and infertile groups is imperative in establishing the usefulness of a mucus penetration assay. In our study[13,14] 32 men who were known to be fertile (who had previously fathered a child) and 18 men who were known to be infertile (with a wife previously pregnant from another partner) were evaluated, using bovine cervical mucus (BCM). Spermatozoa from all of the fertile men penetrated more than 20 mm into the BCM. This result was obtained in 13 of the 18(72%) infertile men (Figure 20–2). Thus, when these 50 men of known clinical status were evaluated as a group to determine the accuracy of the test, the mucus results predicted 74%(37/50) correctly. These results suggest that a negative value is predictive of a fertility problem but a positive result does not guarantee fertility.

In a previous study by Alexander[8] comparing the incidence of pregnancy for individuals with adequate and inadequate penetration, she found that more individuals with good penetration caused a pregnancy. Of 9 couples evaluated for fertility in whom the husband had good penetration, 6 of the wives conceived. Of 18 couples in whom the husband had poor penetration, 4 of the wives conceived.

A different approach to the relevance of mucus penetration to infertility was taken by Matthews and associates.[15] In their study of 132 infertile couples, only 17(13%) of the initial cycles tested had absent mucus penetration. On retesting, 12 of these 17 had normal results. Of the other five, two were not retested and three had a semen factor. The authors suggested that defective sperm penetration was not the explanation for the long-term infertility of these couples.

When bovine mucus penetration is compared for three groups of differing fertilizing potential, overlap of the ranges are seen between the groups (Figure 20–3). In the group with 0% fertilization (penetration in the zona-free hamster egg), the mucus penetration ranged from 3 mm to 56 mm. In the presumably fertile group (penetration ≥ 10%), the range of mucus penetration was 12 mm to 64

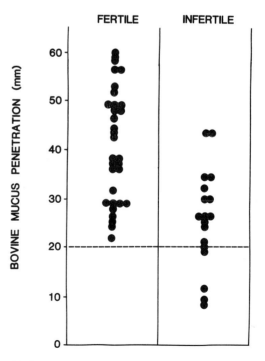

Figure 20–2. Comparison of penetration rates into bovine cervical mucus (BCM) by spermatozoa from fertile and infertile men.

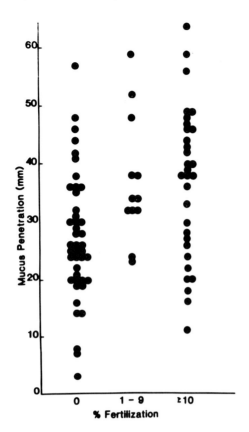

Figure 20–3. Comparison of penetration rates into bovine cervical mucus (BCM) by spermatozoa of different fertilizing potential in the zona-free egg assay. Groups based on penetration rates into zona-free hamster eggs: 0% = subfertile; 1–9% = equivocal range; ≥10% = fertile.

mm. These data suggest that the diagnostic potential of the mucus penetration is not always unequivocal.

Another interesting facet of the mucus-semen interaction is provided by the work of Schats and colleagues[16] with patients who had unexplained infertility. Evidence of impaired cervical mucus penetration was found in nine of the 20 couples. This impairment was found to be due to defective sperm function rather than to the cervical mucus quality.

SPERM MOTILITY

In the evaluation of fertilizing potential, sperm motility is a key attribute of semen quality. Sophisticated techniques have been developed to measure objectively the detailed movement characteristics of human spermatozoa. These techniques include time-exposure photomicrography,[17] videomicrography[18] and cinematography.[19] The level of sophistication of these techniques has evolved considerably in the last seven years.

Two photographic techniques for spermatozoal motility determination which are objective were reported in 1979.[17,20] In the Makler method[20] the percentage of motile sperm is determined, and their average speed and the frequency distribution of their velocities are analyzed ob-

jectively and concomitantly. The samples are analyzed within 30 to 90 minutes by the multiple exposure photography method (MEP) which involves taking still camera photomicrographs after films are exposed for one second while moving spermatozoa are illuminated by six short light pulses. Each of two or three drops from a specimen are inserted into a 10 μm counting chamber having a built-in grid, and the photographs are made in four predetermined corners of the grid. Eight to twelve pictures of 300 to 400 spermatozoa/specimen are obtained. Later, measurements are made manually from film projected on 30 × 20 cm sheets of paper. The following information can be obtained: percentage of motile sperm, average and frequency distribution of spermatozoal velocities and sperm concentration. A photomicrograph of a specimen with a high count and low motility rate (Figure 20–4A) is contrasted with a specimen with a low count and high motility rate (Figure 20–4B). In the high count sample the average speed was 28 μm/second, while in the low count sample the average speed was 43 μm/second. The moving sperm appear as six ringed chains, whereas the nonmotile sperm appear as a more accentuated head.

The second technique developed in 1979 for spermatozoal motility determination was a simple objective method which involves 1-second time-exposure photomicrographs taken with dark field illumination.[17,21] The negatives are projected as a filmstrip and are analyzed on a specially designed console. The authors suggest that the filmstrips can be taken and developed in 15 minutes without darkroom facilities, and that a complete analysis of the film would require an additional 15 to 20 minutes. To determine percentage motility, 50 spermatozoa are examined and movement characteristics are recorded for 15 spermatozoa. The sperm suspension after analysis can be described in terms of percentage motility, mean swimming speed, percentage of progressive spermatozoa, mean swimming speed of progressive spermatozoa, percentage of straight-swimming spermatozoa, percentage of rolling spermatozoa, and percentage of yawing spermatozoa. A print of a photographic negative (Figure 20–5) shows different characteristic patterns of sperm movement.

The first comparison of velocity measurements for fertile and infertile groups done with time-lapse photography appeared in 1980.[22] The infertile group of 50 patients was found to have a statistically significant lower sperm velocity than the 20 patients in the fertile group. The dividing line between the two groups appeared to be approximately 30 mm/sec. The authors concluded that the mean sperm velocity was a more important parameter in assessment of the infertile male than sperm density.

The time-exposure system was largely superseded by videomicrography in 1981.[18,21] Objective quantitative measurements of percentage motility, mean swimming speed, and the percentage of progressive sperm can be made directly from the video image. The basic system is composed of the following instruments which are relatively low-cost and technically simple: a video camera mounted on a microscope, a video cassette recorder, a photographic enlarger timer, and a television monitor.

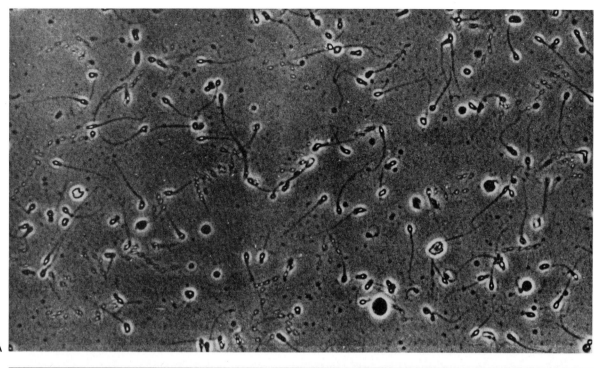

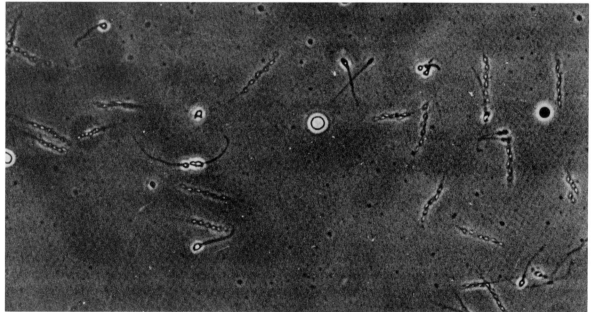

Figure 20–4. Motility determination using the multiple exposure photography method (MEP). A. Sample with high count and low motility has few 6-ringed chains. B. Sample with low count and high motility has many 6-ringed chains. (From Makler and coworkers.[20])

Measurements are made on 10 independent microscopic fields that have been videotaped for 10 seconds each. Swimming speeds are measured with the aid of an analysis transparency consisting of concentric circular arcs. Videotapes have been used to assess sperm motility and morphology in fertile and infertile patients.[23] Morphologically normal sperm were more motile than abnormal sperm in the same ejaculate. In addition, normally-shaped sperm in semen from infertile men were less

likely to be motile than normal sperm in the semen of fertile men.

Functional defects were sought in the motility of sperm from cases of unexplained infertility and oligozoospermia using the technique of time-exposure photomicrography.[24,25] Compared with the fertile group, a majority of movement characteristics were significantly depressed in the group with unexplained infertility. Characteristics significantly related to fertilizing capacity were progressive

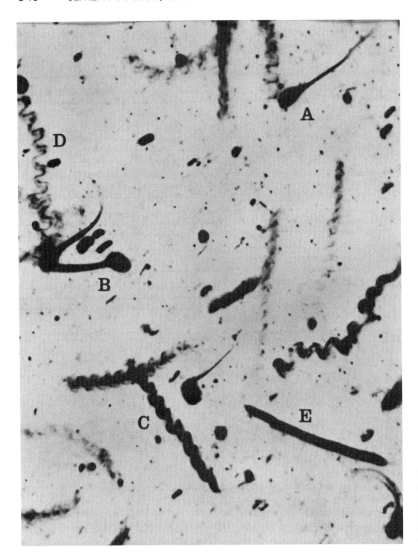

Figure 20–5. Characteristic patterns of sperm movement evaluated by time-exposure photomicrography. (From Overstreet and coworkers.[17]) A. Immotile sperm. B. Stationary sperm with active flagellum. C. Rolling sperm. D. Yawing sperm. E. Straight-swimming sperm.

swimming speed (>25 mm/sec), a straight mode of progression, and a small amplitude of lateral head displacement. Total mean velocity, however, showed a poor correlation with sperm function. In contrast, the total mean velocity of the sperm from the oligozoospermic men was significantly decreased relative to the normal fertile controls.

Multiple exposure photomicrography (MEP) has been used more recently to identify samples in a group presenting for infertility evaluation.[26] Using threshold values which were chosen to allow 96% of the semen samples from the fertile population to be scored as fertile, the MEP technique was able to identify 45% of the samples at the infertility clinic as infertile. This compared to 66% identification of infertile samples by using the sperm penetration assay. As seen in Figure 20–6, the mean track speed of 37 um/sec. gives an 88% specificity. MEP thus has discriminating ability that is valuable in the assessment of male infertility. The MEP technique has been used more recently to compare infertile oligospermic and fertile men.[27] A significant decrease in sperm velocity was observed in infertile oligospermic men as compared to fertile men (45.40 u/sec vs. 38.21 u/sec).

The most recent advances in objective motility evaluation are the automated[28] and semi-automated[29,30] techniques that utilize computer technology. These methods are based on image analysis that records the images of moving sperm, reconstructs the sperm trajectories by the analysis of sequential images, and describes these trajectories. The three types of recording techniques are photomicrography, videomicrography, and microcinematography. A completely automated system requires an automated film reader, an image analyzer, and a minicomputer, in addition to the usual cell, camera, and microscope.

The ultimate question to be answered about quantitative objective motility measurements is: "Do these speed measurements relate to fertility?" An attempt to answer that question was made by comparing speed measurements with the ability of sperm to penetrate both intact human eggs and zona-free hamster eggs.[30] Sperm velocity measurements were found to correlate well with both types of egg penetration. The proportion of slow-swimming cells (<20 um/sec) was found to be a better predictor than mean sperm swimming speed. A conflicting report by Hope[31] did not find a significant difference for

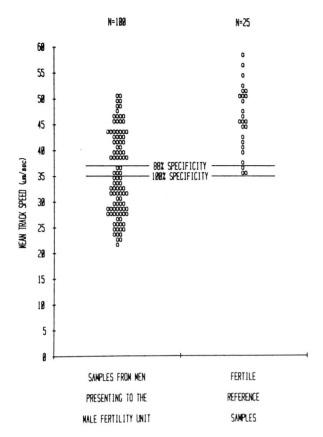

Figure 20-6. Distribution of sperm track speeds in fertile and infertile men. (From Albertsen and coworkers.[26])

sperm swimming speed between fertile and infertile groups. In this study, the two groups were not, however, sufficiently well defined to make a final judgment on the diagnostic potential of swimming speed. The fertile individuals were "presumed" normal and the infertile ones were patients attending an infertility clinic. The objective assessment of sperm movement characteristics does appear to have great potential for an improved semen analysis. The functional property, motility, when evaluated without subjectivity, may become the most readily available diagnostic parameter of spermatozoa.

CAPACITATION AND ACROSOME REACTION

The need for acrosome reaction to take place for successful penetration of an egg makes it a logical candidate to assay in order to determine the fertilizing potential of sperm. This essential prerequisite for fertilization has been monitored in animal species that have large, and thus easily visible, acrosomes such as the guinea pig and hamster. However, human sperm have very small inconspicuous acrosomal caps. Loss of the human sperm acrosomal cap is not discernible at the light microscope level unless sperm are specially stained. The development of a triple-stain technique which allows direct assessment of normal acrosome reaction[32] has provided the tool to

evaluate a potential correlation between acrosome reaction rate and sperm fertilizing ability.

A study by Plachot and coworkers[33] monitored the acrosomal reaction using the triple stain technique after a 17-hour incubation period. The increase of acrosome reaction in living spermatozoa was from 4.2% to 16%. This low level of acrosome reaction did not, unfortunately, correlate with the ability of sperm to fertilize mature oocytes *in vitro*. The staining patterns obtained using the triple stain are shown in Figure 20-7. A staining pattern which shows a white acrosomal region and a light brown postacrosomal region is indicative of the normal live acrosome reaction. The problem with all acrosome reaction studies is the occurrence of a degenerative acrosome reaction associated with sperm death. Often the percentage of "dead" acrosome reaction is greater than the "live" acrosome reaction. In the Plachot study this was also the case. The "dead" acrosome reaction increased from 5.3% to 26%. This complication can be adequately handled using the triple-stain technique since the "live" and "dead" acrosome reactions have a distinguishing postacrosomal region.

In evaluating the relationship of the acrosome reaction to fertilizing ability, only the acrosome-reacted living sperm are important in this correlation. The acrosome-reacted sperm ranged from 1% to 51% after the 17-hour capacitation period.[33] Three categories of acrosome reaction percentages were established to analyze the fertilization data: 3% to 10%, 11% to 20%, and 21% to 51%. The percent of patients demonstrating fertilizing potential in each group was 71%, 80%, and 85%, respectively. The differences were not statistically significant, although the percentage fertilization was highest in the group with most acrosome reaction. A very low level of acrosome reaction (4%) was found to be consistent with optimal fertilization rates. The authors state, "Unfortunately, the scoring of the acrosome reaction of free-swimming spermatozoa does not appear as a useful test in predicting the fertilizing ability of a semen sample."

Another technique has been more recently demonstrated to rapidly and reproducibly assay for acrosome reaction using monoclonal antibodies which are specific to antigens localized in the acrosomal region.[34] This technique was developed to answer questions concerning the relationship of capacitation and acrosome reaction to fertility. Two monoclonal antibodies were found which recognized target antigen restricted to the acrosomal cap. Their disappearance was monitored, using indirect immunofluorescence. Loss of specific antibody binding was correlated with complete acrosomal loss as quantitated by transmission electron microscopy. One drawback to this approach is that a distinction between acrosome reaction in live and dead fixed sperm must be made by concurrent measurements of viability and motility. Alternatively, living motile sperm can be scored directly. The acrosome reaction in the study by Wolf *et al.*[34] was accomplished using the calcium ionophore, A23187,[35] rather than monitoring naturally occurring reactions. They feel that the relationship between acrosomal status and fertility remains an open question and they are continuing work on establishing an assay for human sperm

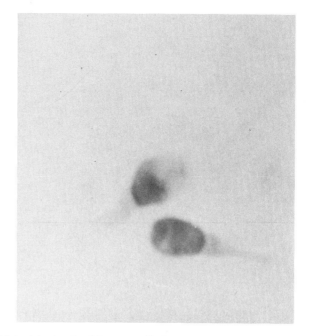

Figure 20–7. Acrosome reaction patterns with the triple stain showing living sperm that are acrosome intact (pink) and acrosome reacted (white), as shown in the Color Plate after page 84. (Provided by Dr. P. Talbot).

capacitation. Their current approach is to contrast the ability of capacitated and noncapacitated sperm to respond to ionophore-induced acrosome reaction.

CUMULUS MATRIX PENETRATION

One of the functions necessary for sperm to reach and fertilize the egg is penetration of the cumulus matrix which holds the cumulus cells together around the egg. The hyaluronic acid molecules in the matrix are acted on by hyaluronidase in the acrosome of the sperm. This enzymatic action allows the sperm to digest a path to the egg. The hyaluronidase released from the sperm appears to be essential for fertilization.[36] The absence of such an essential enzyme or a reduction in quantity could theoretically impair the sperm's fertilizing potential. The measurement of the quantity of hyaluronidase would appear to be an appropriate functional assay for fertilizing potential. Recently,[37] the first report on human sperm hyaluronidase release and extraction appeared. Surprisingly, the hyaluronidase from human spermatozoa is rapidly inactivated upon release. In addition, almost no hyaluronidase could be extracted from frozen thawed human testes and none was detectable in fresh or frozen human seminal plasma. Even though the levels of hyaluronidase could relate to fertilizing potential, the utilization of such an assay must await the development of extraction procedures that prevent inactivation of the enzyme.

ZONA PELLUCIDA PENETRATION

Acrosin, the trypsin-like enzyme which facilitates zona penetration, is thought to be necessary for fertilization

and is thus a potential diagnostic parameter. It has been evaluated in symptomatic and asymptomatic men in fertile couples,[38] as well as in cases of unexplained infertility and oligospermia.[39] The routine semen parameters measured in the 45 asymptomatic men were significantly higher than in the 51 symptomatic men: sperm concentration, 109 vs. 54 million/ml; concentration of motile sperm, 75 vs. 22 million/ml; percent morphologically normal, 74 vs. 39. The values for asymptomatic men showed three times as much total acrosin as those for symptomatic men (106 vs. 35 MIU/10^7 spermatozoa). In comparing fertile donors with unexplained infertility patients and oligospermic patients, the acrosin levels were higher in the fertile donors (18.8 ng/10^6 sperm) than in the unexplained (10.7) or oligospermic (6.7) group. One cannot conclude that the decreased fertilizing potential is directly associated with the lowered acrosin levels. Whatever is causing the reduction in other parameters in the symptomatic men could also be affecting the biochemical properties of the sperm. Another possibility is that reduced acrosin levels could simply be related to more morphologically abnormal sperm forms with less acrosin. It may be, however, that there is an inherent acrosin deficiency in the sperm of the unexplained infertility group. The assay of acrosin activity could be a useful test of functional potential for penetration of the zona pellucida.

SPERM PENETRATION ASSAY

The function of sperm which is directly relevant to fertility potential is the actual penetration of the egg. Using viable human eggs as test eggs is obviously unacceptable because of moral, ethical, and logistical considerations. Even though the penetration of a human egg is the ultimate fertilization test, the substitution of an animal egg is the only feasible approach to *in vitro* fertilization testing. Since cross-species fertilization does not occur naturally, the surrogate egg is specially processed to remove the zona-pellucida which is the site ensuring species specificity during fertilization. At present the animal egg of choice is the zona-free hamster egg. Cross-species fertilization was first demonstrated in 1972[40,41] using zona-free hamster eggs and various animal sperm. The technique was extended to human sperm in 1976.[42] It was then possible to test sperm functionally using human sperm and zona-free hamster eggs. Soon after, in 1979,[43] Rogers' laboratory provided the first fertilization ranges for fertile and infertile men using the zona-free hamster eggs. This functional diagnostic test of sperm fertilizing ability has been widely used since. Recent comprehensive reviews of the procedure and its usefulness[44–48] can be referred to for further detail on the subject. The purpose of this section is to discuss the assay methodology, the relationship of assay results to fertilizing potential in clinical terms, the correlation with other semen analysis parameters and its potential usefulness in diagnosing and treating sperm abnormalities in the infertile male.

The assay methodology for the sperm penetration assay (SPA) as originally described[42,43] is shown in Figure 20–8. The semen sample is collected after at least 48 hours of abstinence, and allowed to liquefy at room tem-

perature for 30 minutes. Processing entails 3 washes at 600 x g for 5 minutes, using BWW culture medium supplemented with 0.3% BSA. The final pellet is ultimately resuspended to a concentration of 10 million spermatozoa per ml and incubated in a 0.5 ml volume in capped Falcon® tubes for 18–20 hours at 37°C in an air incubator.

The simplicity of this method would allow performance of the assay in most clinical laboratories that do routine semen analyses. The basic equipment needed is a microscope, a desk-top centrifuge, and an air incubator.

To prepare the zona-free hamster eggs, the animals are injected with PMS 2 days before the semen is obtained. This is on day 1 of the animal's 4-day-cycle. The hamsters are given an hCG injection on the same day the semen is collected (day 3 of the hamster's cycle) and are sacrificed to recover the oviducts on the day after the semen is collected. Recovering sperm early allows them to preincubate before combining with the eggs.

The rationale for a long preincubation is to allow capacitation and to provide for a flexible protocol that fits into the time constraints of the clinical setting. Patients can be scheduled at various times in the afternoon and technicians are not required to work 10- to 12-hour days. After removal of the oviducts, the tubules are pricked with a needle-pointed probe at the point of cumulus streaming as viewed under a dissecting microscope. The

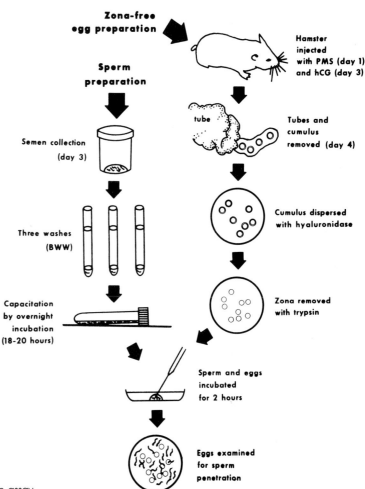

Figure 20–8. Method for performance of sperm penetration assay.

cumulus mass extrudes into the BWW medium in a watch glass or culture dish. The cumulus cells are removed by hyaluronidase (0.1 mg/ml) treatment and the zona-pellucida is removed by trypsin (0.1 mg/ml) treatment. These steps are separated and followed by three wash steps. The trypsin step is extremely critical. The eggs are continuously observed microscopically while in the trypsin to monitor zona dissolution. After zona dissolution (usually about 30 seconds) they are quickly pipetted out of the trypsin. Either too long or too short a period in the trypsin is detrimental to assay results. The preincubated sperm are aliquoted in 100 ul drops into Falcon® culture dishes under mineral oil. Twenty to 25 eggs are placed in one drop. Forty to 50 eggs are examined per patient after a 2-to-3-hour coincubation period. Eggs are placed on a slide covered with a coverslip supported by drops of vaseline-paraffin mixture and examined using a phase contrast microscope. The presence of swollen heads with attached tails is taken as evidence of penetration (Figure 20–9). Percentage of eggs penetrated is recorded as well as the number of swollen heads per egg.

A relationship between the SPA results and true fertilizing potential *in vivo* is best established by evaluating clearly defined groups of fertile and infertile males. When the author (B.J.R.) did this initially,[43] the ranges were 14%–100% penetration for fertile groups and 0–10% for infertile groups. Others[44] have demonstrated similar ranges for groups of different fertility status. At least 18 investigators[44] have published ranges for fertile and infertile samples.

It is disconcerting to find that in many studies there are no clear ranges for discriminating fertile from infertile samples. Much of the problem is due to the establishment of inappropriate groupings to represent fertile or infertile categories. "Men attending an infertility clinic" is not an adequate grouping to establish an infertile category. Other problems associated with establishment of ranges is the existence of false negatives in the bioassay. Men who are truly fertile could score 0% on the assay due to the presence of white blood cells, lack of compliance with abstinence requirements, errors in sample collection, or technical errors in assay performance. Though it is difficult to establish absolute ranges, the preponderance of evidence suggests that the penetration of zona-free hamster eggs correlates very well with fertilizing potential *in vivo*. A positive result is highly diagnostic. A clearly negative result (0%) is diagnostic, if reproducible and without extenuating circumstances such as the presence of numerous white blood cells.

Possible correlation of SPA results with routine semen analysis parameters has been diligently sought by numerous investigators.[44] We initially reported no significant correlation between either sperm concentration or percentage motile sperm and egg penetration results.[43] Conflicting results regarding correlations have been reported. In simplistic terms, count, motility, and morphology may not show significant correlation with SPA results in normal fertile men, but some correlations become significant when looking at groups of oligospermic men or those with unexplained infertility. Morphology and motility characteristics seem to be the most correlated parameters with SPA. The penetration of zona-free eggs appears to be the most successful parameter in predicting infertility, while multiple exposure photomicrography for measuring motility ranks second, and morphology for normal sperm forms ranks third.[44] The SPA is not simply a verification of an abnormal semen analysis. If the penetration results correlated perfectly with semen analysis parameters there would be no point in performing this bioassay. In a group of 616 individuals

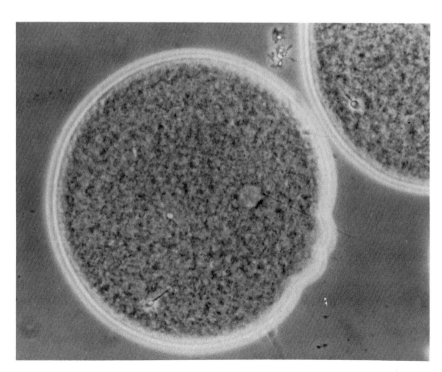

Figure 20–9. Test egg used in sperm penetration assay (SPA). The zona-free hamster egg has been penetrated by one human sperm. The swollen head is visible as a clear area with an attached tail.

with less than 10% penetration, we analyzed the presence of routine semen analysis parameters (concentration, motility, morphology). A subset of individuals (21.1%) had no obvious semen abnormality but had poor penetration in the SPA and were clinically infertile (Figure 20–10). This is the type of individual who would be misdiagnosed in the absence of an SPA. Since routine infertility workups would not include an SPA, these individuals would be most likely detected in an unexplained infertility situation.

The SPA can be useful both in diagnosing and monitoring treatment in the subfertile male, but it is not intended as a routine screen for every infertility work-up. The situations in which the test is most useful appear to be in an equivocal semen analysis or unexplained infertility. The subset of infertile men who are not readily detectable because of abnormal semen parameters can be diagnosed with the SPA. Conversely, men with apparent abnormalities in the routine semen analysis can prove to be penetrators in the SPA and subsequently initiate a pregnancy. Thus the SPA puts a new perspective on sperm pathology with emphasis on functional abilities rather than the traditional evaluation of count, motility, and morphology.

Fertility impairment, once diagnosed, can readily be monitored after treatment is initiated using the SPA. The major problem here is that the treatments available for subfertility are less than encouraging. We have monitored surgical treatments of varicocele,[49,50] the most commonly diagnosed cause of male infertility, as well as Clomid® therapy.[51,52] One of the most relevant findings in both studies was that even though routine semen parameters such as sperm concentration showed improvement, a concomitant enhancement of *in vitro* egg penetration

or pregnancy rates did not occur. In the varicocele study, a high incidence of pregnancy (70%) was observed in those who did improve in the SPA following surgery. The Clomid® results were less encouraging since only one patient had a marginal SPA increase even though half the study group showed a count increase. Any new and innovative treatment protocol can be evaluated reasonably objectively using the SPA without any influence of the female partner on the efficacy of therapy.

IMPROVEMENT OF SEMEN PARAMETERS

Compared with other mammalian species, the human ejaculate is highly heterogeneous in both the kinds and numbers of particulate matter and cells present (Figure 20–11) as well as the functional status of these cells. Motility in apparently normal samples ranges from about 50% to 80%. Given the high heterogeneity of the sample and general low motility in normal individuals, it is not surprising that individuals whose semen analysis is classified as abnormal frequently provide semen samples which are of extremely poor quality. Unless techniques have been used to separate motile and morphologically normal sperm from the remainder of the sample, biochemical and certain other kinds of data obtained on sperm in research laboratories must be questioned simply on the basis of the purity of semen samples used to obtain such data. There is a need for semen samples to be enriched in the population of normal motile sperm, relatively free from contamination, for both research and clinical purposes. With the growing number of *in vitro*

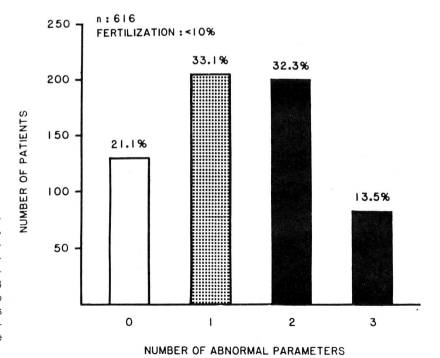

Figure 20–10. Distribution of abnormal parameters in patients who had penetration rates <10% in the SPA. Values that were considered abnormal for the routine parameters were concentration of <20 million/ml, motility of <50% and morphology of <50% normal forms. If all 3 parameters were abnormal, the patient fell into category 3. All combinations of 2 abnormalities were grouped together. Any of the 3 abnormalities occurring alone was categorized in one group.

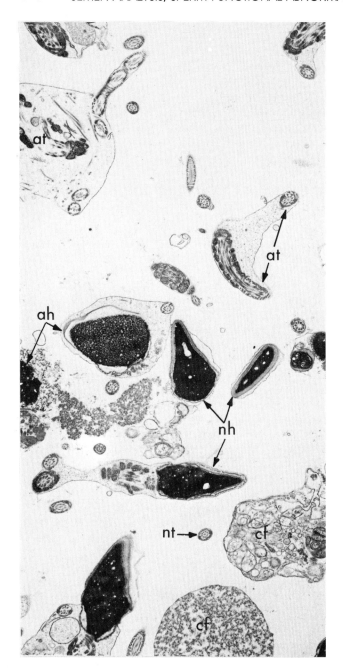

Figure 20–11. Electron micrograph of an unprocessed, pelleted sample. Various abnormal and normal constituents are seen, including several profiles of multiple or folded flagella within a single cytoplasmic boundary.

Key for Figures 20–11 through 16: normal sperm heads = nh; abnormal sperm heads = ah; normal tails = nt; abnormal tails = at; cytoplasmic fragments = cf; cellular elements = ce.

fertilization programs, there is also a definite need to use the best sperm population of a particular sample to achieve fertilization.

Percentage motility, as expressed in traditional semen analyses, and swimming ability, as measured by more sophisticated techniques, are different motility parameters. Given a sufficient number of sperm, the latter mea-

surement is the more useful predictor of sperm function. Sperm motility itself has been used as a basis for separating highly motile sperm from those with little or no motility.[53–56] Separation based on their ability to "swim up" or "rise" in test tube conditions is useful in situations where a small number of highly motile sperm are needed. Different laboratories have slight modifications; the basic sperm rise procedure as done in our laboratory is summarized in Figure 20–12.

In order to compare the effectiveness of the rise procedure we examined individuals who were participating in an *in vitro* fertilization program.[56,57] Semen obtained by masturbation was allowed to liquefy for 30 minutes prior to performing a routine semen analysis and processing for the sperm rise. Several parameters were analyzed as shown in Tables 20–3 to 6. For these data, counts were performed using a hemocytometer, and motility scored using at least 100 sperm. Light microscopic morphology was demonstrated using stained smears in which over 100 sperm were evaluated.

For the rise procedure (shown in Figure 20–12), the semen sample is diluted with an equal volume of insemination medium (IM) which is Ham's F-10 medium containing 7.5% heat-treated fetal cord serum. The sample is washed by centrifugation at 600 g for 10 minutes and the supernatant removed using a Pasteur pipette. The pellet is gently resuspended in 2 ml of IM and washed as before. After removing the supernatant, the pellet is resuspended thoroughly with IM to a final volume of 0.3 ml. This concentrated sperm sample is then underlayered beneath 2 ml of IM in a Falcon® tube taking care to avoid introduction of bubbles. The tube (loosely capped) is placed in a 37°C incubator (5% CO_2 and air) at a 60° angle for 1 1/2 hours to allow the motile sperm to migrate or "rise" into the upper portion of the medium. After 1 1/2 hours, the top 1.6 to 1.8 ml is carefully removed from the tube while it is still held at an angle. Care is taken not to disturb the interface between the concentrated sperm in the bottom of the tube and the upper layer containing the actively motile sperm. The removed sperm are termed the "rise" and the remaining sperm termed the "non-rise."

Both the rise and unprocessed semen samples were analyzed for routine semen parameters in 63 individuals.[57] Table 20–3 shows the semen analysis data as expressed for these individuals. The motility of the rise sample was

Table 20–3. Comparison of Rise and Unprocessed Semen Samples[a]

	Concentration	Motility	Morphology
	(Sperm/ml × 10⁶)	(% motile)	(% normal)
Unprocessed sample	92.8 (±1.00)	51.8 (±0.44)	57.8 (±0.39)
Rise sample	10.2 (±0.36)	89.1 (±0.44)	79.2 (±0.44)
N = 63			

[a] Mean values are represented with standard error in parentheses. $p < 0.001$ for each initial and rise comparison.

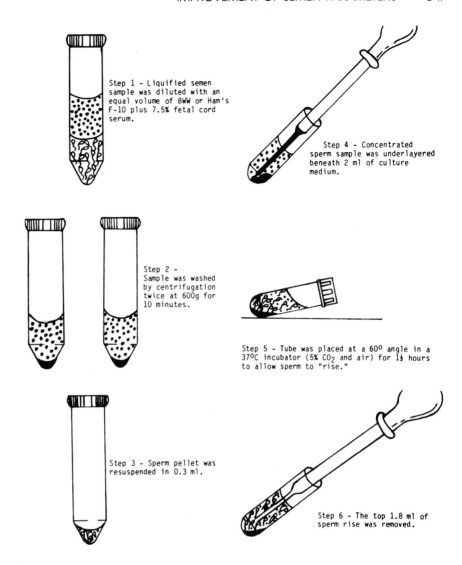

Step 1 - Liquified semen sample was diluted with an equal volume of BWW or Ham's F-10 plus 7.5% fetal cord serum.

Step 2 - Sample was washed by centrifugation twice at 600g for 10 minutes.

Step 3 - Sperm pellet was resuspended in 0.3 ml.

Step 4 - Concentrated sperm sample was underlayered beneath 2 ml of culture medium.

Step 5 - Tube was placed at a 60° angle in a 37°C incubator (5% CO_2 and air) for 1½ hours to allow sperm to "rise."

Step 6 - The top 1.8 ml of sperm rise was removed.

Figure 20–12. Sperm rise procedure.

significantly enhanced from 51.8% to 89.1% (p < 0.001) and the normal morphology from 57.8% to 79.2% (p < 0.001). In a subset of 25 individuals (Table 20–4), where the nonrise portion of the sample was also analyzed, the number of rise sperm represented 5.9% of the total number of sperm in the unprocessed initial ejaculate. The motility was enhanced from 52.4% in the unprocessed sample to 90.3% in the rise sample. An enhancement in normal morphology from 58.0% to 80.8% was recorded for these same groups. The nonrise samples had an even lower percentage of motile sperm and normal forms than the unprocessed sample. This is due to the selective dis-

Table 20–4. Semen Parameters in Rise, Nonrise, and Unprocessed Semen Samples[a]

	Concentration (10⁶ Sperm/ml) [Range]	Total Sperm	% Motile [Range]	% Normal Morphology [Range]
Unprocessed	98.7 (±1.45) [13–215]	293.8	52.4 (±0.71) [25–72]	58.0 (±0.65) [36–71]
Rise	11.5 (±0.59) [0.5–28]	17.5[b]	90.3 (±0.71) [52–99]	80.8 (±0.70) [36–95]
Nonrise N = 25	409.2 (±2.89) [26–809]	233.4	38.5 (±0.78) [13–66]	53.0 (0.62) [37–69]

[a] Mean values are presented with standard error in parentheses.

[b] 17.5 is 5.9% of the unprocessed initial ejaculate and 7.4% of the nonrise sample. p < 0.001 for rise vs. nonrise and rise vs. unprocessed sample.

Table 20–5. Distribution of Various Abnormal Sperm Forms

Abnormality	Unprocessed Mean %	Rise Mean %	Nonrise Mean %
Tapered head[a]	4.1	1.8	5.0
Microcephalic[b]	7.7	6.9	6.6
Macrocephalic[a]	2.8	1.0	3.4
Amorphous[a]	3.6	1.4	3.9
Tail abnormality[a]	9.1	3.1	13.6
Bent midpiece[a]	7.8	2.7	9.1
Cytoplasmic droplet[a]	6.8	1.7	6.0

[a] p < 0.001 for rise vs. either unprocessed or nonrise sample.

[b] p < 0.1 for rise vs. either unprocessed or nonrise sample.

Table 20–6. Morphometric Analysis of Rise and Nonrise Semen Samples[a]

		Nonrise	Rise
$\dfrac{\text{Normal hits of sperm}}{\text{Total hits of particulate and cellular material}}$	× 100	56.4 (±6.0)	92.1 (±2.6)
$\dfrac{\text{Normal sperm head hits}}{\text{Total sperm head hits}}$	× 100	36.2 (±8.0)	86.8 (±6.4)
$\dfrac{\text{Volume density of normal sperm}}{\text{Total volume density of particulate and cellular material}}$	× 100	18.1 (±3.9)	83.4 (±5.5)

[a] Mean values are presented with standard error in parentheses. p < 0.001 for each rise and nonrise comparison.

tribution of motile and normal forms to the rise portion of the sample. Table 20–5 shows the distribution of various abnormal forms, all of which, except the microcephalic category, were significantly decreased in the rise sample. These data are similar to those recently published by McDowell and coworkers.[55]

Surprisingly few normal forms are encountered when a pellet of unprocessed semen is examined with the electron microscope. A study examining sperm from the rise procedure using electron microscopy employed semen samples obtained from nine individuals.[57] Electron microscopy (Figure 20–13) demonstrated that the washed, nonrise sample showed a few normal forms but most were abnormal. The abnormal forms consisted of cellular debris, exfoliated genital tract cells, and abnormal sperm heads and tails. In some nonrise samples virtually all the particulate matter (except most flagella) were abnormal (Figure 20–14). The rise sample is shown in Figure 30–15. Virtually all profiles are of normal appearing sperm. An enlarged normal form typical of the rise sample is shown in Figure 20–16.

Morphometry was performed in the nine individuals in whom rise and nonrise samples were compared (Table 20–6) to examine the quantitative enhancement obtained by the rise procedure.[57] Two hundred hits were scored for a single sample. Profiles of particulate matter seen in micrographs were termed "hits." These hits may be classified as sperm exfoliated cells, immature germ cells, white blood cells, cellular debris, or amorphous debris. The hits of normal sperm, as compared to all hits, rose

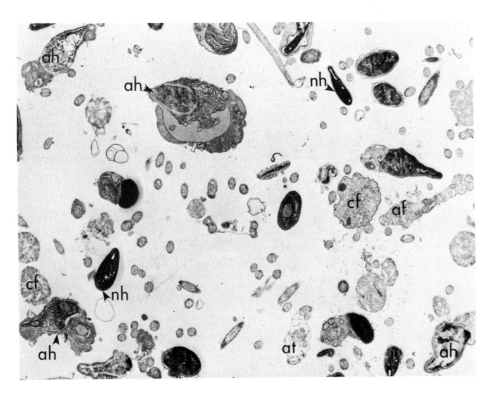

Figure 20–13. Electron micrograph of a non-rise sample. Both normal and abnormal forms are seen. (See Figure 20–11 for key.)

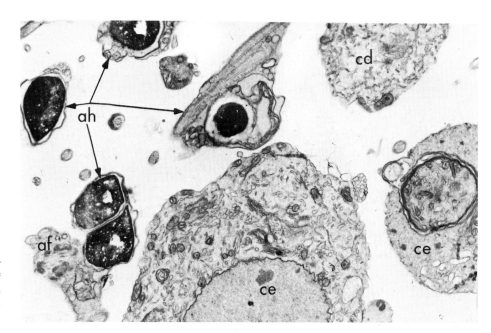

Figure 20–14. Non-rise sample at higher magnification. Virtually all of the sample is composed of elements other than normal appearing sperm. (See Figure 20–11.)

significantly from 56.4% to 92.1% in the nonrise to the rise, respectively. Normal head forms alone increased from 32.6% to 86.8%. With volume density measurements which demonstrated the volume of the sample occupied by normal forms, it was determined that only 18.1% of the volume of the non-rise sample was normal, whereas 83.4% of the rise sample volume was normal.

The rise or swim-up technique produces a population of sperm that is enriched in normal, motile forms. Although only a fraction of the total sperm population is recovered for use either for clinical purposes or for research investigation, this fraction is most likely to provide the most valid results from a functional standpoint, since rise samples give increased penetration in the hamster test when compared with the nonrise samples.[57,58]

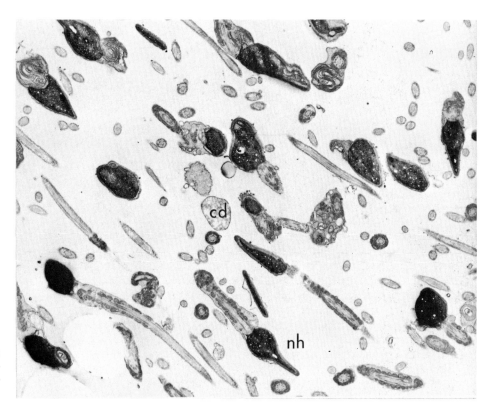

Figure 20–15. Electron micrograph of the rise sample. The sample is enriched in sperm most of which appear normal. (See Figure 20–11.)

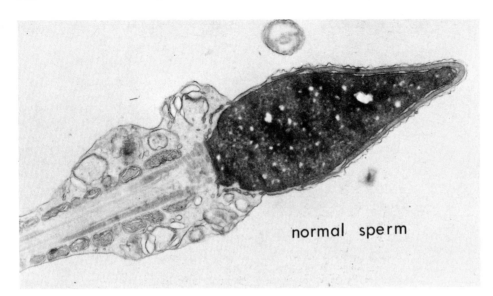

normal sperm

Figure 20–16. Profile of a typical rise sperm. (See Figure 20–11.)

TREATMENT OF SEMEN ABNORMALITIES

Although *in vitro* fertilization (IVF) was designed as a treatment for female infertility, this treatment *may* also have a role in certain kinds of male infertility. In light of the fact that there are few successful approaches available that affect the majority of sperm in a sample which are functionally incapable, an alternative would be to process the sample using the rise technique and to proceed to fertilize eggs *in vitro* or *in vivo*. This would allow for the enrichment of that minority of sperm which are normal (see section above describing rise technique).

Various approaches to correcting semen abnormalities have been used in the past with varying degrees of success. An attempt at modification of the sperm quality can be made either systemically by treating the individual or directly by manipulating the sperm. The systemic approach includes varicocele surgery, Clomid® therapy, hCG administration, Medrol® treatment, antibiotic regimens and other procedures to modify sperm production and quality. The direct approach includes procedures such as washing with buffers containing substances ranging from arginine and caffeine to high albumin concentration and egg yolk. Neither approach has been overwhelmingly successful and thus the treatment of male infertility by these means is generally regarded as frustrating.

Our recommendation would be to use *in vitro* fertilization as an optional approach for male infertility treatment. The rationale for such an approach comes from our IVF experience in which clearly "abnormal" samples produce rise specimens that readily fertilize eggs and initiate pregnancies. Since the rise procedure selects out potentially functionally competent sperm, this technique can work unless there are very few normal sperm in the sample. In our experience, it was impossible to define lower threshold parameters in semen analyses which could predict failure in fertilization. Severely low counts,

motility, and morphology have been consistent with rise samples that can fertilize. Recently Cohen and coworkers[59] also suggested that oligospermia, asthenospermia, teratospermia, and autoimmunity are among the many forms of male infertility which can be treated by IVF. Even though the real IVF success rate continues to be less than 20% in most settings, this procedure may be a default solution for the treatment of male infertility.

References

1. Chong AP, Walters CA, Weinreib SA: The neglected laboratory test: the semen analysis. J Androl 4:280–282, 1983.
2. Belsey MA, Eliasson R, Gallegos AJ, *et al.* (eds). Laboratory manual for the examination of semen and semen-cervical mucus interaction. World Health Organization. Singapore, Press Concern, 1980.
3. Sherins RJ, Brightwell D, Sternthal PM: Longitudinal analysis of semen of fertile and infertile men. *In* P Troen, HR Nankin (eds) New Concepts of the Testis in Normal and Infertile Men. Morphology, Physiology, and Pathology, pp 473–448. New York, Raven Press 1977.
4. Rogers BJ, Bentwood BJ, Van Campen H, *et al.*: Sperm morphology assessment as an indicator of human fertilizing capacity. J Androl 4:119–125, 1983.
5. David MP, Amit A, Bergman A, *et al.*: Sperm penetration *in vitro*: correlations between parameters of sperm quality and the penetration capacity. Fertil Steril 32:676, 1979.
6. Bergman A, Amit A, David MP, *et al.*: Penetration of human ejaculated spermatozoa into human and bovine cervical mucus. Fertil Steril 36:363, 1981.
7. Gaddum-Rosse P, Blandau RJ, Lee WI: Sperm penetration into cervical mucus *in vitro*. II. Human spermatozoa in bovine mucus. Fertil Steril 33:644, 1980.
8. Alexander NJ: Evaluation of male infertility with an *in vitro* cervical mucus penetration test. Fertil Steril 36:201, 1981.
9. Lee WI, Gaddum-Rosse P, Blandau RJ: Sperm penetration into cervical mucus *in vitro*. III. Effect of freezing on estrous bovine cervical mucus. Fertil Steril 36:209, 1981.
10. Mangione CM, Medley NE, Menge AD: Studies on the use of

estrous bovine cervical mucus in the human sperm-cervical mucus penetration technique. Int J Fertil 26:20, 1981.

11. Hayes MF, Segal S, Moghissi KS, et al.: Sperm-cervical mucus interaction: a comparison of the in vitro sperm penetration test using human cervical mucus and bovine estrus cervical mucus with the postcoital test. Fertil Steril 37 (Abstract Supplement):315, 1982.

12. Moghissi KS, Segal S, Meinhold D, et al.: In vitro sperm cervical mucus penetration test. Fertil Seril 36:201, 1981.

13. Rogers BJ, Takemoto F, Wiltbank M, et al.: Comparison of the penetration ability of human spermatozoa into bovine cervical mucus and zona-free hamster eggs. Fertil Steril 39 (Abstract Supplement):437, 1983.

14. Takemoto FS, Rogers BJ, Wiltbank MC, et al.: Comparison of the penetration ability of human spermatozoa into bovine cervical mucus and zona-free hamster eggs. J Androl 6:162–170, 1985.

15. Matthews CD, Makin AE, Cox LW: Experience with in vitro sperm penetration testing in infertile and fertile couples. Fertil Steril 33:187–192, 1980.

16. Schats R, Aitken RJ, Templeton AA: The role of cervical mucus-semen interaction in infertility of unknown etiology. Br J Obstet Gynaecol 91:371–376, 1984.

17. Overstreet JW, Katz DF, Hanson FW, et al.: A simple inexpensive method for objective assessment of human sperm movement characteristics. Fertil Steril 31:162–172, 1979.

18. Katz DF, Overstreet JW: Sperm motility assessment by videomicrography. Fertil Steril 35:188–193, 1981.

19. David G, Serres C, Jouannet P: Kinematics of human spermatozoa. Gamete Res 4:83–95, 1981.

20. Makler A, Itskovitz J, Brandes JM, et al.: Sperm velocity and percentage of motility in 100 normospermic specimens analyzed by the multiple exposure photography (MEP) method. Fertil Steril 31:155–161, 1979.

21. Katz DF, Overstreet JW, Hanson FW: Variations within and amongst normal men of movement characteristics of seminal spermatozoa. J Reprod Fert 62:221–228, 1981.

22. Milligan MP, Harris S, Dennis KJ: Comparison of sperm velocity in fertile and infertile groups as measured by the time-lapse photography. Fertil Steril 34:509–511, 1980.

23. Lewis EL, Katz DF: Simultaneous assessment of human sperm motility and morphology by videomicrography. J Urol 26:357–360.

24. Aitken RJ, Best FSM, Richardson DW, et al.: An analysis of sperm function in cases of unexplained infertility: conventional criteria, movement characteristics, and fertilizing capacity. Fertil Steril 38:212–221, 1982.

25. Aitken RJ, Best FSM, Richardson DW, et al.: An analysis of semen quality and sperm function in cases of oligozoospermia. Fertil Steril 38:705–711, 1982.

26. Albertsen PC, Chang TSK, Vindivich D, et al.: A critical method of evaluating tests for male infertility. J Urol 130:467–475, 1983.

27. Reyes A, Martinez R, Luna M, et al.: Quantitative evaluation of the human spermatozoal motility and acrosome reaction in infertile oligozoospermic and fertile euspermic men. Arch Androl 12:187–194, 1984.

28. Schoevaert-Brossault D: Automated analysis of human sperm motility. Comp Biomed Res 17:362–375, 1984.

29. Makler A, MacLusky NJ, Chodos A, et al.: Rapid microcomputer-based analysis of semen characteristics from photographs taken by the MEP method. Arch Androl 12:91–95, 1984.

30. Holt WV, Moore HDM, Hillier SG: Computer-assisted measurement of sperm swimming speed in human semen: correlation of results with in vitro fertilization assays. Fertil Steril 44:112–119, 1985.

31. Hope E, Blackburn K, Zenick H, et al.: Computerized evaluations of human sperm. Biol Reprod (Suppl I)30:176, 1984.

32. Talbot P, Chacon RS: A triple-stain technique for evaluating normal acrosome reactions of human sperm. J Exp Zool 215:201–208, 1981.

33. Plachot M, Mandelbaum J, Junca A: Acrosome reaction of human sperm used for in vitro fertilization. Fertil Steril 42:418–423, 1984.

34. Wolf DP, Boldt J, Byrd W, et al.: Acrosomal status evaluation in human ejaculated sperm with monoclonal antibodies. Biol Reprod 32:1157–62, 1985.

35. Russell L, Peterson RN, Freund M: Morphologic characteristics of the chemically induced acrosome reaction in human spermatozoa. Fertil Steril 32:87–92, 1979.

36. Perreault S, Zaneveld LJD, Rogers BJ: Inhibition of fertilization in the hamster by sodium aurothiomaleate, a hyaluronidase inhibitor. J Reprod Fertil 60:461–467, 1980.

37. Joyce C, Jeyendran RS, Zaneveld LJD: Release, extraction, and stability of hyaluronidase associated with human spermatozoa: comparison with the rabbit. J Androl 6:152–161, 1985.

38. Goodpasture JC, Zavos PM, Cohen MR, et al.: Relationship of human sperm acrosin and proacrosin to semen parameters. I. Comparisons between symptomatic men of infertile couples and asymptomatic men, and between different split ejaculate fractions. J Androl 3:151–156, 1982.

39. Mohsenian M, Syner FN, Moghissi KS: A study of sperm acrosin in patients with unexplained infertility. Fert Steril 37:223–229, 1982.

40. Hanada A, Chang MC: Penetration of zona-free eggs by spermatozoa of different species. Biol Reprod 6:300–309, 1972.

41. Yanagimachi R: Penetration of guinea pig spermatozoa into hamster eggs in vitro. J Reprod Fertil 28:477–480, 1972.

42. Yanagimachi R, Yanagimachi H, Rogers BJ: The use of zona-free animal ova as a test system for the assessment of the fertilizing capacity of human spermatozoa. Biol Reprod 15:471–476, 1976.

43. Rogers BJ, Van Campen H, Ueno M, et al.: Analysis of human spermatozoal fertilizing ability using zona-free ova. Fertil Steril 32:664–670, 1979.

44. Rogers BJ: The sperm penetration assay: its usefulness reevaluated. Fertil Steril 43:821–840, 1985.

45. Rogers BJ: Hamster egg: evaluation of human sperm using in vitro fertilization. In PG Crosignani, BL Rubin (eds) In Vitro Fertilization and Embryo Transfer, pp 101–144. London, Academic Press, 1983.

46. Yanagimachi R: Zona-free hamster eggs: their use in assessing fertilizing capacity and examining chromosomes of human spermatozoa. Gamete Res 10:187–232, 1984.

47. Blasco L: Clinical tests of sperm fertilizing ability. Fertil Steril 41:177, 1984.

48. Prasad MRN: The in vitro sperm penetration test. Int J Androl 7:5–22, 1984.

49. Mygatt GG, Soderdahl DW, Rogers BJ: In vitro fertilization rates after varicocele repair. J Urol 127:1103–1104, 1982.

50. Rogers BJ, Mygatt GG, Soderdahl DW, et al.: Monitoring of suspected infertile men with varicocele by the sperm penetration assay. Fertil Steril 44:800–805, 1985.

51. Rogers BJ, Maruyama D, Linsenmeyer TA, *et al.:* The effect of clomiphene citrate on oligospermic male infertility as monitored by the sperm penetration assay. J Androl 6:105, 1985.

52. Linsenmeyer TA, Rogers BJ, Maruyama D, *et al.:* The effect of clomiphene citrate on oligospermic male infertility as monitored by the SPA. J Urol. (in press) 1987.

53. Drevius LO: The "sperm rise" test. J Reprod Fertil 24:427–429, 1971.

54. Makler A, Murillo O, Huszar G, *et al.:* Improved techniques for collecting motile spermatozoa from human semen. I. A self-migratory method. Int J Androl 7:61–70, 1984.

55. McDowell JS, Veeck LL, Jones HW: Analysis of human spermatozoa before and after processing for *in vitro* fertilization. J In Vitro Fertil and Embryo Trans 2:23–26, 1985.

56. Rogers BJ, Russell LD: Comparisons of the rise and nonrise samples of human sperm as employed in fertility programs. J Androl 6:60, 1985.

57. Russell LD, Rogers BJ: Improvement in the quality and fertilization potential of a human sperm population using the rise technique. J Androl 8:25–33, 1987.

58. Cohen J, Felten P, Zeilmaker GH: *In vitro* fertilizing capacity of fresh and cryopreserved human spermatozoa: a comparative analysis of freezing and thawing procedures. Fertil Steril 36:356–362, 1981.

59. Cohen J, Edwards R, Fehilly C, *et al.: In vitro* fertilization: a treatment for male infertility. Fertil Steril 43:422–432, 1985.

21. Sperm Ultrastructural Pathology and Infertility

Luciano Zamboni

Electron microscopy has contributed significantly to the understanding of the complex structural organization of the human spermatozoon and the highly specialized functions of its components.[1-5] In turn, knowledge of sperm morphophysiology has been instrumental in elucidating major aspects of the reproductive process, such as capacitation and its structural manifestations, and the mechanisms that facilitate the progression of the sperm through the egg investments and its conjugation with the egg.

Considering that it is through the spermatozoa that men express their reproductive potential, one should expect that the structural integrity and the functional fitness of these cells be evaluated in the diagnostic approach to infertility as critically as they are in basic research. Yet, generally this is not so. In the clinical practice of andrology, in fact, the analysis of the semen, still the most fundamental test for the evaluation of male fertility, is routinely performed, largely by non-specialists, in total unawareness of the progress made in the area of sperm morphophysiology and utilizing inadequate and subjective analytical methods.

This is especially true for the assessment of sperm morphology which is evaluated by examining live or crudely prepared spermatozoa with the light microscope, a tool that does not permit the visualization of the many subcellular components upon which sperm function (and thus, fertility) are so dependent. Consequently, the spermatozoa are assessed as if they simply consisted of a head and a tail, and they are classified and rated on the basis of the size, shape, and overall appearance of these two components exclusively. This may explain why current classifications of sperm morphology[6,7] have not changed from the schemes originally proposed by those[8] who pioneered the concept that sperm abnormalities are a cause of infertility. Such a wide gap separating investigators intent on elucidating the substructural organization of the spermatozoon and comprehending its highly complex and specialized functions and clinicians interested in evaluating the structural integrity and the functional

competence of the very same cell with the objective of assessing its fertility potential, is incomprehensible and hardly justifiable.

In the last few years, the limited armamentarium of the laboratory procedures available for the evaluations of male fertility has been expanded by the introduction of the zona-free hamster egg penetration test.[9] This bioassay, a product of basic research on gamete physiology,[10] has rapidly gained popularity and is being widely utilized in andrology[11] (see Chapter 20). However, the procedure is associated with methodological vagaries, variability of results, inconsistent reproducibility[12] and high cost.

The adoption of this bioassay has further widened the dichotomy between reproductive medicine and the progress made in the area of sperm morphophysiology. In fact, it is difficult to bridge the gap between a simplistic, if not rudimentary, vision of spermatozoa consisting only of "a head and a tail" and a test whose results should be the expression of the structural integrity and functional preparedness of cell organelles playing essential roles in the reproductive process.[13] Practically, this translates into the frequent difficulty of correlating the results of the bioassay with those of the analysis of the semen, especially when the clinician must explain to a patient with a "normal or minimally subnormal semen quality" (as assessed by conventional laboratory methods) the reasons why "he failed the hamster test." It is instead becoming increasingly evident that the spermatozoa of many of these patients, far from being normal or only slightly subnormal, are afflicted with severe defects of their submicroscopic components whose presence fully accounts for the failure to penetrate the denuded hamster eggs. In some cases, the ability to demonstrate these abnormalities is not only of diagnostic but also of prognostic importance.

The ultrastructural pathology of the human spermatozoon has been documented in the literature mostly in the form of isolated case reports. Of the few reviews published on the subject, the most comprehensive are those by Bisson and David,[14] Holstein,[15] Escalier and David,[16] Nistal and Paniagua,[17] and the morphogenetic review by Holstein and Schirren.[18] The task of the pathologist who wishes to provide a systematic classification of the various ultrastructural defects and developmental abnormalities of the human sperm, and to rate them in relation to the patient's fertility, is made arduous by the following prob-

The author wishes to express his gratitude to Ibrahim Hernandez, Dolores Scott, Marilyn Jones and William Lungo for the technical assistance provided to him, and to Maureen Dewey for her patience and skillful assistance in the preparation of the manuscript.

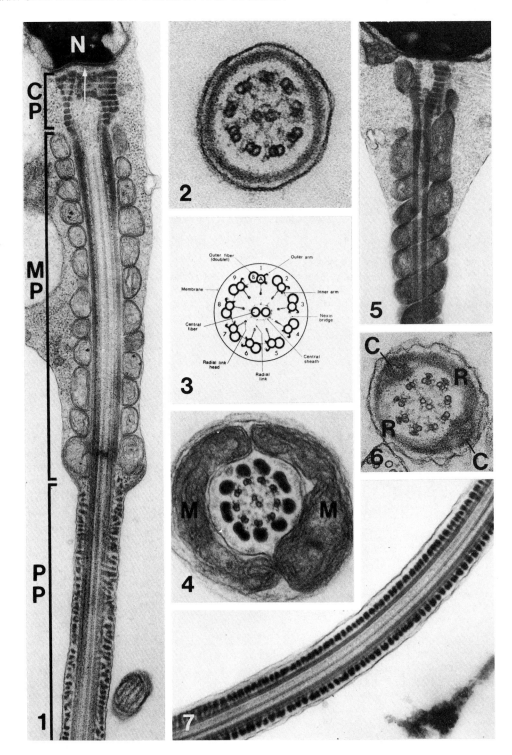

Figure 21–1. The complex ultrastructural organization of the sperm flagellum is shown in this low-power electron micrograph. N, nucleus; CP, connecting piece; MP, mid-piece; PP, principal piece. The arrow points to the implantation fossa.

Figure 21–2. Cross-section of sperm flagellum (principal piece) showing the 9 + 2 system of axonemal microtubules and their accessory structures; for interpretation, see text and the schematic representation of Figure 21–3.

Figure 21–3. Schematic illustration of the 9 + 2 system of axonemal microtubules and accessory structures; compare with Figure 21–2.

Figure 21–4. Cross-section of sperm flagellum (mid-piece) showing the 9 dense outer fibers surrounding the microtubules of the axoneme. In this segment of the tail, the 9 + 9 + 2 system of flagellar fibers and microtubules is encircled by mitochondria, M (see also Figures 21–1 and 21–5).

lems: 1. The well-known pleomorphism of human spermatozoa, which contrasts with the morphologic uniformity of those of other mammals including non-human primates,[19,20,21] makes it difficult to define what constitutes a "normal" model. 2. The organizational complexity of the cell and the large number and variety of anomalies that occur defy attempts to review its ultrastructural pathology without assembling a pedantic list of questionable significance. 3. The frequent occurrence in the same cell of combinations of defects nullifies any otherwise justifiable attempt to organize the ultrastructural pathology of the human sperm on a microanatomic basis. 4. The almost regular presence of variable numbers of abnormal spermatozoa in all semen samples makes it difficult to establish when a specimen is within the "normal range" or when it is clearly abnormal.

To minimize these problems and still provide a reasonably complete overview of the ultrastructural pathology of the human sperm, this review will not only be based primarily on functional perspectives, but will also emphasize only those deviations from the normal that have significant impact on the reproductive capacity of the cell and the fertility potential of the individual. It represents a distillate of the ultrastructural examinations of seminal fluids of about one hundred patients referred to the author over the last few years.

The functions of the human spermatozoon that are of cardinal importance for the reproductive process are the following:

1. The sperm must be capable of the vigorous and progressive motility required to reach the site of fertilization under physiologic conditions. For this function it needs a structurally intact flagellum.
2. The sperm must be capable of penetrating through the egg investments. For this function it must be capable of movement and, especially, it must have been effectively "capacitated" and possess the ability to undergo the acrosome reaction.
3. The sperm must be able to fuse its plasma membrane with that of the egg. For this function the sperm needs to have undergone the acrosome reaction and its plasma membrane behind the acrosome must be intact.
4. The sperm must be capable of normally contributing to syngamy, the fusion of the paternal and maternal genomes which occurs in the activated oocyte and marks the onset of embryonic development. For this function, it must have intact an organization of its nuclear material.

Structural defects impairing any of these functions result in reduction or suppression of the fertilizing capacity of the sperm and constitute either direct causes of infertility, such as those that prevent fertilization (head defects), or indirect causes, such as those that limit motility (flagellar defects).

THE FLAGELLUM

The sperm tail has a highly complex organization and consists of numerous components which altogether constitute a very effective and powerful propelling mechanism (Figure 21–1). None of them is visible with the light microscope. Considering their importance for motility and that, physiologically, there is no fertility without sperm motility, the inability to evaluate these components represents a severe limitation of conventional methods of semen analysis.

Normal Structure

The flagellum implants on a concavity of the posterior surface of the head, the *implantation fossa* (Figures 21–1, 35, 36). Extending throughout its length is the structurally complex system of the axonemal microtubules[22–24] whose organization is best appreciated in transverse sections. The system consists of nine doublet microtubules (known also as doublets), circularly arranged around two central singlet microtubules (known also as singlets), forming the 9+2 microtubular pattern typical of the flagella and the cilia of all eukaryotic organisms (Figures 21–2–4, 6). Each doublet consists of a subunit A, a complete microtubule, and a subunit B, incomplete, c-shaped and attached to the wall of A. The microtubules are made up of heterodimers of *tubulin,* a protein M_2 110,000, organized in protofilaments 3.5 nm in diameter; subunit A of each doublet and the two central singlets consist of 13 dimers, while only 10 dimers make up the incomplete subunits B of the peripheral doublets. The two central singlets are connected at their closest points by 6 nm long bridges organized as the rungs of a ladder, and encircled by a *helical sheath* consisting of a system of filamentous projections departing from their wall (Figure 21–3). Subunit A of each doublet is provided with two *dynein arms,* an outer and an inner, directed in clockwise manner and with slightly diverging courses toward subunit B of the next doublet (Figures 21–2, 3, 4). Dynein is a heterogeneous protein[25] M_2 500,000 possessing ATPase activity; its fraction 1, which accounts for 75% of the total ATPase activity of the axoneme, is localized principally in the arms of the doublet microtubules. A fraction 2, representing 15% of the axonemal ATPase, has also been isolated; indirect evidence suggests that it could be localized in the central singlets.[26,27] Also arising from each subunit A is a system of long, thin filaments, the *nexin links,* traversing the inter-

Figure 21–5. The helicoidal arrangements of the mid-piece mitochondria is evident in this slide.

Figure 21–6. In the principal piece, the axonemal microtubules are encircled by the fibrous sheath consisting of two longitudinally oriented columns (C) and two hemispherical ribs (R).

Figure 21–7. Longitudinal section of sperm flagellum showing the regular distribution of the ribs of the fibrous sheath throughout the principal piece.

doublet space and connecting subunit A of each doublet with the B of the adjacent one,[28] and a *radial spoke,* a hammer-shaped structure attaching to the helical sheath around the singlet microtubules.

The concept that flagella move, just like cilia, as a result of the relative sliding of their microtubules alongside one another was first postulated by Afzelius[29] on the basis of his demonstration of the dynein arms which he compared, structurally as well as functionally, to the crossbridges between the actin and the myosin filaments of striated muscle fibers. His view was subsequently confirmed by numerous studies (reviewed by Haimo and Rosenbaum[30]). These studies demonstrated that flagellar motility requires the presence of an intact plasma membrane and the availability of ATP; that in the presence of Mg^{2+} or Ca^{2+} the dynein arms of the axonemal microtubules hydrolyze ATP, thus converting chemical energy into mechanical movements; and that the radial spokes regulate the sliding movements of the peripheral doublets and transform them into bending waves by becoming alternatively detached from, and reattached to, the helical sheath around the two central singlets.[24,31,32]

The importance of the structural integrity of *all* axonemal elements and of their harmonious functional interrelationship for the normalcy and the effectiveness of sperm movements has been amply demonstrated by experimental studies showing that flagellar mutants which lack the central pair of singlet microtubules or the dynein arms are incapable of movement.[33–35] In the absence of the radial spokes, they can neither regulate the sliding of the peripheral microtubles nor convert sliding movements into bending waves.[36] However, the most vivid demonstration of the key role of the various axonemal structures has been provided in recent years by the severely limiting effects that their pathology has on the motility of human spermatozoa (see below).

For most of their length, the peripheral microtubules are encircled by a system of nine *outer dense fibers* (Figure 21–4), whose presence results in the 9+9+2 flagellar system typical of spermatozoa of all animals characterized by internal fertilization. (They are not present in sperm of aquatic phyla.) Cranially, each fiber fuses with a segmented column of the connecting piece (Figures 21–1, 35, 36) while caudally it terminates, after considerable tapering, by fusing to the wall of its corresponding doublet. The outer dense fibers probably are not contractile elements. Their amino acid profile, which is different from that of contractile proteins,[37] their high cysteine content,[38] and the high number of S-S bonds[39–41] all suggest keratin-like properties.[42] Even though their specific role has not been fully elucidated, the outer dense fibers are considered to be resilient, stiffening elements[2,43–45] that confer an elastic rigidity to the flagellum,[46,47] facilitate forward progressive movement,[5] and, possibly, protect its most sensitive elements from damage during passage through the female reproductive tract.

In the upper segment of the flagellum, or *mid-piece,* the outer dense fibers and the axonemal microtubules are enveloped by mitochondria (Figures 21-1, 4, 5) organized end-to-end (Figure 21–4) in a helix (Figure 21–5) of 12 to 15 gyres with two mitochrondria per gyre.[20] The

mitochondria are the source of the chemical energy that the sperm requires for its mechanical work. Their localization in the uppermost segment of the flagellum favors the downward diffusion of ATP to the axonemal microtubules and their dynein arms.

The *fibrous sheath,* which begins just below the last mitochondrial gyre, surrounds the outer dense fibers and the axonemal microtubules over the longest segment of the flagellum, the *principal piece* (Figures 21-1, 7). It consists of: two *longitudinal columns* (Figure 21–6) situated 180° apart along the circumference of the flagellum and positioned on the plane of the two central axonemal microtubules, and a regular series of circumferentially oriented ribs (Figure 21–7) each encircling one-half of the tail perimeter and attaching onto the longitudinal columns with their extremities (Figure 21–6). The fibrous sheath consists primarily of a single polypeptide M_2 80,000.[48,49] Its function in flagellar movement and sperm motility is not clear. It has been suggested that it may facilitate the planar bending of the tail.[50] As the flagellum becomes progressively thinner along its length, the columns become tapered and the ribs more slender. Shortly before its end, the fibrous sheath abruptly terminates; in the short segment beyond this point, the *end piece,* the flagellum consists only of the axonemal microtubules (the outer dense fibers disappear gradually at different levels along the principal piece) surrounded by the plasmalemma.

Microtubule Defects

Not surprisingly, given the number and structural complexity of its elements, the sperm flagellum often presents with a broad spectrum of abnormalities: distinguishable into numerical aberrations in defect or in excess, topographic derangements, and structural defects. Of the abnormalities of the 9+2 system of the axonemal microtubules, all of which cause ineffective motility or immotility, those of the peripheral doublets are more frequent than those of the two central singlets. The doublets may be present in less than normal numbers (Figures 21–8, 9, 10), or in excessive numbers (Figures 21–10, 11), or they may be replaced by singlets (Figure 21–12), or display lack of parallelism, and/or occur in a non-circular arrangement (Figure 21–13). They can also be completely disorganized (Figure 21–14). These defects do not occur individually. Usually none of them is found to be the sole or the predominant defect in the sperm population of a sample; rather, they occur in different combinations and alongside flagella having a normal axonemal organization, at least on individual planes of sections (Figure 21–10). Identical observations were made by McClure, Brawer, and Robaire[51] in a study of the spectrum of ultrastructural defects associated with sperm immotility. Escalier and David[16], in a detailed and wide-based study on the flagellar pathology of astheno- and teratospermia, reported that the defects of the peripheral microtubules of the axoneme are the most frequent axonemal abnormalities, that they do not affect all the spermatozoa even though they may involve a significant num-

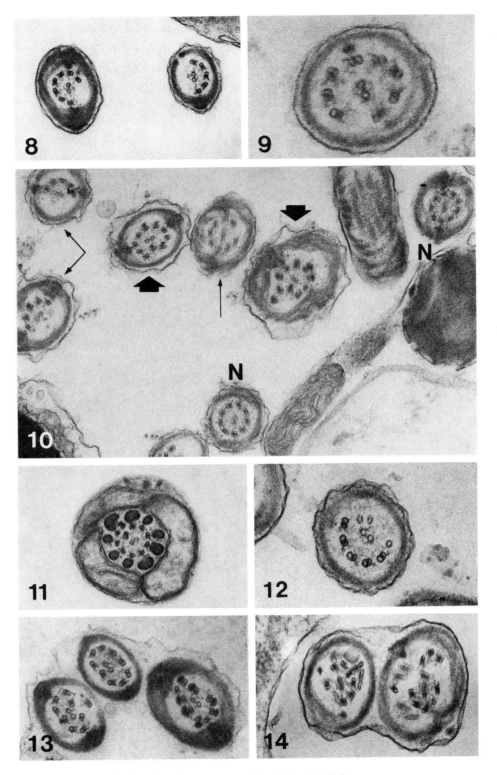

Figure 21–8, 9. Sperm flagella with <9 axonemal doublet microtubules.

Figure 21–10. Sperm flagella with a normal 9 + 2 axonemal organization (N) together with tails provided with <9 (thin arrows) and >9 (thick arrows) axonemal doublet microtubules.

Figure 21–11. Sperm tail (mid-piece) showing an 11 + 2 organization of the axonemal microtubules.

Figure 21–12. Sperm tail defective for axonemal doublet microtubules, some of which have been replaced by singlets.

Figure 21–13. Noncircular arrangement of the 9 + 2 system of axonemal microtubules.

Figure 21–14. Generalized disorganization of the axonemal microtubules.

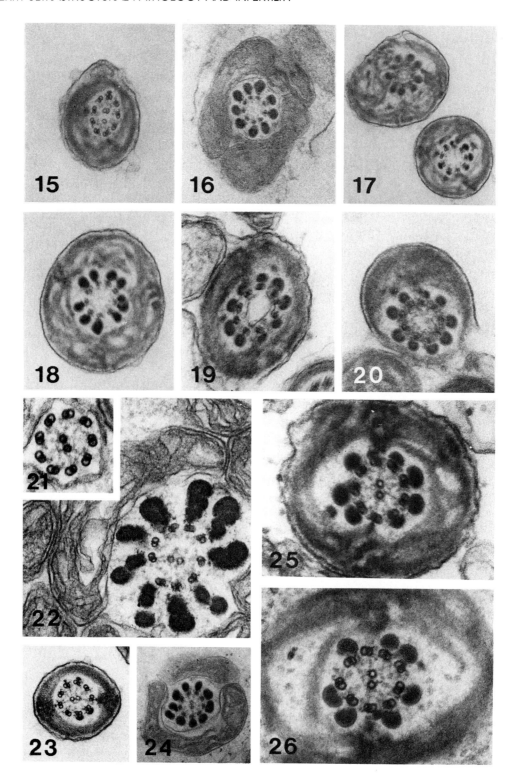

Figure 21–15. Sperm tail with a 9 + 3 organization of the axonemal microtubules. Of the three in central position, one is a doublet.

Figure 21–16–20. Sperm tails with a 9 + 0 axonemal organization. The spermatozoa shown in Figures 21–17–20 also display fibrous sheath defects (multilayering and uneven thickness of the ribs, absence of the longitudinal columns). Ten outer dense fibers are present in the sperm of Figure 21–18. In Figure 21–19, extraneous membranes are present in the center of the axoneme; in Figure 21–20, the peripheral axonemal doublets are masked by dense material which also fills the interdoublet spaces.

Figures 21–21, 22. Complete absence of dynein arms. In the sperm of Figure 21–22, the outer dense fibers have an irregular shape; each consists of two expanded extremities connected by a thin neck.

ber or even the majority of them, and that they occur principally in association with other axonemal defects. The pleomorphism of the doublet microtubule abnormalities suggests complex dysfunctions of the proximal and distal centrioles from which the axonemal elements become assembled during late spermiogenetic stages.[52]

Less frequent numerical aberrations of the singlet microtubules of the axoneme include the very rare occurrence of a supernumerary microtubule in central position (Figure 21–15), the equally rare deletion of a singlet, and the relatively less exceptional absence of both singlets, the so-called 9+0 defect (Figures 21–16 to 21–20). The author has encountered this defect, which is invariably associated with sperm immotility, in four infertile patients. While in three patients the lack of the central microtubules was only one of the several axonemal abnormalities that were noted, in the fourth the 9+0 flagellar organization was universal, i.e., affected all spermatozoa, and was associated with an abnormal organization of the fibrous sheath (Figures 21–17 to 21–20). The absence of the two central singlets as predominant axonemal defect was described also by Nistal et al.[53] in an infertile patient producing spermatozoa with short and thick flagella, and by Baccetti et al.[26,27] Electrophoretic analysis of the sperm flagella of the patients studied by these authors demonstrated presence of dynein fraction 1 but absence of fraction 2, a finding suggesting that the latter could possibly be localized in the central singlets. Absence of the singlet microtubules, together with occurrence of membranous structures in the center of the axoneme (Figure 21–19) and with presence of a ring of dense granular material masking and/or replacing the peripheral doublets and filling the interdoublet spaces (Figure 21–20), have also been noted. Another defect of the singlet microtubules, the so-called 8+2, will be considered together with the flagellar abnormalities of the "ciliary dyskinesis" syndrome.

An extremely rare flagellar defect causing sperm immotility is the absence of all axonemal microtubules. Only one such case has been described in the literature.[54] It involved an infertile man with chronic respiratory tract infections in whom the axonemal microtubules reportedly were absent also in the cilia of the tracheal and bronchial epithelium; the axonemal defect was accompanied by universal absence of the proximal centriole, a finding that underscores the role already mentioned that the centrioles play in the assembly of the elements of the axoneme.

The structural defects of the axonemal microtubules are essentially represented by absence or abnormal organization of the very delicate elements that are associated with them, especially the dynein arms. The most frequent is the absence of both outer and inner arms in all doublets (Figures 21–21, 22) followed by the absence exclusively of the inner or of the outer arms; absence of the outer and inner arms only in some of the doublets can also occur (Figure 21–23). Often these defects are accompanied by other flagellar abnormalities, such as the 9+0 defect or shape deformations of the outer dense fibers (Figure 21–22). Generally, but not universally, these defects result in complete sperm immotility and, as such, represent mediated causes of infertility. That the sterility of these patients results mainly from the incapacity of their sperm to ascend through the female reproductive tract and reach the site of fertilization has been confirmed by the demonstration that their spermatozoa are capable of undergoing the acrosome reaction and penetrating the zona-free hamster eggs.[55]

The absence of one or both dynein arms and the occurrence of dynein arms shorter than normal are the best documented and most frequently occurring ultrastructural abnormalities of sperm flagellar organization.[56–66] Contributing to the general awareness of these flagellar defects is the fact that, in the same patient, they frequently occur together with identical abnormalities of the cilia of the respiratory epithelium, and both form the structural bases of the clinical entity referred to as "immotile cilia syndrome"[59,60,67–69] characterized by chronic ear and sinopulmonary infections and reduced or absent mucociliary clearance. In approximately 50% of these patients, these manifestations occur together with bronchiectasis and situs viscerum inversus, a clinical-anatomic constellation referred to as Kartagener's syndrome.[70] The non-uniform geographical distribution of these defects is well known.[71]

Recently, the structural bases of the immotile cilia syndrome were expanded to include other flagellar and ciliary defects such as the abnormalities of the radial spokes,[72] the transposition of one set of doublet microtubules from the periphery to the center of the axoneme to substitute for the central singlet microtubules that are either very short or absent (the 8+2 defect),[73,74] the absence of the central sheath,[75] and others.[76] Thus, the immotile cilia syndrome is now considered a heterogeneous entity[68,74–76] not only structurally or anatomically, but also from a functional viewpoint. In fact, while the defects responsible for the syndrome usually result in complete ciliary and flagellar immotility, it has been shown that spermatozoa lacking the outer dynein arms but retaining the inner are still capable of some degree of motility.[16,62,65,75] The same is true for cilia and flagella with transposition of the axonemal microtubules.[73,74] The term "immotile cilia syndrome" has thus been replaced by "ciliary dyskinesis" or "dyskinetic cilia syndrome"[78] of

If the latter is not included in the plane of section, the fiber may appear to be "duplicated" (see Figure 20–30).

Figure 21–23. Dynein arm absence in some, but not all, axonemal microtubules characterizes this spermatozoon.

Figure 21–24. Sperm with >9 outer dense fibers.

Figures 21–25, 26. Spermatozoa with <9 outer dense fibers and fibrous sheath abnormalities.

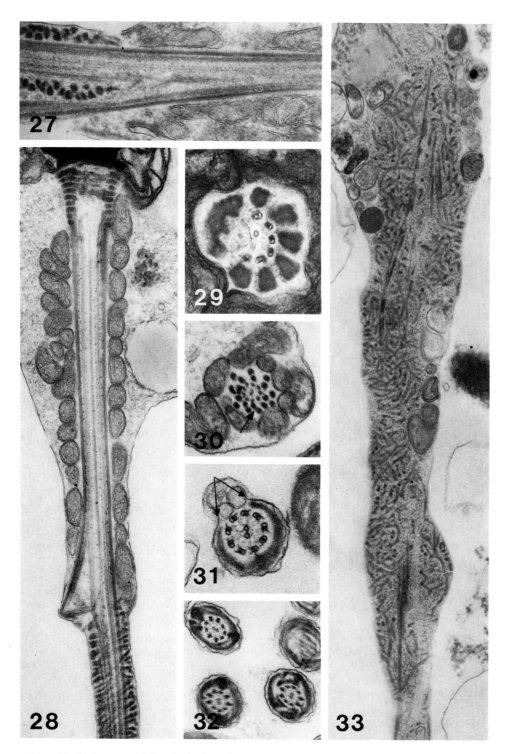

Figure 21–27. Sperm exhibiting lack of parallelism of the outer dense fibers.

Figure 21–28. Sperm with lack of parallelism and sudden deflection of the outer dense fibers from their normal orientation.

Figure 21–29. Sperm showing outer dense fiber fusion.

Figure 21–30. Pseudo-duplication of the outer dense fibers. Eighteen fibers are seemingly present while their actual number is really nine. Their apparent duplication is due to the fact that the fibers are lobated (see Figure 21–22) and each consists of two expanded extremities connected by a thin collar; none of these collars has been included in the plane of section, possibly with the exception of the fiber at the arrow.

Figure 21–31. Sperm with incompletely formed fibrous sheath; the defect is between the two arrows.

which three variants are recognized: Type 1 with defective dynein arms, Type 2 with defective radial spokes, and Type 3 with microtubule translocation.

The structural and functional heterogeneity of the condition has been further underscored by reports of infertile individuals with immotile spermatozoa displaying the classic flagellar defects of the "immotile cilia syndrome" whose cilia, however, are structurally normal and who consequently do not experience any of the clinical manifestations caused by the immotility of these structures.[79] Patients with Kartagener's syndrome with normal ciliary ultrastructure[80] or who have fathered children (reported by Afzelius and Eliasson[81]) have also been reported. A case of Kartagener's syndrome associated with the presence of normal dynein arms in the sperm flagella, sperm motility and, apparently, fertility has also been reported.[82] These observations have led to a revision of the original concept postulating that the same gene was responsible for both the flagellar and the ciliary defects of the immotile cilia syndrome.[74] It is now thought that different genes regulate the production of human dynein.[64,77,83] The view that the 9+2 microtubular organization of sperm flagella and somatic cilia is under the control of different genes also has been corroborated by evidence showing that different axonemal patterns may coexist in the cilia and the flagella of the same animal.[66,84] The complexity of the various issues related to ciliary and flagellar axonemal defects has been compounded even further by the recently demonstrated heterogeneity of the ultrastructural organization of respiratory cilia and sperm flagella of normal men.[85–87]

Outer Dense Fiber Defects

Defects of the outer dense fibers are rare. They consist of numerical aberrations in excess (Figure 21–24) or in defect (Figures 21–25, 26), topographic derangements mostly represented by a lack of parallelism (Figure 21–27) and/or abrupt deflection of one or more fibers from their normal course (Figure 21–28), and structural abnormalities; the fibers may be fused with one another (Figure 21–29), or their shape may be deformed. An example of the latter is shown in Figure 21–22 where the fibers are of abnormal length and appear lobated, i.e., each consists of two dilated segments connected by a thin "neck"; if this is not included in the plane of section, the fibers appear as if they were "duplicated," thus giving the impression of being present in excessive numbers (Figures 21–22, 30). This rare defect is actually referred to that way in the review of Nistal and Paniagua.[17] In spite of the prevailing concept that the outer dense fibers are not contractile elements, experience demonstrates that sperm with these defects are either immotile or dyskinetic. This was recently confirmed by Feneux, Serres and Jouannet[88] who reported that spermatozoa with outer dense fiber defects display a "sliding" pattern of motility and are incapable of penetrating through the cervical mucus.

Fibrous Sheath Defects

The defects of the normal organization of the elements of the fibrous sheath are frequent. They range from subtle ones which may be occasionally noted even in "normal" semen samples, such as the incompleteness of the ribs (Figure 21–31) and/or the absence of the longitudinal columns (Figures 21–17, 18, 19, 20), to very conspicuous ones such as splitting, multilayering (Figures 21–17, 18, 19, 25, 26, 32), and/or complete disorganization (Figure 21–33). These represent major defects. Not only do they involve all or most of the spermatozoa (Figure 21–32), but they also occur together with abnormalities of the dense outer fibers, axonemal microtubules, mitochondria (Figure 21–33), nucleus and acrosome, in different combinations. The occurrence of these associations has been reported also by others. Fibrous sheath defects combined with chromatinic abnormalities were reported by Ross, Christie and Kerr,[89] and Ross, Christie and Edmond,[90] with abnormalities of the acrosome by Pedersen and Hammen[91] and Pedersen, Rebbe and Hammen,[92] with absence of mitochondria and absence or rudimentary development of the mid-piece by McClure, Brawer and Robaire,[51] Ross, Christie and Edmond,[90] Pedersen and Hammen,[91] and Alexandre, Bisson and David,[93] with an exaggerated length of the mid-piece and disorganization of the mitochondria by Pedersen, Rebbe and Hammen,[92] and with disorganization of one or more elements of the 9+9+2 system of flagellar fibers and axonemal microtubules by McClure, Brawer and Robaire,[51] Ross, Christie and Edmond,[90] Pedersen and Hammen,[91] and Alexandre, Bisson and David.[93]

The ultrastructural defects of the fibrous sheath invariably result in sperm immotility; this is intriguing since the fibrous sheath is not thought to be directly involved in sperm movements. The association of abnormalities of the fibrous sheath with defects of other sperm components constitutes a veritable organizational anarchy that Pedersen and Hammen[91] referred to as "complete subcellular derangement." Additional examples of generalized disorganization of sperm ultrastructure will be considered later in this review.

Mitochondrial Defects

The last flagellar defect that needs to be mentioned is the absence of the mitochondria which may occur as sole abnormality (Figure 21–34) or concomitantly with other

Figure 21–32. Generalized multilayering of the fibrous sheath (see Figures 21–17 through 19 and Figures 21–25, 26).

Figure 21–33. Spermatozoon with generalized organizational anarchy of all flagellar components (mitochondria, axonemal microtubules, outer dense fibers, and elements of the fibrous sheath).

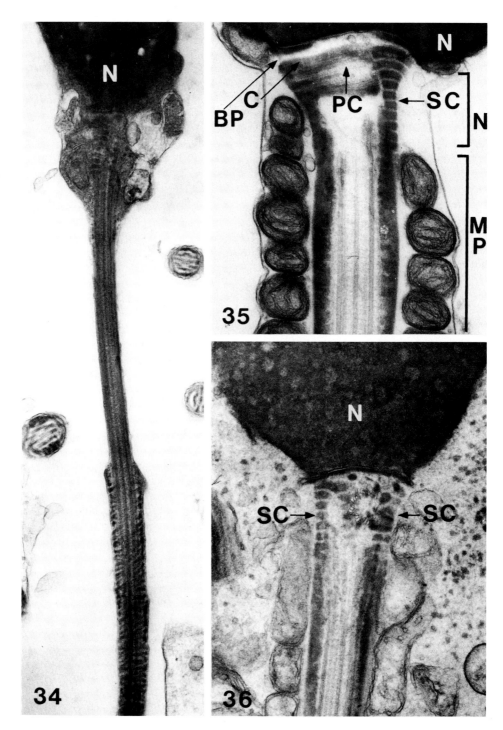

Figure 21–34. Spermatozoon with absence of mitochondria along the mid-piece. N, nucleus.

Figure 21–35. The neck region of the sperm flagellum and the uppermost segment of the flagellar mid-piece (MP) are illustrated in this micrograph. The basal plate (BP) lining the implantation fossa on the posterior surface of the nucleus (N), the capitulum (C), one of the nine segmented columns (SC), and the longitudinally sectioned of proximal centriole (PC) are indicated.

Figure 21–36. The neck region sectioned on a plane orthogonal to that of Figure 21–35. The nine triplet microtubules of the centriole (now sectioned along a transverse plane) and two segmented columns (SC) are discernible. N, nucleus.

aberrations. Absence and/or functional impairment of the mitochondria result in sperm immotility due to the unavailability of the chemical energy necessary for mechanical movements.

THE CONNECTING PIECE

The connecting piece or neck (Figures 21–1, 35, 36) is the most cranial or uppermost segment of the flagellum; it consists of several elements that are of fundamental importance for the maintenance of the connection between the head and tail, the coordination of their movements and, possibly, the generation of motility.

Normal Structure

The most cranial element of the connecting piece is the *capitulum,* a slightly convex articular structure that is accommodated in the concavity of another articular element, the *basal plate,* lining the implantation fossa of the posterior surface of the nucleus. The narrow space between the capitulum and the basal plate contains a faintly discernible, finely filamentous material of relatively high electron density; it has been shown that in rodent sperm this substance can be readily digested with trypsin, chymotrypsin, and pronase with consequent separation of the head from the tail.[94] Just below the capitulum, there is a circular system of nine *segmented columns,* each consisting of a cranio-caudal array of dense segments separated by narrow spaces; at its caudal extremity, each column fuses with a corresponding flagellar fiber.

Just below the capitulum and surrounded by the segmented columns lies the *proximal centriole* (Figures 21–35, 36) consisting of a circular array of nine triplet microtubules oriented perpendicular to the axis of the flagellum. Together with the *distal centriole,* whose presence in the spermatozoa of the rabbit, monkey and man was reported by Zamboni and Stefanini,[95] the proximal centriole plays a key role in the assembly of the axonemal microtubules during the development of the flagellum in the spermatid stage of spermiogenesis.[52] Zamboni[1] and Zamboni and Stefanini[95] identified the proximal centriole also as the sperm kinetic center, i.e., the element responsible for the generation of flagellar movements. This hypothesis, however, needs to be evaluated further since it is known that segments of bull sperm flagella dissected distal to the neck are still capable of wave motion,[96] and that rat spermatozoa, which lack the proximal centriole,[97] move just as those of other mammals in which the existence of this structure was demonstrated (rabbit,[95] guinea pig,[98] boar,[99] bull,[100] rhesus macaque,[95] and man,[95,101]).

Bent Head Defect

An abnormal position of the proximal and distal centrioles along the posterior surface of the spermatid nucleus at the time of incipient development of the flagellum in the seminiferous tubules of the testis (Figure 21–37) appears to be responsible for the "bent head" defect (Figures 21–38, 39), one of the few sperm abnormalities detectable by light microscopy. Not only is the head of these spermatozoa bent, but it is also disconnected from the flagellum; the separation between the two occurs very likely during epididymal transit at the time sperm acquire motility, as a result of the inability of a faulty implantation to maintain them connected to one another. Spermatozoa with the "bent head" defect are characterized by abnormal and ineffective motility due to lack of coordination between the movements of the head and the tail; the defect is almost invariably associated with nuclear and acrosomal abnormalities (Figures 21–38, 39) which further contribute to the functional ineffectiveness of these spermatozoa.

Decapitation Defect

The most severe connecting piece abnormality and, possibly, the most limiting sperm defect is the separation of the head from the tail. This abnormality is generally referred to as "decapitation" or "decapitated sperm defect" and was documented for the first time by Lüders.[102] Patients with this defect, which is irreconcilable with any fertility potential, produce an ejaculate containing exclusively (or predominantly) headless but vigorously motile flagella (Figure 21–40), the heads having become separated in the lumina of the seminiferous tubules or in the epididymis at the time the spermatozoa acquire motility. Ultrastructural examination of these headless flagella (Figure 21–41, 42) discloses interesting aspects. First, their ultrastructural organization is normal; secondly, their uppermost segments are enveloped by, or contained within, a voluminous, elliptical cytoplasmic droplet, an observation that was also made by Perotti, Giarola, and Gioria[103] and by Baccetti, Selmi, and Soldani.[104] On examination with the light microscope, these droplets can easily be interpreted by the untrained eye as small-size heads (Figure 21–40), their presence explaining why these headless tails are frequently classified in semen analysis as "microcephalic" or "pinheaded" spermatozoa.[105] The defect is congenital; it appears to be due to a faulty connection[106] or failure of the proximal centriole and the other elements of the neck to assume the proper location with respect to the spermatid nucleus at the time of flagellar development.[104] The abnormality may be more common than the cases so far described in the literature (four) would indicate. (Four unpublished cases have been collected in the author's laboratory.) Decapitation is, in fact, a common sperm defect in farm animals, particularly bulls; as in man, it constitutes an irreversible cause of sterility.[107–113]

THE HEAD

The sperm head, generally viewed as a single entity, actually consists of at least three essential components for the reproductive process, the nucleus, the acrosome, and the membranous elements of the postacrosomal region.

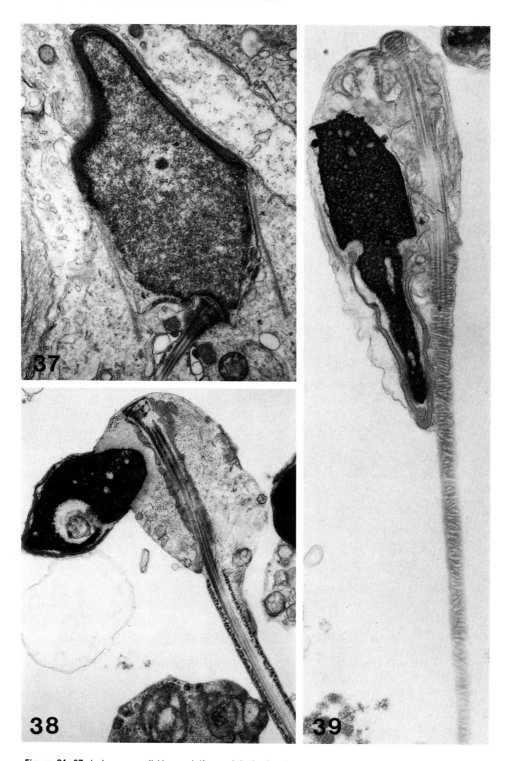

Figure 21–37. Late spermatid in seminiferous tubule showing abnormal implantation of the developing flagellum with respect to the nucleus; this developmental abnormality constitutes the basis of the defects illustrated in Figures 21–38, 39.

Figures 21–38, 39. Spermatozoa with the "bent head" defect. In both cases, not only are the heads flexed over the axis of the flagellum but they are also disconnected from the latter. Nuclear abnormalities such as intranuclear vacuoles (Figure 21–38) and immature patterns of chromatin aggregation (Figure 21–39) are frequently associated with this connecting piece defect.

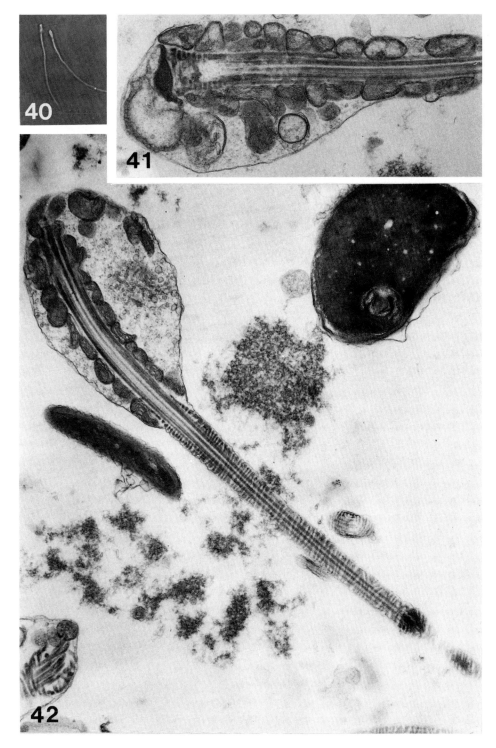

Figure 21–40. Light micrograph of two headless spermatozoa in a fresh semen sample, analogous to those illustrated in the electron micrographs of Figures 21–41, 42. The knob-like extremities of these headless flagella are cytoplasmic droplets; they can be interpreted as representing small-size heads and the defect thus diagnosed as microcephaly or "pin-head" defect.

Figures 21–41, 42. Electron micrographs of two headless flagella. Note the otherwise normal organization of the elements of the tail, and the presence of an elliptical cytoplasmic droplet enveloping the uppermost segment of the latter; these residual cytoplasmic bodies are the knob-like bodies at the cephalic extremities of the two flagella in Figure 21–40.

Normal Structure

The *nucleus,* the repository of the paternal genome, consists of DNA coupled to basic proteins; ultrastructurally, it appears as a uniformly compact, keratinoid mass of chromatin of high electron opacity (Figure 21–43). The organization and appearance of the nucleus of the mature sperm result from profound physico-chemical transformations of the chromatin, occurring in late stages of spermiogenesis simultaneously with nuclear elongation, and continuing during epididymal transit; they include the elimination of the RNA from the nucleus,[114] the replacement of somatic histones by protamines,[115] the formation of disulfide bonds essential for sperm stability,[116,117] and the gradual transformation of the finely granular chromatin of the young spermatid nucleus (Figure 21–44) at first into the more coarsely granular or globular variety of the late spermatid (Figure 21–45) and, ultimately, into the uniformly compact and dense mass of the mature spermatozoon (Figure 21–43).

Normal sperm nuclei are highly resistant to disruption; their DNA can be neither unraveled by sonication nor digested by DNAase,[118,119] and they can be partially decondensed only following the application of detergents,[120,121] even though some success has been reported recently with other methods[122,123] (for a review, see[5]). It has been postulated that such a high degree of unreactivity may serve to protect the genomic patrimony of the sperm from physical or chemical injury during transit through the female reproductive tract.[119,124]

Often enclosed in the dense chromatin mass are one or two small vacuoles appearing as non-membrane-bound areas of rarefaction and containing sparse granular or filamentous material (Figure 21–43); they seem to form as the consequence of uneven processes of chromatin condensation.[1,125] The sperm nucleus is delimited by a double membrane envelope, the inner leaflet of which is hardly visible due to its adherence to the chromatin.

The *acrosome,* referred to by early morphologists as the nuclear cap, is a cytoplasmic organelle covering the anterior three-fourths of the nucleus and constituting the most superficial element of the rostral portion of the sperm, below the plasma membrane (Figure 21–43). It consists of a homogeneous matrix of medium electron opacity, and a single limiting membrane distinguished into an outer acrosomal membrane situated just below the plasmalemma, and an inner membrane running parallel to the outer leaflet of the nuclear envelope. In its posterior fifth, the organelle becomes much thinner and tapered. Since this occurs where the nucleus exhibits its widest diameter, this part of the acrosome is referred to as the *equatorial region.* The acrosome develops from the Golgi apparatus during early stages of spermatid differentiation. Its final shape and appearance are the result of dynamic remodeling processes involving not only the Golgi apparatus but also the spermatid nucleus and, possibly, the array of the cytoplasmic microtubules of the "manchette,"[1,125–127] (Figures 21–44, 45). The matrix and the limiting membrane of the acrosome contain an array of hydrolytic enzymes[5,128,129] of which hyaluronidase and acrosin are noteworthy for the purpose of this discussion.

Due to its origin from the Golgi complex and its enzymatic properties, the acrosome is generally considered analogous to a primary lysosome even though some of its characteristics are different from those of typical lysosomes and more similar to those of a specialized zymogen granule.[130]

The role that the acrosome plays at fertilization has been the subject of numerous studies recently reviewed by Yanagimachi,[131] Bedford,[132] and Moore and Bedford.[133] These studies indicate the capacitation, the preparatory process which expresses the fertilizing potential of the spermatozoon, and physiologically takes place in the female reproductive tract,[134,135] but also can be achieved by various methods *in vitro*,[136] has the primary function of preparing the organelle for the role that it is to perform shortly before sperm conjugation with the egg. The structural manifestation of a "capacitated" state or condition is presently recognized as the ability of the sperm to undergo the acrosome reaction[137] at the time of its penetration through the egg investments. The reaction, which is allegedly characterized by the rapid dismantling of the periacrosomal portion of the plasma membrane and the outer acrosomal membrane, would allow the acrosomal matrix and enzymes to diffuse outside the cell. The liberation of hyaluronidase would bring about the digestion of the mucopolysaccharidic matrix in which the cumulus cells are suspended, and would thus facilitate the progression of the sperm through this investment. By the time the sperm reaches the outer aspect of the zona pellucida, the second periovular investment consisting essentially of glycoproteins,[138,139] the acrosomal matrix would be fully dispersed and the most rostral region of the nucleus would be covered only by the inner acrosomal membrane containing acrosin, a protease-like enzyme. Even though serious doubts about the role of acrosin in sperm penetration through the zona have been expressed,[133] it is still widely accepted that liberation of this enzyme would result in the focal digestion of the zona pellucida material, thus creating a tunnel-like path (the "penetration slit") through which the sperm would be allowed to reach the surface of the egg.

Not involved in the acrosome reaction is the equatorial region which in fully reacted spermatozoa remains intact,[140–142] a behavior that underlies evident (but partially understood) functional dissimilarities between this component and the remainder of the organelle. Bedford, Moore, and Franklin[142] postulated that the lack of participation of the equatorial segment in the acrosome reaction may have the purpose of preserving the integrity of the overlying plasmalemma for the function of initiating the process of gamete membrane fusion; this hypothesis, however, is not consistent with the demonstration that it is in the postacrosomal region that initial contact between gametes becomes established.[143–145]

The acrosome is not clearly visible in live and unstained spermatozoa because of its small size and its translucency. For this purpose several special staining methods have been proposed. Bryan[146] has proposed an eosin-fast green-naphthol yellow mixture. Singer *et al.*[147] advocate the utilization of the Papanicolau stain, while Talbot and Chacon[148,149] have devised special staining

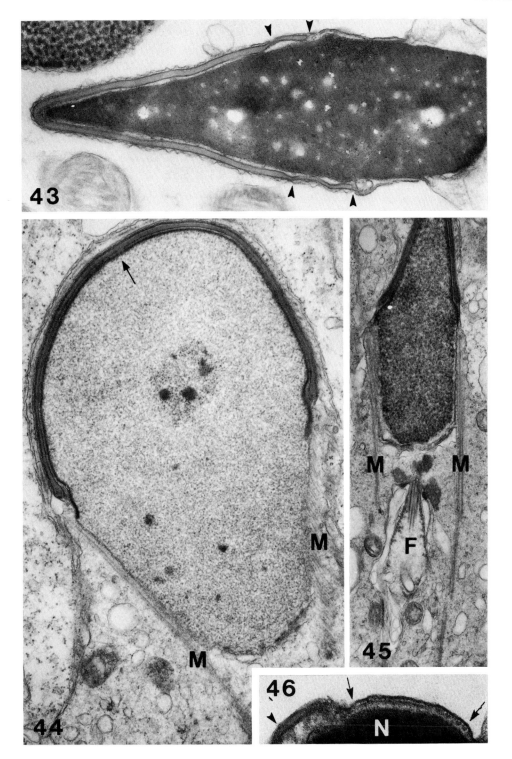

Figure 21–43. Ultrastructural appearance of a "normal" sperm head. Notice the highly compact aggregation of the chromatin, and the acrosome surrounding the rostral portion of the nucleus. Arrowheads point to the equatorial segment of the acrosome.

Figure 21–44. Young spermatid at onset of nuclear elongation; note the uniformly fine granularity of the chromatin. M, "manchette" microtubules; arrow points to the acrosome.

Figure 21–45. Late spermatid stage. The coarsely granular pattern of chromatin aggregation is evident. M, "manchette" microtubules; F, developing flagellum.

Figure 21–46. The limits of the specialized laminar structure covering the postacrosomal region of the sperm nucleus (N) are indicated by the arrows. The arrowhead points to the equatorial region of the sperm acrosome.

procedures that permit the visualization of the changes induced by the acrosome reaction and their differentiation from those occurring as a consequence of sperm death. However, these staining methods are relatively complex and none is routinely applicable. Considering how essential the normalcy, both structural and functional, of the acrosome is for fertilization, the inability to assess its condition is in itself one of the most severe limitations of the conventional methods of semen analysis.

Posterior to the equatorial segment, the nucleus is covered by a laminar structure exhibiting, in favorable but rarely encountered planes of section, a distinct periodicity in the form of cross-striations separated by regular intervals (Figure 21–46). The sperm plasma membrane participates in the composition of this structure so intimately as to be no longer resolvable as a separate entity, forming with it a specialized functional unit which structurally resembles a septate desmosome.[1,20,150] As already mentioned, there is morphologic evidence suggesting that this specialized segment of the membranes covering the sperm head has the function of establishing and maintaining the adhesion between gametes.[143–145]

Differing from the situation prevailing in other primates where uniformity of head shape is the rule,[19–21] the human spermatozoon is characterized by marked variations in the configuration of its head. Ideally, its outline should be elliptical on an antero-posterior plane, and much thinner and tapered in a sagittal direction, since its thickness is considerably less than its width. While in "normal" semen samples, most sperm may indeed display this head configuration, triangular and/or extremely tapered outlines (on an antero-posterior plane as well) are not at all infrequent and may even predominate. These comments are made to emphasize the difficulty of establishing what constitutes a normal head shape and should not be taken to suggest that shape oddities are to be dismissed as unimportant. Particularly when the same shape deviations from the "norm" are observed in the majority or all of the spermatozoa in a sample, they should receive special attention, since they almost regularly indicate underlying structural malformations that need to be precisely evaluation. For example, the cephalic over-elongation (tapering) that is frequently associated with varicocele,[151–155] but is not pathognomonic of this condition,[151,154,155] is due to exaggerated length of the most posterior region of the nucleus as well as to presence of abundant scrolls of redundant membranes (Figure 21–47), an observation reported also by Rouy and Sentein[156] and by Dadoune et al.[157] Considering the importance of the postacrosomal region in establishing contact with the oocyte, the occurrence of shrouds of membranes in this area could very well account for the reduced fertility that often affects men with tapered sperm heads. Variations of head size larger or smaller than the "norm" should also be considered reasons for submitting the ejaculate to methods of morphologic evaluation more accurate than those employed in routine semen analysis. A normal head should average 2 to 3 μm in width and 3 to 5 μm in length.[105] Even though these measurements should be regarded as ideal, since variations in size are not uncommon in spermatozoa of individuals of proven fertility, the possible occurrence of structural defects should be kept in mind when all or most of the sperm in a sample display heads are larger or smaller than the "norm."

Considering the functional importance of its components, the defects of the sperm head are of ominous significance for fertility; they may involve the nucleus and the acrosome individually or in combination, and/or they may occur in isolation or together with abnormalities of the elements of the tail.

Chromatin Abnormalities

Out of the very large variety of ultrastructural head defects which have been documented,[14,15,17,18,91,158–166] one of the most frequent is the abnormal organization of the chromatin, a defect which is invariably associated with a wide range of acrosomal defects as well as other aberrations, such as presence of gigantic intranuclear vacuoles or inclusions (Figures 21–48, 49) and/or occurrence of multiple nuclei joined together by commonly shared acrosomes (Figure 21–50). Most often, the chromatin appears in the coarsely granular, immature aggregational patterns characteristic of the spermatids at the stage of incipient nuclear elongation.[1,125] In extreme examples, a true nucleomalacic condition is evident (Figures 21–51, 52) with the chromatin unraveling into filamentous threads which disperse into the subacrosomal space and/or the cytoplasm around the posterior region of the nucleus. While abnormal chromatin patterns may be seen sporadically in spermatozoa in "normal" semen samples,[120,167] this defect represents one of those most frequently encountered in the seminal fluids of infertile patients where it usually involves most or all spermatozoa (Figure 21–53). While other anomalies, especially those of the acrosome, may contribute to the infertility of these individuals, physico-chemical and chromosomal studies provide compelling evidence that per se this nuclear defect is capable of severely affecting or preventing fertility. Evenson, Darzynkiewicz, and Melamed[168] have reported that the DNA of sperm nuclei with abnormal patterns of chromatin aggregation is principally single- rather than double-stranded and, as such, has a markedly decreased resistance to thermal denaturation as compared to the DNA of normal sperm. Baccetti et al.[127] have shown that chromatin immaturity is associated with lower phosphorus concentrations, higher than normal zinc content, and persistence of variable amounts of lysine, suggesting that in these spermatozoa the somatic histones have not been replaced by basic proteins which are instead rich in arginine and cysteine. This hypothesis is indirectly supported by the finding that the spermatozoa of infertile men frequently contain histones instead of protamines.[169] Finally, a direct correlation between decreased density of chromatin aggregation and chromosomal abnormalities has been reported by Kjessler[170–172] and by Abramsson et al.[173]

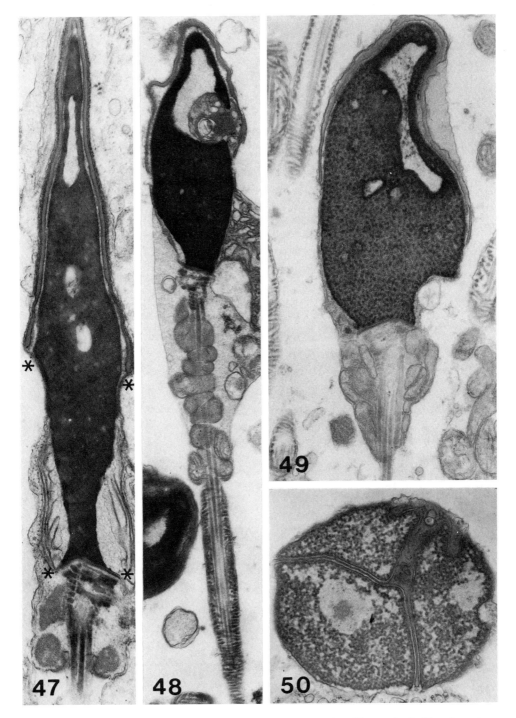

Figure 21–47. Cephalic over-elongation (tapering) of the sperm head in a patient with varicocele. Notice the exaggerated length of the postacrosomal region of the nucleus (between asterisks) and the scrolls of redundant membranes surrounding most of its extension.

Figures 21–48, 49, 50. Three examples of abnormal, immature patterns of chromatin aggregation of increasing severity, the one in Figure 21–48 being the least, and that in Figure 21–50 being the most pronounced. Note the association of this defect with occurrence of large intranuclear vacuoles (Figures 21–48, 49), incompleteness of the nucleus, and intranuclear inclusions (Figure 21–48), and multiple nuclei joined by a commonly shared acrosome (Figure 21–50).

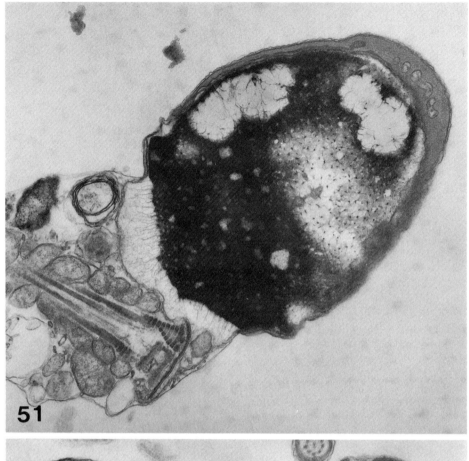

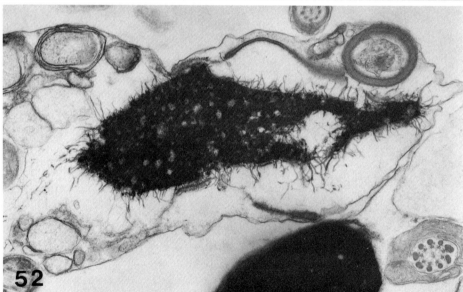

Figures 21–51, 52. Two examples of sperm nucleomalacia. Notice the unraveling of the chromatin into filamentous threads. In the sperm of Figure 21–52, the chromatin disperses in the perinuclear cytoplasm due to absence of a nuclear envelope; this sperm also shows pronounced acrosomal abnormalities.

Intranuclear Vacuoles and Inclusions

Intranuclear vacuoles and inclusions, often large enough to result in conspicuous deformations of the nuclear shape, are not infrequent findings even in normal semen, but in some infertile patients they occur in nearly all the spermatozoa (Figure 21–54) where they are often associated with acrosomal defects and/or with the just described abnormal patterns of chromatin condensation

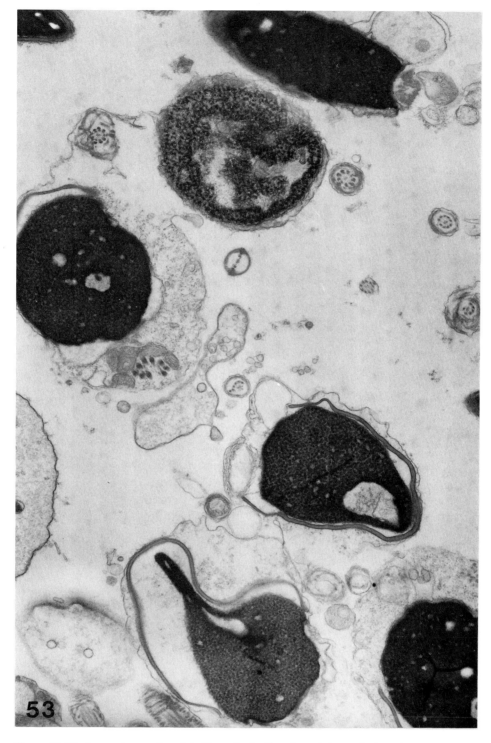

Figure 21–53. Spermatozoa of an infertile patient with universal chromatin immaturity and/or nucleomalacia.

(Figures 21–48, 49, 53). The vacuoles are not membrane-bound and appear as irregular, chromatin "voids." They may be empty, but more frequently they contain pleomorphic inclusions such as membranous structures arranged in whorls (Figure 21–55) or in parallel arrays (Figure 21–56), vesicles of different size (Figure 21–55), and lipid droplets (Figure 21–57). These intranuclear inclusions develop at the spermatid stage of spermiogene-

sis in the course of nuclear elongation and chromatin condensation. Their morphogenesis, which can be traced by examining early (Figure 21–58) and late spermatids (Figure 21–59) in testicular biopsies, was carefully reconstructed by Holstein[15] in a study of 128 patients with a history of subfertility or infertility, and with a variety of andrological disorders characterized by oligo-, terato- or azoospermia. Very recently, analogous nuclear ultrastruc-

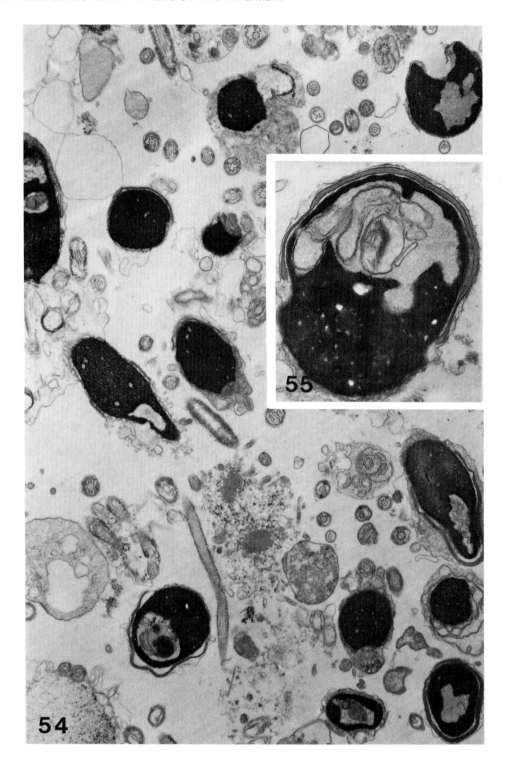

Figure 21–54. Spermatozoa of an infertile patient showing universal presence of gigantic intranuclear vacuoles and pleomorphic nuclear inclusions. A few spermatozoa also display immature patterns of chromatin aggregation.

Figure 21–55. A sperm from the same patient showing a gigantic intranuclear vacuole containing sequestered membranes and vesicles of different size.

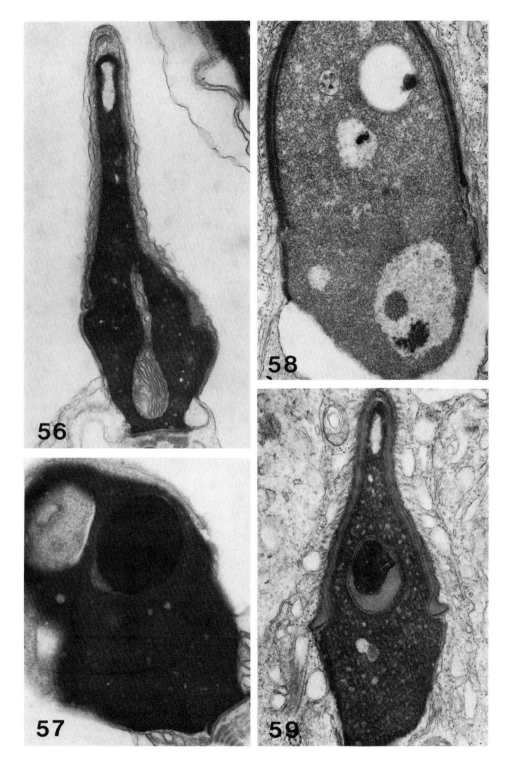

Figures 21–56, 57. Intranuclear vacuoles containing parallel arrays of sequestered membranes (Figure 21–56) and a lipid droplet (Figure 21–57).

Figures 21–58, 59. Two phases of the morphogenesis of intranuclear vacuoles and inclusions in a young, (Figure 21–58) and a late spermatid (Figure 21–59) in the seminiferous tubules of the testis.

tural defects were described in detail by Hrudka and Singh[174] in infertile patients with inflammatory bowel disease; the defects were considered attributable to the disease *per se,* rather than to medication with sulfadrugs, as hypothesized by those who also had noted the association of inflammatory bowel disease with infertility, inferior semen quality, and abnormal sperm morphology.[175-179]

Acrosomal Defects

Acrosomal defects occur just as frequently as the nuclear defects with which they are often associated. Because of their pronounced pleomorphism,[18] a detailed description of the multiplicity of forms under which they occur would not be consistent with the approach of this review. Therefore, the following description will be limited to two main types of acrosomal abnormalities, both constituting important causes of infertility.

The first is acrosomal hypoplasia and fragility. The spermatozoa of patients with this defect have universally thin acrosomes (Figure 21–60). The hypoplasia of the organelle is so pronounced that the differences in size which normally distinguish the equatorial segment are often completely effaced (Figure 21–61). The acrosomes may be of conventional outline (Figure 21–61) but more frequently they have deformed, often bizarre shapes (Figure 21–62) and/or are detached from the nucleus (Figures 21–62, 63). They are often swollen to various degrees (Figures 21–64, 65) with consequent extreme rarefaction of the matrix. The presence of uninterrupted intact plasma membranes over even the most swollen, ballooning acrosomes indicates that the changes are not artifacts. Except for their acrosomal defects, which are not visible by light microscopy, these spermatozoa are normal in appearance, and the only feature detectable in conventional semen analysis is the somewhat reduced size of their heads. The defect has not been given the attention that it deserves, and even in major reviews of sperm pathology[14,17] it is only superficially mentioned under the heading of "microcephaly." Yet it is a direct cause of sterility. This author has frequently encountered it in patients with a long history of infertility whose spermatozoa failed to penetrate the zona-free hamster eggs in spite of repeated semen analyses showing "normal sperm numbers, motility, and morphology." Electron microscopic examination of the semen of these individuals demonstrated unequivocally that the negative results of the "hamster test" and their sterility resulted from the abnormality of their sperm acrosomes which prevented effective capacitation and/or the occurrence of the acrosome reaction.

The second major acrosome defect is the agenesis of the organelle (Figures 21–66, 67, 68). Patients with this defect produce spermatozoa universally lacking the acrosome, and with spheroidal rather than normally elongated nuclei, the latter feature accounting for the term "round head defect" by which this abnormality is conventionally designated. The vast majority of these spermatozoa also have abnormal, immature patterns of chromatin aggregation (Figures 21–66, 68). The triad of agenesis of the acrosome, sphericity of the nucleus and immaturity of the chromatin has been documented in all cases so far described in the literature,[180-185] and has also been demonstrated by all of those who investigated the morphogenesis of the defect studying testicular biopsies by electron microscopy,[15,18,127,186-188] cytochemical analysis,[127,187] and immunohistochemical methods.[189] These studies have concordantly shown that the agenesis of the acrosome results from defective deposition and/or anomalous localization of the proacrosomal material, lack of contact between the Golgi-derived proacrosomal vesicle (the precursor of the acrosome) and the nucleus of the spermatid, and absence or rudimentary development of the microtubular system of the "manchette."

The identification of these morphogenetic mechanisms, and the association of the acrosomal defect with the abnormality of nuclear shape and immaturity of the chromatin reinforces the hypothesis that the structural integrity, shape, and physico-chemical organization of the sperm head are controlled by the same or, if different, concomitantly operating mechanisms. Acrosome-less spermatozoa rarely occur without tail defects; among those most frequently encountered are the wrapping of the flagellum around the nucleus (Figure 21–66), the presence of large cephalic cytoplasmic droplets enveloping the nucleus and the uppermost segment of the flagellum together (Figure 21–68), partial or complete lack of mitochondria (Figure 21–68), and defects of the axonemal microtubules and of the dense outer fibers (Figure 21–66), features suggesting that the agenesis of the acrosome is only the most consistent evidence of a profoundly altered spermiogenetic process.

The defect has a familial trait,[182,184,190] and is congenital. Recently a polygenic rather than a monogenic mode of inheritance has been suggested.[190] The infertility of patients with this defect rests primarily on the inability of their spermatozoa to become capacitated and undergo the acrosome reaction. This is shown also by the demonstrated incapacity of these spermatozoa to penetrate the denuded hamster eggs.[191-193] In routine semen analysis, the defect should be suspected any time large numbers of round-headed spermatozoa are visible, and its actual occurrence should be verified by electron microscopy. While this defect is probably among the least overlooked in the clinical practice of andrology, it is not yet universally recognized that a spheroidal shape of the sperm head signals an irreversible cause of infertility.[185]

Macrocephalic and Multi-tailed Sperm

To complete this review, it is necessary to comment briefly on the ultrastructural features of the few "gross" sperm defects, i.e. those that can be visualized in the course of conventional semen analysis. Multi-tailed, macrocephalic sperm are frequently found in the semen of sterile patients. Studying their ultrastructure, Nistal, Paniagua, and Herruzo[194] and, more recently, Escalier[195] noted that they regularly display acrosomal aberrations

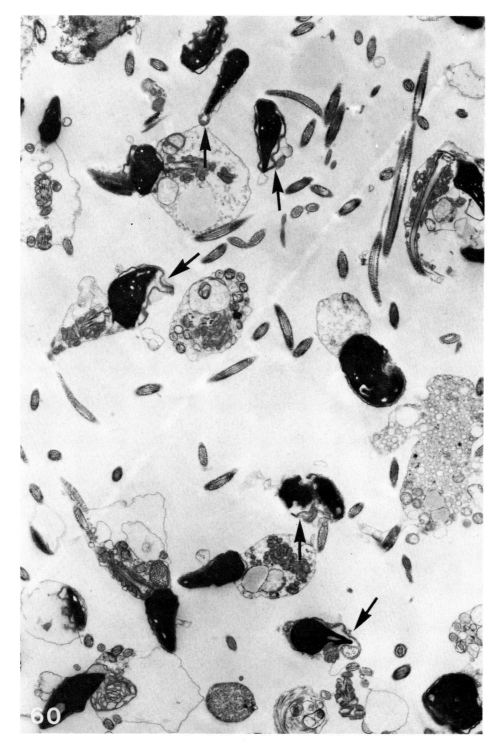

Figure 21–60. Spermatozoa of an infertile patient with hypoplasia of the acrosome. Notice the universal thinness of the organelle, its shape aberrations and detachment from the nucleus (arrows).

and a variety of defects of the axonemal microtubules and other flagellar elements. It is thus the occurrence of these ultrastructural abnormalities, rather than the macrocephaly and the multiplicity of the tails, that accounts for the sterility of these patients.

It is probable that the abnormality of these spermatozoa is the manifestation of a generalized dysfunction of the microtubular system. Functional inadequacy of the microtubules of the "manchette," whose role in the shaping of the nucleus and of the acrosome is strongly suspected, albeit not completely defined,[126,196] could account for the nuclear and acrosomal abnormalities, while the dysfunction of the centriolar microtubules could explain the multiplicity of the tails. The demonstrated presence

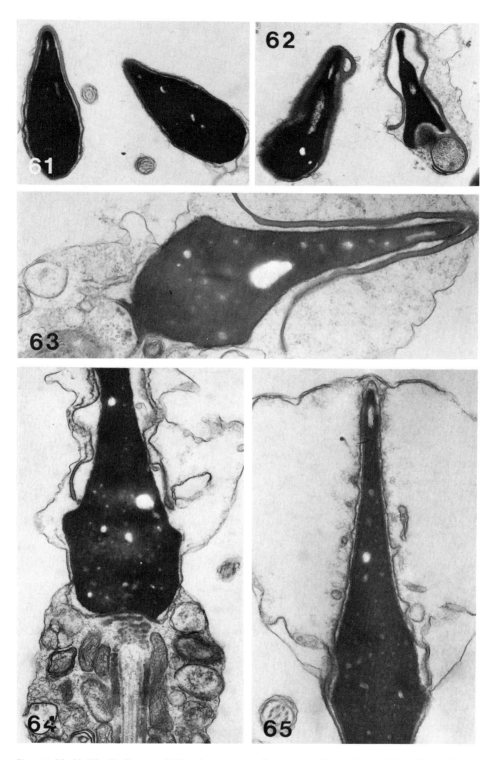

Figures 21–61, 62, 63. Three additional examples of acrosomal hypoplasia. Notice the extreme thinness of the organelle (all micrographs), its deformed shape (Figure 21–62), and its separation from the nucleus (Figure 21–63).

Figures 21–64, 65. Frequently, acrosomal hypoplasia is associated with extreme swelling (ballooning) of the organelle. Notice the continuity of the plasma membrane over the swollen, completely rarefied organelle. These two sperm are from the same patient whose spermatozoa are shown in Figure 21–60.

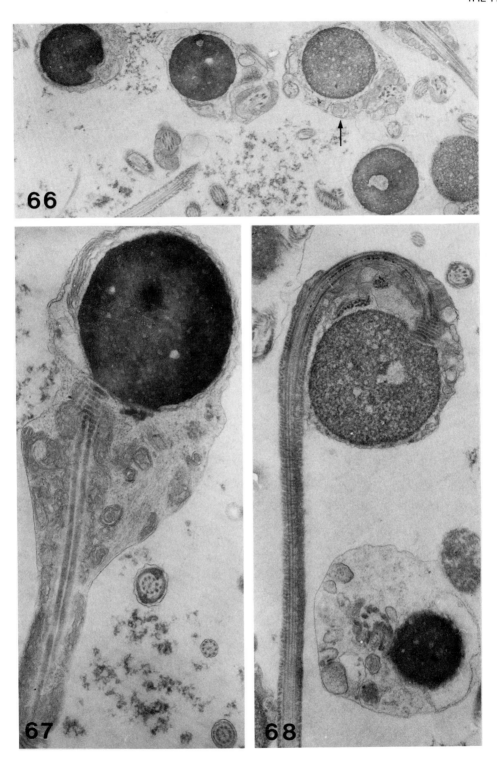

Figures 21–66, 67, 68. Agenesis of the acrosome. Notice the universality of the defect (Figure 21–66) and its association with sphericity of the nucleus and immaturity of the chromatin. Arrow in Figure 21–66 points to a sperm with the tail wrapped around the nucleus and with disorganization of the outer dense fibers. The sperm shown in Figure 21–68 has a pericephalic cytoplasmic droplet enveloping the nucleus and the initial segment of the flagellum together and also displays mitochondrial defects.

in these spermatozoa of excessive amounts of DNA[197] suggests the possibility that their nuclei may have formed from the coalescence of spermatid nuclei that did not become individualized at the appropriate time—another developmental defect attributable to dysfunction of the microtubules—in this case those of the intercellular bridges connecting cells in identical stages of differentiation. The finding that the somatic cells of these patients are polyploid (up to 92 chromosomes have been counted) very likely because of abnormal mitotic regulatory mechanisms, reinforces the hypothesis of a generalized microtubular dysfunction.[17] Analogous sperm abnormalities were noted by Baccetti et al.[198] in the spermatozoa of a hyperprolactinemic patient with pituitary adenoma and similarly ascribed to functional impairment of the mechanisms controlling cell division. Interestingly enough, the abnormalities disappeared following appropriate therapy.[199]

I have intentionally omitted from this review any specific reference to the occurrence of the "cytoplasmic droplets," the portions of residual cytoplasm that remain attached to the spermatozoa at the time they are released into the lumina of the seminiferous tubules. They should ideally be shed, as in other species, during transit through the epididymis, but in men usually are not, as demonstrated by their frequent occurrence in "normal" spermatozoa. The omission is justified by the consideration that the presence of these residual cytoplasmic bodies in itself is neither a defect nor a cause of infertility.

CONCLUSION

Considerable work remains to be done in identifying all the etiologic factors and morphogenetic mechanisms that are responsible for the abnormalities of human spermatozoa. Genetic factors are obviously involved in the development of defects such as agenesis and hypoplasia of the acrosome, decapitation, the 9 + 0 defect, the various defects constituting the structural bases of "ciliary dyskinesis," the derangements of the fibrous sheath, etc. This is reinforced by the well established familial incidence of some of these structural abnormalities and their association with chromosomal aberrations. Other defects are unquestionably caused by physical factors that negatively affect spermiogenesis. One factor is heat; not only is it well established that scrotal heating in farm animals produces acrosomal defects with consequent decrease in fertility,[200–202] but exposure to heat is also frequently found in the clinical histories of patients with one or another of the above described sperm defects.[162] Varicocele as a cause of sperm abnormalities has been already mentioned. The teratogenic effects of cigarette smoking and a correlation between incidence of sperm abnormalities and number of cigarettes smoked per day were first reported by Viczian,[203] and later by Evans, Fletcher, Torrance et al.,[204] who suggested that the sperm defects of smokers could be the expression of genetic damage to the germinal cells, as well as Shaarawy and Mahmoud.[205]

Berry[206] speculated that smoke may affect sperm motility through the same mechanisms that have been shown to damage somatic cell cilia exposed to cigarette smoke in vitro, while Kulikauskas, Blaustein and Ablin[207] have invoked the mutagenic properties of smoke condensates. The teratogenic effect of alcohol and other drugs is well known. Obviously, the etiology of many defects remains unclarified.

This review may provide an up-to-date account of the ultrastructural pathology of the human spermatozoon as a cause of infertility, but it should increase the reader's awareness of the limitations of the conventional semen analysis and of the fact that, of the wide constellation of sperm structural defects and developmental anomalies, only a few can be identified by the methods and the tools employed for the routine evaluation of human semen. Does this mean that an ultrastructural examination of the ejaculate should be considered a routine component of the assessment of the infertile male? Certainly not; however, it should be used as a necessary procedure in special circumstances.

Bisson and David[14] advocated electron microscopic examination as a diagnostic necessity in patients with a history of infertility who produce sufficient numbers of sperm ($>10^6$/ml) characterized, however, by pronounced and predominantly monomorphic teratospermia. Afzelius,[76] and Pedersen, Rebbe and Hammen[92] very appropriately stated that ultrastructural evaluation of semen is also required to establish whether generalized asthenospermia is due to sperm death or to immotility resulting from flagellar abnormalities, as well as to differentiate changes of testicular origin from those occurring during passage through the excurrent ducts. This indeed is an important point since the reliability of the special staining procedures that are used to differentiate live, but immotile, spermatozoa from dead ones is not absolute; in these cases, electron microscopy is of unquestionable help since changes such as the fragmentation of the plasma membrane, the degenerative phenomena of the acrosome, the effacement of the mitochondrial cristae, and the rarefaction of the matrix, the blurring of the axonemal microtubules, etc. are indications of cell death.

In addition, ultrastructural examination of the ejaculate is warranted whenever the results of analysis of the semen fail to account for the patient's infertility and/or do not reconcile with the results of the zona-free hamster egg penetration assay. In these cases, electron microscopic evaluation of the semen very often terminates long months of investigation and/or futile therapy. In our experience, ultrastructural evaluation of the semen has been very beneficial not only for a better definition of semen abnormalities and the pathophysiology of male infertility, but also because it reveals to the physician that the "inferior" quality of a particular semen was not amenable to improvement. This has saved many a patient repeated semen analyses and investment of time and money, has spared him and his partner emotional turmoil, and has permitted the physician to advise the couple in a timely manner on the availability of alternative methods for the resolution of their infertility. One of these alternative methods is in vitro fertilization.[208] There are defects that, while hardly reconcilable with any degree of fertility under physiologic conditions, could still permit the spermatozoa to fulfill their reproductive role under "assisted" conditions. It is obvious, for example, that flagellar defects are likely to be less limiting *in vitro* where the spermatozoa are in direct contact with the egg and its investment, than they are *in vivo*. Thus, an elucidation of the ultrastructural basis of "poor semen quality" could also contribute to providing the infertile couple with alternatives that would not be otherwise available. In any case, it makes sense that, whenever required, the precise evaluation of the structural integrity of isolated cells be performed utilizing "cytologic" methods of analysis.

References

1. Zamboni L: Fine Morphology of Mammalian Fertilization. New York, Harper and Row, 1971.
2. Fawcett DW: The mammalian spermatozoon: a review. Devel Biol 44:394–436, 1975.
3. Pedersen H, Fawcett DW: Functional anatomy of the human spermatozoon. *In* ESE Hafez (ed) Human Semen and Fertility Regulation in Men. St Louis, C.V. Mosby Company, 1976.
4. Setchell BP: Spermatogenesis and spermatozoa. *In* CR Austin and RV Short (eds) Germ Cells and Fertilization. Cambridge, Cambridge University Press, 1982.
5. Bellvé AR, O'Brien DA: The mammalian spermatozoon: structure and temporal assembly. *In* JF Hartman (ed) Mechanisms and Control of Animal Fertilization. New York, Academic Press, 1983.
6. WHO: Laboratory manual for the examination of human semen and semen-cervical mucus interaction. *In* MA Belsey, KS Moghissi, CA Paulsen, *et al.* (eds) World Health Organization Special Programme of Research, Development and Research Training in Human Reproduction. Singapore, Press Concern, 1980.
7. Hargreave TB, Nilsson S: Seminology. *In* TB Hargreave (ed) Male Infertility. Berlin, Springer-Verlag, 1983.
8. MacLeod J: Human seminal cytology as a sensitive indicator of the germinal epithelium. Int J Fertil 9:281–295, 1964.
9. Yanagimachi R, Yanagimachi H, Rogers BJ: The use of zona-free animal ova as a test system for the assessment of the fertilizing capacity of human spermatozoa. Biol Reprod 15:471–478, 1976.
10. Hanada A, Chang MC: Penetration of zona-free eggs by spermatozoa of different species. Biol Reprod 6:300–309, 1972.
11. Yanagimachi R: Zona-free hamster eggs: their use in assessing fertilizing capacity and examining chromosomes of human spermatozoa. Gamete Res 10:187–232, 1984.
12. Lipshultz LI: Beyond the routine semen analysis. Fertil Steril 38:153–155, 1982.
13. Gould JE, Overstreet JW, Yanagimachi H, *et al.*: What functions of the sperm cells are measured by *in vitro* fertilization of zona-free hamster eggs? Fertil Steril 40–344–352, 1983.
14. Bisson JP, David G: Anomalies morphologiques du spermatozoide humain; 2) Étude ultrastructurale. J Gynecol Obstet Biol Reprod 4(Suppl. 1): 37–86, 1975.
15. Holstein AF: Morphologische Studien an abnormen Spermatiden und Spermatozoen des Menschen. Virchows Arch A (Pathol Anat Histol) Berlin, 367:93–112, 1975.
16. Escalier D, David G: Pathology of the cytoskeleton of the human sperm flagellum: axonemal and peri-axonemal anomalies. Biol Cell 50:37–52, 1984.
17. Nistal M, Paniagua R: Testicular and Epididymal Pathology. New York, Thieme-Stratton, 1984.
18. Holstein AF, Schirren C: Classification of abnormalities in human spermatids based on recent advances in ultrastructure research on spermatid differentiation. *In* DW Fawcett, JM Bedford (eds) The Spermatozoon. Maturation, Motility, Surface Properties, and Comparative Aspects. Baltimore, Urban and Schwarzenberg, 1979.
19. Bedford JM: Observations on the fine structure of spermatozoa of the bush baby (*Galago senegalensis*), the African green monkey (*Cercopithecus aethiops*), and man. Am J Anat 121:443–460, 1967.
20. Zamboni L, Zemjanis R, Stefanini M: The fine structure of monkey and human spermatozoa. Anat Rec 169:129–154, 1971.
21. Bedford JM: Biology of primate spermatozoa. Contrib Primatol 3:97–139, 1974.
22. Olson GE, Linck RW: Observation of the structural components of flagellar axonemes and central pair microtubules from rat sperm. J Ultrastruct Res 61:21–43, 1977.
23. Linck RW: Advances in the ultrastructural analysis of the sperm flagellar axoneme. *In* DW Fawcett, JM Bedford (eds) The Spermatozoon: Maturation, Motility, Surface Properties and Comparative Aspects. Baltimore, Urban and Schwarzenbeg, 1979.
24. Gibbons IR: Cilia and flagella of eukaryotes. J Cell Biol 91:1075–1245, 1981.
25. Gibbons IR: Structure and function of flagellar microtubules. *In* BR Brinkley, KR Porter (eds) International Cell Biology. New York, Rockefeller University Press, 1977.
26. Baccetti B, Burrini AG, Maver A. *et al.*: "9+0" immotile spermatozoa in an infertile man. Andrologia 11:437–443, 1979.
27. Baccetti B, Burrini AG, Pallini V, *et al.*: Human dynein and sperm pathology. J Cell Biol 88:102–107, 1981.
28. Baccetti B, Porter KR, Ulrich M: High voltage electron microscopy of sperm axoneme. J Submicrosc Cytol 17:171–176, 1985.
29. Afzelius BA: Electron microscopy of the sperm tail: results obtained with a new fixative. J Biophys Biochem Cytol 5:269–278, 1959.
30. Haimo LT, Rosenbaum JL: Cilia, flagella, and microtubules. J Cell Biol 91:125s–130s, 1981.
31. Gibbons BH: Studies on the mechanisms of flagellar movement. *In* DW Fawcett, JM Bedford (eds) The Spermatozoon. Maturation, Motility, Surface Properties and Comparative Aspects. Baltimore, Urban and Schwarzenberg, 1979.
32. Satir P: Basis of flagellar motility in spermatozoa: current status. *In* DW Fawcett, JM Bedford (eds) The Spermatozoon. Maturation, Motility, Surface Properties and Comparative Aspects. Baltimore, Urban and Schwarzenberg, 1979.
33. Witman GB, Fay R, Plummer J: *Chlamydomonas mutans*: evidence for the role of specific axonemal components in flagellar movement. *In* RD Goldman, TD Polland, JL Rosenbaum (eds) Cell Motility. New York, Cold Spring Harbor, 1976.

34. Witman GB, Plummer J, Sander S: *Chlamydomonas* flagellar mutants lacking radial spokes and central tubules. Structure, composition, and function of specific axonemal components. J Cell Biol 76:729–747, 1978.

35. Huang B, Piperno G, Luck DJL: Paralyzed flagellar mutants of *Chlamydomonas reinhardtii* defective for axonemal doublet microtubule arms. J Biol Chem 254:3091–3099, 1979.

36. Brokaw CJ, Luck DJL, Huang B: Analysis of the movement of *Chlamydomonas* flagella: the function of the radial-spoke system is revealed by comparison of wild type and mutant flagella. J Cell Biol 92:722–732, 1982.

37. Olson GE, Sammons DW: Structural chemistry of outer dense fibers of rat sperm. Biol Reprod 22:319–332, 1980.

38. Baccetti B, Pallini V, Burrini AG: Accessory fibers of the sperm tail. I. Structural and chemical composition of the bull "coarse fibers." J Submicrosc Cytol 5:237–256, 1973.

39. Baccetti B, Pallini V, Burrini AG: The accessory fibers of the sperm tail. II. Their role in binding zinc in mammals and cephalopods. J Ultrastruct Res 54:261–275, 1976.

40. Baccetti B, Pallini V, Burrini AG: The accessory fibers of the sperm tail. III. High sulphur and low sulphur components in mammals and cephalopods. J Ultrastruct Res 57:289–308, 1976.

41. Baccetti B: The evolution of the sperm tail. Symp Soc Exp Biol 35:521–532, 1982.

42. Calvin HI, Hwang FH-F, Wohlrab H: Localization of zinc in a dense fiber-connecting piece fraction of rat sperm tail analogous chemically to hair keratin. Biol Reprod 13:228–239, 1975.

43. Phillips DM: Comparative analysis of mammalian sperm motility. J Cell Biol 53:561–573, 1972.

44. Phillips DM, Olson G: Mammalian sperm motility. *In* BA Afzelius (ed) The Functional Anatomy of the Spermatozoon. New York, Pergamon Press, 1975.

45. Fawcett DW: Unsolved problems in morphogenesis of the mammalian spermatozoon. *In* BR Brinkley, KR Porter (eds) International Cell Biology. New York, Rockefeller University Press, 1977.

46. Bedford, JM, Calvin HI: Changes in S-S-linked structures of the sperm tail during epididymal maturation with comparative observations in submammalian species. J Exp Zool 187:181–204, 1974.

47. Swan MA, Linck RW, Ito S, *et al.*: Structure and function of the undulating membrane in spermatozoan propulsion in the toad, *Bufo marinus*. J Cell Biol 85:866–880, 1980.

48. Olson GE, Hamilton DW, Fawcett DW: Isolation and characterization of the fibrous sheath of rat epididymal spermatozoa. Biol Reprod 14:517–530, 1976.

49. Olson GE: Isolation of the fibrous sheath and perforatorium of rat spermatozoa. *In* DW Fawcett, JM Bedford (eds) The Spermatozoon. Maturation, Motility, Surface Properties and Comparative Aspects. Baltimore, Urban and Schwarzenberg, 1979.

50. Phillips DM: Mammalian sperm structure. *In* DW Hamilton, RO Greep (eds) Handbook of Physiology. Washington, American Physiology Society, 1975.

51. McClure RJ, Brawer J, Robaire B: Ultrastructure of immotile spermatozoa in an infertile male: a spectrum of structural defects. Fertil Steril 40:395–399, 1983.

52. Fawcett DW, Phillips DM: The fine structure and development of the neck region of the mammalian spermatozoon. Anat Rec 165:153–184, 1969.

53. Nistal M, Paniagua R, Herruzo A: Absence de la paire centrale du complexe axonémique dans une tératospermie avec flagelles courts et épais. J Gynaecol Obstet Biol Reprod 8:47–50, 1979.

54. Baccetti B, Burrini AG, Pallini V: Spermatozoa and cilia lacking axoneme in an infertile man. Andrologia 12:525–532, 1980.

55. Aitken RJ, Ross A, Lees MM: Analysis of sperm function in Kartagener's syndrome. Fertil Steril 40:696–698, 1983.

56. Pedersen H, Rebbe H: Absence of arms in the axoneme of immotile human spermatozoa. Biol Reprod 12:541–544, 1975.

57. Afzelius BA, Eliasson R, Johnsen O, *et al.*: Lack of dynein arms in immotile human spermatozoa. J Cell Biol 66:225–232, 1975.

58. Baccetti B, Burrini AG, Pallini V, *et al.*: The short-tailed human spermatozoa. Ultrastructural alterations and dynein absence. J Submicrosc Cytol 7:349–359, 1975.

59. Afzelius BA: A human syndrome caused by immotile cilia. Science 193:317–319, 1976.

60. Eliasson R, Mossberg B, Camner P, *et al.*: The immotile cilia syndrome. A congenital ciliary abnormality as an etiologic factor in chronic airway infections and male sterility. N Engl J Med 297:1–6, 1977.

61. Baccetti B, Burrini AG, Dallai R, *et al.*: The dynein electrophoretic bands in axoneme naturally lacking the inner or the outer arm. J Cell Biol 80:334–340, 1979.

62. Camner P, Afzelius BA, Eliasson R, *et al.*: Relation between abnormalities of human sperm flagella and respiratory tract disease. Intern J Androl 2:211–224, 1979.

63. Terquem A, Dadoune JP: Les anomalies de structure dans les troubles de la mobilité du spermatozoide humain a propos de 60 cas d'asthenospermie. Bull Assoc Anat 64:567–576, 1980.

64. Lungarella G, Fonzi L, Burrini AG: Ultrastructural abnormalities in respiratory cilia and sperm tails in a patient with Kartagener's syndrome. J Ultrastruct Res 3:319–323, 1982.

65. Jouannet P, Escalier D, Serres C, *et al.*: Motility of human sperm without outer dynein arms. J Submicrosc Cytol 15:67–71, 1983.

66. Walt H: Untersuchungen an Spermieflagellen und Zilien mit pathologischer Motilität und Ultrastruktur. Schweiz med Wochenschr 114:1442–1450, 1984.

67. Afzelius BA: The immotile-cilia syndrome and other ciliary diseases. Int Rev Exp Path 19:1–43, 1979.

68. Afzelius BA: Genetic disorders of cilia. In HG Schweizer (ed) International Cell Biology 1980–1981. Berlin, Springer-Verlag, 1980.

69. Afzelius BA, Mossberg B: Immotile cilia. Thorax 35:401–404, 1980.

70. Kartagener M: Zur Pathogeneses der Bronchiektasien: Bronchiektasien bei Situs viscerum inversus. Beitr Klin Tuberk 83:489–501, 1933.

71. Waite D, Steele R, Ross I, *et al.*: Cilia and sperm tail abnormalities in Polynesian bronchiectatics. Lancet 2:132–133, 1978.

72. Sturgess J, Chao J, Wong J, *et al.*: Cilia with defective radial spokes. A cause of human respiratory disease. N Engl J Med 300:53–56, 1979.

73. Sturgess J, Chao J, Turner P: Transposition of ciliary microtubules. Another cause of impaired ciliary motility. N Engl J Med 303:318–322, 1980.

74. Sturgess J, Chao J: Ultrastructural features of a human genetic defect of cilia. Prog Clin Biol Res 80:7–12, 1982.

75. Afzelius BA, Eliasson R: Flagellar mutants in man: On the heterogeneity of the immotile-cilia syndrome. J Ultrastruct Res 69:43–52, 1979.

76. Schneeberger EE, McCormack J, Issenberg HJ, et al.: Heterogeneity of ciliary morphology in the immotile-cilia syndrome in man. J. Ultrastruct Res 73:34–43, 1980.

77. Afzelius BA: Genetical and ultrastructural aspects of the immotile cilia syndrome. Am J Hum Genet 33:852–864, 1981.

78. Rossman CM, Forrest JB, Less RMKW, et al.: The dyskinetic cilia syndrome. Abnormal ciliary motility in association with abnormal ciliary ultrastructure. Chest 80:860–865, 1981.

79. Walt H, Campana A, Balerna M, et al.: Mosaicism of dynein in spermatozoa and cilia and fibrous sheath aberrations in an infertile man. Andrologia 15:295–300, 1983.

80. Herzon FS, Murphy S: Normal ciliary ultrastructure in children with Kartagener's syndrome. Ann Otol Rhinol Laryngol 89:81–83, 1980.

81. Afzelius BA, Eliasson R: Male and female infertility problems in the immotile cilia syndrome. Eur J Resp Dis 64(suppl 127): 144–147, 1983.

82. Jonsson MS, McCormick JR, Gillies CG, et al.: Kartagener's syndrome with motile spermatozoa. N Engl J Med 307:1131–1133, 1982.

83. Chao J, Turner JAP, Sturgess JM: Genetic heterogeneity of dynein deficiency in cilia from patients with respiratory disease. Am Rev Respir Dis 126:302–305, 1982.

84. Baccetti BA, Burrini AG, Pallini V: Different axoneme patterns in cilia and flagella of the same animal. J Submicrosc Cytol 13:479–481, 1981.

85. Fox B, Bull TB, Barden GB: Variations in the ultrastructure of human nasal cilia including abnormalities found in retinitis pigmentosa. J Clin Pathol 33:327–335, 1980.

86. Rossman CM, Lee RMKW, Forrest JB, et al.: Nasal cilia ultrastructure and function in patients with primary ciliary dyskinesia compared with that in normal subjects and in subjects with various respiratory diseases. Am Rev Respir Dis 129:161–167, 1984.

87. Wilton LZ, Teichtahl H, Stemple-Smith PD, et al.: Structural heterogeneity of the axonemes of respiratory cilia and sperm flagella in normal men. J Clin Invest 75:825–831, 1985.

88. Feneux D, Serres C, Jouannet P: Sliding spermatozoa: A dyskinesia responsible for human infertility? Fertil Steril 44:508–511, 1985.

89. Ross A, Christie S, Kerr MG: An electron microscope study of a tail abnormality in spermatozoa from a subfertile man. J Reprod Fertil 24:99–103, 1971.

90. Ross A, Christie S, Edmond P: Ultrastructural tail defects in the spermatozoa from two men attending a subfertility clinic. J Reprod Fertil 32:243–251, 1973.

91. Pedersen H, Hammen R: Ultrastructure of human spermatozoa with complete subcellular derangement. Arch Androl 9:251–259, 1982.

92. Pedersen H, Rebbe H, Hammen R: Human sperm fine structure in a case of severe asthenospermia-necrospermia. Fertil Steril 22:156–164, 1971.

93. Alexandre C, Bisson JP, David G: Asthenospermia totale avec anomalie ultrastructurale du flagelle chez deux frères stériles. J Gynecol Obstet Biol Reprod 7:31–38, 1978.

94. Edelman GM, Millette CF: Molecular probes of spermatozoan structures. Proc Nat Acad Sci 68:2436–2440, 1971.

95. Zamboni L, Stefanini M: The fine structure of the neck of mammalian spermatozoa. Anat Rec 169:155–172, 1971.

96. Lindeman CB, Rikmenspoel R: Sperm flagella: autonomous oscillations of the contractile system. Science 175:337–338, 1972.

97. Woolley DM, Fawcett DW: The degeneration and disappearance of the centrioles during the development of the rat spermatozoon. Anat Rec 177:289–302, 1973.

98. Fawcett DW: The anatomy of the mammalian spermatozoon with particular reference to the guinea pig. Z Zellforsch 67:279–296, 1965.

99. Nicander L, Bane A: Fine structure of boar spermatozoa. Z Zellforsch 57:390–405, 1962.

100. Blom E, Birch-Andersen A: The ultrastructure of the bull sperm. II. The sperm head. Nord Vet Med 17:193–212, 1965.

101. Pedersen H: Further observations on the fine structure of the human spermatozoon. Z Zellforsch 123:305–315, 1972.

102. Lüders G: Ein Defekt der Kopf-Schwanz-Verknüpfung beim menschlichen Spermatozoen. Andrologia 8:365–368, 1976.

103. Perotti ME, Giarola A, Gioria M: Ultrastructural study of the decapitated sperm defect in an infertile man. J Reprod Fertil 63:543–549, 1981.

104. Baccetti B, Selmi MG, Soldani P: Morphogenesis of "decapitated" spermatozoa in a man. J Reprod Fertil 70:395–397, 1984.

105. Zaneveld LJD, Polakoski KL: Collection and physical examination of the ejaculate. In ESE Hafez (ed) Techniques of Human Andrology. Amsterdam, Elsevier/North Holland Biomedical Press, 1977.

106. LeLannou D: Tératospermie consistant en l'absence de tête spermatique par défaut de connexion tête-col chez l'homme. J Gynecol Obstet Biol Reprod 8:43–45, 1979.

107. Hancock JL, Rollinson DHL: A seminal defect associated with sterility of Guernsey bulls. Vet Rec 61:742–743, 1949.

108. Hancock JL: The disintegration of bull spermatozoa. Vet Rec 67:825–826, 1955.

109. Jones WA: Abnormal morphology of the spermatozoa in Guernsey bulls. Br Vet J 118:257–261, 1962.

110. Williams G: An abnormality of the spermatozoa of some Hereford bulls. Vet Rec 77:1204–1206, 1965.

111. van Rensburg SW, van Rensburg SJ, de Vos WH: The significance of the cytoplasmic droplet in the disintegration of semen in the Guernsey bull. Anderstepoort J Vet Res 33:169–184, 1966.

112. Settergren I, Nicander L: Ultrastructure of disintegrated bull sperm. Proc 6th Int Congr Anim Repr Artif Insem (Paris), 1968.

113. Blom E, Birch-Andersen A: Ultrastructure of the "decapitated sperm defect" in Guernsey bulls. J Reprod Fertil 23:67–72, 1970.

114. Monesi V: Chromosome activities during meiosis and spermiogenesis. J Repr Fertil Vol Suppl 13: 1–14, 1971.

115. Bellvé AR: The molecular biology of mammalian spermatogenesis. In CA Finn (ed) Oxford Reviews of Reproductive Biology. London, Oxford University Press, 1979.

116. Bedford JM, Calvin HI: The occurrence and possible functional significance of S-S- crosslinks in sperm head with particular reference to Eutherian mammals. J Exp Zool 188:137–156, 1974.

117. Saovaros W, Panyim S: The formation of disulfide bonds in human protamines during sperm maturation. Experientia 35:191–192, 1979.

118. Meistrich ML, Reid BO, Barcellona WJ: Changes in sperm nuclei during spermiogenesis and epididymal maturation. Exp Cell Res 99:72–78, 1976.

119. Fawcett DW: The Cell. Philadelphia, WB Saunders, 1981.

120. Evenson DP, Witkin SS, de Harven E, et al.: Ultrastructure of partially decondensed human spermatozoal chromatin. J Ultrastruct Res 63:178–187, 1978.

121. Gusse M, Chevailler P: Electron microscopic evidence for the presence of globular structures in different sperm chromatins. J Cell Biol 87:280–284, 1980.

122. Tanphaichitr N, Sobhon P, Chalermisarachai P, et al.: Acid-extracted nuclear proteins and ultrastructure of human sperm chromatin as revealed by differential extraction with urea, mercaptoethanol, and salt. Gamete Res 4:297–316, 1981.

123. Sobhon P, Chutatape C, Chalermisarachai P, et al.: Transmission and scanning electron microscopic studies of the human sperm chromatin decondensed by micrococcal nuclease and salt. J Exp Zool 221:61–79, 1982.

124. Bustos-Obregon E, Leiva S: Chromatin packing in normal and teratozoospermic human ejaculated spermatozoa. Andrologia 15:468–478, 1983.

125. Holstein AF: Ultrastructural observations on the differentiation of spermatids in man. Andrologia 8:157–165, 1976.

126. Fawcett DW, Anderson WA, Phillips DM: Morphogenetic factors influencing the shape of the sperm head. Devel Biol 26:220–251, 1971.

127. Baccetti B, Renieri T, Rosati F, et al.: Further observations on the morphogenesis of the round-headed human spermatozoa. Andrologia 9:255–264, 1977.

128. Zaneveld LJD: The acrosomal enzymes of mammalian spermatozoa. In ESE Hafez, CG Thibault (eds) The Biology of Spermatozoa. Transport, Survival and Fertilizing Ability. Basel, Kanger, 1975.

129. Mann T, Lutwak-Mann C: Male reproductive function and semen. Berlin, Springer-Verlag, 1981.

130. Friend DS: The organization of the spermatozoa membrane. In M Edidin, MH Johnson (eds) Immunology of Gametes. London, Cambridge University Press, 1977.

131. Yanagimachi R: Mechanisms of fertilization in mammals. In L Mastroianni, D Biggers (eds) Fertilization and Embryonic Development in Vitro. New York, Plenum Publishing, 1981.

132. Bedford JM: Significance of the need for sperm capacitation before fertilization in eutherian mammals. Biol Reprod 28:108–120, 1983.

133. Moore HDM, Bedford JM: The interaction of mammalian gametes in the female. In JF Hartmann (ed) Mechanisms and Control of Animal Fertilization. New York, Academic Press, 1983.

134. Austin CR: Observations on the penetration of sperm into the mammalian egg. Aust J Sci Res Series B 4:581–592, 1951.

135. Chang MC: Fertilizing capacity of spermatozoa deposited in the fallopian tubes. Nature 168:697–698, 1951.

136. Rogers BJ: Mammalian sperm capacitation and fertilization in vitro: A critique of methodologies. Gamete Res 1:165–223, 1978.

137. Barros C, Bedford JM, Franklin LE, et al.: Membrane vesiculation as a feature of the mammalian acrosome reaction. J Cell Biol 34:C1–C5, 1967.

138. Merriono AR, Wright RW: Characterization of porcine oocyte zonae pellucidae by polyacrylamide gel electrophoresis. Proc Soc Exp Biol Med 160:449–452, 1979.

139. Bleil JD, Wassarman PM: Structure and function of the zona pellucida: identification and characterization of the proteins of the mouse oocyte zona pellucida. Devel Biol 76:185–202, 1980.

140. Bedford JM: Ultrastructural changes in the sperm head during fertilization of the rabbit. Am J Anat 123:329–358, 1968.

141. Bedford JM: An electron microscopic study of sperm penetration into the rabbit egg after natural mating. Am J Anat 133:213–254, 1972.

142. Bedford JM, Moore HDM, Franklin LE: Significance of the equatorial segment of the acrosome of the spermatozoon in eutherian mammals. Exp Cell Res 119:119–126, 1979.

143. Stefanini M, Ōura C, Zamboni L: Ultrastructure of fertilization in the mouse. 2. Penetration of sperm into the ovum. J Submicrosc Cytol 1:1–23, 1969.

144. Yanagimachi R, Noda YD: Ultrastructural changes in the hamster sperm head during fertilization. J Ultrastruct Res 31:465–485, 1970.

145. Yanagimachi R, Noda YD: Physiological changes in the postnuclear cap region of mammalian spermatozoa: A necessary preliminary to the membrane fusion between sperm and egg cells. J Ultrastruct Res 31:486–493, 1970.

146. Bryan JHD: An eosin-fast green-naphthol yellow mixture for differential staining of cytologic components in mammalian spermatozoa. Stain Technol 45:231–236, 1970.

147. Singer R, Sagir M, Barnet M, et al.: Head abnormalities. Assessment of sperm in the routine laboratory. Andrologia 13:236–241, 1981.

148. Talbot P, Chacon R: A new procedure for rapidly scoring acrosome reaction of human sperm. Gamete Res 3:211–216, 1980.

149. Talbot P, Chacon R: A triple stain technique for evaluating normal acrosome reactions of human sperm. J Exp Zool 215:201–208, 1981.

150. Fawcett DW, Ito S: The fine structure of bat spermatozoa. Am J Anat 116:567–582, 1965.

151. MacLeod J: Seminal cytology in the presence of varicocele. Fertil Steril 116:735–757, 1965.

152. Paulsen CA: The Testes. In RH Williams (ed) Textbook of Endocrinology. Philadelphia, Saunders, 1974.

153. Glezerman M, Rakowszky M, Lunenfeld B, et al.: Varicocele in oligospermic patients: Pathophysiology and results after ligation and division of the internal spermatic vein. J Urol 115:562–571, 1976.

154. Rodriguez-Rigau LJ, Smith KD, Steinberger E: Varicocele and the morphology of spermatozoa. Fertil Steril 35:54–57, 1981.

155. Panidis D, Brozos G, Margaritis M, et al.: The contribution of sperm morphology to the diagnostic approach to varicocele. Acta Endocr 107(Suppl 265):20–21, 1984.

156. Rouy S, Sentein P: Particularités ultrastructurales des spermatozoides humains a tete allongée. Pathol Biol 25:691–697, 1977.

157. Dadoune JP, Fain-Maurel MA, Guillaumin M, et al.: Scan-

ning electron microscopic morphometry of a discriminated population of elongated human spermatozoa. Intern J Fertil 25:18–27, 1980.

158. Fujita T, Miyoshi M, Tokunaga J: Scanning and transmission electron microscopy of human ejaculate spermatozoa with special reference to their abnormal forms. Z Zellforsch 105:483–497, 1970.

159. Renieri T: Submicroscopical observations on abnormal human spermatozoa. J Submicrosc Cytol 6:421–432, 1974.

160. Bisson JP, David G, Magnin C: Étude ultrastructurale des anomalies de l'acrosome dans les spermatozoïdes à tête irrégulière. Bull Assoc Anat 59:345–356, 1975.

161. Holstein AF, Mauss J: Licht- und elektronenmikroskopische Untersuchung fehlgebildeter Spermatiden in zwei Fällen von Teratozoospermie. Hautarzt 26:144–148, 1975.

162. Brun B, Clavert A. Modifications morphologiques de l'acrosome chez un homme exposé à la chaleur. J Gynecol Obstet Biol Reprod 6:907–912, 1977.

163. Aughey E, Orr PS: An unusual abnormality of human spermatozoa. J Reprod Fertil 53:341–342, 1978.

164. Camatini M, Chiara F, Franchi E, et al.: Acrosomal cap abnormalities of spermatids from infertile men. In A Fabbrini, E Steinberger (eds) Recent Progress in Andrology. London, Academic Press, 1978.

165. Sun CN, White HJ: The variety of abnormal spermatozoa from patients with fertility problems. An ultrastructural study. II. Mature forms. Cytologia 43:551–554, 1978.

166. Söderström KO: An acrosomal abnormality in spermatids from infertile men. Arch Androl 7:275–278, 1981.

167. Bedford JM, Bent MJ, Calvin H: Variations in the structural character and stability of the nuclear chromatin in morphologically normal human spermatozoa. J Reprod Fertil 33:19–29, 1973.

168. Evenson DP, Darzynkiewicz Z, Melamed MR: Relation of mammalian sperm chromatin heterogeneity to fertility. Science 210:1131–1133, 1980.

169. Silvestroni L, Frajese G: Abnormal structure of "spermatozoa" in infertile oligospermic men. In A Fabbrini, E Steinberger (ed) Recent Progress in Andrology. London, Academic Press, 1978.

170. Kjessler B: Karyotype, meiosis, and spermatogenesis in a sample of men attending an infertility clinic. Monogr Hum Genet 2:10–19, 1966.

171. Kjessler B: Facteurs génétiques dans la subfertilité male humaine. Fecondité et stérilité du mâle. Acquisitions Récentes. Paris, Masson, 1972.

172. Kjessler B: Chromosomal constitution and male reproductive failure. In RE Mancini, L Martini (eds) Male Fertility and Sterility. London, Academic Press, 1974.

173. Abramsson L, Beckman G, Duchek M, et al.: Chromosomal aberrations and male infertility. J Urol 128:52–53, 1982.

174. Hrudka F, Singh A: Sperm nucleomalacia in men with inflammatory bowel disease. Arch Androl 13:37–57, 1984.

175. Levi AJ, Fisher AM, Hughers L, et al.: Male infertility due to sulphasalasine. Lancet 2:276–278, 1979.

176. Toth A: Reversible toxic effect of salicylazosulfapyridine on semen quality. Fertil Steril 31:538–540, 1979.

177. Traub AL, Thompson W, Orville J: Male infertility due to sulphasalazine. Lancet 2:639–640, 1979.

178. Toovey S, Hudson E, Hendry WF, et al.: Sulphasalazine and male infertility: Reversibility and possible mechanism. Gut 22:445–451, 1981.

179. Hudson E, Dore C, Souter C, et al.: Sperm size in patients with inflammatory bowel disease on sulphasalazine therapy. Fertil Steril 38:77–84, 1982.

180. Holstein AF, Schirren C, Schirren CG: Human spermatids and spermatozoa lacking acrosomes. J Reprod Fertil 35:489–491, 1973.

181. Pedersen H, Rebbe H: Fine structure of round-headed human spermatozoa. J Reprod Fertil 37:51–54, 1974.

182. Kullander S, Rousing A: On round-headed human spermatozoa. Intern J Fertil 20:33–40, 1975.

183. Anton-Lamprecht I, Kotzur B, Schopf E: Round-headed human spermatozoa. Fertil Steril 27:685–693, 1976.

184. Nistal M, Herruzo A, Sanchez-Corral F: Teratozoospermia absoluta de presentación familiar. Espermatozoides microcéfalos irregulares sin acrosoma. Andrologia 10:234–240, 1978.

185. Tyler JPP, Boadle RA, Stevens SMB: Round-headed spermatozoa: A case report. Pathol 17:67–70, 1985.

186. Schirren CG, Holstein AF, Schirren C: Über die Morphogenese rundköpfiger Spermatozoen des Menschen. Andrologia 3:117–125, 1971.

187. Castellani L, Chiara F, Cotelli F: Fine structure and cytochemistry of the morphogenesis of round-headed human sperm. Arch Androl 1:291–297, 1978.

188. Nistal M, Paniagua R: Morphogenesis of round-headed human spermatozoa lacking acrosomes in a case of severe teratozoospermia. Andrologia 10:49–51, 1978.

189. Florke-Gerloff S, Krause W, Topfer-Petersen E, et al.: On the teratogenesis of round-headed spermatozoa: Investigations with antibodies against acrosin, an intra-acrosomally located acrosin-inhibitor, and the outer acrosomal membrane. Andrologia 17:126–138, 1985.

190. Florke-Gerloff S, Topfer-Petersen E, Muller-Esterl W, et al.: Biochemical and genetic investigation of round-headed spermatozoa in infertile men, including two brothers and their father. Andrologia 16:187–202, 1984.

191. Weissenbergh R, Eshkol A, Rudak E, et al.: Inability of round acrosomeless human spermatozoa to penetrate zona-free hamster ova. Arch Androl 11:167–169, 1982.

192. Syms AJ, Johnson AR, Lipshultz LT, et al. Studies on human spermatozoa and round head syndrome. Fertil Steril 42:431–435, 1984.

193. Jeyendrau RS, Van der Ven HH, Kennedy WP, et al.: Acrosomeless sperm. A cause of primary male infertility. Andrologia 17:31–36, 1985.

194. Nistal M, Paniagua R, Herruzo A: Multi-tailed spermatozoa in a case with asthenospermia and teratospermia. Virchows Arch B Cell Path 26:111–118, 1977.

195. Escalier D: Human spermatozoa with large heads and multiple flagella: A quantitative ultrastructural study of 6 cases. Biol Cell 48:65–74, 1983.

196. Baccetti B, Afzelius BA: The Biology of the Sperm Cell. Basel, Karger, 1976.

197. German J, Rasch EM, Huang CY, et al.: Human infertility due to production of multiple-tailed spermatozoa with excessive amounts of DNA. Am J Hum Gen 33:64A, 1981.

198. Baccetti B, Fraioli F, Paolucci D, et al.: Double spermatozoa in a hyperprolactinemic man. J. Submicrosc Cytol 10:249–260, 1978.

199. Baccetti B, Fraioli F, Paolucci D, et al.: High prolactin level and double spermatozoa. Gamete Res 2:193–199, 1979.

200. Howard B: Fertility in the ram following exposure to elevated ambient temperature and humidity. J Reprod Fertil 19:179–185, 1969.

201. Braden AWH, Mattner PE: The effect of scrotal heating in the ram on semen characteristics, fecundity, and embryonic mortality. Aust J Agric Res 21:509–519, 1970.

202. Williamson P: The fine structure of ejaculated ram spermatozoa following scrotal heating. J Reprod Fertil 40:191–195, 1974.

203. Viczian M: Ergebnisse von Spermuntersuchungen bei Zigarettenrauchern. Z. Haut Geschlechtskr 44:183–187, 1969.

204. Evans HJ, Fletcher J, Torrance M, *et al.*: Sperm abnormalities and cigarette smoking. Lancet 21:626–629, 1981.

205. Shaarawy M, Mahmoud KZ: Endocrine profile and semen characteristics in male smokers. Fertil Steril 38:255–258, 1982.

206. Berry EM: Sperm abnormalities and cigarette smoking. Lancet 21:1159, 1981.

207. Kulikauskas V, Blaustein D, Ablin RJ: Cigarette smoking and its possible effect on sperm. Fertil Steril 44:526–528, 1985.

208. Cohen J, Edwards R, Fehilly C, *In vitro* fertilization: A treatment for male infertility. Fertil Steril 43:422–432, 1985.

Index